Monica DiFonzo.
009026659.

W9-DGX-957

NURSING
MANAGEMENT
IN CANADA

NURSING MANAGEMENT IN CANADA

SECOND EDITION

JUDITH M. HIBBERD
DONNA LYNN SMITH

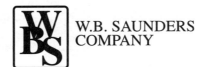

W.B. SAUNDERS
COMPANY

A Harcourt Canada Health Sciences Company

Toronto Montreal Fort Worth New York Orlando
Philadelphia San Diego London Sydney Tokyo

Copyright © 1999 W.B. Saunders Canada,
a Harcourt Canada Health Sciences Company.

All rights reserved. No part of this publication may be reproduced or transmitted in any form or by any means, electronic or mechanical, including photocopy, recording, or any information storage and retrieval system, without permission in writing from the publisher. Reproducing passages from this book without such written permission is an infringement of copyright law.

Requests for permission to photocopy any part of this Work should be sent in writing to: College Licensing Officer, Cancopy, 1 Yonge Street, Suite 1900, Toronto, ON, M5E 1E5. Fax: (416) 868-1621. All other inquiries should be directed to the publisher.

Every reasonable effort has been made to acquire permission for copyright material used in this text, and to acknowledge such indebtedness accurately. Any errors or omissions called to the publisher's attention will be corrected in future printings.

Canadian Cataloguing in Publication Data
Main entry under title:

Nursing management in Canada
2nd ed.
first edition written by Judith M. Hibberd and Mavis E. Kyle.
Includes index.
ISBN 0-920513-32-8

1. Nursing services – Canada – Administration. I. Hibberd, Judith M. (Judith Mary), 1934–   . II. Smith, Donna Lynn, 1945–   .

RT89.H53 1998   362.1'73'068   C97-932823-3

Acquisitions Editor: Heather McWhinney
Developmental Editor: Martina van de Velde
Senior Production Coordinator: Sue-Ann Becker

Copy Editor: TypoGraphics, Inc.
Cover and Interior Design: The Brookview Group Inc.
Typesetting and Assembly: TypoGraphics, Inc.
Cover Art: Karyn Percival, *Compassion* (1996), watercolour/dry colour on 300 lb. paper, 22" x 22". Reproduced with the permission of the artist.
Printing and Binding: Webcom Limited

Harcourt Canada
55 Horner Avenue, Toronto, ON, Canada M8Z 4X6
Customer Service
Toll-Free Tel.: 1-800-387-7278
Toll-Free Fax: 1-800-665-7307

This book was printed in Canada.
2 3 4 5 6   03 02 01 00 99

TO OUR PARENTS

Hilary and Gerald Hibberd   Sylvia and Percy Smith

Preface

▼▼▼▼▼▼▼▼▼▼▼▼▼▼▼

In times of rapid change, leaders and managers face a particular challenge. What is the relevance of what they have learned and done in the past to their current environment and responsibilities? How can the latest organizational fad or passing trend be distinguished from innovations that will be of lasting importance or value? How can leaders establish and work toward developing and implementing a vision, when it is increasingly difficult to predict with certainty what the future will hold for the health system and for particular health organizations? This edition of *Nursing Management in Canada* was conceived and written with an acute awareness of the ambiguity and uncertainty that faces professional practitioners, leaders, and administrators at all levels of the health system today.

When the first edition of this book was published in 1994, the Canadian health system had already entered a period of unprecedented turbulence. When the time came to consider a second edition, it was obvious that an updated version of the original would not suffice. Therefore, this edition, while indebted to its predecessor in many ways, is also very different from it. The differences are attributable not only to changes in the health system, but also to changes in the intuitions and values of the authors and editors of the book.

The health systems of all western countries are undergoing dramatic structural changes. Hospitals continue to be recognized for their importance but in the last several years, other sectors of the health system such as continuing and community care, mental health, and health promotion have gained increasing prominence. In the past, the literature on health-system administration has focussed primarily on hospitals. This second edition of *Nursing Management in Canada* has been consciously reoriented to address issues of leadership and management in a variety of health-service sectors and agencies.

Nursing Management in Canada was originally written to meet the need for a text and reference book for nurses who were learning about, or practising in, first-line or middle management roles. In the last several years, organizations of all kinds have been "restructured," "downsized," "rightsized," "decentralized," "flattened," and "redesigned." Understanding the meaning of these terms, and their implications, is often only possible within a particular organizational context. Position titles have changed and now vary so widely that they are no longer useful in making generalizations and comparisons across organizations. However, some trends can be identified as common to various countries, and to a variety of health sectors and organizational types. One common development is a reduction in the number of middle-management positions and corresponding changes in the roles of first-line leaders. A second is the increasing importance attached to teamwork—within and among health disciplines, and within and among health-service organizations. These two developments have made it more difficult to address the "audience" for this book, as its members are likely to come from a variety of disciplines, and to occupy a host of different positions.

We created a book that is intended to continue to be of value to those first-line and middle managers whose roles have remained relatively stable, while at the same time meeting the needs of nurses and other health professionals who are preparing for, or practising in, "redesigned" leadership and management roles. This has been accomplished through the addition of a number of new chapters, and a refocussing of some of the chapters that appeared in the first edition of the book.

It has become popular in recent years to distinguish between "leadership" and "management," and to portray the former role as the more important and challenging of the two. The planning and writing of this book was in part an affirmation of our belief that leaders who lack management skills are as much a liability to modern organizations and the communities they serve as are managers who lack the vision of leadership. We encourage readers of this book to value, and to develop knowledge and skills in, both management and leadership.

AN OVERVIEW OF THE BOOK

The content of the second edition of *Nursing Management in Canada* reflects our belief in the importance of acquiring knowledge regarding the historical contexts, analytical frameworks, principles, and processes upon which effective leadership and management are founded. A number of the chapters, including some that students may find challenging initially, were designed intentionally to provide this kind of reference framework. The chapters on management theory and on the social, political, and economic forces shaping the health-care system are examples. The focus of other chapters is on providing current information, or on supporting the development of skills that can be put to immediate and practical use in leadership roles. The chapters in section five are all of this type, as are many of the chapters in sections two, three, and four.

This second edition has been shortened to thirty chapters. Only nine of the thirty-six original chapters, all of them updated, have been retained. All chapters in this edition follow a standard format that includes learning objectives and a summary of key points. Many chapters contain additional learning aids and resources, such as case studies and annotated lists of suggested readings.

The first section presents the broad context for health services in Canada through a series of reference chapters dealing with the political, social, and economic forces shaping the health system; demographic and epidemiological issues; the legal framework for health services; and health economics.

The second section deals with the structure and organization of the health system. This section begins with a chapter on management theory that acts as an important reference point for the chapters that follow it, which deal with recent and current approaches and trends in delivering health services, structuring organizations, and the work of health professionals.

In the third section, issues of professional leadership are explored from a number of different perspectives. Moreover, these chapters address topics that are unique to the administration of professional disciplines: professional governance and peer review, research, ethics, and setting and maintaining standards, for example.

The fourth section focusses on the management of human and material resources, including recruiting, selecting and developing staff, allocating resources, and preparing business plans and budgets.

The final section of the book has been structured as a "tool kit," focussing on a number of skill areas that are of current and continuing importance in carrying out leadership and management roles.

The contributors to this second edition come from across Canada and from all sectors of the health system. They are, or have been, leaders and managers in the real world. Through their contributions to this book, they act as mentors and models for emerging leaders in the Canadian health system. We hope that this book will encourage excellent leaders to aspire to be excellent managers as well; and we encourage excellent managers to assume the full challenges and responsibilities of leadership. Our health system needs both.

ACKNOWLEDGEMENTS

We are indebted to many people for their assistance in preparing this second edition of *Nursing Management in Canada*. We thank our friends and colleagues, who lead and practice in the turbulent world of nursing and health-care administration, for contributing their experiences and perspectives. Colleagues at Canadian universities who used the first edition as a textbook provided us with valuable feedback and suggestions that helped to shape the new edition. Heather McWhinney, Senior Acquisitions Editor at Harcourt Brace & Company, Canada, and Martina van de Velde, Developmental Editor, have actively supported our vision for the second edition, and have provided collegial advice and support as it evolved.

Mavis Kyle, co-editor of the first edition, retired from the School of Nursing, University of Saskatoon, in 1997. However, she has remained involved as a scientific reviewer and consultant for this edition, and we thank her for these contributions.

We also thank the following friends and colleagues who have contributed to the book as reviewers of chapters: John Church, PhD, Assistant Professor, Public Health Sciences, University of Alberta; Dallas Cullen, PhD, Associate Professor, Business Faculty, University of Alberta; John B. Dossetor, OC, BM, BCh(Oxf), PhD; Albert R. Haskell, BCom, ISP; Jenny Medves, RN, MN, PhD candidate; Richard C. Fraser, QC, BA, LLB, LLM; Noela Inions, BScN, LLB, LLM, CHE; Nancy Rowan, BScN, MHSA; and Deanna Williamson, RN, PhD, Assistant Professor, Faculty of Nursing, University of Alberta. We appreciate the advice of Sue Russel, BScN, MN with respect to the practice environment, and the assistance of Jane E. Smith, BScN, MN who provided valuable editorial and research support.

Glennis Zilm was the outstanding copy editor of the first edition and we were fortunate to have the benefit of both her nursing and editing knowledge and experience as the second edition developed and progressed. We acknowledge with gratitude the work of Mary W. Walters of Edmonton, who joined our team as copy editor to assist in the completion of the book.

We thank our colleagues and students in the Faculty of Nursing at the University of Alberta for contributing to an environment where work of this kind can flourish. Finally, and most importantly, we thank the book's contributors for the knowledge, objectivity, goodwill, and teamwork that helped to make the second edition of *Nursing Management in Canada* a reality.

—JMH & DLS

Statistics Canada information is used with the permission of the Minister of Industry, as Minister responsible for Statistics Canada. Information on the availability of the wide range of data from Statistics Canada can be obtained from Statistics Canada's Regional Offices, its World Wide Web site at http://www.statcan.ca, and its toll-free access number 1-800-263-1136.

A NOTE FROM THE PUBLISHER

Thank you for selecting *Nursing Management in Canada,* Second Edition, edited by Judith M. Hibberd and Donna Lynn Smith. The authors and publisher have devoted considerable time to the careful development of this book. We appreciate your recognition of this effort and accomplishment.

We want to hear what you think about *Nursing Management in Canada*, Second Editon. Please take a few minutes to fill out the stamped reader reply card at the back of this book. Your comments and suggestions will be valuable to us as we prepare new editions and other books.

Contents

▼▼▼▼▼▼▼▼▼▼▼▼▼▼▼▼

Environmental Context for Health Services in Canada

Chapter 1

▼▼▼▼▼▼▼▼▼▼▼▼

Political, Social, and Economic Forces Shaping the Health-Care System

JANET L. STORCH AND CARL A. MEILICKE

KEY OBJECTIVES

In this chapter, you will learn:

- Major forces and events that shaped the health-care system from Pre-Confederation days to the close of the 1990s.
- Division of powers between federal and provincial governments in relation to health-care services.
- The Act of Parliament that originally established and continues to influence jurisdiction for health services in Canada.
- The five principles upon which the Canadian health-care system is founded.
- Influential reports that affected development of health and social welfare programs in Canada, and their significance for social policy.
- Legislation that has had major impacts on development of the health-care system.
- The main reasons provincial and federal governments in the 1990s are promoting reform of the health-care system, and recent developments at the provincial level.

INTRODUCTION

In this chapter, the Canadian health-care system is briefly described, with attention to political, social, and economic forces that have shaped the system. To trace the causes and consequences in the development of the Canadian health-care system, a historical-analytical approach is adopted, beginning with the period predating Confederation. The chapter concludes with a discussion of current issues and trends, and future policy implications relative to the Canadian health-care system.

NATURE OF THE CANADIAN HEALTH-CARE SYSTEM

Knowing the general types of health-care systems across the industrialized nations assists in placing the Canadian health-care system in context. Four general types ("ideal types") of health-care systems are apparent, ranging from those in which governments play a residual role in a system governed by a market orientation (private health insurance systems), to the opposite extreme in which governments define health care as an essential service (socialized health-care systems) (Najman & Western, 1984). In private health insurance systems, preservation of the autonomy of physician, health institution, and client take priority. The fact that a substantial minority of people might be without health care in such a system is viewed as unfortunate but unavoidable. In socialized health-care systems, minimal autonomy of health provider or client is accepted, since the goal of the health-care system is to preserve the collective good by ensuring optimal productivity of citizens.

Between these two opposite types of health-care systems are two other approaches to the delivery of health care. In one of these system types, the role of government in health services is viewed as a necessary vehicle for reasonable social distribution of resources (national health service). Health services are seen to be a natural resource that should be available to all based on need, not ability to pay. Physician, institution, and client autonomy are secondary to public need. In the final general type of health-care system, government attempts to balance autonomy with the collective good through public insurance programs (national health insurance). In this type of system, physician, institution, and client autonomy are preserved, but within a context of equitable access to health services for all citizens.

If the private health insurance system is typified by the general approach to delivering health care in the United States, and the national health service system is typified by the approach of the United Kingdom, then the Canadian health-care system (the national health insurance system) can be viewed as a blend of American and British approaches. By encouraging autonomy for health professionals and health agencies while ensuring relatively equal access to health care by all individuals regardless of their ability to pay, two important values in Canadian society are protected.

PRINCIPLES OF CANADIAN HEALTH CARE

In attempting to protect and preserve autonomy and equity, the Canadian health-care system has been built upon five main principles: universality, accessibility, comprehensiveness, portability, and public administration. Provincial tax revenues and, to a declining degree, federal tax revenues fund medical and hospital service delivery in all provinces so long as the five essential principles are honoured. Only two provinces (Alberta and British Columbia) levy premiums to assist with costs of health services and, for the most part, there are no user charges/extra billing for services considered medically necessary because such fees are seen to violate the principle of accessibility. Thus, coverage of basic hospital care (including X ray, medications, and diagnostic testing) and physician care is provided "free" to all Canadian citizens. Private health insurance (e.g., Blue Cross and other insurers) covers only supplemental benefits, such as private accommodation, ambulance, out-of-country costs not covered under the public plan, and other health benefits.

The Canadian health-care system is part of a broader network of social security programs that developed over time. This network of programs, made accessible to all, is a remarkable achievement for a relatively young nation. Although the phrase "Canadian health-care system" is commonly used, it is important to remember that Canada does not have a federal health-care system; it has ten provincial health-care systems, plus two territorial systems. The federal government plays a more direct role in care in the northern territories, although the territories also are moving toward more autonomy.

The range of social programs reflects basic values that evolved over more than 200 years. Some of the most notable commitments developed in the early part of the twentieth century, particularly in Saskatchewan, where a number of innovative approaches to health care occurred. These innovations became part of the background for establishing a national blueprint of Canadian social security in the mid-1940s. The values underlying these innovations continue to shape health-care policy and programs in the 1990s. As Deber and Vayda (1992) note, "Historically, Canadians have accepted government intervention in social programs and have welcomed sponsorship of health care" (p. 3).

Understanding how this network of programs took shape is critical to understanding the strengths and challenges of the system in the 1990s. Therefore, this historical perspective on the system outlines six main eras of health policy and program development and highlights the nature and dynamics of the changes that shaped its evolution. Each era is characterized by distinctive concerns and activities. Eras span: days of the earliest settlements until Confederation in 1867, Confederation to the mid-1940s, mid-1940s to mid-1960s, mid-1960s to mid-1970s, mid-1970s to 1990s, and 1991 toward the future. The time periods are approximate; multidimensional historical dynamics defy precise categorization into uni-dimensional time periods.

ERA ONE: PRE-CONFEDERATION

In the young and developing Canadian nation predating Confederation, self-reliance was valued; self-reliance involved providing for the necessities of life, looking after one's family, and providing health care. The natural outcome of this focus on self-reliance was the belief that there should be limited government involvement in social security, other than a modicum of services for the sick, the mentally ill, and delinquents (Cassidy, 1947; Splane, 1965). Typical examples of the limited legislation and existing programs were acts (dating from the early 1700s) to control the sale of meat, establish quarantine stations, deal with foundlings, and make provision for sick and disabled seamen (Heagerty, 1934; Gregoire, 1962; Gelber, 1973). Buildings were provided for the insane (lunatic asylums), provisions were made for care of lepers, and procedures were implemented to handle epidemics of cholera, typhus, and smallpox. The procedures for dealing with epidemics were ad hoc measures, with no permanent boards of health. This ad hoc approach was typical; governments chose not to develop proactive policies as these might be viewed as interfering with self-reliance. Instead, governments reacted only to the major crises of the day. As Wallace (1950) notes, Canada's population was primarily rural, and problems that might now be defined as social problems were then viewed as problems for families, local communities, or the church to address, rather than the state.

These were among the reasons the *British North America Act* (*BNA Act*), one of the constituting acts of Canada, made provision only for residual needs; the authors assumed that the family, community, or church were capable of handling the major concerns. Thus, Section 91 of the *BNA Act* outlines federal responsibilities as the raising of money by a mode or system of taxation, provision for census and statistics, provision for quarantine and establishment and maintenance of marine hospitals, and responsibility for Indians and for lands reserved for Indians.

The only items relevant to health care are in Section 92, which outlines provincial responsibilities. These are responsibility for "establishment, maintenance, and management of hospitals, Asylums, charities, and eleemosynary institutions in and for the province, other than marine hospitals," and "generally all matters of a merely local or private Nature in the Province" (Van Loon & Whittington, 1976, p. 483). This short-sighted delineation of legal responsibilities left virtually all health service provision in the hands of the provinces, which had an insufficient tax base to support such extensive services to meet the needs of the Canadian public. "The fathers of Confederation proved to be poor prophets. The resulting imbalance between fiscal resources and constitutional responsibilities has made federal-provincial relations the primary concern of Canadian politics" (Deber & Vayda, 1992, p. 3).

Since the *BNA Act* contained such limited provisions for determining federal and provincial responsibilities in matters of health and welfare, and with the lion's share of responsibility resting with the provinces, only three options were open later to federal or provincial governments to deal with this anomaly: (1) they could go ahead on their own; (2) they could push for a constitutional amendment; or, (3) they could enter into cost-shared programs (Taylor, 1987). All these strategies are evident in the system that unfolded during the ensuing years.

It is important to note that the division of powers and the use of these strategies are not only historically interesting but also important in understanding the Canadian health-care system of today, since these same provisions prevail. In 1982, the *BNA Act* became part of the constitutional package under the *Constitution Act* (1982), which added the Canadian Charter of Rights and Freedoms and a domestic amending formula.

ERA TWO: CONFEDERATION TO THE MID-1940S

The second era was characterized by growing awareness that organized action was necessary to deal with the social security needs of an increasingly urbanized and industrialized nation. This awareness led to extensive developments in governmental and voluntary programs and eventually to a profoundly important clarification of federal versus provincial authority in matters relating to social security. The era is characterized by increasing government involvement and a slow but steady progression from reactive and ad hoc programming to beginning efforts to effect planned change.

Between Confederation (1867) and 1920, municipal and provincial programs in health and social security were considerably expanded and many important voluntary organizations were formed. For example, organizations now known as the Toronto Children's Aid Society (1891), Red Cross (1896), Victorian Order of Nurses (1897), Canadian Mental Health Association (1918), Canadian Institute for the Blind (1918), and Canadian Council of Social Development (1920) were organized during this time (Armitage, 1975).

Growth in municipal and provincial government activities during this period occurred because the *BNA Act* was silent on matters of health and welfare services, reflecting the conviction that these matters, insofar as they were the responsibility of government, were of proper concern only to local and provincial authorities (Splane, 1965; Wallace, 1950). Representative of such activities was the substantial expansion of welfare services in Ontario, implementation of municipal doctor plans and union hospitals in Saskatchewan, an income-support plan for widowed mothers in Manitoba, and municipal hospital plans in Manitoba and Alberta (Gelber, 1966; Morgan, 1961; Rorem, 1931; Splane, 1965; Taylor, 1949).

These municipal and provincial developments proceeded apace through to the 1940s. At that time, the federal government, in response to growing public demand for social services, as well as to the social disruptions caused by World War I (1914–1918) and the Great Depression (1930s), began to consolidate its health responsibilities and to respond to new needs deemed to require federal assistance. These initiatives were largely reactive rather than planned (e.g., grants-in-aid scheme for venereal disease control, *Soldiers' Settlement Act* of 1920), and relatively few programs were actually established. One program, however (the *Old Age Pensions Act* of 1927), was significant in being Canada's first nation-wide income support plan and the first major, continuing, federal-provincial cost-shared social security program (Bryden, 1974; Cameron, 1962; Morgan, 1961). Various ad hoc unemployment measures were also undertaken by the federal government during the Depression of the 1930s because thousands of individuals could no longer be self-sufficient and self-reliant, and neither municipal nor provincial governments were capable of financing the relief programs required (Bellamy, 1965; Gelber, 1973).

The problems inherent in an ad hoc approach were dramatized in 1937, when the *Employment and Social Insurance Act* of 1935, designed to provide an extensive federal program for dealing with the economic and social problems created by unemployment, was declared unconstitutional because the federal government did not have the power to levy direct premiums on provincial residents for health and welfare programs (Taylor, 1987). A commission was established to deal with this first major federal-provincial controversy and was charged with determining areas of federal-provincial jurisdiction in a wide variety of fields, including social security. In this case, the strategy of pressing for a constitutional amendment was employed, but was not effected until 1940 when federal responsibility for unemployment insurance was added to Section 91 of the *BNA Act*.

The end of Era Two was dominated by federal government efforts to evolve a planned approach to long-range policy and program development based on a careful definition of national needs, a plan which was to founder on the problem of federal versus provincial authority. Passage of the *Unemployment Insurance Act* in 1940 permitted the federal government to implement a compulsory, contributory insurance program at the national level. A wide variety of pressures, including serious concerns about social and economic dislocations caused by the Depression and World War II (1939–1945) as well as commitment to the Atlantic Charter of 1941 (which stressed the concept of individual freedoms and rights), further stimulated federal government action. Two major reports were undertaken by the federal government, commonly known as the Marsh Report and the Heagerty Report (Collins, 1976; Heagerty, 1943; Marsh, 1975).

The Marsh report, prepared in 1943, has been cited as the "single most important document in the development of the post-war social security system in Canada" (Collins, 1976, p. 5). It took a long-range perspective and outlined a comprehensive national plan for social security for Canada. The Marsh plan recommended social insurance for interruptions of earning capacity (such as unemployment insurance), for occasions requiring special expenditure (such as major accidents or illness), and for greater continuous budgetary needs than the family income could accommodate (such as chronic poverty). Marsh also emphasized the need for integration of social security programs.

The Heagerty report was more limited in scope than the Marsh report, but more specific in its proposals. Heagerty considered it essential that everyone in Canada should be provided with health insurance, but that no compulsion should be placed on provinces other than that all indigents be included in the plan. Health program benefits were to be broad in scope, including medical, dental, and pharmaceutical benefits, and additional program grants to the provinces were proposed, including grants for tuberculosis, mental health, and professional training. Heagerty stressed integration of public health and medical care as well, with the goal of "raising and maintaining the standard of health care of the Canadian people" (Heagerty, 1943, p. 5).

The only apparent immediate result of these remarkably prescient reports, however, was the passage, in 1944, of the *Family Allowance Act*. It provided for payment by the federal government of monthly allowances for every child under sixteen years of age. The prime reason that even this program went forward was the perceived urgent need for its expected economic stabilization effects through income redistribution (Bellamy, 1965; Lindenfield, 1959). The challenges inherent in federal versus provincial responsibilities meant it would be many years before the Marsh and Heagerty concepts could be realized. Ultimately, a great deal of the leadership came from the provinces rather than from the federal government.

The Marsh and Heagerty reports formed the basis for a major document considered at the Dominion-Provincial Conference on Reconstruction in 1945. Proposals in the document stressed the need for co-operation among all levels of government and groups in the country to attain high levels of employment, increased welfare, and security. The proposals also outlined strategies to address three main gaps in the present system: health insurance, national old age pensions, and unemployment assistance (Dominion-Provincial Conference on Reconstruction, 1945).

Because the social security proposals were part of larger proposals relating to financial matters upon which there was no provincial consensus, the innovative concept of comprehensive, integrated, co-ordinated, national programming for social security was eventually abandoned. This unfortunate outcome impelled the federal and provincial governments to independently seek ways in which to influence health policies.

However, the extensive investigations and discussions associated with the conference had established political and social pressures for action that were not to be denied (Taylor, 1987). This pressure toward action in integration of health and welfare services led to amalgamation of health and welfare under one common federal department in 1944. The minister of the new Department of Health and Welfare now had responsibility for "all matters relating to the promotion or preservation of the health, social security, and social welfare of the people of Canada over which the Parliament of Canada has jurisdiction" (Cameron, 1962, p. 1).

ERA THREE: MID-1940S TO MID-1960S

The third major era in development of social security policy and programs in Canada was marked by consolidation of a dominant government role in social security and by remarkable progress made at both the federal and provincial levels in establishing a wide range of new programs and in improving those that already existed (Taylor, 1956). With one outstanding exception, it was a period of what is termed "disjointed incrementalism"; the order in which new programs were implemented and the relationships between them were not guided by a formal, rational plan, such as had been conceived at the federal level through the Marsh and Heagerty plans.

The one exception to this disjointed approach was in Saskatchewan, which was to lead health-care planning and programming for all of Canada during the next twenty years. In 1944, the Co-operative Commonwealth Federation (CCF) party came to power. This democratic-socialist agrarian protest movement put forth a platform promising a "complete system of socialized health services" (Sigerist, 1944, p. 3). Dr. Henry Sigerist of Johns Hopkins University was engaged to develop the plan that would guide health policy and program development in Saskatchewan.

The most dramatic immediate action of the Saskatchewan government was the establishment, on January 1, 1947, of a Hospital Services Plan. This was the first compulsory and comprehensive hospital insurance plan in North America. During the next three years, provincial plans were also implemented in Alberta, British Columbia, and Newfoundland (Taylor, 1987). As a result of these developments, the provinces requested that health insurance be placed on the agenda of the 1955 federal-provincial conference. Subsequent federal-provincial negotiations resulted in federal proposals to pay approximately 50 percent of the costs of insured hospital services, based on a cost-sharing formula (Taylor, 1973). By 1958, the federal *Hospital Insurance and Diagnostic Services Act* was implemented in five provinces; the remaining provinces had all joined the plan by 1961.

Several other important federal programs were also developed during this time. In 1948, National Health Grants were introduced. These grants had been part of the Proposals on Reconstruction and were designed to enable the provinces to establish the foundations for comprehensive health insurance. Public health, tuberculosis control, mental health care, venereal disease control, crippled children's diseases, cancer control, professional training, and public health research were targeted by this grants-in-aid program, as were hospital construction and health survey capability (Martin, 1948). A number of positive modifications were also made to income security programs during this era.

In 1962, Saskatchewan again took the lead in health care when, on July 1, 1962, a medical insurance plan was introduced. It faced adamant opposition from the medical profession, opposition that resulted in the famous "doctor's strike" (Badgely & Wolfe, 1967; Meilicke, 1967; Tollefson, 1964). The fact that public opinion moved against the striking doctors ensured that medical insurance plans could be introduced in other provinces and, eventually, at the federal level.

In 1964, the Report of the Federal Royal Commission on Health Services, headed by Chief Justice Emmett Hall (the first "Hall Commission") was released. It recommended the federal government enter into agreements with the provinces to assist them in introducing and operating a "comprehensive, universal, provincial program of personal health services" (Royal Commission, 1964, p. 19). This led, in 1968, to the federal *Medical Care Act*, which provided for federal sharing of approximately 50 percent of costs of a provincial medical insurance plan if it incorporated comprehensive medical coverage, a universally available plan, portable benefit coverage, and public authority administration (four of the five principles of medicare).

Several other federal programs began in the 1960s: National Welfare Grants in 1962; Youth Allowance Program in 1964; Canada Pension Plan in 1965; Canada Assistance Program in 1966 (a comprehensive program for federal sharing of provincial expenditures for public assistance and for welfare services on a conditional cost-sharing basis similar to that in health); and *Health Resources Act* (federal payments over a fifteen-year period for construction, acquisition, and renovation of facilities for training health-care workers and for research in health fields) (Hacon, 1967).

In only twenty years, Canada had moved from what had been described as a "backward position in welfare state development by international standards" (Collins, 1976, p. 6) to a point where at least the major social security programs necessary for a modern industrial nation were in place. The speed of progress and the scope and range of the programs generated a vast array of new problems; these problems were to become the focus of the next era.

ERA FOUR: MID-1960S TO MID-1970S

The ten-year period from the mid-1960s to the mid-1970s was characterized by the commissioning of special inquiries and reports. These examined the numerous and complex social security programs established in the previous twenty years, reassessed needs, and made recommendations for improvements in services, organization, financing, and cost control. One of the most ambitious investigations began in Quebec in 1966 with establishment of the Commission of Inquiry on Health and Social Welfare (the Castonguay-Nepveu Commission). Ontario established the Committee on the Healing Arts and the Ontario Council of Health in that year. In the years following, almost every province instituted one or more mechanisms of inquiry into general or specific aspects of their respective social security services. For an extensive listing of these and other reports see Storch and Meilicke (1979), and for a summary and comparison of six of the most significant provincial and federal government-sponsored reports see Browne (1980).

At the federal level, a range and variety of inquiries were established: Task Force on the Cost of Health Services (National Health and Welfare Canada: 1969), which attempted to suggest ways to restrain health-care costs; Report of the Special Senate Committee on Poverty in Canada (1971), which highlighted the finding that poverty is reflective of a social attitude translated into economic and political policies; and Report of the Community Health Centre Project (Hastings, 1972), which suggested establishment of people-centred primary care centres. Federal Health Minister Marc Lalonde issued *A New Perspective on the Health of Canadians* (Lalonde, 1974), which maintained that a new emphasis on human biology, environment, and lifestyle, equal to the traditional emphasis on health-care delivery, was necessary to improve the health of Canadians. He also issued a *Working Paper on Social Security* (Lalonde, 1973), which upheld proposals similar to those of the Marsh Report of 1943 (i.e., need for an employment strategy, a social-insurance strategy, an income-supplementation strategy, a social and employment services strategy, and a federal-provincial strategy).

An extremely important reappraisal process began in December 1970, when the federal government initiated discussions regarding new federal-provincial cost-sharing formulas. Dialogue between the federal and provincial governments continued sporadically and, in 1975, the federal government served notice of its intent to terminate the existing formula for hospital cost sharing. After drawn-out negotiations with the provinces, this led, on April 1, 1977, to the *Established Programs Financing Act*, whereby federal cost sharing for both hospital and medical insurance was changed from a conditional grant to a modified block grant system. The intent of this change was to provide greater provincial flexibility and facilitate the containment of costs to the federal treasury (Van Loon, 1978).

The fourth era in the development of the Canadian social security program was a time of extensive reappraisal. Although few definitive solutions were found, many problems and issues were more clearly identified and a rich variety of ideas and proposals were generated. Among the themes most frequently heard were that a comprehensive and integrated approach to planning, organizing, administering, and evaluating social security was required, that costs must be controlled, and that quality had to be better defined and controlled.

ERA FIVE: 1977 TO 1991

The fifth era was characterized by federal government attempts to uphold the principles of health care while reducing its cost commitments to the health enterprise. Still operating within the context of the provisions in the *BNA Act*, the federal government's only real enforcement mechanism to maintain the principles of accessibility, universality, comprehensiveness, portability, and non-profit administration was the power to withhold grant monies to coerce conformity. With the change in funding involving block grants and tax point transfers, the financial transfer to the provinces became less valuable than that realized during the period of conditional cost sharing. Thus, even the threat of withholding a portion of the block grant was not as serious as it might have been.

In 1984, the federal government introduced the *Canada Health Act*; this was intended to replace the *Hospital Insurance and Diagnostic Services Act* and the *Medical Care Act* and to re-establish the five principles. The *Canada Health Act* was bitterly opposed by the provinces and by organized medicine. The provinces resented intrusion into what they considered their constitutional domain. So, too, did organized medicine. The penalty for lack of adherence to the Act, by allowing extra billing for example, was the ability to withhold funds from the block grant transfer on the basis of one dollar for every dollar the provinces allowed to be paid through user fees or balance billing. The medical profession opposed these constraints, contending that user fees and balance billing represented a means for raising health revenues and for exercising physicians' professional freedom (Taylor, 1987). There were numerous challenges to this Act, with a particular challenge from within Ontario in the form of a physicians' strike in 1986.

Public opinion moved against the doctors in this strike, and the medical profession failed to sustain a united front. Ontario banned extra-billing, and the last province holding out for extra-billing (Alberta) banned the practice five weeks later.

During this era, numerous government commissions and inquiries examined ways in which health care might be delivered in a more cost-effective manner. The growing cost constraint brought about by a downturn in the economy forced the provinces to a deeper level of consideration of the structure of the health-care system and the necessity for major reforms to effect an affordable system. *The Rainbow Report* in Alberta and the *Closer to Home* report from British Columbia are only two of numerous reports produced at this time calling for fundamental changes in the delivery of health care, stronger emphasis on health promotion and primary care, and care delivered outside institutions.

ERA SIX: INTO A NEW MILLENNIUM

By the early 1990s, a dramatic change had occurred in the way health services were to be planned and financed. The federal government basically restricted its role to maintenance of the five medicare principles, and the provincial governments were left with the main responsibility for funding. In the face of growing budget deficits, this placed immense pressure on provincial and territorial governments to economize on health expenditures. In turn, this created a climate for change in the organization and management of health services that transcended anything since the foundation for the current system was completed more than 25 years ago.

Changes evident throughout the system included mergers, amalgamations, and regional planning. There was growing activity to refine the operational mission and role of health-care organizations and to minimize costs associated with inappropriate or unnecessary distribution and utilization of resources. Provincial and territorial funding agencies moved to funding systems that more directly encouraged efficient management of resources, such as funding hospitals on severity of illness measures (Meilicke, 1990) (see also Chapters 4 and 15). There were also modifications made to narrow the definition of basic health services under the *Canada Health Act.*

Running parallel to these activities were efforts to rationalize technology assessment and distribution and to improve hospital information systems. This was considered essential to allow more precise definitions of intra-institutional responsibility, to improve the appropriateness of patient placement relative to care alternatives, and to develop guidelines for clinical decision making in physician practice. To some extent, health promotion and prevention activities were also expanded, although the investment of funding to elevate the status of these activities was still modest. Changes in delivery systems were beginning, with the intent of focussing on community-based services.

Different patterns of governance, such as regional planning agencies and area health authorities, were discussed, planned, and/or implemented in most provinces. In Saskatchewan, for example, plans were underway to replace the existing 400 separate boards with 30 autonomous health district boards to administer the province's health-care budget. Such planning for health districts was reminiscent of the work of the Sigerist Commission in the mid-1940s (Sigerist, 1944).

Accepting their fundamental responsibility for health, the provincial ministers of health and their deputies began meeting to share their approaches to health-care reform and to unite in their common struggle for cost containment. The intensity of these deliberations was similar to meetings preceding the Dominion-Provincial Conference on Reconstruction in 1945. The agenda had changed, however, from one requesting federal government assistance in funding health care to one that assumed greater provincial responsibility, and that designed to provide mutual support and consultation to effect health-care reform.

The common fundamentals of governmental reform for this modern era are:

- to improve the health status of all Canadians;
- to reaffirm the principles of the *Canada Health Act*;
- to ensure a more cost-effective system; and
- to provide a continuum of services characterized by a shift from institution-based to community-based services, by healthy public policy, and by an emphasis on health promotion (*Background Paper...*, 1992).

A prime example of unity across the provinces and territories was evident in the commissioning of a study on physician resources in Canada (Barer & Stoddart, 1991). Not only were the provinces instrumental in examining the numbers of physicians in the system and entering the system, but they also took action to deal with several recommendations of the report, such as reductions in medical-school enrollment.

By 1993, there were clear signals that health-care restructuring with a view to health-care reform was more than rhetoric and that virtually all policies and services were vulnerable to change. As the provinces accepted increasing responsibility for health care, they began to reconsider consumers' needs in a more orderly manner—needs for first access care, for continuity of care, for care in emergency, for community care, and for social welfare. In many respects, a return to ideals promoted in the Marsh and Heagerty reports and reiterated in the plethora of reports issued during the fourth era was becoming evident.

In late 1994, shortly after a Liberal government was returned to power, Prime Minister Jean Chretien established the National Health Forum to involve and inform Canadians and advise the federal government on innovative ways to improve the health of the people of Canada and the health-care system (National Health Forum, 1997). The Forum focussed attention in four key areas:

1. Values (exploring core values Canadians connect to the health-care system;
2. Striking a Balance (examining health resource allocation);
3. Determinants of Health (identifying actions to address population health and non-medical aspects of health);
4. Evidence-Based Decision Making (considering how policy-makers, practitioners, and individuals can have the best access to and use of evidence upon which to base their decisions).

The report, released in early 1997, concluded that Canadians had inherited an excellent health-care system, which had been developed over four decades and which continued to enjoy strong support from the people of Canada. It was deemed to be essential to protect that legacy by preserving what had been acquired, and by developing more integrated systems of care and broader approaches to promoting health.

Also released in 1997 was *A Renewed Vision* (Provincial/Territorial Ministers of Health, 1997) from the Conference of Provincial/Territorial Ministers of Health, which represented a consensus of all provinces and territories except Quebec. This report recommended a new administrative mechanism to secure the future of the *Canada Health Act*. An expert advisory panel was to serve as a reference body to make recommendations on disputes and issues referred by either the federal government or the provinces/territories. This panel's duties would include clarification and interpretation of the Act and its five principles, and review of provincial/territorial application and adherence to the principles. With the return of the Liberal government to a second term in June 1997, the potential for preserving the values of the current system sounded promising.

Meanwhile, most provinces were devolving authority relative to health and social services to regional levels, with the intent to control costs, increase responsiveness and flexibility, better integrate services, and improve health outcomes. Five provinces led the way in these initiatives: Quebec, New Brunswick, Saskatchewan, and Prince Edward Island (all of which commenced implementation prior to 1994), and Alberta (which implemented regional health authorities so rapidly that it came to be regarded as one of the leaders in health-care restructuring) (Lomas, Woods, & Veenstra, 1997a).

In Alberta, the severity and rapidity of reduction and restructuring, with closure of several major urban hospitals, led to serious questioning of government motives by many citizens and by health providers. Critics claimed that reduction and restructuring were informed more by political ideology than by rational planning. At least two commentators suggested that the rapid changes, based upon the argument that health-care costs were out of control, could not be justified. They claimed that this argument was a clever foil for those attempting to privatize Canada's health-care system, and a mask for the real cause of provincial deficits, namely massive subsidies to the private sector, not public expenditure on health (Nelson, 1995; Taft, 1997).

CONCLUSION

Toward the turn of the century, tensions characterizing regionalization efforts are common in almost every province. These include tensions between provincial roles and regional roles (particularly in regard to budgetary control), between regional authorities and health-care professionals and providers, and between regional authorities and the public they were intended to serve (Lomas, Woods, & Veenstra, 1997b). At the core of these tensions is a fundamental questioning of whether devolution of health care is a good thing for Canadian health care and for the health status of the Canadian people. With the Ontario government proceeding with major restructuring of both health and welfare, distribution of financial responsibility for health and welfare characteristic of the 1940s looms as a distinct possibility for the future. In 1940, for example, municipalities paid 22.3% of public health and welfare costs, the province paid 41.5%, and the federal government contributed 36.2% (Cassidy, 1945).

Such redistribution of fiscal and moral responsibility threatens the concept of a national health-care (and social-service) system. Further, as Stingl (1996) noted, "the current health reform debate in Canada is not just about the kind of health system we want for ourselves and our family members. At a deeper and more far-reaching level, it is about the kind of society we want to live in, one that feels an obligation to care for its sick and injured or one that does not" (p. 17).

Although history rarely repeats itself exactly, it is clear that similar problems in health-care delivery frequently emerge in different contexts across the years. Knowledge of the past, therefore, allows a respect for history and can contribute a useful degree of wisdom in the creative search for new solutions while avoiding repetition of past mistakes.

A thorough knowledge of the development of Canadian health-care delivery is critical to understanding the social, political, and economic forces that have shaped the system, and that will continue to influence future changes within it.

SUMMARY

- Division of powers relative to health care between the federal and provincial governments (under the *British North America Act*) has been a major factor in shaping the Canadian health-care system.
- Current health-care restructuring programs to control costs, increase responsiveness and flexibility, better integrate services, and improve health outcomes have their roots in past reports and commissions.
- Canadians generally support the five principles upon which the Canadian health-care system is founded.
- Although significant restructuring is in progress, there is as yet limited evidence of reform.

FURTHER READINGS AND RESOURCES

Angus, D.E. (1991). *Review of significant health care commissions and task forces in Canada since 1983–84*. Ottawa: Canadian Nurses Association and Canadian Medical Association. Using a report style format, Angus provides a synopsis and analysis of major government commissions and task forces within Canada. Following a discussion of the central themes, directions, and trends, he reviews major commissions in each province and nationally. For each commissioned report, he outlines terms of reference and major recommendations, creating a handy and useful reference to documents published between 1983 and 1990.

Meilicke, C.A., & Storch, J.L. (Eds.). (1980). *Perspectives on Canadian health and social services policy: History and emerging trends*. Ann Arbor, MI: Health Administration Press. This book of previously published articles is a collection of historical perspectives on the development of the Canadian health and social services policy. Perspectives include those of government bureaucrats, journalists, academics, and agency personnel, who collectively provide a rich review of policy and practice in health care and social welfare. Integration of the numerous articles is provided through an introduction and brief commentaries on each section.

Taylor, M.G. (1987). *Health insurance and Canadian public policy: The seven decisions that created the Canadian health insurance system and their outcomes* (2nd ed.). Montreal: McGill-Queen's University Press. This book contains an interesting and brilliant analysis of the critical steps in development of Canada's health insurance system, and of policy-making at federal and provincial levels of government. Featuring three federal and four provincial key decisions, Taylor describes the inputs to those decisions as well as immediate and long-term outcomes.

REFERENCES

Angus, D. E. (1991). *Review of significant health care commissions and task forces in Canada since 1983–84*. Ottawa: Canadian Hospital Association.

Armitage, A. (1975). *Social welfare in Canada: Ideals and realities*. Toronto: McClelland & Stewart.

Background paper on health care reform initiatives. (1992). Health Reform Paper for Provincial Health Ministers Meeting in Newfoundland. Regina, SK: Saskatchewan Health Planning and Policy Development Branch.

Badgely, R. F., & Wolfe, S. (1967). *Doctors strike*. Toronto: Macmillan of Canada.

Barer, M. L., & Stoddart, G. L. (1991). *Toward integrated medical resource policies in Canada*. Winnipeg, MB: Manitoba Health.

Bellamy, D. (1965). Social welfare in Canada. In *Encyclopedia of Social Work*. New York: National Association of Social Workers.

Browne, J. (1980). Summary of recent major studies of health care in Canada. In C. A. Meilicke & J. L. Storch (Eds.), *Perspectives on Canadian health and social service policy: History and emerging trends* (pp. 293–305). Ann Arbour, MI: Health Administration Press.

Bryden, K. (1974). *Old age pensions and policy-making in Canada*. Montreal: McGill-Queen's University Press.

Cameron, G. D. W. (1962). The department of national health and welfare. In R. D. Defries (Ed.), *The federal and provincial health services in Canada* (2nd ed.). Toronto: Canadian Public Health Association.

Cassidy, H. M. (1945). *Public health and welfare reorganization: The post-war problem in the Canadian provinces*. Toronto: Ryerson Press.

Cassidy, H. M. (1947). The Canadian social services. *Annals of the Academy of Political and Social Science, 253*, 191–198.

Collins, K. (1976, January-February). Three decades of social security in Canada. *Canadian Welfare, 51*, 5–7.

Deber, R., & Vayda, E. (1992). The political and health care systems of Canada and Ontario. In R. Deber (Ed.), *Case studies in Canadian health policy and management* (Vol. 1) (pp. 1–16). Ottawa: Canadian Hospital Association Press.

Dominion-Provincial Conference on Reconstruction. (1945). *Proposals of the Government of Canada*. Paper presented at the meeting of the Dominion-Provincial Conference on Reconstruction. Ottawa, ON: Queen's Printer.

Gelber, S. M. (1966, June). The path to health insurance. *Canadian Public Administration, 9*, 211–220.

Gelber, S. M. (1973). *Personal health services in Canada: The early years*. Address to the Association of University Programs in Hospital Administration, Faculty Institute, Ottawa.

Gregoire, J. (1962). The ministry of health of the province of Quebec. In R. D. Defries (Ed.), *The federal and provincial health services in Canada* (2nd ed.). Toronto: Canadian Public Health Association.

Hacon, W. S. (1967, October 28). Improving Canada's health manpower resources. *Canadian Medical Association Journal, 97*, 1104–1108.

Hastings, J. E. F. (1972). *The community health centre in Canada: Report of the community health centre project to the health ministers* (Vol. 1.). Ottawa: Information Canada.

Heagerty, J. J. (1934). The development of public health in Canada. *Canadian Journal of Public Health, 25*, 54–56.

Heagerty, J. J. (1943). *Report of the advisory committee on health insurance*. Ottawa: Queen's Printer.

Lalonde, M. (1973). *Working paper on social security*. Ottawa: Government of Canada.

Lalonde, M. (1974). *A new perspective on the health of Canadians: A working document.* Ottawa: Government of Canada.

Lindenfield, R. (1959). Hospital insurance in Canada. *Social Service Review, 33,* 149.

Lomas, J., Woods, J., & Veenstra, G. (1997a). Devolving authority for health care in Canada's provinces: 1. An introduction to the issues. *Canadian Medical Association Journal, 156* (3), 371–377.

Lomas, J., Woods, J., & Veenstra, G. (1997b). Devolving authority for health care in Canada's provinces: 3. Motivations, attitudes and approaches of board members. *Canadian Medical Association Journal, 156* (5), 669–676.

Marsh, L. (1975). *Report on social security for Canada: 1943.* Toronto: University of Toronto Press.

Martin, P. (1948). A national health program for Canada. *Canadian Journal of Public Health, 39,* 220–223.

Meilicke, C. A. (1967). The Saskatchewan medical care dispute of 1962: An analytical social history. Unpublished doctoral dissertation, University of Minnesota.

Meilicke, C. A. (1990). International perspectives on healthcare: Canada. *Healthcare Executive, 5* (4), 25–26.

Morgan, J. S. (1961). Social welfare services in Canada. In M. Oliver (Ed.), *Social purpose for Canada.* Toronto: University of Toronto Press.

National Health Forum. (1997). *Canada health action: Building on the legacy. Final report of the National Health Forum* (Vols. I and II). Ottawa: Minister of Public Works and Government Services.

Najman, J. M., & Western, J. S. (1984). A comparative analysis of Australian health policy in the 1970's. *Social Science and Medicine, 18* (1), 949–958.

National Health & Welfare Canada: Task Force on the Cost of Health Services in Canada. (1969). *Report: Summary* (Vol. 1). Ottawa: National Health & Welfare.

Nelson, J. (1995, January-February). Dr. Rockefeller will see you now: The hidden players privatizing Canada's health care system. *Canadian Forum,* pp. 7–12.

Provincial/Territorial Ministers of Health. (1997). *A renewed vision for Canada's health system: A report of the Conference of Provincial/Territorial Ministers of Health.* Ottawa: Health Canada.

Rorem, R. C. (1931). *The municipal doctor system in rural Saskatchewan.* Chicago: University of Chicago Press.

Royal Commission on Health Services. (1964). *Report: Royal Commission on Health Services* (Vol. 1). Ottawa: Queen's Printer.

Sigerist, H. E. (1944). *Saskatchewan Health Services Commission: Report of the Commissioner.* Regina: King's Printer.

Special Senate Committee on Poverty. (1971). *Poverty in Canada: Report of the Special Senate Committee on Poverty.* Ottawa: Information Canada.

Splane, R. B. (1965). *Social welfare in Ontario: A study of public welfare administration.* Toronto: University of Toronto Press.

Stingl, M. S. (1996). Equality and efficiency as basic social values. In M. Stingl & D. Wilson (Eds.), *Efficiency and equality: Health reform in Canada.* Halifax: Fernwood Publishing.

Storch, J. L., & Meilicke, C. A. (1979). Health and Social Services Administration: An annotated bibliography. Ottawa: Canadian College of Health Service Executives.

Taft, K. (1997). *Shredding the public interest.* Edmonton: University of Alberta Press.

Taylor, M. G. (1949). The Saskatchewan hospital services plan. Unpublished doctoral dissertation, University of California, Berkeley.

Taylor, M. G. (1956). The administration of health insurance in Canada. Toronto: Oxord University Press.

Taylor, M. G. (1973, January-February). The Canadian health insurance program. *Public Administration Review, 33,* 35.

Taylor, M. G. (1987). *Health insurance and Canadian public policy: The seven decisions that created the Canadian health insurance system* (2nd ed.). Montreal: McGill-Queen's University Press.

Tollefson, E. A. (1964). *Bitter medicine: The Saskatchewan medical care dispute.* Saskatoon: Modern Press.

Van Loon, R. J. (1978, Winter). From shared cost to block funding and beyond. *Journal of Health Politics, Policy and Law, 2,* 460.

Van Loon, R. J., & Whittington, M.S. (1976). *The Canadian political system: Environment, structure and process* (2nd ed.). Toronto: McGraw-Hill Ryerson.

Wallace, E. (1950). The origin of the social welfare state in Canada, 1867–1900. *Canadian Journal of Economics and Political Science, 16,* 384.

Chapter 2

▼▼▼▼▼▼▼▼▼▼▼▼▼▼

Using Demographics and Epidemiological Information in Management

L. JANE KNOX

KEY OBJECTIVES

In this chapter, you will learn:

- Basic demographic and epidemiological trends used by health-care managers to plan and evaluate health care.
- How to set priorities and target services to groups with the greatest health needs.
- How to identify and explain significant issues in the health status of Canadians.
- Sources of information about the health of Canadians.

INTRODUCTION

Accurate prediction of future health needs is both fascinating and essential for effective health care. Like other research-based activity, predicting health needs demands curiosity, imagination, and an understanding of community values or ethics. It also requires nurses and other health managers to use demography and epidemiology. More effective care results when health managers use these tools to ensure that health care makes a difference to the health of the population.

This chapter reviews basic Canadian demographic and epidemiologic facts, and identifies areas where these facts should influence change in Canada's health-care system. The chapter shows how population growth and health status of population groups (infants, children, youth, adults, and aboriginal people) should influence health care. Using this information, nurse managers can lead multidisciplinary teams to plan and evaluate health services that respond to identified health needs in communities.

Effective nursing actions improve health. Effective nursing management improves the health of whole communities.

POPULATION HEALTH AND MANAGEMENT'S ROLE

Population health is an approach to health care. It considers all factors influencing health, and plans strategies affecting large groups of people. Tools such as epidemiology and demography help to identify health issues affecting many people.

Epidemiology is the study of patterns of injury, disease, and determinants of health in specific populations for the purpose of controlling health problems and improving health. **Demography** is the study of population growth, age distribution, migration, births and deaths, and the interaction of these factors with social and economic conditions.

Today's policy makers and successful health managers use the tools of epidemiology and demography to assess key health needs and allocate resources in response to those needs. Health managers also use community values to ensure acceptance of their program decisions by the people they hope to serve.

Nurse managers help assess health needs by sharing their knowledge about health behaviour, and injury and disease patterns. They can use and inform others about Statistics Canada publications on national health surveys, and the *Report on the Health of Canadians*, by the Federal, Provincial and Territorial Advisory Committee on Population Health (abbreviated FPT ACPH) (1996). Nurse managers need to involve communities in setting health priorities. As well, nurse managers must recognize that communities do not act independently to resolve problems they do not recognize. Setting health goals and objectives also brings nurse managers and community members together.

Recognizing all the determinants of health is important to help identify health goals. **Determinants of health** are key factors influencing health, including personal risk factors (e.g., age, sex, genetics, health practices, coping skills) and environmental factors (e.g., living conditions, working conditions, physical surroundings, health services).

In 1996, Canada's Ministers of Health used a simple "windmill" framework (see Figure 2.1) to describe key factors creating health or harm for a target group (FPT ACPH, 1996, p. 4). Like a windmill, the framework's arms are each important but do not work alone. When health determinants work together, they have an unexpectedly powerful impact.

Senior nurse managers work with the governing board to set specific objectives so that the board can tell the public its plans. Nurse managers then set achievable performance targets based on health-status indicators. These targets provide clear direction for the staff, who develop action plans. Clear objectives and performance targets also allow evaluation of program effectiveness based on health outcomes. Evaluations are useful when management acts on the findings.

F i g u r e   2 . 1

WINDMILL OF DETERMINANTS OF HEALTH

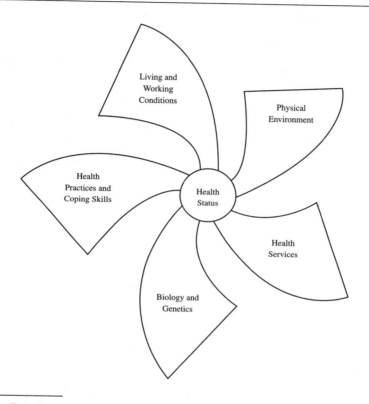

Source: From *Report on the Health of Canadians,* Health Canada, Federal, Provincial and Territorial Advisory Committee on Population Health (FTP ACPH), 1996, p.4. Reproduced with permission of the Minister of Public Works and Government Services Canada, 1998.

Nurse managers can use a six-step process to guide the health system and improve health, as shown in Box 2.1. Every step requires nurse managers to use demographics and epidemiology. This process makes health services more effective by responding to real population health needs.

DEMOGRAPHICS OF POPULATION GROWTH

Both immigration and births contribute to growth in a population. Since 1981, Canadian fertility rates have been below the replacement level of two children per woman (Statistics Canada, 1996b, p. 61). Despite this, Canada's population continued to grow during the 1980s and early 1990s

---

B o x   2 . 1

PROCESS TO GUIDE THE HEALTH SYSTEM AND TO IMPROVE HEALTH

To contribute to improving population health, nurse managers:

- Assess health needs, including all determinants of health and community views;
- Analyze health problems by comparing local needs assessments with provincial or national data on health behaviours and disease or injury patterns;
- Help develop achievable health goals and objectives for the population with short—and long-term performance targets;
- Design health programs to meet goals and objectives, focussing on primary health needs in target populations;
- Identify health status indicators to monitor significant changes in population health; and
- Evaluate the success of health programs in improving population health

---

because of a large proportion of childbearing-age women. Three major factors will influence Canada's demographic patterns in future: aboriginal demographics, immigration, and the aging of the "baby-boom" generation.

ABORIGINAL DEMOGRAPHICS

Demographic patterns for aboriginal people differ from the national picture. The population is very young and is growing rapidly. Basic needs like housing, clean water, and education may be less accessible. For example, in 1991, only 43 percent of aboriginal Canadians had completed high school, compared with 60 percent of people in Newfoundland and 83 percent in British Columbia (FPT ACPH, 1996, *Technical Appendix*, pp. 35–36).

Birth rates, death rates, and the proportion of youth in aboriginal populations, all have important differences from national averages. For example, the birth rate of aboriginal women was twice the rate for all Canadian women in 1991. Fifty-five percent of aboriginal mothers were less than twenty-five years old, compared with 28 percent of non-aboriginal mothers (Hanvey et al., 1994, p. 136). In 1991, 38 percent of aboriginals were under age fifteen, compared with 21 percent in the Canadian population (Statistics Canada, 1996b, p. 74; Hanvey, Avard, Graham, Underwood, Campbell, & Kelly, 1994, p. 2).

The aboriginal population is growing rapidly. The special needs of aboriginal people are an urgent priority for many sectors, and a challenge for all health services. By working effectively with aboriginal people, nurse managers may be able to assist in the search for creative and culturally acceptable solutions to these challenges.

IMMIGRATION

Immigrants consistently represent about 16 percent of Canada's population and tend to live in large cities in Ontario, British Columbia, Alberta, and Manitoba (Badets, 1993). New Canadians bring creativity, cultural richness, and hope for economic growth and stability to the country. They may also bring dietary and other cultural habits which increase risk of disease. To plan effective care, nurse managers consider six factors influencing health behaviour: communication, space, social organization, time, environmental control, and biological variations (Giger & Davidhizar, 1990, p. 199).

During the 1990s, immigration policies favoured the acceptance of wealthy and/or well-educated adults to Canada to take jobs requiring their unique skills. In 1991, most came from Asia (53 percent), followed by Europeans (20 percent), and those born in the Caribbean and Central or South America (17 percent) (Hanvey et al., 1994, p. 3). Immigration policies are sensitive to public opinion, and may change as Canadians continue to experience workforce adjustments and unemployment.

AN AGING POPULATION

The final trend influencing Canada's population demographics is the aging of the "baby-boom" generation. Canada's "baby boom" occurred primarily between 1946 and 1966 (Statistics Canada, 1996b, p. 60–61). In 1996, the first wave of "boomers" turned 50. Canada's population of seniors will triple between 1993 and 2041. This startling fact already shapes the health-care system. It also contributes to health policies that promote mobility and general well-being rather than institutionalization. In general, the elderly welcome this change as a quality-of-life issue. Policy makers accept it as a cost-saving measure. Nurse managers recognize it as a shift that improves health and also changes the nature of nursing work.

In planning for an aging population, many factors require attention. First, the proportion of elderly people will vary across the country and within provinces. Second, the nature of the older population is changing: many seniors are informed, assertive, and less deferential to health professionals than ever before. They increasingly take charge of their health. Third, seniors often choose to live in small rural communities where transportation problems limit access to health-care services. Fourth, there will be many more elderly women than men, especially over age 75. The health system has been unresponsive to this pattern, perhaps because unisex warehousing of the elderly was the focus of seniors' health care throughout the 1970s and 1980s. Finally, many of Canada's caregivers are "baby-boomers." As the population ages, caregivers will be aging too.

Nurse managers can plan services that respond to the health needs of people. They can involve seniors in decision making about their health at the individual, group, and community levels. They can look for ways to address transportation and other issues hindering access to health services.

They can be alert to the health needs of older women when designing health programs, and they can plan to support mobility and independence. They can take transfer and lift programs seriously, and help staff and at-home helpers avoid back injuries and other risks to their health.

HEALTH STATUS OF POPULATION GROUPS

Within the overall population, health-care managers focus on the needs of various age groups, as they do in the case of seniors as discussed above. Other population groups requiring attention to their changing health-care needs include infants, children, youth, adults, and aboriginal peoples.

INFANTS

One useful measure of a population's health is the infant mortality rate. Infant mortality has declined steadily in Canada since the late 1960s, but there still is room for improvement. Many countries do better than Canada's 1990 rate of 6.8 deaths per 1,000 infants (Hanvey et al., 1994, p. 18). This rate varies among the provinces, but the differences are smaller than during the 1980s (FPT ACPH, 1996, p. 32). In some provinces, northern populations and aboriginal people experience more than double the national infant mortality rate. Perinatal causes (e.g., premature births) and congenital anomalies account for 72 percent of all deaths under age one, but sudden infant death syndrome is also a leading cause of death (Wilkins, 1995).

Another indicator of population health is the rate of low birth weight babies (less than 2500 grams at birth). Low birth weight babies are at risk for infant death or health problems throughout life. The effects of low birth weight are usually irreversible (Millar, Strachan, & Wadhera, 1993). They include cerebral palsy, learning disabilities, visual and auditory defects, and other deficits in physical and mental development. The cost to the individual, the family, and society is high.

In 1993, 5.7 percent of live babies born in Canada were low birth weight babies (FPT ACPH, 1996, p. 11). This pattern has changed little since the 1980s. The critical factors in the mother that are associated with low birth weight infants include poor nutrition, use of tobacco, alcohol or drugs, multiple births, and low socio-economic status (Millar et al., 1993). Nurse managers must speak out about these factors and provide information for policymakers and future parents. Nurse managers can also promote parent-to-parent messages about the negative impact of smoking on infant health. This strategy may be more effective than pamphlets and posters.

Most Canadian children are remarkably healthy, but some infants require hospitalization, usually for injuries or respiratory illnesses or injuries. Respiratory illnesses in children can be reduced by encouraging families to limit second-hand smoke and to breast-feed their babies. Correct use of child restraints could also reduce the numbers of hospital admissions. A Transport Canada survey (cited in Hanvey et al., 1994, p. 36) found that only 33 percent of infants were properly restrained in the correct car seat for their age. Community studies (e.g., in Saskatoon) often show that even fewer infants are correctly protected. Nurse managers need to consider enabling and motivating strategies to help parents use child restraints correctly. Planning for emergency care is not enough.

CHILDREN

Statistics Canada (1996a, p. 17) reports that in 1994–95, children aged 0 to 11 years comprised 16 percent of the Canadian population, compared with 30 percent in 1971. About 84 percent of children lived in two-parent families in 1994–95; about 15 percent lived in one-parent families; less than 1 percent lived with other relatives/guardians (Statistics Canada, 1996a, pp. 28–29). Of the 15 percent living in one-parent families, almost 93 percent lived with a single mother. The 8.6 percent who were stepchildren most often lived in families with their own mother and siblings, and a stepfather.

In Canada, 18 percent of children born in the early 1980s saw their parents separate by age six. This statistic is still increasing. These young children face emotional stress, conflict, and confusion. Alert nurse managers consider this group at risk, and plan programs to help prevent mental health problems for children dealing with parental separation. Lack of social support (e.g., friends, relatives, stable day care) is an important indicator of health risk.

Preschoolers and School-Age Children

Preschoolers are beginning to walk, run, jump, and climb. Their constant motion increases their risk of injury. Injuries are the leading cause of death for children aged one to four, followed by birth defects (Hanvey et al., 1994, p. 44). Motor vehicle accidents, burns, or drowning most often cause these preventable injuries and deaths.

In 1990, school-age children (5 to 14 years) died of injuries at the rate of eight per 100,000 children (Hanvey et al., 1994, pp. 61–62). Motor vehicle accidents caused most of these deaths, including children who were occupants in cars, pedestrians, and bicyclists. For every school-age child killed by motor vehicles, 87 are injured (Hanvey et al., 1994, p. 65). Equally alarming, the second leading cause of death for children aged 10 to 14 is intentional injury or suicide (Hanvey et al., 1994, p. 64). Parents and professionals alike must accept responsibility for studying the causes of these tragic injuries and deaths, and for finding ways to prevent them.

For example, many children still do not wear seat belts or bicycle helmets, or make use of other readily available methods of preventing injury. Failure to use bicycle helmets is also common among teenagers. In an Alberta study of 500 teens (average age 15.8 years), MacMillan and Jantzie (1993) found that only 17 percent of males and 11 percent of females reported helmet use. Nurse managers can stimulate community action toward vigorous multi-sector strategies to prevent disabilities and deaths caused by "accidents."

Disabled Children

In 1991, 7.2 percent of children aged 0 to 19 living in Canadian households were disabled, with Alberta and Saskatchewan having rates over 9 percent (Hanvey et al., 1994, pp. 151–155). Of these children, 85 percent had "mild" disabilities; however, almost 18 percent required technical aids, and 8.5 percent had difficulty getting together with friends their own age.

The most common disabilities were learning disabilities, emotional or mental disabilities, sensory difficulties, and mobility or agility disabilities. Although the families of these children often develop remarkable coping skills, they deserve recognition, support, and liberal access to respite care. Nurses and other health managers can be supporters of, and powerful advocates for, families with disabled children.

Violence, Poverty, and Working Parents

Young Canadians tend to be aggressive in their relationships. A study by King and Coles (1992, p. 96) showed that they experience more bullying than children in European countries. When the results of this study were released, many Canadian educators examined interventions designed to increase respect and understanding. By 1995, some Saskatchewan schools used planned discussions and posters to help children learn to respect each other and themselves. Parents, coaches, youth leaders, and nurse managers all have important roles to play in this area.

An increasing number of Canadian children live in poverty. In 1994, 18 to 24 percent of children under 18 lived in poverty in most provinces (FPT ACPH, 1996, p. 60). Nation-wide, in one-parent families from 58 percent of children in Alberta up to 70 percent of children in Manitoba are poor. Family income is one of the most powerful determinants of health. Poor children have lower birth weights, more infant deaths, higher rates of death from injuries, more exposure to second-hand smoke, more chronic health problems, and less school success (Hanvey et al., 1994, pp. 122–124).

Poor children do not necessarily suffer more violence. Canada does not have accurate data on child abuse, but does have data on violence against women. For example, an alarming 60 percent of women over eighteen in Alberta and British Columbia reported they had experienced violence severe enough to be considered a criminal offence (FPT ACPH, 1996, pp. 60–61). These provinces also have high family incomes and high levels of latchkey children who spend time alone while their parents work (Hanvey et al., 1994, p. 71). Newfoundland had the highest proportion of children in low-income families, but women over eighteen in that province reported the lowest level of physical or sexual violence (30% in 1993) (FPT ACPH, 1996, pp. 60–61). Newfoundland also had the lowest proportion (13%) of latchkey children, suggesting there were fewer families where both parents worked away from home (Hanvey et al., 1994, p. 71).

Alert nurse managers know that the poor have many health needs. They lobby for supportive environments like smoke-free spaces and safe play areas. Nurse managers try to ensure that the poor have easy access to services. They watch for barriers to access caused by location, language, or issues related to timing, such as hours during which services are available. They monitor access using demographics, and check the percentage of the target group that is using key services.

T E E N S

Most teenage deaths can be prevented. Motor vehicle accidents kill over 40 percent of the youth who lose their lives as teens. Suicide is also a high risk. In 1993, suicide was the stated cause of death for 23 percent of male and 13 percent of female deaths among those 15 to 19 years old (Wilkins, 1995, p. 36). The rate of suicide for young men is six times higher than for young women (Hanvey et al., 1994, p. 97). More than ten times the number of young people who actually commit suicide must be hospitalized as a result of attempting it, particularly among younger teens (Hanvey et al., 1994, pp. 75, 97). It is a concern that Canada admits to these statistics but has few plans to address the problem.

Physical Activity

Physical activity is essential for mental and physical health, and for the management of stress. Hanvey and colleagues (1994, pp. 79, 104) reported that a 1988 study found that 90 percent of 10- to 14-year-old girls and boys participated in three or more hours of physical activity weekly. By age 15 to 19, the proportion of children with high levels of physical activity dropped to 75 percent for boys and 66 percent for girls. Only 60 percent of boys and 40 percent of girls expected to be involved in physical activity at age 20 (King & Coles, 1992). Figure 2.2 shows that their expectations may be all too accurate.

Many strategies are needed to address this complex problem. Physical activity is essential throughout life, and it is especially critical that young people have enough weight-bearing activity to enhance bone density throughout the growing years (Bailey & Martin, 1994). Physical activity may also be an effective strategy for building self-esteem. Research reviewed by Quinney, Gauvin, and Wall (1994) reports the strong impact of active living on health and well-being.

Public-policy approaches and supportive environments can help young people to maintain levels of physical activity into their adult years. School-board policies regarding sports need to be monitored to ensure that sports excellence for a few does not take precedence over continued participation and free access to activity areas. Healthy public policy supports active living for all.

Figure 2.2

PREVALENCE OF LIFESTYLE RISK FACTORS

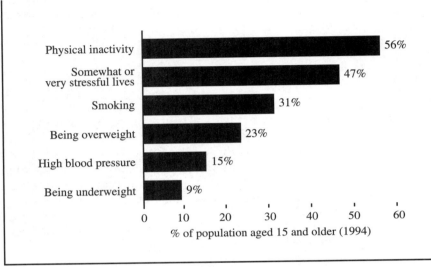

1991-1994

Source: Statistics Canada, *Canada Year Book, 1997*, Catalogue No. 11–402, p. 103. Reproduced by authority of the Minister of Industry, 1998.

Interpersonal Relationships, Sexual Activity, AIDS, and Pregnancy

One way teens develop self-esteem is by building an identity, values, and lifestyle separate from their parents. Bibby and Posterski (1992) studied the values and views of more than 3,500 Canadian teenagers. They found teens emphasized the individual over the group, and also placed reduced value on interpersonal relationships. However, friendships and music still ranked high as sources of enjoyment. Friendship is now understood as a significant determinant of health in Canadian society (FPT ACPH, 1996, p. 3).

Considering the threat of AIDS, it is alarming that sexual activity "has become fairly commonplace among Canadian young people" (Bibby & Posterski, 1992, p. 27), especially in Quebec where young people were most likely to approve of both petting (95 percent) and sexual intercourse (70 percent) after a few dates. Differences between young men and young women were pronounced, however; about 75 percent of males approved of sex after a few dates, while only 40 percent of females agreed. Bibby and Posterski emphasized they found "virtually no change in attitudes over the past decade for either males or females" (1992, p. 28).

Teen pregnancies declined during the 1970s and 1980s. Approximately 85 percent of Canadian teens (15 to 19 years) have taken sex education courses and 90 percent believe that they are "fairly knowledgeable about birth control" (Bibby & Posterski, 1992, p. 38). Nonetheless, in 1991 the Canadian rate of teen pregnancy was 41 per 1,000 (Hanvey et al., 1994, p. 102). In some communities the rate is much higher. Both pregnant teens and their infants may be at risk of ill health in both the short and long term (Jacono, Jacono, St. Onge, Van Oosten, & Meininger, 1992).

Although teens reported increased awareness of AIDS, few altered their sexual habits as a result. Only half of sexually active teens use condoms for 'safe sex' (Bibby & Posterski, 1992, p. 47). The danger of exposure to HIV is very real for these teens. HIV has entered the Canadian adolescent population, particularly among intravenous drug users (Remis & Sutherland, 1993).

Not all sexually active teenagers are willing participants in sex. A 1990 survey of more than 3,000 youth aged 13 to 16 found that almost 1 in 5 young women and 1 in 10 young men had been sexually abused (Holmes & Silverman, 1992, p. 19). Denial and silence about sexual abuse contribute to the harm. Nurse managers can be alert to this issue during analysis of health-needs assessments. Programs that enhance self-esteem through physical activity and peer support may be useful, especially if the community is not ready to confront abuse more directly.

Alcohol and Tobacco

King and Coles report that "by age 15 over a quarter of Canadian youths drink alcohol at least once a week, and 60 percent have been drunk at least once" (1992, p. 95). Alcohol use is a risk factor for both motor vehicle accidents and suicide, the leading causes of death in this age group. The use of non-medicinal drugs and tobacco declined during the 1980s, but 24 percent of boys and 29 percent of girls said they smoked by age 15 (Pederson, 1993, p. 92). Experimenting with tobacco, which is addictive, often starts as young as age 12. Young people need anti-smoking information long before they reach puberty, where they encounter additional peer pressures. Nurse managers can form powerful partnerships with elementary schools and youth organizations to address these risk factors.

The strong links among health risk behaviours suggest the need to create supportive environments for health, and then to focus health programs for particular target groups. King and Coles (1992) emphasize that many teen smokers are also drinkers and substance abusers, and are less likely to be physically active, and more likely to have poor diets. They may have poor self-esteem, difficulties in relationships with parents, and poor adjustment to school. King and Coles believe "this pattern contributes to the formation of peer groups alienated from school and home ... [and] behaviours that put them at risk" (1992, p. 96). High-risk groups clearly have interrelated health-risk factors. In addition, powerful group forces exist among young people. Effective programming requires careful planning and many partnerships.

ADULTS

In 1995, cancer was the leading cause of death among Canadian adults (Statistics Canada, 1995, p. 118). After decades as the biggest killer, heart disease took second place, followed by cerebrovascular disease (FPT ACPH, 1996, pp. 19–20). The pattern shown in Figure 2.3 illustrates this change. Heart disease killed fewer and fewer people each year throughout this century until deaths dropped below the fairly stable cancer death rate. Also note the pattern is different if heart disease is defined to include cerebrovascular disease. Nonetheless, if the present pattern continues, cancer will be Canada's leading killer in the next century.

Cancer

Cancer is an important health problem for all Canadians. It is the leading cause of premature death, resulting in more potential years of life lost than from injuries. More than one in three Canadians develop some form of cancer in their lifetimes. However, there are variations in the trends for major types of cancer.

Among women, new cases of lung and breast cancer are increasing rapidly (FPT ACPH, 1996, p. 17). Breast cancer now affects 1 in 9 Canadian women during their lifetime. For men, there are more new cases of prostate and colorectal cancers and, especially, melanomas. New cases of lung cancer in men levelled off in the mid-1980s and declined slightly in the early 1990s (FPT ACPH, 1996, p. 17).

Rising cancer rates may be due to an aging population, as repeated exposure increases risk over time. In addition, early detection in screening programs may create a false impression of more disease. Death rates are stable, due in part to earlier detection, new drugs, and improved treatment technologies. Overall, more people are living with cancer rather than dying from it. This adds to the expense of cancer care.

Not all cancers are preventable due to genetic risks. Nonetheless, nurse managers can act strongly against proven risk factors like smoking and diet. Vigorous action could reduce suffering and loss of life from this disease as well as help to control rising costs of cancer care. In addition to strategies for reduced tobacco use and limited sun exposure, nurse managers could draw attention to the potential protective effects of physical activity and diets high in vegetables, fruits, and fibre.

Heart Disease

Heart disease results from a combination of risk factors. In the early 1990s, about 68 percent of Canadians aged fifteen and over were not physically active, 26 percent smoked daily, 20 percent had high blood pressure, and 15 percent had high cholesterol (Millar, 1992; FPT ACPH, 1996, pp. 12, 44). By 1994, over 20 percent of men aged 18 to 74, and almost as many women, reported being overweight. Current trends predict that more women will be overweight in future (FPT ACPH, 1996, p. 12).

Figure 2.3

AGE STANDARDIZED DEATH RATES
IN CANADA, 1950-1995
(DEATHS PER 100 000 POPULATION)

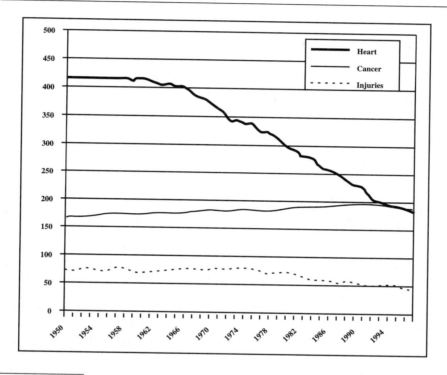

Source: Unpublished graph and ordinals provided March 10, 1998 by Francois Nault, Senior Analyst, Vital Statistics, Statistics Canada.

Although heart disease continues to kill many Canadians, the heart disease death rate has dropped every year since 1970. This decline is due in part to improved treatment and better survival rates. Risk factors are also being reduced. In spite of these improvements, not all Canadians recognize key risk factors: a high fat diet, physical inactivity, hypertension, and oral contraceptive/estrogen therapy. Smoking is a risk factor Canadians do recognize (*Cardiovascular disease in Canada,* 1993).

In 1994, the smoking rate among people with less formal schooling was more than double the rate among the well-educated (Millar, 1996, p. 13). One-third to one-half of smokers with elementary education or less reported trying to quit without success. They tend to live and work in environments that do not prohibit or discourage smoking. This group of people states they identify health professionals as an information source. They are less likely to use pamphlets or the media than are the well-educated (Millar, 1996, p. 16).

New strategies are needed for hard-to-reach groups. Supportive environments, community action, and peer-to-peer programs may all be useful. Nurse managers with demographic and epidemiologic awareness can use a comprehensive approach. They promote health in the context of social and environmental factors influencing people's choices and use long-term, multi-sector approaches. They are able to target positive health messages at specific groups. Some managers focus on fun, physical activity, and nutrition.

Alcohol, Accidents, and Suicides

Accidents, assaults, and suicides are also major causes of death and hospital admission among adult Canadians. Alcohol abuse is a significant risk factor associated with these events. Canadians are generally not heavy drinkers but alcohol's toll on society is high. Single, Robson, Xie, and Rehm (1996) estimate that 1.15 million days of hospitalization per year resulted from alcohol-related falls, motor vehicle accidents, and alcohol dependence syndrome. They assessed the 1992 total cost to society for items such as health care, workplace losses, and law enforcement at $265 per capita—almost as much as for smoking-related costs.

Too many Canadian drivers die in motor vehicle accidents. In 1990, Transport Canada tested 80.5 percent of fatally injured drivers for blood-alcohol concentration (1992). Of these, 49.6 percent of male drivers and 28 percent of female drivers had been drinking. The highest proportion of alcohol impairment (48.7 percent) occurred among those 26 to 35 years old (Transport Canada, 1992, p. 2). Alcohol use was much higher among fatally injured truck or van drivers and motorcyclists than among automobile drivers. Fortunately, the overall trend has been generally downward.

Adult deaths due to suicide fluctuate across the country, but are stable from year to year. In 1993, an average of 12 Canadians per 100,000 died in this way. Suicides by young adult men tend to be violent (firearms, strangulation). The highest suicide rates for women occur in the 50 to 54 age group and more commonly involve medication or vehicle exhausts (Beneteau, 1990).

Chronic Conditions

About 55 percent of adult Canadians responding to the 1994–95 National Population Health Survey reported at least one chronic condition. The conditions most commonly named were allergies (20 percent), back problems (15 percent), arthritis/rheumatism (13 percent), and high blood pressure (9 percent) (Statistics Canada, 1996b, p. 100). In addition, migraine headaches and asthma each affect more than 5 percent of the population. In more rigorous provincial Heart Health Surveys (1986–1992), more than 20 percent of those aged 18 to 74 had high blood pressure and 30 percent reported themselves overweight (FPT ACPH, 1996, p. 12).

Of Canadians aged 65 and over, 8 percent reported Alzheimer's or other forms of dementia in a 1991 survey (FPT ACPH, 1996, p. 19). This means that factors such as safe wandering areas are essential in long-term care. As the baby-boom population ages, the number of people with chronic conditions and dementia will increase greatly (Burke, Lindsay, McDowell, & Hill, 1997). For example, between 1990 and 2013, the number of Canadians over age fifty-five will increase by 80 percent.

Nurse managers can help to slow the rapid rise of chronic respiratory conditions. Advocating for clean air will help. Major Canadian cities made tremendous progress toward clean air in public places and restaurants during the mid-1990s. Interdisciplinary and multi-sector partnerships make progress easier. This is also true for more specific strategies to prevent asthma and allergies. Nurse managers can be more effective by working with partners in the community. Ernst, Fitzgerald, and Spier (1996) explain the views of Canadian experts about prevention and control of asthma.

AIDS

Most Canadians with AIDS live in Ontario, Quebec, and British Columbia. The majority are men aged 20 to 49 who are in homosexual or bisexual relationships. An increasing number are intravenous drug abusers, particularly in British Columbia (FPT ACPH, 1996, p. 14). This points to the risk of AIDS spreading into younger heterosexual populations. Multi-sector initiatives could prevent an epidemic of AIDS in Canada. Health managers cannot afford to ignore this risk. Death from AIDS can be a long process, using all of a family's resources and extensive health services.

Experience in countries where the AIDS epidemic is in full force shows that this disease attacks young people. They are exposed to HIV as teenagers or young adults, diagnosed with AIDS in their early thirties, and die before age forty-five. This disease may leave young children without both parents. Future costs in human suffering, health care, and social assistance may be very high if society does not work to decrease its spread.

Nurse managers may wish to invite the AIDS community to initiate support groups and help its members accept the need to prevent infection of others. This is an unavoidable burden for those with a deadly and communicable illness. Nurse managers can also involve youth in planning preventive strategies such as peer support groups that support positive health messages. Youth are creative in finding interested community partners.

ABORIGINAL ISSUES

For many Canadian health professionals, the most significant cultural group is the aboriginal population. Canada's Inuit, Métis, and Status and non-Status Indian people suffer much more illness than other Canadians. It is important to note that aboriginals are not a homogeneous people. Often disease rates are different for Inuit and Indians. Within the Status Indian population there may be significant differences between northern and southern parts of provinces (MacMillan, MacMillan, Offord, & Dingle, 1996).

In an extensive review of research published between 1989 and 1995, MacMillan and colleagues (1996) found that specific aboriginal populations have increased risk of death from pneumonia, suicide, alco-holism, and homicide compared with other Canadians. Infant mortality rates are two to three times higher than national rates (FPT ACPH, 1996, p. 30).

Disability

The disability rate among the adult aboriginal population is an alarming 31 percent compared with the 13 percent national rate (Ng, 1996). Accidents and violence are underlying causes of aboriginal disabilities, along with poor community conditions and housing. The rates for disabilities are slightly higher for women. Disabilities and chronic conditions may differ across the country. For example, about 2 percent of Canadians have dia-betes, compared with 8.7 percent of aboriginals in the Atlantic region, 1.6 percent of aboriginals in British Columbia, and 1.2 percent in the Yukon (MacMillan et al., 1996).

Tuberculosis

Aboriginal people across the country suffer nine times as much tuberculo-sis as the Canadian average. This difference is influenced by the current rate of infection in the population, poverty, crowding, environmental pollutants such as tobacco and wood smoke, and, possibly, nutritional problems (MacMillan et al., 1996). Waldram, Herring, and Young (1995, p. 262) em-phasize that genetic factors do not play a part.

Heart Disease and Cancer

Aboriginal women have higher death rates for ischemic heart disease and stroke, and for uterine and cervical cancer (Mao, Moloughney, Semenciw, & Morrison, 1992) than do Canadian women on average. During the 1980s, some of these differences began to disappear, but the rate of is-chemic heart disease among aboriginal women continues to climb. Risk fac-tors for heart disease, including smoking, obesity, diabetes, and high blood pressure, are higher among many aboriginal groups (*Cardiovascular Disease in Canada,* 1993, p. 9). Aboriginal participation in cancer prevention pro-grams may be as much as 30 percent lower than for other Canadians (His-lop, Deschamps, Band, Smith, & Clark, 1992). Nurse managers cannot afford to ignore these danger signals, which show that the health system is not meeting the needs of aboriginal women.

Suicide

Suicide rates are much higher than the national average for Canada's abo-riginal people. MacMillan and colleagues (1996) report that in the late 1980s, Canadian Indian and Inuit suicide rates were two to three times higher than the rate for non-aboriginals. One risk factor strongly associ-ated with suicide is poverty (MacMillan et al., 1996).

Aboriginal youth are five times more likely to die of suicide than the total Canadian youth population. The highest risk period for aboriginal suicide is age 15 to 29 (Statistics Canada, 1996b, p. 74) and the current aboriginal population is very young.

Canadians can act together as a society to support healing, or become part of the cause of even higher suicide rates in the next century. This is a huge challenge for nurses, for health managers, for aboriginal people, and for society. The tragedy of suicide among aboriginal people requires co-operation and urgent action from all sectors. Economic strategies and healthy public policy may be more effective than direct health care. Health-care professionals cannot afford to ignore any potentially effective strategy.

Strategies for Improving Aboriginal Health

It is the responsibility of Canadian health professionals to learn more about aboriginal health. Nurse managers can work with aboriginal people to address inequalities. Health managers must be patient and listen, they must plan carefully to ensure that the right programs are offered to the right people at the right time, and they must emphasize strategies that suit the local community.

Multiple strategies are necessary to change health behaviours in any group. Health behaviours are closely associated with self-esteem and peer-group membership (King & Coles, 1992, p. 96). Ineffective attempts to change behaviour can result in frustration, disappointment, and defence mechanisms, all of which can make individuals and groups more difficult to reach on subsequent attempts. Sharing knowledge is not helpful by itself. Skills, resources, and motivation are required for sustained behaviour change (Green & Simons-Morton, 1991). Culturally appropriate health promotion and care are critical.

Self-government

Perhaps the primary cultural issue for aboriginal health is governance. Since 1984, Canadian policy makers have aimed to strengthen Native autonomy, with Native communities governing themselves. The control of health-care decision making has become a significant goal for First Nations people. This is particularly true where aboriginal peoples represent up to 20 percent of the population, as in the Northwest Territories, the Yukon, and parts of Saskatchewan and Manitoba. Politicians and nurse managers of all cultural backgrounds are challenged to find ways to increase aboriginal involvement in decision making and control of health services.

Waldram, Herring, and Young (1995, p. 270) take a broad view of what is necessary to improve aboriginal health in future. They insist upon action in five basic areas: a co-operative public-health approach, cultural sensitivity, control of service delivery at the community level, affirmative action with employment equity, and an overall improvement in the socio-economic status of aboriginal Canadians. This is a tall order, but effective health planners and managers take it seriously.

IMPLICATIONS: EFFECTIVE STRATEGIES FOR ACTION

As early as 1974, Canada's Minister of Health told policy makers about the need for a broad approach to improving health (Lalonde, 1974). Awareness that many factors influence health did not improve health much in the intervening quarter of a century. Success in improving the health of Canadians requires that all health managers and policy makers *act* differently.

ROLE OF NURSE MANAGERS

Nurse managers, in particular, must act. All nurse managers can assess health needs, use effective action strategies, and evaluate the impact of these strategies on health. The future requires the integration of population health approaches. Hundreds of community nurse managers have expertise in this field.

Nurses are the largest group of health professionals in the country and their individual and collective actions influence the health system. More than any other group, nurse managers decide whether the health system improves health or is a financial drag on the economy. It is vital that they recognize that power and use it well.

ROLE OF COMMUNITIES

Involving communities in identifying health needs and in selecting strategies is essential. The Health Policy Conference (1992) points out that citizens must define equitable access to health care. Societal values influence whether people believe care to be appropriate and accessible. A community of First Nations people, for example, may see things differently than a nurse manager from a different community.

After a review of six health promotion programs, Goodman, Steckler, and Hoover (1993) recommended the importance of an initial assessment of the community's capacity to manage change. This simple first step would save many dollars and avoid considerable frustration. Too often, nurse managers try to address a health priority without realizing that community focus is on another issue.

Goodman and his colleagues also recommend that health-needs assessments be analyzed and shared quickly with communities in a useful format. Goodman encourages getting technical assistance, staying flexible, and using local ideas, co-ordination, and capacity building for future success. The use of multiple interventions is strongly encouraged. The list concludes by stressing that effective health promotion approaches are integrated into ongoing community programming in a way that ensures continuation and sustainability over time.

The First National Conference on Chronic Diseases in Canada identified seven major strategies (Edwards, 1989, pp. 13–18). These strategies include developing and evaluating prevention goals and increasing the use of preventive measures, particularly for disadvantaged and high-risk groups. Clearly this work requires nurse managers to use demographics and epidemiology.

CONCLUSION

The role of nurse managers is not only to offer quality health care. They have opportunities to improve the health of the population. The health-care system will contribute more effectively to improved health if all nurse managers:

- Use the determinants of health to analyze health needs.
- Invite community participation to assess health needs, analyze priorities, select goals and objectives, and choose strategies for action.
- Make program decisions based on epidemiologic and demographic trends as well as community values.
- Evaluate on a regular basis whether health services improve health by monitoring the achievement of specific objectives using health-status indicators.

The ultimate goal would be to have Canadians begin to reap benefits in improved health status.

SUMMARY

- Many of Canada's major health problems are preventable.
- Determinants of health and specific risk factors often combine to create complex health issues that require multidisciplinary, multi-sector solutions.
- Cancer is an increasingly important health issue as the population ages and heart disease declines.
- Disabilities and dementia will increase sharply in the next two decades as the population ages. Reducing accidents reduces disability.
- Aboriginal health is a major challenge in Canada and requires multi-sector, culturally sensitive solutions.
- By using demographics and epidemiology to plan and evaluate care, nurse managers help improve the health of Canadians.

FURTHER READINGS AND RESOURCES

Federal, Provincial and Territorial Advisory Committee on Population Health (FPT ACPH). (1994). *Strategies for population health: Investing in the health of Canadians.* Ottawa: Health Canada. This report contained a framework for action encompassing all the major influences on health including: living and working conditions; physical environment; personal health practices and coping skills; and health services. Strategic directions in the report were adopted by federal, provincial, and territorial Ministers of Health at their meeting in Halifax, September 1994.

Federal, Provincial and Territorial Advisory Committee on Population Health (FPT ACPH). (1996). *Report on the health of Canadians.* Ottawa: Health Canada. Communications and Consultation Directorate. This report contains valuable information on trends in the population's health status and on factors that influence health. See also the *Technical Appendix* to this report.

Miller, A.B. (1992, January/February Supplement). Planning cancer control strategies. *Chronic Diseases in Canada, 13*(1). This whole supplement is a valuable resource for nurses who wish to take action against rising cancer rates.

See also the most recent, various annual reports provided annually by Statistics Canada, such as those listed in the references for this Chapter. These reports provide excellent resources and should be reviewed regularly by all nurse managers. The Canadian Council on Social Development also publishes many reports useful to nurses, including *The Progress of Canada's Children 1996*, by K. Scott.

REFERENCES

Badets, J. (1993, Summer). Canada's immigrants. *Canadian Social Trends, 29,* 8–11.

Bailey, D., & Martin, A.D. (1994). Physical activity and skeletal health in adolescents. *Pediatric Exercise Science, 6,* 330–347.

Beneteau, R. (1990). Trends in suicide. In C. McKie & K. Thompson (Eds.), *Canadian social trends* (pp. 93–95). Ottawa: Minister of Supply and Services.

Bibby, R.W., & Posterski, D.C. (1992). *Teen trends: A nation in motion.* Toronto: Stoddart.

Burke, M.A., Lindsay, J. McDowell, I., & Hill, G. (1997, Summer). Dementia among seniors. *Canadian Social Trends, 45,* 24–27.

Cardiovascular disease in Canada. (1993). Ottawa: Heart and Stroke Foundation.

Ernst, P., Fitzgerald, J.M., & Spier, S. (1996). Canadian consensus conference: Summary of recommendations. *Canadian Respiratory Journal, 3* (2), 89–100.

Edwards, P. (1989). *Summary report, first national conference—chronic disease in Canada: Challenges and opportunities.* Ottawa: Canadian Public Health Association.

Federal, Provincial and Territorial Advisory Committee on Population Health (FPT ACPH). (1996). *Report on the health of Canadians.* Ottawa: Health Canada. Communications and Consultation Directorate. (see also *Technical Appendix*)

Giger, J.N., & Davidhizar, R. (1990). Transcultural nursing assessment: A method for advancing nursing practice. *International Nursing Review, 37* (1), 199–202.

Goodman, R.M., Steckler, A., & Hoover, S. (1993). A critique of contemporary community health promotion approaches: Based on a qualitative review of six programs in Maine. *American Journal of Health Promotion, 7* (3), 208–220.

Green, L.W., & Simons-Morton, D. (1991). Education and life style determinants of health and disease. In W. Holland, R. Detels, & G. Knox (Eds.), *Oxford textbook of public health* (2nd ed.). London: Oxford University Press.

Hanvey, L., Avard, D., Graham, I., Underwood, K., Campbell, J., & Kelly, C. (1994). *The health of Canada's children: A CICH profile*. Ottawa: Canadian Institute of Child Health.

Health Policy Conference (5th). (1992). *Beyond 'equitable access': New perspectives on equity in health care systems*. London, ON: McMaster University Centre for Health Economics and Policy Analysis.

Hislop, T.G., Deschamps, M., Band, P. R., Smith, J.M., & Clark, H.F. (1992). Participation in the British Columbia cervical cytology screening programme by native Indian women. *Canadian Journal of Public Health, 83* (5), 344–345.

Holmes, J., & Silverman, E.L. (1992). *We're here, listen to us!: A survey of young women in Canada*. Ottawa: Canadian Advisory Council on the Status of Women.

Jacono, J.J., Jacono, B.J., St. Onge, M., Van Oosten, E., & Meininger, E. (1992). Teenage pregnancy: A reconsideration. *Canadian Journal of Public Health, 83* (3), 196–199.

King, A.J.C., & Coles, B. (1992). *The health of Canada's youth*. Ottawa: Minister of Supply and Services.

Lalonde, M. (1974). *A new perspective on the health of Canadians*. Ottawa: Minister of Supply and Services.

MacMillan, H.L., MacMillan, A.B., Offord, D.R. & Dingle, J.L. (1996). Aboriginal health. *Canadian Medical Association Journal, 155* (11), 1569–1578.

MacMillan, S., & Jantzie, D. (1993). Young adults: Attitudes toward community health. *Wellspring, 4* (2), 1, 7.

Mao, Y., Moloughney, B.W., Semenciw, R. M., & Morrison, H. I. (1992). Indian reserve and registered Indian mortality in Canada. *Canadian Journal of Public Health, 83* (5), 350–353.

Millar, W. (1992, Spring). A trend to healthier lifestyles. *Canadian Social Trends, 24* (supplement).

Millar, W.J., Strachan, J., & Wadhera, S. (1993, Spring). Trends in low birth weight. *Canadian Social Trends, 28*, 26–29.

Millar, W.J. (1996, Autumn). Reaching smokers with lower education attainment. *Health Reports, 8* (2). Ottawa: Statistics Canada.

Ng, E. (1996). Disability among Canada's aboriginal peoples in 1991. *Health Reports, 8* (1), 25–31.

Pederson, L.L. (1993). Smoking. In T. Stephens & D. F. Graham (Eds.), *Canada's health promotion survey 1990: Technical report* (pp. 92–101). Ottawa: Minister of Supply and Services.

Quinney, H.A., Gauvin, L., & Wall, A.E.T. (1994). *Toward active living*. Windsor, ON: Human Kinetics.

Remis, R.S., & Sutherland, W.D. (1993). The epidemiology of HIV and AIDS in Canada: Current perspectives and future needs. *Canadian Journal of Public Health, 84*, supplement 1, S34–S38.

Single, E., Robson, L., Xie, X., & Rehm, J. (1996). *The costs of substance abuse in Canada*. Ottawa: Canadian Centre on Substance Abuse.

Statistics Canada. (1995). *Births and deaths, 1995*. Ottawa: Minister of Industry.

Statistics Canada. (1996a). *Growing up in Canada: National longitudinal survey of children and youth*. Ottawa: Minister of Industry.

Statistics Canada. (1996b). *Canada year book, 1997*. Ottawa: Minister of Industry. Cat. 11–402.

Transport Canada. (1992). *Alcohol use by drivers fatally injured in motor vehicle accidents: 1990 and the past ten years*. Ottawa: Road Safety Division.

Waldram, J.B., Herring, D.A., & Young, T.K. (1995). *Aboriginal health in Canada: Historical, cultural, and epidemiological perspectives*. Toronto: University of Toronto Press.

Wilkins, K. (1995). Causes of death: How the sexes differ. *Health Reports, 7*(2).

Chapter 3

▼▼▼▼▼▼▼▼▼▼▼▼▼▼

Legal Framework for Health-Care Services

Leah Evans Parisi

KEY OBJECTIVES

In this chapter, you will learn:

- The basic structure of the Canadian legal system, and the differences between constitutional law, statutory law, civil law, and professional regulation.
- Ways health-care providers can be involved with criminal proceedings and inquests or inquiries.
- Elements the plaintiff must demonstrate in a negligence action.
- Two ways—battery and negligence—in which a plaintiff can bring a claim regarding lack of informed consent, and the elements required for each.
- Requirements for an employment contract, and how such contracts may differ in union and non-union environments.
- Information on the legal doctrine of vicarious liability and how it may apply to health-care providers.
- How professional regulating bodies protect the public interest.
- The purpose of risk management.
- How documentation may influence the nurse's ability to provide evidence of care.
- Legal concepts that apply to delegation.

INTRODUCTION

The intent of this chapter is to provide an overview of legal issues important to nurses in staff, leadership, and management roles. It is not all-inclusive and is not intended as legal advice or as a substitute for legal advice. The information is meant to increase awareness and to highlight areas important to practice and policy development. Particular attention should be given to case law and to individual provincial or territorial statutes, regulations, and standards, which provide the details for each jurisdiction, as well as to the policies of the employing agency or institution.

The Canadian Constitution addresses government definition and regulation while the Charter of Rights and Freedoms, which is a part of the Constitution, sets forth fundamental rights of Canadians. These documents are the highest law of Canada, and other laws must comply with them to be enforceable. Canadians are also subject to statutory law, made by Parliament and provincial legislatures, and common law made by judges. In Quebec, the Quebec Civil Code takes precedence over common law and most other statutes. Ministers may allocate responsibility for developing regulations, which further define statutes such as those related to professional regulation, to professional regulatory bodies. Additionally, health-care providers must comply with professional standards and institutional or agency policies. Each of these is discussed in more detail in this chapter, and some advice is offered related to risk management.

CONSTITUTIONAL LAW

The Canadian Constitution (1982), which includes the Charter of Rights and Freedoms (1982), forms the highest law of the land. With few exceptions, laws must conform with the Constitution and Charter to be enforceable. The Constitution addresses predominantly the definition and regulation of government, while the Charter addresses the fundamental rights of Canadians, such as the freedoms of expression, peaceful assembly, association, religion, the right to vote, mobility rights, the right to life, liberty, and security of the person, and equality before the law without regard to race, sex, national or ethnic origin, colour, religion, age, and mental or physical disability.

The Constitution assigns the power to make statutory law to both the federal and provincial governments, each in designated areas. Any areas not assigned to provinces are reserved for the federal Parliament.

There are two legal systems in Canada, one derived from the English legal system, which is used by the federal government and all provinces except Quebec, and one based on the French Civil Code, which is used in Quebec.

For the most part, health care is a provincial responsibility, although the federal government retains jurisdiction in health care for the armed forces, veterans with related disabilities, Native people, the Royal Canadian Mounted Police, quarantine, federal inmates, and occupational health for federal civil servants (*Constitution Act*, 1867). Figure 3.1 provides a brief overview.

STATUTORY LAW

There are three branches of Canadian government: the legislative branch, consisting of the federal Parliament and provincial legislatures, which make

Figure 3.1
BASIC STRUCTURE OF THE CANADIAN LEGAL SYSTEM

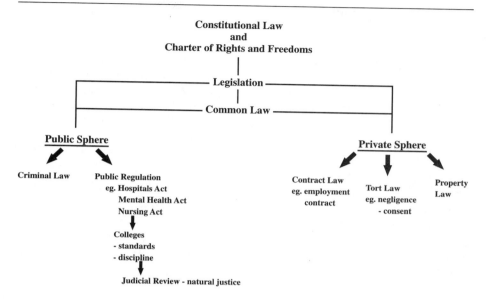

statutory law; the executive branch, consisting of the Queen and Ministers who are responsible for law enforcement; and the judicial branch, or courts, which resolve disputes and create common law or case law.

The federal Parliament consists of two houses: the House of Commons representing the people, and the Senate representing the Queen. In contrast, provincial legislative assemblies have only one house, which represents the people. The laws made by Parliament and the provincial legislatures are called acts or statutes. Statutes take precedence over common law, or judge made law, although the latter is often used to clarify application of statutes.

After a bill passed by Parliament or a provincial legislature receives Royal Assent and is proclaimed and published, it becomes law. All citizens are deemed to know the law as of the date on which it takes effect. Because of this presumed knowledge, laws become enforceable.

An example of a federal statute that affects health care is the *Canada Health Act,* which was passed in 1984. This Act requires that each province provide care which is universal, publicly administered, inter-provincially portable, and comprehensive. The *Canada Health Act* also prohibits provinces from charging user fees or allowing extra billing by physicians. The federal government may withhold health care transfer payments from the province as the penalty for violation of this statute.

Because statutes cannot provide for all circumstances, regulations may be passed by an administrative body to further define the law. Examples include regulations made pursuant to provincial nursing acts.

COMMON OR CASE LAW

Common law is derived from principles set forth in judicial opinions. Under the doctrine of *stare decisis*, lower courts must follow previous appellate decisions of the same jurisdiction, as well as those of the Supreme Court of Canada. If a party asserts that a past court decision has been misapplied by the court, or if a change in a previous holding is needed to comply with changing societal values, an appellate court may hear the case and determine whether the law should stand, or be changed.

QUEBEC CIVIL CODE

The *Quebec Civil Code* (*Code Civil du Quebec*, 1991) is a detailed, comprehensive statute that defines legal rules and principles to be followed in the province. In Quebec, judicial precedent is followed by courts, but it is secondary to the Civil Code. The Civil Code also takes precedence over other statutes unless specifically stated otherwise. Additionally, Quebec judges refer to legal doctrine (scholarly writings of experts) to determine the application and interpretation of the Civil Code.

CRIMINAL LAW

The *Criminal Code of Canada* (1985), a federal statute, defines criminal offences and sets forth the procedures to be used in determining criminal conduct. Other federal statutes (e.g., *Controlled Drugs and Substances Act,* 1996, and *Food and Drugs Act,* 1985) supplement the *Criminal Code,* as does relevant case law.

Nurses are rarely charged with a criminal offence. However, they are commonly involved in criminal proceedings as witnesses (Grant & Ashman, 1997, p. 109).

INQUIRIES AND INQUESTS

Both federal and provincial statutes establish a process for inquiry into events that relate to good government, such as events involving investigation of deaths or policy matters in health care. An inquiry familiar to most nurses is the *Royal Commission of Inquiry into Certain Deaths at the Hospital for Sick Children* (Grange, 1984). The issue pertained to 35 deaths that occurred on two wards of the hospital within one year. It was alleged that digoxin given by a nurse had caused some of the deaths. There was not sufficient evidence presented in the preliminary hearing to support a murder charge against the nurse, however, and subsequently a Commissioner was appointed to conduct a public inquiry. The nurse was ultimately exonerated (Nelles v. Ontario, 1989).

Inquiries and inquests are handled differently by each of the provinces. Alberta, Manitoba and Nova Scotia have passed *Fatalities Inquiries Acts* (1980, 1989-90, and 1989). Each establishes an office of the Medical Examiner and a Board, which determines whether a public inquiry will be conducted by a judge. In Newfoundland, judges conduct inquiries under the provincial *Summary Proceedings Act* (1990). In contrast, in the remaining provinces, the traditional coroner's investigation and inquest, if required, is held pursuant to provincial *Coroner's Acts* (please see citations in reference list) and the *Causes and Circumstances of Death Act* in Quebec (1983).

During a coroner's investigation or fatality inquiry, an autopsy may be conducted, the site of death investigated, witnesses and others interviewed, and medical records examined. Caregivers should make every attempt to preserve evidence for investigation. After death, a body must be transported with tubes, needles, and dressings in place to allow differentiation of invasive procedures required for care from injury resulting from other cause(s). Other potential evidence arriving at the hospital with the deceased or victim (such as clothing and personal belongings) should be preserved in the manner received, if at all possible, since it will most likely be used as evidence.

In contrast to criminal and civil trials, which are adversarial in nature, an inquiry or inquest is inquisitorial. The rules of evidence may not be as strict as in a court proceeding. The purpose of the hearing is to determine the identity of the deceased and when, where, how, and by what means death occurred (Grant & Ashman, 1997, p. 79). The final report may lead to recommended policy changes, but will not lead to a civil or criminal finding. However, either criminal charges or civil allegations may result in further court proceedings after the inquiry or inquest.

A nurse may be called to testify in an inquiry or inquest, and in usual circumstances the hospital defence counsel may provide necessary legal advice. It is normal that the nurse may not recall some or all of the events related to the issue. The record may be reviewed to refresh recollection, and will be used as evidence, as will any other relevant documentation. The nurse must tell the truth and answer the questions that relate to the issue. Although patient confidentiality rights may be waived or limited for the purpose of the hearing, the nurse should assure that testimony given is factual and pertains specifically to points at issue. Thus, confidentiality of unrelated health matters may be preserved.

CIVIL LAW

In contrast to criminal law where the public is represented by the Crown Attorney, civil law involves two or more private parties who retain their own separate lawyers. Tort law, property law, and contract law are the primary types of civil law. Although all three types may have implications for nurses, tort law as it relates specifically to negligence, and contract law, as it relates to employment, will be discussed here.

TORT LAW — NEGLIGENCE

In relation to nursing, negligence may be defined as doing or failing to do something that the reasonable nurse, in similar circumstances, would do or would not do. In order to prevail in a negligence action, the plaintiff (party bringing the action) must show, by a preponderance of the evidence, that each of the following elements existed between the patient and nurse:

1. A duty of care.
2. A breach of that duty.
3. A causal connection between the act and the injury.
4. Resulting damages.

Each of these elements will be discussed more fully.

Duty of Care

In most employment circumstances, there is an established duty of care. For example, a nurse working as an employee on a ward in a hospital is responsible for all patients under his or her care by virtue of employment. In contrast, a nurse in private enterprise may have the option of deciding whether to accept a patient for care, thus the duty is incurred when the patient is accepted.

Breach of Duty

To prevail in relation to this element, the plaintiff must show that the nurse acted, or failed to act, in a manner in which other reasonable nurses would have acted in the same or similar circumstances. This is established by examination of nursing notes and the entire health record, hospital or agency policies, professional standards of practice, and testimony of expert witnesses. The practice is measured against that of similar nurses, unless the nurse undertakes a practice outside the usual nursing role in the circumstance; in such an instance, the nurse may be held to a higher standard in accordance with the amount of extra training and experience required and previously accomplished by the nurse.

Relationship Between a Nurse's Actions and an Injury — Causation

For the plaintiff to prevail, there must be a causal connection between the nurse's actions and the injury. Even if the nurse was negligent, if the negligent action did not contribute materially to the injury, there should be no compensation.

The plaintiff has the burden of proving causation in two ways: (1) whether the defendant's conduct was the actual (factual) cause of the injury; and (2) whether the defendant's conduct was the legal (proximate) cause of the injury.

Actual causation is evaluated by using the "but for" test; would the injury not have occurred "but for" the defendant's conduct. Actual causation is often difficult to prove since effect of the underlying medical condition must be differentiated from injury caused by the acts of the defendant. Expert testimony is often useful in arriving at a conclusion.

Proximate causation is a legal principle based on the premise that, to be liable for conduct, the injury or damage must have been "foreseeable" to a reasonable person in the defendant's position. In other words, a reasonable physician or nurse would have foreseen that this injury could have resulted from his or her action, and the injury is not a remote result of the conduct. Again, expert testimony is useful in making this determination (Picard, 1996, p. 228).

Damages

To prevail, the plaintiff must incur damage due to breach of the standard of practice by the nurse. For example, a nurse administers acetaminophen, as opposed to aspirin as ordered, to a child with a fever. No harm results. Even though the nurse had a duty to the child and breached the standard of care by administering the incorrect medication, no injury was caused by the error. Thus there is no injury for which compensation should be made.

Contributory Negligence

A finding of contributory negligence indicates that the plaintiff, as well as the defendant, contributed in some way to the injury. In such a case, the amount of damages awarded may be reduced by the amount that the plaintiff contributed to the injury.

CONSENT

There are two ways in which a plaintiff can assert a claim based on lack of informed consent: battery and negligence. Battery occurs: when treatment is given which has been refused; when consent has not been obtained (except in an emergency situation); when treatment given is beyond the scope of consent; or when consent was obtained by misrepresentation (Picard, 1996, p. 114). For example, in the Ontario case of *Malette* v. *Shulman* (1990), an unconscious patient arrived in the emergency department following a motor vehicle accident. A card found in her purse stated that she was a Jehovah's Witness and did not consent to receive blood. The card was signed but not dated or witnessed. Dr. Shulman questioned whether the card reflected the patient's current wishes given the circumstances of her condition and, in his opinion, the medical need for transfusion. In an attempt to save her life, the physician gave blood. The patient survived and prevailed in a claim of battery. The court found that the card represented her wishes and held that patient wishes that are known and documented must be respected. Thus this case established, in Ontario, that a patient who understands the potential consequences of the decision has the right to choose whether or not to have treatment regardless of the potentially serious nature of the outcome of the decision.

Plaintiffs may also allege negligence in relation to consent claims. If a claim is brought in negligence the plaintiff must show that the health-care provider failed to properly inform the patient of information which the reasonable person in the circumstances of the patient would want to know prior to giving consent to treatment (*Reibl* v. *Hughes*, 1980).

The elements of formal consent include the nature of treatment proposed, risks of that treatment, alternative treatments and associated effects and risks, and the effects and risks of no treatment. Additionally, the patient's questions regarding the treatment must be answered. The patient must be able to understand the risks and the alternatives to the decision of whether or not to have the treatment, and consent must be voluntarily given, without coercion.

The actual consent is the affirmation given by the patient after hearing the explanation of the proposed treatment or procedure given by the care provider. The consent should be documented in a note by the provider who explained the treatment or procedure to the patient. It may be further documented, in accord with hospital or agency policy, on a consent form. The nurse may ask the patient to sign this form. When the nurse witnesses such a form, the nurse is witnessing the fact that the patient signed the form. If the nurse questions whether the patient is able to understand the information provided, or whether the patient actually understands the information, the issue should be raised with the practitioner who explained the procedure to the patient or, if that person is unavailable, with another similarly qualified professional who can assist with clarification.

Consent may be withdrawn at any time. The patient's latest wishes prevail, although if consent is withdrawn during a procedure, the procedure may be continued to a point where it is safe to terminate.

In an emergency situation involving an incompetent patient, where there is immediate danger to the patient's life or health, treatment may proceed; the patient should consent to ongoing treatment when capacity is regained, however. It is important to document why consent could not be obtained and why the situation was an emergency.

Ontario emphasized the importance of the patient's right to consent by enacting the *Health Care Consent Act* (1995). This statute codified and further defined the common law consent principles, thus emphasizing the right of the competent patient to refuse or consent to treatment.

Allegations of lack of informed consent are most frequently raised in conjunction with allegations of negligence. The plaintiff claims that, if the risk of injury had been understood, he or she would not have consented to the procedure. Individuals may not recall exactly what was explained prior to surgery, especially if injury resulted, therefore documentation of what was told to the patient, and to the family, is especially important to the defence.

EMPLOYMENT CONTRACTS

Nurses, whether in independent practice or as employees, have employment contracts. A contract is defined as "An agreement between two or more persons which creates an obligation to do or not to do a particular thing" (Black, 1979, p. 291). For a contract to exist, each party entering the contract must be competent, must understand the subject matter and obligations of the contract, and must have obligations and benefit derived from the contract, and legal consideration must create inducement to contract. In the case of employment, legal consideration may be that the employer provides work to do and the pay for that work, and the employee provides the work. At minimum, all employment contracts must meet the standards set forth in provincial and federal labour standards and codes.

Employment contracts may be oral, written, or implied. If an employer offers a job to a nurse either in writing or orally, and the nurse accepts, there is a contract that may be enforced. If no union is involved, the nurse and the employer may negotiate an individual employment contract; this sets forth the rights and obligations of each party. In an individual contract, terms and conditions may vary for each employee although, in actual practice, hospitals and agencies tend to have similar contracts for all employees in a given job classification. Terms and conditions may be set forth in detail, or the contract may be simple with few conditions stated. In a unionized organization, the terms and conditions of employment are those of the union contract with the employer.

Verbal employment contracts are often more difficult to enforce than written contracts, because of the problem of providing proof of the terms negotiated. Thus, the nurse in a non-union position may be wise to have important terms put in writing. Such terms may include duration of the contract, issues regarding probation, negotiated time off, notice of termination, and job description.

Employment is regulated by federal and provincial employment statutes, common law, industry standards, accreditation standards, human rights legislation, and institutional policies, as well as by employment and union contracts. All contracts must meet legal conditions to be enforceable. In the event of a contract dispute, the resolution will most likely be based on evidence of the intent of the parties at the time of the contract. Written evidence of contract terms is important; behaviour and usual practice of the parties may assist, however, in demonstrating intent.

In all employment contracts, the employee has an expectation of reimbursement and the employer has the expectation that the employee will perform the expected work and follow professional standards of practice and any additional policies set by the institution. Limits on the employer's right to manage may arise from common law, provincial or federal employment standards, codes, and contracts.

In a union environment, the terms and obligations of the contract are negotiated between the employer and the union, who are the parties to the contract. All employees within a given bargaining unit of the union are subject to the same terms and conditions of employment.

Discipline

In the non-union workplace, discipline is subject to statutory and common law requirements. The employee disciplinary procedure is usually progressive, consisting first of counselling, then a verbal warning, followed by a written warning that becomes part of the employment record, and, finally, written notice that further discipline will lead to discharge. (See also Chapter 26.)

Performance appraisals may be used as a method of performance documentation, and should often be supplemented by anecdotal notes that are discussed with the employee and kept as a part of the employee record. The employee is usually required to sign the performance appraisal or anecdotal note as evidence that he or she has seen it and that discussion has taken place. The signature does not indicate the employee's agreement with the content of the appraisal or note. (See also Chapter 20.)

Unless stated in the employment contract or policies of the institution, there is no specific procedure for discipline in a non-union facility, other than procedures required by common law or applicable employment standards or codes.

In a union environment, discipline must follow labour relations laws, prior arbitration decisions, and the collective agreement grievance procedure. Arbitration is the binding means of determining the outcome, although few cases proceed that far. Both the employer and the union representing the employee must follow the terms of the contract (collective agreement) in resolution. In rare instances, particularly when mistakes are alleged in relation to the resolution procedure, the case may proceed to the judicial system after an arbitration decision.

Employment Termination

In a non-union environment, the employer may dismiss an employee at will subject to the statutory and common law principles of reasonable notice or, alternatively, compensation for the required notice period. If there is just cause (e.g., taking narcotics from the employer), reasonable notice is not necessary. The length of the notice period usually depends upon the length of employment; pay must continue during the notice period.

The remedy in regard to wrongful dismissal is usually monetary damages based on what would have been earned during the notice period or for the period of the contract if the duration of employment is defined. The employee is usually expected to try to find new work, and the award may be reduced if new employment is found. Alternatively, an employee is also expected to give the employer notice of termination pursuant to the employment contract and employment standards.

In a union environment, dismissal is governed by the collective agreement, which must meet the requirements of law and which usually sets forth specific procedures to be followed by each party. In times of downsizing, layoffs or terminations must follow the collective agreement, which usually means that seniority governs which union members retain employment. Each union agreement, however, may have specific terms, particularly in regard to specialty nursing. Collective agreements also usually set forth the procedures to be used in relation to termination for just cause.

Labour relations statutes protect employers from illegal strikes and certain behaviors by employees or unions. These statutes require that notice and bargaining obligations be met prior to strike. Some also preclude strikes by essential employees such as nurses. Remedies for illegal work actions may include injunction, back-to-work orders, and fines (Morris, 1991, p. 185).

Vicarious Liability

The legal doctrine of *vicarious liability* applies to employment relationships. Under this doctrine, the principle of *respondeat superior* leads to the employer being indirectly responsible for acts of the employee committed within the scope of employment (Picard, 1996, p. 353). Thus, the employer has indirect liability while the employee has direct liability. This concept is based on the premise that the employer is able to conduct business because of the employee's work, and thus obtains the benefits of conducting the business. Additionally, the employer usually has what is referred to as the "deep pockets"—access to greater financial resources than the employee, usually through insurance. Thus, the employer is responsible for the costs of defence and any award to the plaintiff. For example, in the case of *Joseph Brant Memorial Hospital* v. *Koziol* (1978) a patient died from aspiration following back surgery. The nurse had not roused him to cough or deep breathe and the record did not document care. The nursing care was found to be below the standard and the hospital was held vicariously liable.

For the doctrine of vicarious liability to apply, the nurse must be an employee acting within the scope of practice of the profession and in the role specified by the employing agency. For example, a nurse who is certified to start an intravenous treatment on one unit may not be permitted to do so on another unit, pursuant to hospital policy. Thus, nurses working in several hospital locations or at several jobs must be clear as to their roles and responsibilities and scopes of practice at each. An emergency situation may provide a possible exception; for example, provision of CPR if there is no DNR order even if that is not within the specific job description.

The majority of nurses are employed, and thus benefit from the doctrine of vicarious liability while practising within the employment relationship and within the job description. Nurses in independent practice are usually directly responsible for their own actions and thus must be personally insured for potential legal costs.

PROFESSIONAL REGULATION

Provincial statutes and regulations govern nursing as one of the regulated professions. The primary purpose of regulation is public protection. The regulatory body is given the power by the provincial or territorial government to set criteria for practice. These criteria include requirements to enter and continue to practice the profession, methods of handling complaints and disciplinary procedures, and development of codes of ethics and practice standards. Each nurse practising in the province or territory must be on the current register of the regulatory body, and thus must meet all criteria set forth as membership requirements. In this way the public is assured that each nurse has met minimum criteria against which performance can be measured.

Regulatory bodies, often called colleges, which act in the public interest, must be differentiated from professional associations (e.g., Canadian Nurses Association) or unions (e.g., British Columbia Nurses Union), which act in the interest of members.

COMPETENCY AND DISCIPLINARY ACTIONS

Each provincial or territorial regulatory body has its own specific procedures for handling complaints against registrants. Managers must be familiar with the requirements of their jurisdictions. Some jurisdictions impose specific reporting responsibilities on the employer or regulated professional. For example, the Ontario *Regulated Health Professions Act* (1991) requires that any registered health professional file a report if he or she has reasonable grounds, obtained in the course of practising his or her profession, to believe that another member of the same or a different regulated profession has sexually abused a patient.

Although jurisdictions vary as to specific procedures, the complaints received by professional regulatory bodies are all subject to similar general processes. When a written complaint is filed, the named nurse is notified that the complaint was received and of the allegations. She or he may be advised to seek legal counsel. The professional association or union may also provide assistance. An investigation then ensues. At this stage, there is usually no mandate that witnesses speak with investigators, but cooperation is generally encouraged. Witnesses should limit discussion to their personal knowledge of facts. While issues are under investigation or during a disciplinary proceeding, the issues should not be discussed apart from discussion required for the proceeding. After investigation, the investigator's written report is reviewed by the appropriate body and either the action is dismissed, a warning is issued, or the complaint is referred for negotiated resolution or disciplinary hearing. If the complaint proceeds to disciplinary hearing the governing body must demonstrate, in an adversarial legal process, that the nurse is guilty of professional misconduct. Such proceedings are more informal than proceedings in a court of law and usually follow similar, but less stringent, rules of evidence. If the nurse is found guilty, penalties vary from revocation, limitation, or suspension of registration to a fine or reprimand. There may also be requirements imposed on continuing registration, such as successful completion of certain continuing education courses. An appeal to a court of law may be available following a disciplinary proceeding on a matter of law or fact or both. Details regarding the appeal process vary with provincial legislation.

Although confidentiality is usually maintained during disciplinary procedures, the regulatory body will verify whether the member has a valid license. Employers should obtain evidence of valid licensure for all registered employees. Those who do not document current registration, or who do not independently investigate claims of professional misconduct in their institution or agency, may be subject to claims of negligent hiring or employment if an unregistered nurse is hired and causes injury.

RISK MANAGEMENT

Risk management is defined as the "identification, assessment or analysis and treatment (reduction or elimination) of the risk of financial loss" (Stock & Lefroy, 1988, p. 22). Risk management is concerned not only with potential malpractice, but also with "loss of physical and human resources, security, occupational health and safety, environmental and administrative areas ... and the hospital's reputation" (Stock & Lefroy, 1988, p. 22). Risk management is a well-developed practice in industry, but its application to health care did not begin until the 1970s, when the practice was initiated in the United States in response to increasing malpractice claims. In Canada, risk management was not commonly implemented until the 1980s (Stock & Lefroy, 1988, p. 21).

Risk management is a proactive process (see Figure 3.2). It may be a part of the quality management process, although it differs in that its purposes are to prevent or minimize foreseeable risks and to achieve an acceptable standard of care. In contrast, quality management is concerned with constant improvement toward an optimal standard of care.

INCIDENT REPORTS

Incident reports are tools of both quality assurance and risk management. They are used to identify, and then modify, systems issues to prevent or decrease injury to patients, staff, organizations, visitors, and property. Most institutions have policies requiring that such reports be completed following any unusual occurrence. The documentation on these reports should be

Figure 3.2
THE RISK MANAGEMENT PROCESS

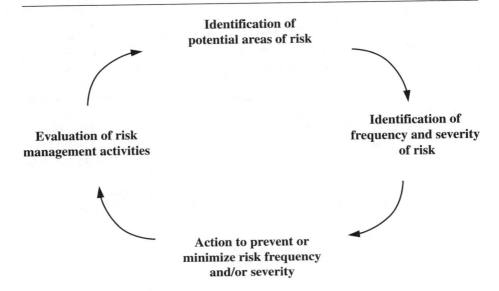

concise but complete, accurate, and non-opinionated. The report should be completed by the employee involved in or witnessing the event—in other words, by the person with first-hand knowledge of the incident. Since the purpose of these reports is administrative (i.e., to identify areas of risk), they should not be a part of the medical record. However, like medical records, incident reports may be introduced as evidence at trial, and therefore should contain only factual information. Supplementary documents prepared later, after a lawsuit has been filed, for the specific purpose of submission to the hospital lawyer who is preparing the case, may be protected by privilege and thus may be inadmissible at trial (Rozovsky & Rozovsky, 1992, p. 169).

DOCUMENTATION

Standards related to what is required in documentation and how long records must be kept are derived from provincial statutes, professional standards, and local policy. Documentation must be carried out as an integral part of care. It facilitates communication between health care team members and assists with care continuity. In addition, records are used to demonstrate accountability, provide quality assurance, and facilitate research.

Forms used for documentation may incorporate any of the many recognized approaches to charting. Charting may be either inclusive or by exception, as long as it is consistent for each professional group, department, or procedure and meets requirements of the standard of care. Forms should facilitate documentation, allowing care to be documented in an accurate, inclusive, and timely manner. As far as possible, charting should be carried out immediately after care is provided and notes should be made in chronological order. If it is necessary to make a late entry, it should be marked as such and the time of entry should be noted; such entries should be limited to situations of absolute necessity.

In the Ontario case of *Kolesar* v. *Jeffries* (1976), a post-operative patient was found dead. The last nursing note had been made five hours previously. It was the routine that nurses charted near the end of the shift, and assisted each other to recall the events to be recorded. In this instance, there was no proof that the patient had been assessed for five hours. Even if assessment had occurred, the practices of late charting and discussion with others calls accuracy of the records into question. The court stated, "One is always suspicious of records made after the event." Therefore, the care provider who actually provides care, or who witnesses the event, should chart what was done or seen immediately, or as soon after the event as possible.

In the British Columbia case of *Meyer* v. *Gordon* (1981), a newborn infant suffered brain damage during birth. It was alleged that two nurses who attended the mother were negligent in their care. The admitting nurse did not obtain an adequate obstetrical history (which included rapid labour) and there was evidence that charting was incomplete and inaccurate. It also appeared that information had been added to the chart after the delivery to make the record seem more complete. In finding against the hospital, the court said that the nurses' observations and care were insufficient. The judge wrote that the chart contained alterations and additions "which compelled me to view with suspicion the accuracy of many of the observations which are recorded. The chart also contained at least one entry which was discovered during the trial to have been made after the fact" (*Meyer* v. *Gordon*, 1981). This case emphasizes the need for nurses to chart in a timely manner, never alter records, and limit late entries to necessary situations.

It is recognized that in situations such as cardiac arrest or trauma care, care providers cannot both chart and care for the patient. Therefore a recorder, whose role is to chart, is designated. In such cases, it is recommended that the recorder note the name of each caregiver involved and that each caregiver initial documentation of his or her own actions at the conclusion of the procedure. By doing so, not only is an accurate record provided, but if a legal action should arise, each care provider can speak about the care he or she directly provided.

Charting should be clear, concise, and accurate. Opinions must be avoided unless related to nursing or medical diagnosis. Significant statements by the patient and family should be quoted accurately. The record of observations should state exactly what was observed, and should include changes from previous assessments. If conclusions relating to care are included, the evidence on which the conclusions were based should be documented.

A nurse should chart so that, if called to testify several years later, after reading the chart he or she can recall what occurred and give credible evidence of the care provided and the events that occurred. Legal cases may take approximately five years to come to court. Because memory is likely to fade during that period, the record may provide the only evidence of the events. The record can be relied on during testimony and is admissible as evidence. Complete, accurate, precise, and timely charting will allow the nurse to convey information included in the record, even if he or she has no direct memory of the case.

ADMINISTRATIVE COMMUNICATION AND DOCUMENTATION

Communication is an important management function and requires a significant portion of a manager's time. Direct verbal communication, written memos, proposals, reports, electronic mail, and telephone conversations all provide means of communication. Care providers are conscious of the importance of care documentation; for managers, however, documentation of management issues such as counselling, performance appraisal, staffing issues, and budget preparation and requests are also important. Clear, accurate, and complete documentation is essential, not only for communication but also as a record of action.

Managers must be aware of confidentiality issues in regard to communication and store confidential materials safely. Particular note should be made in regard to fax transmission and electronic mail, as these methods of communication are not private. Only non-confidential information should be transmitted through these means.

TELEPHONE ADVICE

Some nurses are now involved in providing telephone advice as a part of their care. This practice leads to unique issues with potential legal implications since the nurse is relying on what the caller says to give advice. The history and symptoms should be charted exactly as stated by the caller. Questions asked, advice given, and referrals made, as well as the caller's stated decision regarding follow-up should also be accurately and completely recorded. The patient's name, caller's name and relationship to the patient, address, and telephone numbers should be recorded with the date and time. Institutional policies regarding telephone advice must be followed, both in taking calls and in documenting conversations.

DELEGATION

Increasingly, nurses are working with unregulated care providers. Legal questions are often raised in relation to assigning and delegating. Many provincial regulating bodies and professional associations have developed guidelines specific to each jurisdiction, and these should be followed. Provincial statutes, regulations, and professional standards may address the scope of practice of regulated workers and specify acts that may not be delegated. For example, in Ontario the *Regulated Health Professions Act* (1991) and the *Nursing Act* (1991) specify controlled acts that are authorized to nurses. Those acts must be performed by a person registered with a College authorized to perform the act unless the performance has been delegated to another by a registered person, or unless the performance falls under another exception stated in the Act. Unregulated care providers may, in Ontario, provide care that is not restricted to nurses but that may be a usual part of nursing practice (e.g., skin care), and controlled acts that are delegated. The *Regulated Health Professions Act* (1991) also states that "no person, other than a member treating or advising within the scope of practice of his or her profession, shall treat or advise a person ... in circumstances in which it is *reasonably foreseeable* that serious physical harm may result from the treatment or advice or from an omission from them" (emphasis added). Thus, the nurse must assess each client situation to determine the appropriateness of delegation, must assess the knowledge, skill, and ability of the person to whom the task will be delegated, and must follow up with evaluation of the care and client condition. The nurse must also be competent to carry out the task and to teach and evaluate the competence of the care provider.

Many institutions have developed policies regarding what may be delegated to unregulated providers. They have also developed policies for teaching and ongoing measurement of the competence of those providers. Nurses should become familiar with those policies and be actively involved in their development and change.

The College of Nurses of Ontario (1996) identifies the following expectations for a registered nurse (RN) assigning responsibility for care to an unregulated care provider (UCP):

- assess the care needs of the client(s);
- know that the UCP is competent and has the necessary authority to meet the client needs;
- establish the parameters for performing the procedure (e.g., how to seek assistance and report outcomes);
- provide ongoing client assessment and evaluation;
- take action if the UCP's competence is questionable in the given situation.

The employer makes overall staffing decisions, but the individual nurse must objectively evaluate and communicate information regarding the performance of co-workers, be they other nurses, students, or unregulated workers. Management issues regarding less-than-optimal individual performance should be separated from concern about delegation to a specific group of unregulated employees. Nurses who delegate to another care provider must be sure that the other provider is competent to carry out the task. This may be done, according to institutional policy, either through a specified organizational monitoring system or through individual knowledge.

Limits must be set on what the alternative provider may do, and the parameters for reporting back to the nurse must be clear.

Laws addressing delegation usually provide general guidance; regulations are more specific. Institutional or agency policy should give the most specific direction regarding delegation. This allows each institution or agency to meet individual staffing needs within the law.

Nurses have the educational foundation to assess, plan, and evaluate care. They can effectively co-ordinate care and assign tasks to others, but they cannot delegate the assessment, planning, and evaluation; these are essential to the practice of nursing (Hansten & Washburn, 1996).

SUMMARY

- All nurses, and especially nurses in management, should be aware of the structure of the Canadian legal system, and of the differences between constitutional law, statutory law, civil law, and professional regulation, and of methods of risk management.
- Governments may conduct inquiries or investigations related to deaths or health-care policy matters. This is a fact-finding, as opposed to an adversarial, procedure, although a civil or criminal proceeding may follow. Nurses may be called as witnesses in such proceedings.
- A plaintiff who brings a suit alleging negligence must show by the preponderance of the evidence that: 1) the defendant owed him or her a duty of care; 2) the defendant breached that duty; 3) there was a causal connection between the act and the injury; 4) damages resulted. The standard of proof is what the reasonable person (nurse) would have done, or not done, in similar circumstances.
- A claim alleging lack of informed consent may be brought in battery or negligence. Prior to consent, a patient must be told the nature of the proposed treatment, the risks, and the available alternatives with the associated risks and benefits. For consent to be valid, the patient must be competent and voluntarily give consent. The patient may withdraw consent.
- Employment contracts may be written, oral, or implied. In a non-union workplace, the contract is subject to related statutory and common law. In the union workplace, the contract is negotiated between union and employer and applies to all union members. The contract or collective agreement must comply with relevant law.
- Risk management is a proactive process and may be a part of quality management. It involves identification and assessment of potential areas of risk that may lead to financial loss. Incident reports are one means of identifying areas of risk and preventing or reducing such occurrences. Like patient records, they may be used as evidence in a court proceeding.
- Documentation is an integral part of care and management. It should be carried out immediately after care or action to provide the most cred-

ible record. It should be clear, concise, and accurate, and state facts as opposed to opinions or perceptions.

• Although nurses may assign or delegate tasks to others, they cannot assign or delegate nursing assessment, planning, and evaluation.

REFERENCES

Black's Law Dictionary (5th ed.). (1979). St. Paul, MN: West Publishing.
Canada Health Act (1984) R.S.C. C–6.
Canadian Charter of Rights and Freedoms, *Constitution Act* (1982) Part 1.
Causes and Circumstances of Death Act (1983) R.S.Q. C.R–0.2.
Code Civil du Quebec (1991) L.Q., C–64
College of Nurses of Ontario. (1996) *College Communique* 21(2) 14–19.
Constitution Act (1867) U.K. 30 & 31 Vict., c. 3; R.S.C. (1970) App. II, No. 5; *Constitution Act* (1982).
Controlled Drugs and Substances Act (1996) C–19
Coroner's Act (1979) R.S.B.C., C–68
Coroner's Act (1973) R.S.N.B., C–23
Coroner's Act (1988) R.S.N.W.T., C–30
Coroner's Act (1990) R.S.O., C–37
Coroner's Act (1988) R.S.P.E.I. C–25
Coroner's Act (1978) R.S.S., P–38
Coroner's Act (1986) R.S.Y., C–35
Criminal Code of Canada (1985). R.S.C., C–46
Fatalities Inquiries Act (1980) R.S.A., P–29
Fatalities Inquiries Act (1989–90) S.M. C–30
Fatalities Inquiries Act (1989) R.S.N.S., C–164
Food and Drugs Act (1985) R.S.C., F–27
Grange, G. (1984). Report of the Royal Commission of inquiry into certain deaths at the Hospital for Sick Children and related matters. In J. Morris (1991), *Canadian nurses and the law.* Toronto/Vancouver: Butterworths.
Grant, A., & Ashman, A. (1997). *A nurse's practical guide to the law.* Aurora, ON: Aurora Professional Press.
Hansten, R., & Washburn, M. (1996). Why nurses don't delegate. *Journal of Nursing Administration, 26*(2), 24–28.
Health Care Consent Act (1995) S.O.
Joseph Brant Memorial Hospital v. Koziol (1978) 2 C.C.L.T. 170 (S.C.C.).
Kolesar v. Jeffries (1976) 9 O.R. (2d) 41, 59 D.L.R. (3d) 367.
Malette v. Shulman (1990) 67 D.L.R. (4th) 321, 72 O.R. (2d) 417, 37 O.A.C. 281, 2 C.C.L.T. (2d) 1.
Meyer v. Gordon (1981) 17 C.C.L.T. 1, B.C.S.C.
Morris, J. (1991). *Canadian nurses and the law.* Toronto/Vancouver: Butterworths.
Nelles v. Ontario (1989) 2 S.C.R. 170, 60 D.L.R. (4th) 609, 98 N.R. 321, 71 C.R. (3d) 358
Nursing Act (1991) S.O. C–32.
Picard, E. (1996). *Legal liability of doctors and hospitals in Canada* (3rd ed.). Toronto: Carswell.
Regulated Health Professions Act (1991) S.O. C–18.
Reibl v. Hughes (1980) 2 S.C.R. 880.

Rozovsky, L., & Rozovsky, F. (1992). *Canadian health information* (2nd ed.). Toronto/ Vancouver: Butterworths.

Stock, R., & Lefroy, S. (1988). *Risk management: A practical framework for Canadian health care facilities*. Ottawa: Canadian Hospital Association.

Summary Proceedings Act (1990) R.S.N., P–38.

CASE STUDIES

Case Study #1

Maria Ashton, a nurse in the intensive care unit for fifteen years, is respected for her professional expertise. She has always been reliable and has started to volunteer for extra shifts. She also frequently volunteers to relieve others for breaks. Her excellent care has continued, but it appears that patients under her care often require greater amounts of narcotics than those cared for by other nurses. She states that she wants to assure the comfort of her patients. On several recent occasions, the narcotic count has been inaccurate. Co-workers and the manager are beginning to suspect that Ms. Ashton may be using narcotics. Today, a ventilator became disconnected and Ms. Ashton did not quickly notice as would be expected.

1. How should the co-workers and manager address the issue if Maria Ashton is not a union member/is a union member?
2. Do the consequences potentially differ if Ms. Ashton is found to have taken narcotics from the hospital, as opposed to using narcotics acquired outside of the workplace?
3. Do the issues potentially differ for Maria Ashton and/or the hospital if the patient suffers damage as a result of the ventilator being disconnected? How?
4. If allegations are brought, which tribunal(s) may hear the case? Explain.

Case Study #2

Jim Burke is a nurse in the emergency department. Recently, a new program has been implemented that allows registered nurses to give telephone advice to persons calling the department. Mr. Burke is part of a team that will write the policy pertaining to giving telephone advice. Considering issues that may arise when giving nursing telephone advice and the elements of potential negligence:

1. What would you include in the policy?
2. What should be included in the policy in regard to documentation?
3. Would Jim Burke have additional issues to address if he owned an independent agency of nurses who offer a telephone advice service, as opposed to giving such advice as a part of his job as a nurse in the hospital? Describe the potential differences.

Case Study #3

A registered nurse on a surgical ward has been asked to have a patient sign a consent form for surgery. It is the usual practice of the surgeon to discuss the procedure with the patient during an office visit prior to admission.

1. When the nurse asks the patient to sign the hospital consent form, and signs as a witness, what does the nurse's signature imply?
2. If the patient says that he or she understands the procedure and does not have questions, what is the role of the nurse?
3. Does the nurse's responsibility change if the patient voices concerns about undergoing the procedure?

Case Study #4

A nurse is offered a job by a hospital and begins to work there. There is no written contract signed by the parties.

1. Does a contract for employment exist? Why or why not?
2. What differences regarding the contract, and obligations of the parties exist if the hospital is unionized/non-unionized?

Case Study #5

Sue Edwards, a registered nurse, is assigned to work with Helen French, a new health care aide. Ms. French has not worked in the hospital before. Her job description states that she may assist with patient care responsibilities at the discretion of the registered nurse.

1. What are the expectations of Sue Edwards when working with Helen French?
2. What aspects of her practice must Sue Edwards reserve for herself or another registered nurse?
3. Ms. Edwards is a member of a committee set up to develop policies regarding the role of health care aides. What should be included in such policies? Why?

Chapter 4

▼▼▼▼▼▼▼▼▼▼▼▼▼▼▼

Health Economics and Health-Care Reform

PHILIP JACOBS

KEY OBJECTIVES

In this chapter, you will learn:

- Three functions of a health-care system: finance, funding, and delivery.
- Traditional ways of funding medical and hospital care in the Canadian health-care system, and effects these funding methods have had on care in recent years.
- Relationships between the traditional funding methods and the call for reform in Canada.
- Reforms that have been proposed: 1) to replace fee-for-service funding of physicians; and 2) to develop better linkages between hospital and community care.
- Effects such reforms may have.

INTRODUCTION

At the beginning of the 1990s, Canada, along with many other countries, was faced with a deep financial problem. Health-care expenditures per person were increasing annually at an alarming rate. As shown in Figure 4.1, total per-person expenditures had risen from $911 in 1980 to $2,200 in 1990 (Health Canada, 1997). Federal and provincial governments were distressed with this growth, because governments paid roughly 75 percent of total health expenditures. Government deficits were growing, and health care was one contributing factor. Also adding to this alarm was a steadily aging population, which could only add to the growth, because older people generate more health-care expenditures. Finally, a widespread "evidence-based" movement was under way; there was a growing feeling that many health-care practices (especially inpatient care) were unproved in terms of how they influenced health *status*, which is the presumed outcome of health *care*.

These factors led to calls for "health reform" in Canada. Governments put the brakes on health-care spending during the 1990s, and these expenditures levelled out (see Figure 4.1). The prior growth in health-care expenditures caused governments and health-care analysts to scrutinize the health care system, beyond merely looking at the levels of expenditures. Many analysts concluded that, because of the way it was structured, the health-care system contained inflationary incentives, and fundamental changes needed to be made. Most provinces began making reforms to their health-care systems, at varying degrees of speed.

Economics is the science that deals with how scarce means are allocated among competing ends. This is a broad definition, and one can better see what kinds of subjects are tackled by looking at the three general types of studies that economists conduct:

- economists can describe what is happening. Providing "intelligence" is a most important component of economics because one needs good data to know what is going on;
- economists can explain what is happening or predict what will happen. This task is important because one needs to know how health-care systems will react to incentive changes; and
- economists can evaluate interventions that have been implemented. This is important because one needs to be able to rank alternative policies and interventions on a "better" or "worse" basis.

Health economics is a branch of economics; it deals with the use of resources to achieve the goal of health. As a discipline, it can address the subjects of health-care reform and health-care incentives. Using health economics, one can explain how a health-care system works, in effect by pushing resources in one direction or another. In this chapter, you will be introduced to the science of economics as it can be applied to understanding health-care resource use. The chapter begins with a description of the traditional health-care system, then discusses the incentives inherent in that system, and finally examines how "health reform" is being envisaged to alter the system.

THE TRADITIONAL HEALTH-CARE SYSTEM

Any health-care system can be characterized as having three main functions—a finance function, a funding function, and a delivery function. Sometimes these functions are combined.

The **finance function** refers to the manner in which money is transferred from consumers and taxpayers (the ultimate payers) through to providers (e.g., doctors, hospitals), either directly or via intermediaries (e.g., insurers and regional health authorities). Payments can be in the form of taxes (e.g., income taxes or general sales taxes), insurance premiums, or direct out-of-pocket payments.

Figure 4.1

PER CAPITA EXPENDITURES ON HEALTH CARE

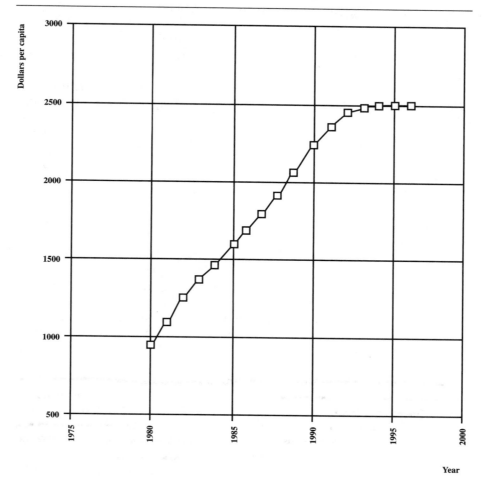

Source: Adapted from Health Canada, *National Health Expenditures in Canada, 1975-1996.*
Fact Sheets, Table 1. Internet: http://www.hc-gc.sc.ca. Reprinted by permission of the Minister
of Public Works and Government Services Canada, 1998.

When the system is government funded, most finance is in the form of taxation. When private health insurance is a major form of finance, the consumers or their employers pay insurance premiums. Finally, consumers can pay directly, out of pocket, for health care. The type of payment has implications in terms of how much different groups pay. Income taxes increase with income, so the average contribution via income taxes is higher for higher-income families. Insurance and health-plan premiums do not vary with income, on the other hand, so as incomes increase, the average contribution falls.

Figure 4.2 depicts the financial flows of the traditional Canadian health-care system. As can be seen from this diagram, all three forms of finance are used in Canada. Most health care is financed through the government-run health insurance programs. In this program plan, individuals and companies pay taxes to both the federal and provincial governments. The federal government transfers funds to the provincial governments to enable the provincial governments to operate health-care insurance programs. These programs cover "medically necessary services" for the general population.

"Medically necessary services" include medical (physician) and hospital care. "Necessary" is a term related to what is essential, but in fact this term has never been clearly defined. Transfers from the federal to the provincial governments cover roughly one-half of the cost of the provincial medicare programs. Additionally, provincial health programs cover professional home care, long-term (nursing home) care, public health, and some outpatient drugs (the latter for welfare recipients and the elderly). Outpatient drugs for the remainder of the population are covered through private insurance (for which individuals or employers pay insurance premiums) or directly, out of pocket.

The **funding function** refers to the manner in which provincial health plans pay the providers of care. The prime form of funding for doctors has been a "fee for service," by which doctors are paid separately for each service provided. Hospitals have been funded on an overall "global budget," a lump-sum payment to the hospital adjusted annually on the basis of numbers of bed days, or numbers and types of cases treated. Other providers have been funded by budgets (public health), fee per service (home care), or fee per day (nursing home care).

The **delivery function** has traditionally been organized in a manner that deals with each type of provider separately. Doctors were organized privately, like businesses. Hospitals were operated by boards of governors; they were organized separately from nursing homes and home care (which had their own governing boards). Institutional providers were, for the most part, not-for-profit; however, a number of for-profit providers have existed in the nursing-home sector. Outpatient drugs were prescribed by doctors, but funded separately.

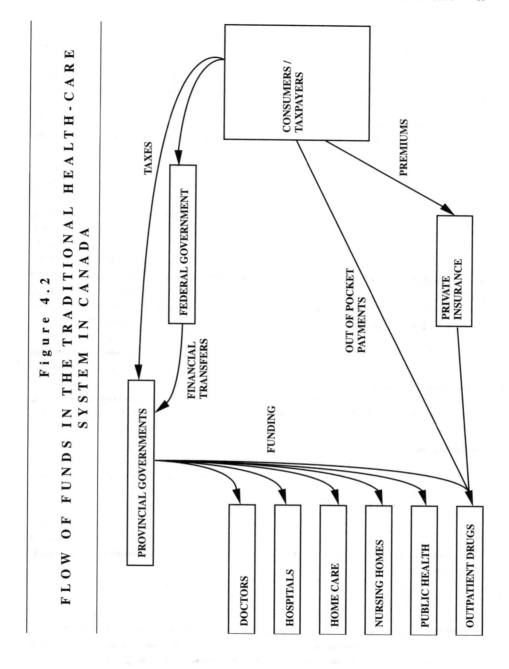

Figure 4.2

FLOW OF FUNDS IN THE TRADITIONAL HEALTH-CARE SYSTEM IN CANADA

INCENTIVES AND THE CALL FOR REFORM

Many aspects of this traditional health-care system created an inflationary orientation. Under the *Canada Health Act* of 1984, which consolidated a number of previous government acts, consumers were guaranteed free physician and hospital services, (i.e., they paid nothing out of pocket). At a zero out-of-pocket price, there was no incentive for patients to cut back their usage.

Consumers will reduce their usage of the health-care system when they pay for some of their care out of pocket. The Canadian health-care insurance program discourages such payments, and so creates a tendency to more use of services. There are reasons why such incentives have been built into the system. When the insurance programs were established, there was a desire to encourage medical care usage, not discourage it. Recently, however, there has been discussion about trying to discourage usage, especially unnecessary usage. Some out-of-pocket payments will discourage usage, though it is not known for certain whether the usage that is discouraged will be "necessary" or not. Additionally, the poor may be disadvantaged more than the rich when out-of-pocket payments are required. It is largely for this reason that out-of-pocket financing has not been used in Canada.

In addition to consumer incentives, there are provider incentives that may influence the system's economic performance. One of these is the fee-for-service basis for the payment of physicians.

Each provincial government has set up a medical-insurance plan, which developed a list of services (e.g., a complete physical examination, a hysterectomy, a complete blood count). For each of these services, there is a fixed fee. Each time a physician provides a service, he or she bills the provincial health-insurance plan. This system has been identified as encouraging the provision of services, since additional services generate additional revenue for the physicians. In response, most provinces have placed a cap on the total fees to be paid annually for a specific service: when doctors in the province reach this cap, no physician is funded for additional services. With or without the cap, there is an issue of whether fee-for-service funding might encourage provision of some unnecessary services, though the term "necessary" is difficult to quantify.

Another provider incentive has been the payment to hospitals on the basis of a fixed global (overall) budget. Provincial governments usually needed to adjust these budgets annually for each hospital. Initially, provinces used the number of days, in total, in which patients were treated. However, this "per diem" payment system encourages hospitals to keep patients in longer because they get more money for doing so, with little extra cost. With hospitalization costs running anywhere from $300 to $600 per day, this was an expensive activity.

In the early 1990s, several provinces, including Ontario and Alberta, switched to a "weighted case mix" system, which was akin to the Diagnosis Related Group (DRG) system developed in the United States a decade earlier. According to these new case-mix funding mechanisms, hospital budgets were adjusted on a per-case basis, with the adjustment amount depending on the average degree of severity or "case mix" of the patients. For example, a hospital would be funded less for a patient admitted for routine medical observation than for one admitted for a heart transplant. The case-mix system provided hospitals with incentives to reduce length of stays, but it also encouraged admission of more cases. This is because hospitals received additional revenue for treating more cases, but no additional revenues for having patients stay longer. This created a major change in incentives for those provinces that instituted case-mix funding.

In addition to drawing attention to the inflationary incentives inherent in the individual components of the health-care system, sweeping world-wide changes in medical care organization raised issues about the organization of the health-care *system*. In the United States, a new form of health-care provision has been emerging since the 1950s: the Health Maintenance Organization (HMO). The HMO is responsible for provision of several different types of services, including physician services, hospital services, and outpatient drugs. Incorporation of all of these services into one single organization is very different from the separate-unit organization style. It makes it easier for services to be co-ordinated, with potential reduction in hospitalizations. HMOs eventually paved the way for "managed care," in which the providing organization can monitor and "manage" how physicians treat their patients (including how much hospitalization takes place). HMOs are not paid for each service provided; rather they are paid by the numbers of members they enrol. This introduction of a "per capita" funding system destroyed the automatic link between payment and services provided, offering an incentive to reduce service use per person.

In Canada, co-ordination was also lacking, not only between physicians and hospitals, but also between hospitals and types of care that could substitute for (and perhaps be less costly than) hospital care, notably community care. The disconnected organizational structure hampered co-ordination between units, and created barriers to the substitution of community care for hospital care.

The disconnected Canadian system was criticized on several other grounds. First, it did not address inequities among populations and regions within a province. No mechanism existed (other than a very inadequate political process) to ensure that populations within a province were treated equally. The disparate system, with fees for service and global budgeting, was not designed to address that issue. It was designed to pay for "production," but did not address who in the population received services. Second, the disparate system was focussed on treatment of the sick, not on prevention of illness. Providers were paid when individuals became sick; there was little incentive in the system to prevent sickness and poor health from occurring.

It should be stressed that the lack of incentives should *not* be equated with a lack of concern among providers for good health. Providers, by and large, are interested in treating patients to help them get better, but the system encourages them to do this by addressing existing illnesses, rather than preventing them. As a result, an enormous industry arose that was geared to diagnosis and treatment of illness, rather than to prevention of illness.

HEALTH REFORM

There is no one single idea of health reform. A number of different groups have embraced the term, and have promoted their own changes as "reform." As a result, the term can mean almost anything. To look at the idea of reform in an orderly manner, it is necessary to return to the initial three functions of the health-care system—finance, funding, and delivery—and to analyze the concept of reform for each of these categories.

The *reform of finance* can mean several things. First, it can mean privatizing care—making patients pay more of the total cost of care directly, rather than through taxation. This would mean decreasing the government share of the pie to less than its mid-1990s level of 75 percent. Some groups have proposed that this be done, largely through "de-insuring" (a nasty word in some circles) certain "less-than-necessary" services currently covered by the health-care insurance plans. A lack of agreement about "necessary" services has hampered the spread of this notion, although some services (e.g., routine eye exams for non-retired adults) have been de-insured in some provinces.

The reform of finance can also mean changing the basis in terms of which the federal government transfers money to the provinces for insured health care. Indeed, the means of transferring funds has changed considerably since the Canadian parliament instituted medical and hospital insurance plans, which began in the early 1960s (see Chapter 1). Initially, provinces were paid roughly half of whatever they spent. Through the years the federal government, recognizing that this encouraged provinces to spend more, moved to a form of finance with a fixed payment per resident, much akin to the capitation payment discussed below. There is a great deal of discussion as to what form this contribution should take.

The *reform of funding* also has a number of different meanings, and in some instances cannot be separated from the *reform of delivery*. Many critics call for the reform of fee-for-service payment to physicians. Because fee for service does encourage the generation of more services (useful or not), many commentators have been looking for another type of payment method, and have been inspired by per capitation funding models. Per capitation funding, used by HMOs in the United States, is a fixed sum of money paid to providers per individual resident, per year. The provider then is responsible for providing all the defined care to the individual during that year. If the provider is an HMO, which includes doctor, hospital, and drug care, this can create a powerful incentive to reduce hospitalization (again, useful or not).

In Canada, discussion about capitation funding has largely involved the payment to primary-care physicians of a fixed sum per person, per year, to provide all primary-care services. Under such a system, each primary-care practitioner would have a roster of patients, and would be required to provide all primary-care services for those patients. Because the budget per person would be fixed for the year (which is the meaning of capitation) there would be an incentive to minimize services provided to each person and to recruit patients who are likely to use fewer services. This is a very different set of incentives from fee-for-service or case-mix funding, which encourage the expansion of services.

Introduction of capitation to primary-care practitioners would require a clear definition as to what is primary care and what is not and, consequently, what services are to be included in the capitation payment. If the primary-care practitioner is not responsible for hospital expenses, for example, then he or she would have an incentive to refer sicker patients to hospitals, rather than have the patients continually visit the practitioner (and thereby increase office costs). A lack of clear specification of covered services might also allow the primary-care practitioner to refer sicker patients to specialists (who would not be covered under the capitation fees). Although it would be a matter of judgement as to when a patient could legitimately be referred to a specialist, such referral would be encouraged under a capitation system as it would reduce the primary-care provider's expenses. Such cost shifting would be a major problem under capitation; indeed, in countries where capitation systems are in place, such as the United States, cost shifting poses a major problem.

Reform of primary care has been an important issue in the United States, where 75 percent of all physicians are specialists. In Canada, specialists represent only about 50 percent of physicians, and primary care, at least for the general population, is more readily available. Nevertheless, primary-care reform has had some attention in Canada, though this is probably because of an aversion on the part of some analysts to fee-for-service medicine.

Reform of fee-for-service medicine has had its proponents for specialized care as well. Recently, the Queen's University medical faculty has changed its funding mechanism from fee for service to a global budget for the entire faculty. The faculty is responsible for dividing up the total budget among its individual clinical practitioners, many of whom are specialists. One concern with such reforms would be that the incentive to generate services would be reduced under a pure global budget, and therefore availability of specialized services might be reduced.

Several western provinces have engaged in funding and delivery reform of institutional services. Saskatchewan was the first to do so; in 1993 Saskatchewan eliminated all hospital, nursing home, and public health boards and placed these institutions under the control of regional health authorities (RHAs). Thirty regions were created, and each had an RHA that was jointly responsible for hospital care, home care, nursing-home care, and public-health services. These regional organizations, as can be seen in Figure 4.3, were akin to HMOs in that they combined several different forms of delivery inside one single organization (drawn inside the dashed lines). This allowed RHAs to address the lack of connection between acute care and post-acute care services, as mentioned above. However, Saskatchewan's RHAs did not include doctors, and so were not the same as HMOs.

Funding to RHAs was set according to a "needs based" per capita payment. Each region received a set fee for each resident, based on the provincial average cost of services used by individuals in given age and gender groups. Needs-based funding addressed the inequity issue, in that individuals in each age group would get the same funding, regardless of the region in which they lived. Each region was responsible for providing care to all individual residents within the region, and was required to provide for this care out of capitation funding from the province.

Some people in each age and gender group are healthier than others, and therefore "needs," even among individuals of the same age and sex, will differ. To address this point Saskatchewan, following British practice, introduced an additional needs-based supplement, by which regions with less healthy populations would receive a needs-based adjustment in addition to the age-based and sex-based capitation payments. Among the bases for making these adjustments were the mortality rate, the number of elderly who lived alone, and the premature birth rate for the region. All such groups "need" more care, and regions with more of these individuals received needs-based bonuses.

However, the concept of "need" is a subjective one. "Need" may be defined as the minimum amount of health-care services that should be provided to bring an individual to a desired level of health. To assess "need," therefore, analysts should know what that desired state of health is to be, and what minimum level of services would bring individuals to that level. Further, select target health levels for different groups may differ, since it may not be feasible to make everyone completely healthy. In fact, no one yet knows what should go in to a "needs-based" funding formula. A better description of this plan is that it is "equity based."

The regional capitation system itself is not incentive-free. Residents of one region, a rural area for example, may travel to other regions to receive medical services. If the capitation payments are made to the RHA where the individual resides, then some way must be made to fund the RHA that provides the services. It has been said that "the money should follow the patient."

Incentives under such a system can work in several different ways. Flows of payments for service between regions can be established; however, such payments provide incentives for regions to try to attract patients from outside the region, in order to enhance their budgets. At the same time, if a region notices that a patient in its region is prohibitively expensive, then there is an incentive for it to refer the patient out to other regions (called "dumping" in the United States). This is particularly likely to occur where the inter-regional settlement will not cover the treatment costs. Thus capitation funding has incentives of its own, and these must be addressed.

A final type of reform is privatization. In Alberta, a number of privately owned clinics and hospitals have been opened or proposed, and these have been encouraged on the basis that the public sector should be

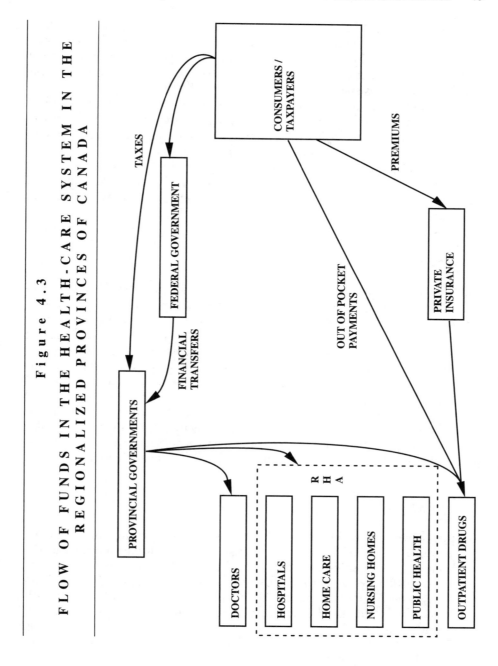

Figure 4.3

FLOW OF FUNDS IN THE HEALTH-CARE SYSTEM IN THE REGIONALIZED PROVINCES OF CANADA

able to compete with the private sector, even in health care. Some of these privately operated establishments have been promoted on the basis of their potential export value, or the ability of the organizations to market their services to full-paying, non-resident patients—perhaps even relieving the pressure on the government health-insurance systems.

The ability of doctors to sell services to private clients and public clients simultaneously raises some concerns. A doctor who practices in both sectors has an incentive to build up queues in the public sector so that public patients will move to the doctor's private clinic.

The original health-care insurance acts prohibited a "two-tier" system, but private clinics owned by practising doctors are now operating, and there is a "reform" element in Canada that seeks to expand privatization in this direction.

CONCLUSION

The Canadian health-care system has gone through considerable changes in the 1990s, and reform continues. Health-care reforms are responses to several decades of rising costs; however, they vary in their intent. Some are attacks on fee-for-service medicine. Others are attacks on full-service coverage. And still others are attacks on government-funded health care.

The incentives created by these reforms are not well understood at this time. It is not clear by how much utilization will be reduced as a result, and it is even less clear whether health promotion and disease prevention will increase. Overall, the reforms may reduce costs, but they should not be judged on the basis of cost alone. Changes in outcomes, in terms of health status, must also be assessed. All practices—whether new or existing—should be judged on the basis of solid evidence of their effectiveness.

SUMMARY

- Economics is a science that is used to describe, predict, and evaluate events related to the scarcity of resources. Health economics is the branch of economics that deals with health-related events.
- The health-care system has three functions: finance, funding, and delivery. The finance function is the mechanism by which funds are collected from the public via insurance premiums, taxes, and direct charges. The funding function is the means of paying providers of care. The delivery function is the means by which health-care services are provided to the public.
- In the traditional health-care system, physicians were funded by fees for services. Hospitals were funded through global budgets.
- Fee-for-service funding has been perceived as increasing the number of health-care services, and has therefore been linked to growing health-care expenditures.

- Both fee-for-service funding of physicians and global budgeting for hospitals have been perceived as relating to services, rather than to people or needs.
- A number of separate concepts for health reform have been proposed. These include the privatization of health care, per capita funding for hospitals, and the dismantling of fee-for-service funding for physicians.
- Reforms are being instituted in Canada, including regionalization of health-care providers and funding of providers on a per capita basis. These systems are new, and should be subjected to careful scrutiny. As with their predecessors, they will have drawbacks as well as benefits.

FURTHER READINGS AND RESOURCES

Angus, D.E., Auer, L., Cloutier, J.E., & Albert, T. (1995). *Sustainable health care for Canada.* Ottawa: University of Ottawa Economic Projects. This concise book is the synthesis report of an ambitious research project launched in 1991 by the Economic Council of Canada. The Canadian health system is discussed in the light of economic data contained in a number of technical documents. Factors accounting for the increase in health-care costs are examined, and four scenarios are developed from economic data that illustrate the impact of various policy and administrative approaches to downsizing in the Canadian health system. Four sectors of the health system are then considered separately: institutional services (primarily hospitals), continuing-care services, health professionals, and pharmaceuticals. Cost drivers and incentives that operate within each of these sectors are discussed, and policy options for achieving significant cost savings are considered.

Jacobs, P. (1995). Economics of health care. In G.L. Deloughery (Ed.), *Issues and trends in nursing* (pp. 97–124). St. Louis, MO: Mosby. This chapter is written primarily for U.S. audiences as the author describes economic relations between various types of insurers, and the economic characteristics of health maintenance organizations (HMOs) and preferred provider organizations (PPOs). It contains a detailed explanation of the role of incentives in directing resources to alternative uses in health care. Although this chapter provides a good overview of the topic, it is likely to be more relevant for graduate than undergraduate courses.

National Forum on Health (1997). *Canada health action: Building on the legacy.* Volume I, Final Report, and Volume II, Synthesis Reports and Issues Papers. Ottawa: Minister of Public Works and Government Services. These easy-to-read reports are the result of two years work by an advisory body established by the Prime Minister of Canada in 1994. The mandate was to involve and inform Canadians and to advise the federal government on innovative ways to improve both the health system and the health of Canada's people. Volume I is an executive summary and Volume II contains synthesis reports to the Forum from various working groups. These include, for example, reports on striking a balance in relation to limited resources, on determinants of health, and on evidence-based decision making. One of the main conclusions was that Canada spends enough money on health care, but that more efficient and effective ways of using resources must be found.

REFERENCES

Canada Health Act (1984) R.S.C. C-6.

Health Canada. (1997). *National health expenditures in Canada, 1975–1996*. Fact Sheets, Table 1. Ottawa: Minister of Public Works and Government Services. http://www.hc-sc.gc.ca.

PART TWO

Structure &
Organization

Chapter 5

▼▼▼▼▼▼▼▼▼▼▼▼▼

Management Theory: Critical Review and Application

Carl A. Meilicke

KEY OBJECTIVES

In this chapter, you will learn:

- Basic theoretical concepts of strategic management theory, including open and closed models and rational and natural approaches to planning.
- Six key peripheral concepts that influence a management approach.
- Relationships that exist among the total organization, the nursing department, and the nursing unit as "systems."
- Application of these basic theoretical concepts in a practical situation.

INTRODUCTION

Nursing services are almost always delivered in the context of a formal organization and this has a profound effect on the quality of these services. Because of this, all nurses should be competent at analyzing the efficiency and effectiveness of formal organizations, and nursing administrators should be highly competent at modifying and managing them.

This chapter provides an overview of organization design theory and discusses how to make use of that knowledge in everyday practice. The first and second sections will introduce basic theoretical concepts. The third section will provide a conceptual framework for strategic management that will help the reader to apply these theoretical concepts to practical situations. The fourth section will show how to use the conceptual framework to analyze a practical nursing management situation and provide a theory-based critique of what happened in that situation. A postscript briefly highlights recent changes. The brief annotated bibliography identifies useful background readings for health-care managers.

INTRODUCTION TO ORGANIZATION DESIGN THEORY

Evolution of contemporary organization theory began at the turn of the century, and the most important developments have occurred since the 1930s. By the late 1970s, the large and varied store of useful ideas that had been developed could be grouped under two general perspectives—open and closed—and, under each of these, could be divided into two distinct approaches, rational and natural, as is shown in Table 5.1. Each of these four approaches offered many valuable insights but, as the "Limitations" section of Table 5.1 shows, none offered a complete answer to the question of how to create and maintain an efficient and effective organization. Since the 1970s, a new approach has emerged—strategic management theory (not to be confused with the strategic contingencies approach). Strategic management theory provides a way to integrate the prior perspectives and approaches into a more or less coherent whole.

This section contains a brief description and critical assessment of the original four approaches. In addition, some supplementary concepts are introduced that are useful to those who are applying theoretical concepts. The section that follows contains a description of strategic management theory.

The basic assumptions underlying each of the four approaches are dramatically different. These assumptions reflect either a closed or open system perspective on organizations and, within each of these two options, a rational or a natural approach. The closed versus open system perspectives reflect the degree to which it is believed that the external environment of the organization must be taken into account when managers make decisions. The rational versus natural approaches reflect the degree to which management is perceived to involve (rational) pre-planning of objectives and the means to achieve them, as opposed to a more (natural) dynamic process of ongoing adaptation to changing circumstances.

The result of these differences in basic assumptions is that each approach leads to dramatically different solutions. Table 5.1 shows how these four approaches affect seven key organizational issues. For example, both closed system perspectives tend to support the idea that there is a "one best way" to manage, but this is largely the result of discounting or ignoring the impact that a wide variety of factors in the environment can have upon the organization. To illustrate, classical bureaucratic theory may seem to be the best way to deal with the control of cost and quality in a situation where the management issues are complex and the consequence of error is high. It is difficult to defend this position, however, if one recognizes that many employees have strong negative feelings about rigid authoritarianism because of attitudes they bring to the work situation from outside the organization. The human relations school recognizes that workers often prefer more participation in decision making (and therefore concludes that the one best way to manage is an approach that encourages worker involvement in decision making); it fails to recognize, however, that many workers do not wish to accept the responsibility that comes with partici-

Table 5.1

SUMMARY OF THEORETICAL
PERSPECTIVES ON
ORGANIZATIONAL ISSUES

Organizational Issues	Closed System	
	Rational Approaches	Natural Approaches
	Classical bureaucratic theory (Taylor, 1911; Gulick & Urwick, 1937; Weber, 1947; Mooney, 1947; Gouldner, 1954)	The "human relations" school (Barnard, 1938; Roethlisberger & Dickson, 1939; McGregor, 1960; Argyris, 1966; Likert, 1967)
Efficiency	Classical/Bureaucratic Theory Position May be obtained through application of work-study methods and predetermined principles of "good" management. Maximized through a hierarchically ordered chain of positions and specified procedures for operation.	Human Relations Position Best brought about by integrating individual aspirations with organizational goals. Involve workers in their job through participatory decision making, job enlargement, job enrichment, etc.
Effectiveness	As above.	In addition to profit, growth, and quality, individual member satisfaction in the organization is viewed as a major goal in its own right.
Conflict	Should be avoided. This can be accomplished by constructing appropriate departmentalization, chains of command, and span of control. Minimize potential for conflict by having a rule or procedure for everything.	Is generally viewed as dysfunctional, but should be managed and confronted openly when it occurs.
Change (innovation)	Handle by means of rational accommodation and intervention, establishment of new rules and procedures.	Must be accommodated through changes in the informal structures of the organization as well as the formal structures.

pation because of commitments and interests they have outside of the organization.

By the early 1960s, the open system perspective had gained prominence because researchers began to recognize the undeniable importance of environmental variables. It was not long before a large number of technical, political, and social factors were considered to be potentially important to any

Table 5.1 (continued)

Open system	
Rational Approaches	**Natural Approaches**
(Burns & Stalker, 1961; Woodward, 1965; Lawrence & Lorsch, 1967; Thompson, 1967; Perrow, 1967; Katz & Kahn, 1966; Becker & Gordon, 1966; Hage, 1965, 1980; Khandwalla, 1974; Shortell, 1977; Simon, 1965; Cyert & March, 1963; Alexis & Wilson, 1967)	(Hickson et al., 1971; March & Olson, 1976; Meyer & Rowan, 1977; Hannan & Freeman, 1977; Pfeffer & Salancik, 1978; Tushman & Nadler, 1978; Aldrich, 1979)
Contingency/Decision Theory Position May be attained in several ways depending on the nature of the tasks involved, the people involved, and external circumstances. Depends on the quality of the decisions made under uncertainty.	**Strategic Contingencies/Political Negotiation/Resource Dependence/ Population Ecology Position** Overall objective is not efficiency per se but system survival. As such, political as well as economic transactions become important.
As above. In addition, one way that organizations survive is by expanding or changing their goals to meet new demands from the environment. Emphasis is on goal attainment.	As above. Emphasis is not on goal attainment but on obtaining resources and balancing internal political considerations of those vying for power in order to survive.
Not necessarily viewed as dysfunctional. Can promote creativity and innovation. The problem is to minimize disruptive conflict. Attending to different goals at different times may be helpful.	Viewed as a natural consequence of internal negotiations over power, given the strategic contingencies the organization faces.
Can occur either from within or without the organization. Again, depends on nature of tasks, people, and environment. Some evidence to indicate that more loosely structured organizations are more innovative in an "inventive" sense but that more tightly structured organizations may be better at implementing and diffusing the innovation. Ability to change or innovate is also a function of organizational learning over time.	Comes about both through external demands and internal political adjustments to those demands. Those who can most influence the type, pace, and direction of change at one point in time may not be most influential at another point in time as the organization's environment changes and its need for different kinds of expertise changes accordingly.

given organization. These insights initially led to the idea of a contingency approach to dealing with organizational issues. This means that there is no one best way to manage and the most appropriate management action is seen to be contingent upon the particular combination of environmental variables that act upon each specific organization at a given point in time. Within this open systems perspective, proponents of the rational approach argue that one can assess the environment and develop a plan to cope with its effects.

Table 5.1 (continued)

Organizational Issues	Closed System	
	Rational Approaches	**Natural Approaches**
Social Integration/ Motivation	Can be attained through appropriate structural mechanisms (unity of command, span of control, etc.). Little attention given to the individual.	Achieved through the informal system of relationships among workers. Emphasis on nonpecuniary rewards, such as intrinsic job satisfaction and opportunities for personal expression and growth.
Coordination	A primary goal of the organization. May be achieved through appropriate departmentalization, hierarchy, and specification of rules and procedures.	Little attention given to it. Again, emphasis is on the informal work group as a coordinative mechanism.
Maintenance (adaptation to environment)	Essentially not considered.	Essentially not considered.

	Limitations	**Limitations**
	1. Incomplete motivational assumptions.	1. Many of the studies upon which the theory is based have been poorly designed.
	2. Little appreciation of nature or role of conflict.	2. Limited view of human motivation—assumes all individuals want more participation and involvement.
	3. No consideration of the limitations of individuals as information-processing beings.	3. Essentially no consideration of the environment.
	4. Essentially no consideration of the environment in which organizations function.	4. A "one best way" approach.
	5. A "one best way" approach: the "only way" to manage.	

In the early 1970s, the open natural approach emerged, when some researchers came to believe that environmental complexity and rate of change are so great that the organization cannot plan for environmental changes and can only respond in an ad hoc fashion. There is a troubling aspect to this approach: the assumption that the environment dominates rather than shapes the organization can lead to a dysfunctional organization, as is evidenced by the response to issues such as effectiveness, conflict, and social integration when using this approach (see Table 5.1). The approach can also be used by a dishonest or incompetent management team to justify otherwise unacceptable behaviour by allowing the managers to argue that the environment is too complex to be properly dealt with.

Needless to say, each approach has some degree of usefulness, depending on the circumstances. The rational, pre-planned, and centralized

---

Table 5.1 (continued)

Open system	
Rational Approaches	**Natural Approaches**
May be achieved in a variety of ways including both intrinsic and extrinsic factors contributing to job satisfaction. The emphasis is on role—getting people to function in their role and understanding each other's roles.	Is achieved through internal accommodation among competing groups that agree to go along with the dominant coalition at the time because it is in their best interest to do so.
The more specialized the organization and the greater the degree to which tasks are interdependent, the greater the need for coordination. May be achieved through committees and task forces as well as informal organization.	Primary reliance is placed on informal and emergent processes rather than on formal rules, procedures, or committees. Coordination is achieved through negotiation and bargaining.
Crucial to understanding organizational behavior. The organization must "negotiate" its environment by engaging in search procedures, dealing with uncertainty, and structuring itself to meet the demands of the environment.	Of primary importance. Those in leadership positions must manage the organization's environment as well as the internal structures and processes. Leaders must seek to "enact" their environments in addition to simply "reacting" to them.
Limitations A conceptually sound approach for the study of organizations, but requires much more research to replicate some of the early findings and define further the nature of the interaction between an organization and its environment. Problem of measuring the environment; perceptual versus nonperceptual measures.	Limitations There has been little empirical study to date of the open natural systems approach. The approach may also be somewhat of an overreaction to the rational contingency approaches. A middle ground would suggest that organizations survive in the long run through some degree of goal attainment in which certain kinds of organizational designs and processes provide a structural framework for channeling internal political negotiations. In brief, some degree of goal attainment would appear necessary in order for the organization to maintain sufficient credibility to continue to attract needed resources.

Source: From *Health Care Management: A Text in Organizational Theory and Behavior*, by Stephen Shortell and Arnold Kaluzny (New York: John Wiley & Sons, 1983), pp. 26–29. Reprinted with permission of the authors.

authority techniques of scientific management (a subset of classical bureaucratic theory) are often of great value when the work is highly repetitive and routine, as it is on an assembly line. At the same time, some aspects of participative management will almost always enhance employee morale and some degree of contingency planning is necessary to protect the organization from sudden external changes (as would be the case, for example, if advances in robotic technology rendered much of the assembly line obsolete, or a change in employee attitudes caused them to begin resisting a tradition of highly centralized decision making).

This "mix and match" approach to management leads to many different options, depending on circumstances specific to the management situation. It is helpful to think of these options as falling on a continuum that extends from mechanistic to organic, with the intermediate range of the continuum being described as ambidextrous. A mechanistic style emphasizes rules, procedures, a clear hierarchy of authority, centralization, and a task-oriented approach to employee morale. It tends to incorporate many elements of the closed system orientation. An organic style emphasizes flexibility, individual initiative, decentralization, and encouragement of individual creativity. It tends to reflect many elements of the open system approach. Management approaches found at or near the midpoint of the continuum incorporate elements of both approaches and are described as ambidextrous.

Recognition of the open system concept and the organic/mechanistic concept represented a breakthrough in the utility of management theory, but the price of this progress was complexity and ambiguity. An enormous number of environmental variables potentially require analysis. There are also a large number of management options to consider. Furthermore, environmental variables keep changing, and this often changes the nature of a suitable management response. It became quite clear that good management decision making was much more complex, and had to be much more adaptable to changing circumstances, than had been previously recognized. By the early 1980s, it was clear that a new theoretical framework was necessary—one that would deal more effectively with the complexity and ambiguity of the new insights.

Strategic management theory is what emerged. Although it is based on the open system, rational approach, it allows a wide range of environmental and managerial options to be taken into account much more easily. It also provides a way to make selective use of all of the prior perspectives and approaches in a more or less integrated fashion.

PERIPHERAL CONCEPTS

Before examining the exciting new perspective of strategic management theory, it is useful to review six important peripheral concepts that have emerged from the research since the turn of the century. These supplementary ideas are not central components of any perspective, approach, or theory but, as with the concept of ambidexterity, they are useful rhetorical tools when it comes to applying theory.

1. HISTORY OF THE ORGANIZATION AND PERSONALITY OF ITS ACTORS

The history of the organization and personality of its members are the key factors to consider. Two important historical considerations are the size and life cycle of the organization. It is obvious that as an organization grows in size it will tend to develop more mechanistic characteristics in the form of rules, regulations, policies, impersonality, and so on. What is not quite so obvious is that organizations go through cycles of change depending on changes in the environment or on ways in which the organization undertakes to respond to environmental constraints and opportunities. For example, steady growth in the complexity and instability of the environment usually creates significant new challenges in maintaining an ambidextrous balance between mechanistic elements of management (which are necessary for effective co-ordination and control) and organic elements (which increase the speed with which the organization can adapt to a changing environment).

Changes in leadership and personality of managers can also create a new cycle, because different individuals assess the environment, and respond to it, in different ways. Some managers are highly skilled in this regard, and some are not; some learn and improve with experience, some do not; and, finally, some are emotionally stable personalities who can deal with ambiguity in a mature fashion, and some are not. All managers are *not* created equal.

2. DEFINITION OF A SYSTEM

One automatically thinks of the total organization as a "system," but it is made up of many systems (work teams, units, departments, divisions, and so on) and it is only a small part of larger systems (for example, a hospital is a sub-set of the acute-care system, which is a sub-set of the health-care system). Organization design theory can be used with regard to any level (subsystem) of the organization but the nature of the environmental factors bearing upon each subsystem is likely to be different, and therefore different management solutions may be appropriate at different levels of the organization. The technical, political, and cultural environments of importance to the manager of a pediatric ward, for example, are quite different from those relating to a geriatric ward, and both are different from the overall division of nursing. Accordingly, the best combination of organic and mechanistic components of a management solution may be quite different within and between different levels of the organization.

3. DESCRIBING THE ENVIRONMENT

The third of the six key ideas concerns a way of summarizing the data about the nature of the environment. This is most commonly done in terms of two dimensions, each of which is a continuum: simplicity/complexity and stability/instability. Generally speaking, the more simple and stable the environment, the more mechanistic the organization can be—because the need for adaptability is less. Conversely, the more complex and unstable the environment, the more organic the organization can and should be. In the past few years, for example, the environment of most health organizations has become dramatically more complex and unstable and managers have responded by trying to make the organization more organic in the hope that it can thereby adapt more quickly to change. One example of this is the widespread effort to decentralize authority for decision making and thereby encourage more participation in the decision process.

4. DESCRIBING TECHNOLOGY

The fourth idea is a way of summarizing data about technology. Technical variables involve relatively tangible and inanimate factors, such as money supply, number and types of workers, and the types of knowledge, material, and equipment. The nature of relevant technology is an unusually important environmental variable because it frequently establishes rigid limitations on the options available to managers. Again, two sub-concepts, complexity and interdependence, are basic. Technological complexity is defined by the number (variety) of exceptions to the "normal" case that is indicated by the technology and, given that technology, by how easy it is to define (analyze) an appropriate way to handle these exceptions. High variety (many exceptions) and low analyzability (difficulty in defining the best solution to the exceptions) are described as non-routine technology and tend to call for more organic forms of management. Low variety and high analyzability represent routine technologies and lend themselves to more mechanistic approaches. Looking only at this aspect of technology, for example, one might well expect a relatively organic management style to be used in a psychiatric ward because the knowledge (theory) underlying psychotherapy allows for many exceptions to the normal case and many variations on how to treat each individual case. Conversely, a more mechanistic style might be appropriate on a ward dealing with uncomplicated surgery.

The other sub-concept has to do with the degree of interdependence created as a result of the technology, especially with other work groups, professions, departments, and so on. Interdependence can range from pooled (very low, as between a nursing unit and the accounting office), to sequential (the output of one unit is input for another, such as admitting and nursing), to reciprocal (where outputs flow back and forth, such as a surgical ward and the surgical suite).

Nursing technology, for example, creates high levels of interdependence with a wide variety of diagnostic, clinical, and support groups or units. The higher the level of interdependence, the greater the need for attention to communication and co-ordination. Accordingly, the need for good communication and co-ordination techniques within nursing subsystems, and between them and other subsystems, is greater than in many other components of the hospital. This generally requires more organic styles of management so that rapid adaptability is made easier. At the same time, many of the interdependencies of nursing are pooled or sequential, so that both mechanistic and ambidextrous styles are also often appropriate.

5. RECOGNIZING DILEMMAS

The concept of organizational dilemmas is the fifth key idea. Many of the most important decisions in management involve balancing requirements that are in many ways incompatible but must be provided for if the organization is to survive. For example, both co-ordination and communication are essential for an organization to survive. Communication is usually improved if hierarchy is minimized (which can be done, for example, by reducing the number of supervisors and decentralizing authority), but these measures will almost always make co-ordination more difficult because co-ordination is heavily dependent upon hierarchy, especially in larger organizations. Many other examples could be given, but they can be generally summarized in terms of an organic/mechanistic dilemma. Both styles have merit, and all organizations must have elements of each, so the challenge is to achieve and maintain an ambidextrous style that creates an appropriate balance between them. These dilemmas cannot be avoided, they can only be endured. As a result, they are one of the major challenges, and one of the major responsibilities, facing managers.

Health organizations face a number of unusual dilemmas. One of the more important is the need for high reliability in areas where the cost of error is so high that extraordinary means must be taken to minimize mistakes. The degree to which an organization must require high reliability varies within the organization, and within each subsystem, along a continuum. When a nurse is assisting with transplant surgery or injecting intravenous chemotherapy, for example, there is a need for high reliability. With many other nursing functions, the need may be much lower. High reliability creates a dilemma for the organization because, on the one hand, an organic style of management may encourage the sense of individual responsibility that is needed to minimize errors but, on the other hand, a mechanistic style is more likely to ensure that controls are in place to prevent ill informed or irresponsible behaviour. Professionalization of a work group, incidentally, is an expensive but effective way to increase reliability in work situations, such as nursing, where it is difficult to use mechanistic controls.

The growing emphasis on patient expectations has created a similar dilemma. It is important to be attentive to the preferences and personal satisfaction of the patient, and this is compatible with an organic style that allows front-line workers more flexibility in decision making. On the other hand, the organization as a whole has both a legal and moral responsibility for the acts of its employees and agents, and this requires certain mechanistic elements if their behaviour is to be properly monitored and controlled.

6. ETHICAL ACCOUNTABILITY

A sixth key concept relating to organization design theory concerns ethical implications of management decision making. It is unfortunate that this most important concept has yet to receive the attention it deserves from either organization theorists or management practitioners. It is fortunate, however, that an open system/rational approach is well suited to deal with the complex problems presented by ethical issues in management. The open system orientation requires that the ethical milieu of the organization be considered by management in terms of both its impact on the organization and the impact the organization has on the environment. The rational approach requires that due and deliberate consideration be given to all relevant management variables, and there is no justification for arguing that ethical issues are not relevant in delivering health services. Furthermore, the organic/mechanistic concept facilitates analysis of the extremely important ethical issues related to determining how the organization can best fulfil its responsibility for the actions of its staff.

Two important ethical questions will be dealt with later in this chapter. The first is the responsibility of the health organization to rationalize existing patterns of physician decision making and of inter-institutional competition, in the face of the evidence that, in their current form, both of these compromise efficient and effective use of health resources. The second deals with the question of how organic health organizations can and should be managed, given the moral and legal responsibility of senior management for the actions of their staff.

STRATEGIC MANAGEMENT

The problem of designing and implementing a management theory that was better able to deal with complexity and ambiguity led to the idea of strategic management. Strategic management involves four steps:

Step 1. Assess the environment;

Step 2. Devise an overall management strategy based on this assessment;

Step 3. Make day-to-day decisions based on the overall management strategy; and

Step 4. Modify the management strategy on an ongoing basis in response to changes in the environment and feedback from the daily decision-making process.

It is important to note that this theory provides a way to integrate all of the earlier perspectives and concepts. Looking again at Table 5.1, for example, we can see that this approach incorporates the open system perspective (Step 1), including either of the rational or natural approaches (Steps 2 and 3), and recognizes the associated need for adaptability due either to a changing environment or to actual experience associated with implementing the strategy (Step 4). It similarly allows for easy accommodation of the ideas from the closed system perspective as well as peripheral concepts, such as the six outlined above.

There is no overall consensus about the details of strategic management theory, but a framework developed by Noel Tichy (1983) is useful in addressing this problem (See Table 5.2), and his TPC Model (an acronym for Technical, Political, and Cultural) has been adapted for use in this chapter. In the following discussion, the nine cells in the TPC model will be referred to by number, from left to right, starting in the upper left-hand corner. Thus, the technical system will include cells 1, 2 and 3; the political, cells 4, 5, and 6; and, the cultural, cells 7, 8, and 9.

Tichy's framework incorporates four important assumptions. First, organizations are affected by three major categories of environmental variables: technical, political, and cultural. (Tichy's ideas are sometimes described as TPC Theory.) Technical variables involve relatively tangible and inanimate factors, such as money supply, number and types of workers, and different types of knowledge, material, and equipment. Political variables basically involve the distribution of power in the environment, such as that held by government, professional associations, unions, pressure groups, and even individuals. Cultural variables include the values and beliefs of individuals and groups, such as attitudes regarding women's rights, professionalism, and commitment to a work ethic. (It thus reflects an open systems perspective.)

Second, in response to these environmental variables, organizations must develop three internal systems: technical, political, and cultural. The technical system deals with how managers plan for and organize the technical resources that are available from the environment (Cells 1, 2, and 3 of Table 5.2). The political system deals with how they distribute power within the organization (Cells 4, 5, and 6). The cultural system deals with how they manage attitudes and values, including both adjusting to the employee culture and attempting to change it (Cells 7, 8, and 9). In developing these systems, managers can draw on the entire range of ideas incorporated in Table 5.1 about how to respond to organizational issues, whether from the open or closed perspectives.

Third, it is important that the three systems be in alignment or, put another way, be mutually supportive. For example, if the political system emphasizes staff involvement and decentralization of authority, the technical system should place relatively less emphasis on detailed position descriptions or on rules and regulations. If this is not done, there is misalignment and, in this case, employee cynicism could result from the discrepancy between how the work is actually done, and how work roles are formally defined.

Fourth, managers have three basic tools they can use to ensure that alignment occurs: mission and strategy (Cells 1, 4, and 7), structure (Cells 2, 5, and 8), and human resource management, which is referred to in Table 5.2 as "process" (Cells 3, 6, and 9). All of the ideas in Table 5.1 can be made part of this "tool kit."

The following brief example will demonstrate how this theory can be applied to a real situation. Many health organizations have reduced the

Table 5.2

MANAGERIAL TOOLS FOR STRATEGIC MANAGEMENT

Managerial Areas	Mission and Strategy	Organizational Structure	Processes
Technical System	(1) · Assessing environmental threats and opportunities. · Assessing organizational strengths and weaknesses. · Defining mission and fitting resources to accomplish it.	(2) · Differentiation: organization of work into roles (production, marketing, etc.). · Integration: recombining roles into departments, divisions, regions, etc. · Aligning structure to strategy.	(3) · Fitting people into roles. · Specifying performance criteria for roles. · Measuring performance. · Staffing and development to fill roles (present and future). · Matching management style with technical tasks.
Political System	(4) · Who gets to influence the mission and strategy. · Managing coalitional behaviour around strategic decisions.	(5) · Distribution of power across the role structure. · Balancing power across groups of roles (e.g., sales vs. marketing, production vs. research and development, etc.).	(6) · Managing succession politics (who gets ahead, how do they get ahead). · Decision and administration of reward system (who gets what and how). · Managing the politics of appraisal (who is appraised by whom and how). · Managing the politics of information control and the planning process.
Cultural System	(7) · Managing influence of values and philosophy on mission and strategy. · Developing culture aligned with mission and strategy.	(8) · Developing managerial style aligned with technical and political structure. · Development of subcultures to support roles (production culture, R&D culture, etc.). · Integration of subcultures to create company culture.	(9) · Selection of people to build or reinforce culture. · Development (socialization) to mould organizational culture. · Management of rewards to shape and reinforce the culture. · Management of information and planning systems to shape and reinforce the culture.

Source: Adapted from *Managing Strategic Change: Technical, Political and Cultural Dynamics*, by Noel M. Tichy (New York: John Wiley & Sons, 1983), p. 119. Reprinted by permission of John Wiley & Sons, Inc.

number of supervisors (a change in Cell 2 of the technical system; in this case, a change in the organization chart). Many of these organizations have also moved to change the cultural system by modifying the mission and strategy (Cell 7) in such a way that staff are encouraged to exercise their own values, attitudes, and judgement regarding their work (in other words, decentralizing authority). These two changes can be described as a shift to a more organic and less mechanistic management process.

Unfortunately, the above changes often result in a misalignment with the political system. Encouraging staff autonomy tends to reduce the power of middle managers and this is exaggerated by extra work demands imposed on supervisors as a result of reduction in their numbers. This type of misalignment can create many problems, but one of the most dangerous is the blurring of accountability, particularly with regard to high reliability functions. One way to rectify the problem is to modify the policies and procedures (Cell 2 of the technical system) in such a way that the parameters of supervisory authority are more clearly defined and there is less ambiguity about when participatory management techniques are acceptable for planning, co-ordination, and quality control, and when they are not. In other words, the solution involves moving the balance point toward the mechanistic side of the organic/mechanistic continuum. Achieving the correct balance, of course, can be exquisitely difficult in this type of situation.

When used in the foregoing fashion, Tichy's model can help to substantially reduce the complexity of strategic management because it provides a relatively uncomplicated set of guidelines regarding what variables should be examined and how the interaction effects between them can be planned for. The steps in strategic management now become:

Step 1. Assess the environment in terms of technical, political, and cultural variables;

Step 2. Devise an overall management strategy that includes: (a) planning and design of technical, political, and cultural systems appropriate in terms of the environmental variables; and, (b) planning and implementing of management strategies involving goals, structure, and process that will establish and maintain alignment;

Step 3. Establish a process whereby day-to-day management decision making is based on the above overall management strategy; and

Step 4. Establish a process whereby management strategy can be modified on an ongoing basis in response to changes in the environment and feedback from daily decision-making experiences.

These steps can be used to describe or to assess an existing organization and, as well, to develop a strategy for change.

APPLYING STRATEGIC MANAGEMENT THEORY

A critical assessment of some management changes that occurred in many Canadian nursing departments during the 1980s and 1990s illustrates how strategic management theory is used. Nursing departments in tertiary care hospitals are used as an example because this type of organization is among the most complex in modern society, and therefore offers a larger variety and magnitude of strategic management problems for examination than any other health organization. Details of the discussion are based entirely on the personal observations and opinions of the author. Not all events happened in all hospitals, but the described events are representative of general developments in health-care environments and in organizational responses across Canada during this time period.

The main purpose of the discussion is to show readers how to apply TPC theory to their own personal experiences, their own knowledge of management theory and research, and the environmental and institutional realities of their own organizations. A secondary purpose is to try to define some of the main management challenges facing acute-care nursing in Canada.

STEP 1: ENVIRONMENTAL ASSESSMENT

The first step in strategic management is to assess the environment in terms of technical, political, and cultural variables. The focus in this section is on the nursing division in its totality as the "system"; therefore, the "environment" includes all relevant external variables, whether they exist within or outside of the hospital.

In the technical arena of the hypothetical hospital described in this example, there had been rapid and continuing growth in the variety and complexity of the knowledge, skills, and equipment that related to hospital operations, and especially to medical and nursing practice. The changes in nursing were particularly important because they reflected a rapid growth in the profession's foundation of research-based knowledge. The overall impact of these changes had been to increase costs but, at the same time, external funding agencies had steadily become more determined to reduce the rate of increase in hospital funding; technological change had in effect created a severe cost-revenue crisis. The crisis was particularly acute in nursing for two interconnected reasons. First, senior management (that is, the chief executive officer and the board, who are ultimately responsible for all management policy and decisions) had not developed effective techniques for planning and controlling acquisition and use of technology by physicians, which had a substantial impact on nursing budgets. Second, newer nursing workload and output-measurement technologies provided valuable information, but this was largely ignored by senior management because the data indicated the nursing budget was increasingly inadequate and senior management did not wish, largely for political reasons, to divert funds away from the priorities of physicians.

In the political environment, there had been rapid growth in the influence of nursing unions, a parallel growth in the technical sophistication as well as the professional self-esteem of nurses, and a slow but steady erosion of traditional medical dominance. Nevertheless, nurses continued to have relatively low political credibility, inside or outside of these hospitals, in great part because of the disunity caused by major differences in their education, work assignments, and career expectations and the much greater social prestige of physicians. This credibility was improving as the profession gained more experience in pressure-group tactics and became more highly educated, but a major constraint on this progress was the continuing strength of chauvinistic attitudes directed at nurses, the stubborn myth that nurses were physicians' handmaidens, the fact that most nurses were female, and the mistaken belief that the nurturing elements of the nursing role are a low-skill activity based more on maternal instinct than on professional expertise. A further constraint was the aforementioned rejection of the information system as a means for providing objective data about workload, output, and productivity.

The cultural environment was dominated by changes in the attitudes of nurses toward work and the nature of their organizational commitment. The advent of the "me generation," feminism, single parenting, unionization, research-based professionalization, different patterns of entry-level education, two-income families, and extensive experience with staff cutbacks had dramatically reduced the traditional willingness of many nurses to accept an authoritarian work environment or to invest a strong personal commitment in a specific organization. These changes were further exaggerated by changing expectations of patients, who tended to be more knowledgeable and demanding, and the growing militancy of nursing-union leaders, who were frustrated by the amount of effort required to move toward equity in pay and conditions of work.

The overall degree of environmental instability and complexity (turbulence) in the hospital had increased rapidly during the past few years and the rate of increase was continuing. The single most significant outcome was a growing cost-revenue crisis, to which nursing was particularly vulnerable because the main cause was utilization decisions made by physicians, and nursing was not able to influence these decisions.

STEPS 2 AND 3: DEVELOPMENT AND IMPLEMENTATION OF A MANAGEMENT STRATEGY

Steps Two and Three require nursing departments to describe and assess the development and implementation of a management strategy in terms of technical, political, and cultural systems.

Although the hospitals frequently had formal statements of mission and strategy (Cell 1), usually these had been approved but never truly accepted by senior management. Senior management's mission, as opposed to the formal statement, was to respond to changes driven by the new technologies requested by physicians and approved in a relatively ad hoc decision-making process. Implementation had depended on the resourcefulness of middle-management nurses in nourishing the individual and collective commitment of nursing staff to needs of patients and quality of care. The lack of comprehensive planning by senior management had precipitated a long series of "add-on" services, such as transplant services and trauma units, which dramatically increased operating costs and management complexity as well as workload and stress at all levels of the nursing hierarchy.

Technical structures (Cell 2) usually reflected the foregoing pattern. A traditional hierarchy mainly based on clinical service units had been expanded over the years as new services were added. Absolute numbers of middle and senior managers and support staff (including educators and clinical specialists) had increased significantly in response to increasing environmental turbulence, exponential growth in research findings relevant to nursing practice, ad hoc expansion of services, and myriad problems associated with growing pressures on the budget. Although these nursing departments were well integrated internally, with extensive formal and informal mechanisms for planning and co-ordination, their cross-departmental linkages had not kept pace with their growing interdependence with other departments, particularly medicine. This was due partly to preoccupation with cost-revenue problems on the part of nursing managers but, most importantly, it was due to a lack of initiative and support from senior management, who did not understand the growing importance of nursing/physician liaison.

The technical aspect of process (Cell 3) was relatively ambidextrous but was under steady pressure to become more mechanistic. Selection criteria for middle managers emphasized leadership ability, teamwork skills, and commitment to quality care. There had been a tradition of extensive consultation with staff nurses but, in response to the cost-revenue pressures, the process was becoming increasingly centralized. The rapid rate of change and growth in technology, for example, had required the development of policy and procedure manuals, orientation programs, and in-service education activities; the sheer volume of this workload meant that the process had become more centralized. In response to the growing competition for funds, a nursing information system had been implemented in an effort to develop objective workload and output data. It included patient classification, quality assurance, various aspects of cost analysis and, in an effort to reduce costs, a variable staffing component that required some nurses to "float" between wards and services depending on the workload of the unit. These measures also increased the centralization of staffing decisions, as well as the time spent on data collection activities at the unit level, which caused some morale problems among staff nurses and criticism from the union.

The political and cultural systems had been in reasonably good alignment with the technical system, but this was beginning to show signs of breakdown. Politically, there had been a tradition of wide involvement among department members in formulating strategy, and these dialogues resulted in effective coalition management and minimum conflict over the distribution and balancing of power within and between the nursing subsystems. The associated cohesive spirit within the nursing department, which had served in the past to enhance its shaky credibility, was rapidly deteriorating. As a result, there was unhappiness with the growing centralization, staff disenchantment with workload (caused by ad hoc expansion of services in the absence of adequate funding), and consequent growth in the militancy of the union. Succession politics, appraisal, and reward systems were still strongly based on teamwork skills and commitment to quality care, but it was necessary for managers to put more and more emphasis on the formal union contract as a framework for relationships with their staff. The most important emerging misalignment, however, was the growing gap between the high technical need and the low political feasibility of a coalition with medicine for the planning of cost and quality control mechanisms.

Surmounting the challenges imposed by contradictory requirements of the technical and political systems had traditionally depended heavily on the professional commitments that derived from the occupational socialization experiences of nurses and a cultural structure and process within the organization that supplemented and sustained these commitments. This too had begun to degenerate as differences in educational backgrounds, work assignments, and career expectations of nurses increased and the values of unionism became more influential. The relationships between nursing managers and staff nurses were steadily becoming more difficult at the very time when cohesion and commonality of purpose was of increasing importance.

STEP 4: MODIFYING THE STRATEGY

Although the problems facing nursing were the result of a normal evolution in the face of a turbulent and hostile environment, they reached a point where corrective action was required. In general theoretical terms, these departments had been using an open system, rational approach, to management but the style of management, which had been highly ambidextrous, had slowly moved under the pressure of rapid change toward the mechanistic side of the continuum. In terms of the strategic management process, senior nursing management had been forced into a reactive posture by limited influence over the acquisition and use of new medical technology. Nursing management needed to move from this reactive strategy, which had been necessary during the period of rapid growth, to a proactive strategy, formulated and implemented in close co-operation with the medical department and oriented to restraint and cutbacks. Nursing management also needed to return to a more organic style of management and to reinvigorate the commitment of staff nurses to the professional values of nursing.

Based on the case evidence presented here, the necessary changes were quite clear. At least three were needed in the technical system. The first was the need for the nursing departments to develop a strong strategic management program, with a major emphasis on mission definition and strategy formulation, and to do this in close co-operation with a comparable program in medicine at all levels of the two departmental structures. This was the most important priority because until this rationalization of the management process was underway, the remaining two priorities could not be accomplished.

The second priority was to streamline the structure of middle management and support personnel, which would allow some reductions in their number as a result of the rationalized strategy process. The third was to reduce the labour intensity of the information system, improve its reliability and validity, and better integrate it with operating-cost data, because this data would become especially important as the hospital moved toward more rational planning and increased budgetary restraint.

The highest priority changes in the political and cultural systems related to the top and middle managers in nursing. The remarkable complexity and turbulence of the environment, and of the organization itself, had vastly increased their importance as technical experts, political actors, and cultural leaders. Politically, the most important issue was the need to strengthen their prestige and influence in the eyes of both their staff and the physicians. In terms of the cultural system, it was becoming increasingly urgent to re-emphasize their leadership role in demonstrating the validity of professional nursing values, reconciling these values with the complementary aspects of the union priorities, and establishing constructive ways of reconciling the differences.

Implementing these changes would have required substantial initiative and support from senior management. In particular, changing the pattern of medical decision making and renewing the prestige and flexibility of middle managers, while simultaneously reducing their numbers, would require a great deal of creativity, courage, and skill on the part of the chief executive officer and the board.

WHAT WAS DONE

The cost-revenue problem reached crisis proportions for this typical hospital when senior management was impelled to implement massive reductions in costs. Given the magnitude and persistence of the growth in government deficits, and in the costs of medical technology, it had become quite clear that the two most important elements of a solution lay outside of the nursing department: rationalization of both physician utilization decisions and inter-institutional competition for services and programs. This would require a major redefinition of the mission and goals of the hospital but would result in major cost reductions and improved quality of care. Senior management were either unwilling or unable to confront directly either of these issues and chose to focus change on structure and process in other services and programs.

Nursing was poorly positioned for the ensuing interdepartmental competition for funds. The nursing department was accountable for the largest single component of the total hospital budget and it was an area of rapid and continuing growth in costs. Because neither its strategic plan nor its information system had credibility at the senior levels of management, the perception had been created that nursing had little objective policy or data with which to justify its priorities and little ability to rectify this problem. Nursing lacked sufficient inherent political power to overcome these deficits and its weakness was compounded by the cultural divisions within the department, particularly the growing split between nursing management and the union, as well as the lack of active support from medicine.

In the above context, in many hospitals, senior management frequently took direct control of nursing. Typically, the head of the nursing department was replaced by an incumbent willing to represent senior management to nursing, rather than nursing to senior management. Control of mission and strategy decisions for nursing then could be controlled at the most senior level by persons who were not nurses. In many Canadian hospitals at this time, the senior executive nursing position was simply eliminated. Staff members responsible for the information system were disbanded, and variable staffing was terminated. Many middle management and support staff positions were eliminated, including evening and night supervisors, specialized clinical teams (such as those to administer IVs), and most nursing researchers and educators. A policy of decentralizing responsibility to the staff nurse level was instituted. This compromised the authority and stature of remaining managers so severely that many began to question the relevance of their roles. Those who questioned or who failed to actively support the management changes were dismissed; many of those let go were among the most experienced and professionally committed managers, and the threat implicit in these terminations was clearly understood by those who remained. Large reductions were also made in the staff nurse complement and this, in conjunction with the decentralization of responsibility for a good deal of day-to-day decision making to the staff nurse level, substantially increased nursing workloads. In such situations, senior management often undertook to introduce a "new" corporate culture, and established a separate group of staff to initiate and maintain its acceptance.

Decisions relating to the technical system were now controlled by lay administrators who were unencumbered by objective data regarding quality or workload. Politically, the nursing department had been purged of its management leadership; the illusion that nursing power had been increased was created through decentralization but, in the absence of an effective nursing hierarchy, it meant that staff nurses and their immediate supervisors now had increased accountability but little authority and influence. It also meant that the union was now the main voice for nursing as a collectivity, and that the power for all major policy decisions regarding nursing was vested with senior management. By introducing a new corporate culture, senior management also had undertaken to define what was considered appropriate in terms of values and philosophy. The litany of popular management buzz words that were introduced, such as empowerment, shared governance, coaching, customer (for patient), and total quality management, created the illusion that the new management strategy was more organic and that a new and better "vision" of institutional values had been created. In reality, the policy decision process for the department was more centralized and arbitrary than ever before. In addition, by discounting the inherent dependency of patients in a complex technological milieu, important moral and legal issues involved in determining how the organization and the individual professional should share their joint responsibility for each patient had been trivialized.

CRITIQUE

The fourth step, modifying the strategy, had been guided primarily by the open, natural approach, rather than the open, rational approach. As a result, relatively few elements of a reasoned and responsible management strategy were evident. Nursing departments had been precluded from developing a proactive strategy guided by the requisites for maximizing quality of care. Close co-operation in strategic management between medicine and nursing had not been facilitated. The nursing information system had been abandoned. The move to a more organic style of management, through an exaggerated form of decentralization, had seriously compromised the remaining prestige and influence of middle managers. The new vision of cultural values was based more on superficial popular interpretations about management in Japanese automobile factories than on a science-based assessment of the complex professional realities of nursing in the Canadian cultural environment and in high tech/high touch health-care organizations. In addition, the formal responsibility for professional leadership had been removed from middle managers in nursing, which further reduced their prestige and influence.

Senior management had misdiagnosed what was appropriate for the hospital and for nursing—and most of all for patients—and had failed to anticipate negative consequences of their decisions.

A serious error was committed when senior managers failed to focus on rationalizing physician decision making and inter-institutional competition. Part of the reason was their failure to understand that the modern hospital had entered a new phase in its life cycle—one in which the environmental changes were so great that the basic mission and strategy of the organization had to be drastically changed if it were to cope adequately with its current and future cost-revenue problems. Part of the reason was a failure to acknowledge their moral responsibility to know, understand, and act on information that traditional patterns of institutional autonomy and of resource utilization by physicians resulted in grossly inefficient use of social resources and unnecessary levels of ineffective service.

Senior management also had failed to recognize that rapid advances in the technology of nursing, especially in educational levels and the profession's research base, had created a need for a stronger, not weaker, administrative presence on the part of the nursing department. They had failed to understand that a proactive nursing management strategy, not subordinated to but in co-operation with the medical department, was essential if the hospital were to be assured that the benefits of the burgeoning professional expertise of nursing would be delivered to patients. They had also dismissed the importance of an information system at a time of drastic restraint and cutbacks when objective data regarding nursing workload and output had reached a new level of importance.

In the political and cultural arenas, senior management had seriously underestimated the need to support strong professional and administrative leadership at the senior and middle levels of nursing management. As a result, they overreacted to the need for a more organic style of management and reduced the number and the power of nursing managers and support staff to the point where they were dangerously limited in their ability to fulfil their responsibilities for political and cultural leadership.

At a more general level, senior management failed to understand the concept of organizational dilemmas and the negative potentials associated with them. In many important ways, along with subscribing to the disadvantages of the open natural approach, they had also incurred the disadvantages inherent in a "one best way" approach to management. In their rush to enhance communication by massive decentralization and management dismissals they had seriously hampered co-ordination. In an effort to reduce traditionalism by introducing a "new" corporate culture, they had undermined important professional values and norms. In an effort to stimulate individual initiative by staff empowerment, they damaged the ability of the organization to properly fulfil its moral and legal responsibility for the acts of its employees and agents in delivering high-reliability services.

An additional important oversight was in the area of managerial ethics. Even though the clinical professions had been active in the definition and resolution of ethical issues involving patients, senior management had failed to grapple with the ethical issues surrounding development and implementation of management policy regarding budget restraint and cutback. Termination of life, the right to information, and the right to respect, for example, were now recognized as important issues that required careful assessment regarding patients, but the same standards were not applied to employees. Careers were terminated with impunity, planning information was withheld from key actors, and little respect was shown for the integrity, judgement, or experience of middle managers when the time came for planning and implementing how budget reductions would be effected. Senior management repeatedly ignored its ethical duty to know the relevant facts of the situation, to be objective in the analysis of these facts, and to be fair in responding to these facts.

It is unlikely that the management strategy described in this example will persist; it creates too many problems. Inadequate utilization of nursing technology will result in increased patient complaints, more lawsuits, and lowered staff morale. The reduced number of middle managers and the increased degree of decentralization will lower administrative efficiency to unacceptable levels. The organization will be under great pressure to modify its approach in the direction of a more mechanistic style, and to place more emphasis on professional values and norms.

Unfortunately, there are two major constraints on the degree and rate of change. First, until the mission of the institution is rationalized, there will be insufficient funds available for more than minor improvements. In nursing, as in other sectors of the health-care system, optimizing the range and quality of service will be dependent on much more progress in rationalizing physician decision making and inter-institutional competition. Second, change will be heavily dependent on the skill and vigour with which nurses pursue efforts to increase their power within the institution. Power is not a sufficient cause of sound management, but it is a necessary cause and, in the final analysis, inadequate intraorganizational power is the root cause of the problems facing this nursing department.

POSTSCRIPT

One positive change that began to emerge in the mid-1990s is the result of a decision by provincial governments. They have imposed institutional integration through various forms of regionalization, and these regional structures have begun the process of rationalizing physician decision making. It is too early to tell how successful this will be; for the most part, the implementation process has been rushed and the consequent problems of political unrest and sheer administrative logistics have impeded adequate planning for these changes. Unfortunately, thus far there seems to be little recognition of the need to reinvigorate the profile and involvement of nursing.

It seems that the adaptation of the health-care system to its contemporary environmental challenges has yet to be accomplished and will be a major component of the responsibilities assumed by caregivers and their leaders in the future.

CONCLUSION

In this chapter, a representative example of acute-care nursing management problems in Canadian hospitals in the 1990s has been analyzed in the context of organization design theory. Insofar as this interpretation is valid, it is clear that the public has not been well served by those assigned stewardship for these hospitals; in particular, the vitally important contribution of nursing to efficient and effective care has been diminished, not enhanced.

This is a serious problem because nurses are engaged in one of the most complex, difficult, and important professional roles in society. Nurses provide their services when patients are highly vulnerable. Their relationship with patients is intimate, intense, and often continuous for long periods. They must be skilled in dealing with the physical, social, emotional, and spiritual needs of patients and, often, of relatives and friends as well. They are responsible for a knowledge base that is growing rapidly in all of these areas. They routinely deal with profound ethical problems. They function in a technical, political, and cultural environment that is one of the most complex in society, and one that is often hostile to both their personal and their professional needs and potentials.

It is not possible for nursing to fulfil its immense potential for improving the efficiency and effectiveness of hospital services without support; nursing must and should enjoy superior leadership from senior management. Nurses must also accept and vigorously pursue new responsibilities.

Nursing has made substantial progress in enhancing the research foundation that underpins its professional status and in establishing a powerful union movement that protects the wages and conditions of work of its members. The benefits of this progress to both the patient and the individual nurse will continue to be threatened, however, if nurses do not recognize the importance of the nursing administrator role and undertake to support it vigorously.

In the final analysis, the value of the example used to illustrate strategic management theory is not in the interpretation of the outcome, but in the analytic framework that is presented, the issues that are raised, and the intellectual stimulus that is provided to those who have a responsibility to deal with similar situations. If this framework and example helps the reader to be a better manager, or contribute to better management, even by stimulating and guiding an analysis that refutes the propositions and conclusions that have been presented here, it will have served its purpose.

SUMMARY

- Open and closed systems represent two useful perspectives for understanding the development of organization design theory.
- Open versus closed perspectives reflect the degree to which it is thought that the external environment must be taken into account when making management decisions about an organization.
- Two distinct approaches within these perspectives (rational and natural) reflect the degree to which management is perceived to involve pre-planning of objectives and means, as opposed to a more dynamic process of ongoing adaptation to changing circumstances.
- Three categories of environmental variables identified by Tichy (1983) are assumed to play a critical role in the design of efficient and effective organizations; these are technical, political, and cultural factors. Corresponding subsystems in organizations must be developed and maintained in alignment with each other.
- A series of supplementary ideas need to be taken into account when applying theory (e.g., describing the organization's technology and recognizing inherent dilemmas in organizational design).
- Managers have three basic tools to assist them in keeping the three subsystems of an agency in alignment: mission and strategy; organization structure; and processes.

- A contingency perspective results in management styles that range on a continuum from mechanistic (i.e., rule-oriented), through ambidextrous, to organic (i.e., flexible).
- Strategic management theory provides a four-step process to assist managers in identifying the relevant variables to consider when designing organizations that can operate efficiently and effectively in an increasingly complex and ambiguous environment.
- Strategic management theory can be used to analyze and explain the dissolution of nursing organizations in large tertiary-care hospitals in the 1980s and 1990s in Canada.
- For nursing to fulfil its potential for improving the efficiency and effectiveness of hospital services, it must have superior leadership and support from senior management.

ACKNOWLEDGEMENT

Although the content of this chapter is solely my responsibility, I wish to thank several people who provided invaluable assistance: Bruce Finkel, Felicity Hey, Don Juzwishin, Dave Reynolds, Ginette Rodger, and Janet Storch. A special thanks to my three favourite nurses: Beth, Dorothy, and Jacqueline.

FURTHER READINGS AND RESOURCES

The following dozen readings represent a significant list for nurse managers in Canada. Some of them are old, but all are classics related to the understanding of the problems in the management of health-care agencies in Canada at the turn of the century.

Angus, D.E. (1991). *Review of significant health care commissions and task forces in Canada since 1983–84.* Ottawa: Canadian Hospital Association, Canadian Medical Association, Canadian Nurses Association. A thoughtful and accurate summary of recommendations from major studies done during this time period.

Blau, P.M., & Scott, W.R. (1962). *Formal organizations.* San Francisco: Chandler Publishing. This is "an oldie but a goldie." Blau and Scott synthesized a good deal of the contemporary research and contributed a number of valuable interpretations and insights, including the concept of organizational dilemmas.

Daft, R.L. (1992). *Organization theory and design* (4th ed.). St. Paul, MN: West Publishing House. There are many excellent introductory textbooks in organization design and this is one of them. It provides much more detail on theory and research than was possible in this chapter.

Growe, S.J. (1991). *Who cares: The crisis in Canadian nursing.* Toronto: McClelland & Stewart. A brilliant analysis of the problems and the promise facing Canadian nurses. This is essential reading for anyone with an obligation to understand the nursing profession.

Juzwishin, D.W.M. (1993). *Ethical issues in health services administration: Canadian health care management* (pp. 12.1–12.12). Toronto: MPL Communication. Juzwishin was one of the first to recognize and write about ethical issues in management. An excellent overview of the existing literature and the major issues.

Perrow, C. (1973, Summer). The short and glorious history of organizational theory. *Organizational Dynamics, 2* (1), 2–15. Written more than 25 years ago, this short article is still one of the best available critiques of modern organization theory. The annotated bibliography is also useful.

Rachlis, M., & Kushner, C. (1994). *Strong medicine: How to save Canada's health care system.* Toronto: HarperCollins. This is a second highly readable book from the authors of the 1989 successful *Second opinion: What's wrong with Canada's health care system and how to fix it.* Toronto: HarperCollins. The authors continue their critical appraisal of the system, conclude that fundamental structural reform is essential, and propose some radical changes.

Shortell, S.M., & Kaluzny, A.D. (1983). *Health care management: A text in organizational theory and behaviour.* New York: John Wiley & Sons. A collection of commissioned articles of core topics in both organization behaviour and design as applied to health organization. Unusually high quality but designed for expert readers.

Spirn, S., & Benfer, D.W. (1982). *Issues in health care management.* Rockville, MD: Aspen Systems Corporation. An invaluable collection of classical articles tailored for the use of health-services managers.

Storch, J.L. (1982). *Patients rights: Ethical and legal issues in health care and nursing.* Toronto: McGraw-Hill Ryerson. Storch was a pioneer in the area of ethical issues in health care and this is still one of the best overviews of the topic that is available. The bibliography is also excellent. (See also Chapter 18.)

Tichy, N.M. (1983). *Managing strategic change: Technical, political, and cultural dynamics.* New York: John Wiley & Sons. A detailed exposition about the origins and substance of TPC Theory. Only recommended for the advanced reader.

Tichy, N.M., & Devanna, M.A. (1986). *The transformational leader.* New York: John Wiley & Sons. The authors use the TPC framework to discuss the planning and implementation of organizational change. Examples and cases from American business management are used extensively to provide practical and realistic insights.

REFERENCES

Shortell, S.M., & Kaluzny, A.D. (1983). *Health care management: A text in organizational theory and behaviour.* New York: John Wiley & Sons.

Tichy, N.M. (1983). *Managing strategic change: Technical, political and cultural dynamics.* New York: John Wiley & Sons.

Chapter 6

▼▼▼▼▼▼▼▼▼▼▼▼

The Trend Toward Regional Governance

P. SUSAN WAGNER

KEY OBJECTIVES

In this chapter, you will learn:

- Differences between governance and management of an organization.
- Reasons governing boards exist in health-care organizations.
- Roles of site- or service-specific boards compared with roles of a regional health board.
- Advantages and disadvantages of regional governance.
- Ways provincial policies affect functioning of regional health boards.
- Relationships between regional health boards and first-level nurse managers in relation to the board's strategic directions, monitoring, and linkage with stakeholders.

INTRODUCTION

In this chapter, differences between the governance and management of health-care boards are described. Reasons for use of governing boards in health care, and for the trend toward regional boards in Canada will be explored. Different models of regional governance are presented, with current examples from Canadian provinces. The role of traditional site—or service-specific boards is contrasted with the role of regional health boards in relation to scope of governance, membership, and the relationship between the boards and the organizations. The influence of provincial policies on regional health boards is described.

Nurse managers are affected by regional health boards, and also have opportunities to influence boards. A goal for the reorganized system is the two-way exchange of information for the common goal of effective planning of health-care services for the future.

MOMENTUM TOWARD CHANGE

A revolution is taking place in Canadian health care and the impetus is coming from governments, health organizations, professionals, and consumers. With health reform as the goal, there is widespread restructuring and reorientation of health-care delivery systems. Pressure for increased effectiveness and efficiency of health-care services has stimulated exploration and implementation of new structures and options in care delivery. Most provinces have begun to implement regionalization of health-care governance in response to fiscal pressures. Each approach is different, for health is within provincial jurisdiction. There are constant developments across the country requiring regular and close attention of all those involved with health care.

GOVERNANCE AND MANAGEMENT

There is widespread confusion about the difference in meaning between "governing" and "managing," which is further complicated by the fact that dictionaries use the words "control" and "direct" in both definitions. The secondary meanings provide more assistance. To "govern" means to "exercise a directing or restraining influence over" (de Wolf, Gregg, Harris, & Scargill, 1997, p. 666). To "manage" means to "succeed in accomplishing" (de Wolf et al., 1997, p. 912). A board of directors governs an organization and decides what it should do and should not do. Management exists to accomplish those activities.

Many organizations in business, health care, non-profit volunteer work, and advocacy have boards of directors at the helm. Boards are common in both public and non-profit organizations. Generally, the public view is that organizations with boards tend to be less self-interested than if only one person is responsible. A board of directors distributes responsibility for decisions related to an organization across a variety of different individuals.

If there were no boards of directors, decisions would be made by single individuals, as is done in privately owned companies. A single individual may not possess all of the information or perspectives that are necessary to make informed decisions, and judgement may be influenced by subjectivity. If, for example, the actions of an individual decision maker are driven by the prospect of monetary gain, the impact on clients, staff, or the mission of the organization may not be adequately considered.

Groups of people tend to make better decisions than individuals, for the discussion is balanced and informed by various opinions. A group will also tend to take more risks than a single person, so innovation is more likely to be encouraged.

Almost without exception, boards of health-care organizations are established under provincial or national legislation, such as the *Non-profit Corporations Act* or the *Cooperatives Act*. These boards are required to have bylaws or constitutions that articulate rules for the governance of the organization. Such rules include the purpose of the organization, role of the board and its officers, qualifications required for membership on the board, terms of office, methods of attaining a board seat, and expectations of board members. In some organizations, representatives of the users of the services are board members. Sometimes people perceived to have a conflict of interest are prohibited from being board members (e.g., an employee of the organization or an owner of a company that does contract work for the organization). Other items addressed in the official board documents include conflict-of-interest guidelines, expectations for financial reporting to the supervisory body, and processes for dissolution or amalgamation.

Accountability is clearer if a group has an approved set of rules of conduct, and attempts to make its decision-making processes open to members and the public. Because most organizations are created under provincial or federal legislation, their boards of directors are legally responsible. The group of people acting as the board is accountable not only for all board decisions and actions, but also for decisions and actions of all of staff and volunteers within that organization. Board members as individuals and the board as a group can be held liable by parties who feel wronged. Most boards take out liability insurance to protect individual board members from financial loss. The member is protected if he or she acted with the best interests of the board in mind. Then, if a lawsuit is successful, the assets of the board or organization will be affected rather than those of the individual.

ROLE OF THE BOARD

The board of directors establishes what services will be offered, to whom, and at what cost. According to Carver (1990), a board of directors for any organization has several roles:

- to make decisions on the strategic direction of the organization;
- to monitor activities of both management and the board itself;
- to establish and maintain linkages with stakeholders; and
- to develop and review policies to guide itself and the organization.

The board's primary responsibility is to articulate a purpose and vision for the future of the organization. It sets the strategic direction for the organization, establishing goals and budget allocations. To fulfill these goals, most organizations hire a Chief Executive Officer (CEO) as manager of the organization.

The second important function of a board is to monitor the performance of the CEO, to ensure that the organization is fulfilling its vision and goals, and that the policies of the board are followed. The board also must monitor its own ability to function and follow board policies. The third function of a board is to establish linkages with other organizations offering similar or complementary services, and linkages with the owners. The owners could be public taxpayers who may be users of the service in the future. The final function of a board is to develop policies, and to review and revise them as necessary. Relationships between boards and nurse managers are based on these functions, and will be discussed later in the chapter.

ROLE OF MANAGEMENT

The primary responsibility of management personnel is to implement the goals and vision of the board. In doing so, the CEO is expected to keep within board policy, and to accomplish the work within the framework of relevant provincial and federal legislation and regulations. It is important that the board and the CEO have a similar understanding of their respective roles and responsibilities. For example, they should agree that it is a board's responsibility to establish goals, but it is the CEO's responsibility to decide how to attain them. Board members should not be involved in operational activities or decisions that relate to implementation of board decisions, such as hiring particular people, choosing colours of carpet, or creating personnel policies. In the same way, CEOs should not control the agenda for board meetings, determine the direction of the organization, or maintain relationships with boards of other organizations.

Because the boundaries of these roles merge and often are difficult to identify, CEOs and boards must continually explore role expectations with one another. Effective governance relies upon similar understandings of roles. The board informs the organization of its strategic directions, managers within the organization report activities so the board can monitor success, and there is two-way communication about linkages with other community providers. Organizations that have problems are often those with poor communication between the board and the CEO.

TRADITIONAL HEALTH-CARE BOARDS

Traditionally, most governing boards in health care have been responsible for a single organization that delivers only one type of service, or a variety of services from only one site (see also Chapter 4). Boards of such organizations have little difficulty in defining the services they deliver, to whom, and how, because the role of the organization or facility determines the board's purpose.

SCOPE OF GOVERNANCE

Most hospitals in Canada are owned by provincial governments or by private non-profit groups. Both public and private non-profit types of ownership use boards to govern the affairs of the hospital. Indeed, most provincial health legislation requires that there be boards of directors, and specifies certain responsibilities for ensuring quality care and stewardship of the human and financial resources within the organization. No private for-profit hospitals existed in Canada until 1997, when the first one was established in Calgary.

Long-term-care facilities in Canada are a mix of publicly owned, private non-profit, and private for-profit organizations. Provincial or municipal governments are usually the owners of the public facilities. In recent years, the federal government has divested itself of direct ownership of most of its health-care facilities; hospitals and long-term-care homes built for veterans have been transferred to provincial or local control. Religious groups or community-based groups frequently own private, non-profit facilities, as in the case of long-term-care facilities owned by such groups as the Lutherans, Seventh Day Adventists, Jews, and various orders of the Catholic faith.

Both publicly owned and private non-profit facilities are managed by boards of directors, who are accountable for the nature and scope of services and for the stewardship of the resources within the organization. For-profit facilities, particularly if they are small operations, will likely be governed and managed by a single owner. In the for-profit facilities, one person or a family may own a group of similar organizations (usually small) and govern them directly without a board, although they may hire managers. For-profit long-term-care facilities are more likely to have a board of directors if they are owned by a large corporation that is involved with several branches or facets of the business. Extendicare, for example, is a large corporation that owns both long-term-care facilities and community-service agencies across Canada, and it is governed by a board of directors that acts on behalf of the owners.

The major advantages of governing boards for site- or service-specific organizations include: an expertise with a particular site or service, or with the client population served; a clear identity that is a source of pride for both staff and clients; and an ability to attract both volunteers and donor dollars. A variety of providers in a community or region add depth and breadth to the network of social and health supports available, and can strengthen the civic pride of local citizens in their community. Smaller organizations may also be able to respond more quickly to client or community needs, provide more personalized care, and be more creative.

A main disadvantage of having governing boards for site-specific or service-specific agencies is that a multiplicity of boards will cost taxpayers or clients more because there are multiple administrations. As well, there are often duplications in client programs (e.g., several maternity services within one local area) or in support services (e.g., several laundry or purchasing departments). Furthermore, governing boards of extremely small site- or service-specific organizations often face challenges in attracting and maintaining competent managers and staff, because these individuals may have fewer opportunities for career advancement. Another disadvantage is the human tendency to guard territory and expand both influence and control (e.g., empire-building). This tendency means that commitment of both board members and staff may be directed to enhancing the status, the number of clients served, or the budget of the organization. It follows that the vision of that organization is often restricted to the site, the service, or the specific client group involved, and that broader goals of the collective good for the community or the region may not be considered. The resulting competition is accentuated if each governing board has access to the Minister of Health for funding. This tendency to be self-serving as organizations discourages co-operation, increases fragmentation of care for clients, and does not address gaps within the larger health service system.

Because of these disadvantages, most provinces are moving away from the traditional site- or service-specific model for health-care agencies. At the time of this writing, the traditional site- or service-specific model still exists in only one province, Ontario.

BOARD MEMBERSHIP

Membership on many health-care boards is open to anyone who expresses an interest. Boards often look for balanced representation, ensuring that membership includes both men and women, people from a variety of ages, professions, and work-experience backgrounds. Board members with an admirable community reputation may be desirable if fundraising is a major activity of the board. Boards that anticipate vacancies among their membership will often canvas friends and acquaintances for those who may be interested in contributing to the good work of the organization by volunteering to be a board member. When a list of interested people is obtained, the selection will be made according to the bylaws or constitution, by board vote, or by a vote of the general membership of a non-profit corporation. Sometimes the board of a provincial health-care organization is appointed by the Minister of Health, through an order-in-council of the provincial cabinet. There are so many boards involved in the governance of health, social service, and sports organizations in Canadian communities that many boards consider themselves lucky to have the required number of members, regardless of particular ability and experience.

The vast majority of these traditional boards are established as volunteer boards, without any financial compensation for the work or time given to the organization. Some of the organizations are so small and short of funds that board members actually perform the work of the organization for no pay. As an organization grows, it begins to assign responsibilities to employed staff, although the board role usually continues to be volunteer. Health-care boards that have honoraria available for board members tend to be larger organizations with a high profile in the community, such as university teaching hospitals.

RELATIONSHIP BETWEEN BOARDS AND MANAGEMENT

Many traditional health-care boards govern small organizations, some with annual budgets of less than $100,000 and only one or two staff members.

In these organizations, it is almost impossible for the board not to become involved in operational details. In fact, board members may be required to do the work. The board may hire a CEO as the only employee, and then the board members will follow the CEO's instructions and do the work of the organization themselves. Roles between board and management personnel blur, become confused, and create many emotional and organizational problems. As the organization becomes larger, there are more staff members and more activities, and it becomes more difficult for board members to know all of the details of daily operations. It is then easier for the board to focus on vision and goals, and easier to give the CEO the independence required to get the daily work done without interference. Differences in size do not, however, determine the quality of the relationship between boards and management. Small organizations are just as likely to have good—or poor—governance as larger ones.

REGIONAL HEALTH-CARE BOARDS

In recent years, provincial commissions examining health-care costs have recommended establishment of health regions, governed by lay health boards. These boards are responsible for delivery of all community-health services offered in the region, including acute care, long-term care, ambulance services, home care, mental health's and substance-abuse programs. (See Figure 4.3 in Chapter 4.) These new boards are intended to increase efficiency and reduce health-care costs by avoiding duplication in care, and by reducing bed usage in both acute care and long-term care (Wagner, 1996, p. 251). Another mandate of these new regional boards is promotion of local community services and increased illness-prevention initiatives, both of which improve the health of the population—hereby increasing the effectiveness of all local health programs. The purpose of a regional board approach is to achieve more integration, and to be more responsive to community and district needs as well to client needs (Wagner, 1996, p. 251).

SCOPE OF GOVERNANCE

There are six basic configurations for regional health boards across Canada, using "scope of governance responsibilities" as the key variable. Although different names are used across the provinces, the governance structures can still be compared. It is assumed for each model of regionalization that the provincial government has the major responsibility for funding health-care services. It is also assumed that the funding of physician services and drug plans remains a provincial responsibility in all models, and that there are some services, such as cancer services, delivered outside the regional system. The major difference among the models of regional health-care governance is the number of organizations that receive funding and power directly from the provincial government.

Figure 6.1

MODEL 1: SECTOR-REGIONAL
HEALTH BOARDS

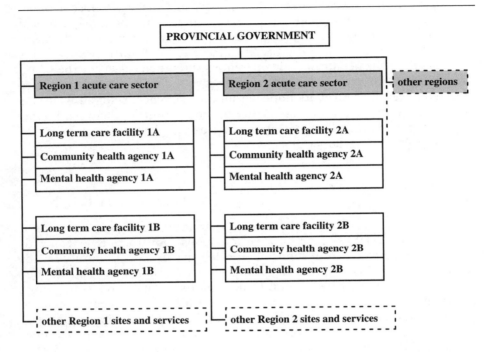

Model 1: Sector-specific Regional Health Boards

The type of regional health board closest to the traditional site- or service-specific structure is the sector-based regional board. Within health care, sectors are clearly defined settings for service delivery. Major health sectors are acute-care institutions, long-term-care institutions, community-based services, and mental-health services. A regional health board that is sector-specific governs more than one site, but includes all services provided in that sector of health care (see Figure 6.1). A variation would involve a regional board with responsibility for more than one sector in several sites.

For example, New Brunswick began a sector-based regional hospital corporation in 1992; all home-care services were delivered through the Extra-mural Hospital, which had a separate governance structure with province-wide jurisdiction. In 1996 this provincial home-care program was divided into parts and became the responsibility of the regional hospital corporations. Long-term-care facilities, mental-health agencies, and other services in other sectors are still governed separately.

Figure 6.2

MODEL 2: PARALLEL REGIONAL SECTOR BOARDS

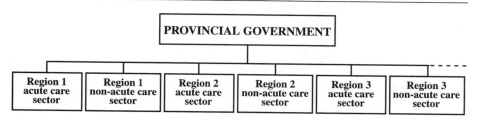

Model 2: Parallel Regional Sector Boards

The next type of regional health board on the continuum is a parallel structure of regional boards by sector or type of service within the province (see Figure 6.2).

Newfoundland has established this system for the province, in an attempt to give each health-care sector independence in working out the difficulties of amalgamation under geographically based regional boards. At the time of this writing, there is one provincial board for community care, one for institutional care across the province (both acute- and long-term-care facilities), and two boards for the St. John's area—one for acute-care hospitals, and one for long-term-care facilities. Labrador and the north are excluded from this structure. The sector-specific regional boards negotiate linkages and common goals for the common client populations who require co-ordination of services from both sectors.

Model 3: Combined Model

The third type of regional health-care governance is the combined model, where there is a mixture of types of authorities (see Figure 6.3). There may be site- or service-specific boards as well as regional health boards that receive funds from the provincial government, as in Nova Scotia. There may be two types of regional authorities, as in Manitoba and British Columbia.

Nova Scotia has a combination of traditional site- or service-specific boards and regional boards. The traditional model of health-care governance is used by four "non-designated organizations," which have been created as mergers of the largest acute-care centres in the province. These four have individual boards funded directly by the provincial government. Boards of these "non-designated organizations" communicate extensively with the regional boards, and staff work closely with regional staff to plan and deliver client care.

There are four geographic regional boards, with a planned wide jurisdiction over the full range of health services, including acute, long-term,

Figure 6.3 (a)

MODEL 3: COMBINED MODEL

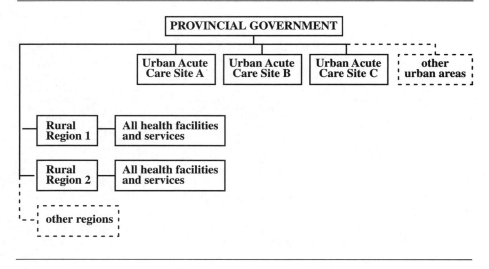

Figure 6.3 (b)

MODEL 3: COMBINED MODEL

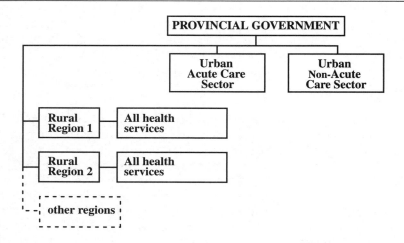

and community care. At the time of this writing, mental-health and home-care services had not yet been transferred from provincial jurisdiction. Community health boards have been added to the structure in Nova Scotia. These are smaller local boards, responsible for conducting needs assessments, doing public consultation and education, and providing advice to the regional health boards on health-service planning and evaluation.

Manitoba has a different sort of combined model for governance of health-care services, using single health authorities and parallel sector boards. After talking about it for two or three years, the government established rural health authority boards in 1996 with control over several health sectors. In Winnipeg, which has two thirds of the province's population, there will be a parallel sector model of health-care governance. Until both the Winnipeg Hospital Authority board and the Winnipeg regional authority for community services and long-term-care institutions are established, site- and service-specific health-care boards will continue.

A nesting model (see Model 4 below) was initially planned in British Columbia, with 82 "community health council" governing boards that were to receive funds for community and long-term-care services from twenty regional boards. In November 1996, after an extensive review, the structure was changed to reduce duplicate administrations and recognize differences between urban and rural areas. As a result, B.C. now resembles the combined model. Health services in urban centres will be governed by eleven regional health boards, and those in discrete geographical areas, mostly rural, will be governed by 34 community health councils. The regional health boards will have responsibility for tertiary acute-care services, long-term-care institutions, and public-health, mental-health, and continuing-care services formerly delivered by the province. The community health councils will have responsibility for acute-care and long-term care institutional services in their local areas. Public-health, mental-health, and continuing-care services outside the major urban centres will be governed by regional community health society boards, serving several community health council jurisdictions. All three types of boards are autonomous, so the system will be a combination of parallel-sector boards with different sizes of jurisdiction and single health authorities. Some regional boards have created community health committees to provide advice on local needs.

Model 4: Nesting Model

In a nesting model, one regional board with governance responsibility for a wide range of health-care services allocates money to another board that governs one sector of health services in that region (see Figure 6.4).

After community health and social service centres (Centres local de santé communautaire, or CLSCs), were established in the mid-1970s, Quebec had a system similar to the parallel regional board system (Model 2). The geographic areas for the CLSCs were smaller than the regions for the hospitals, but the two tried to work together for the benefit of the client. The scope of governance of the CLSCs went beyond health to include social services. In 1991, legislation passed in Quebec created new regional boards with control over both the hospital regional boards and the CLSC boards (Pineault, Lamarche, Champagne, Contandriopoulos, & Denis, 1993). Thus, Quebec has a nesting model, because two levels of governance

Figure 6.4

MODEL 4: NESTING MODEL

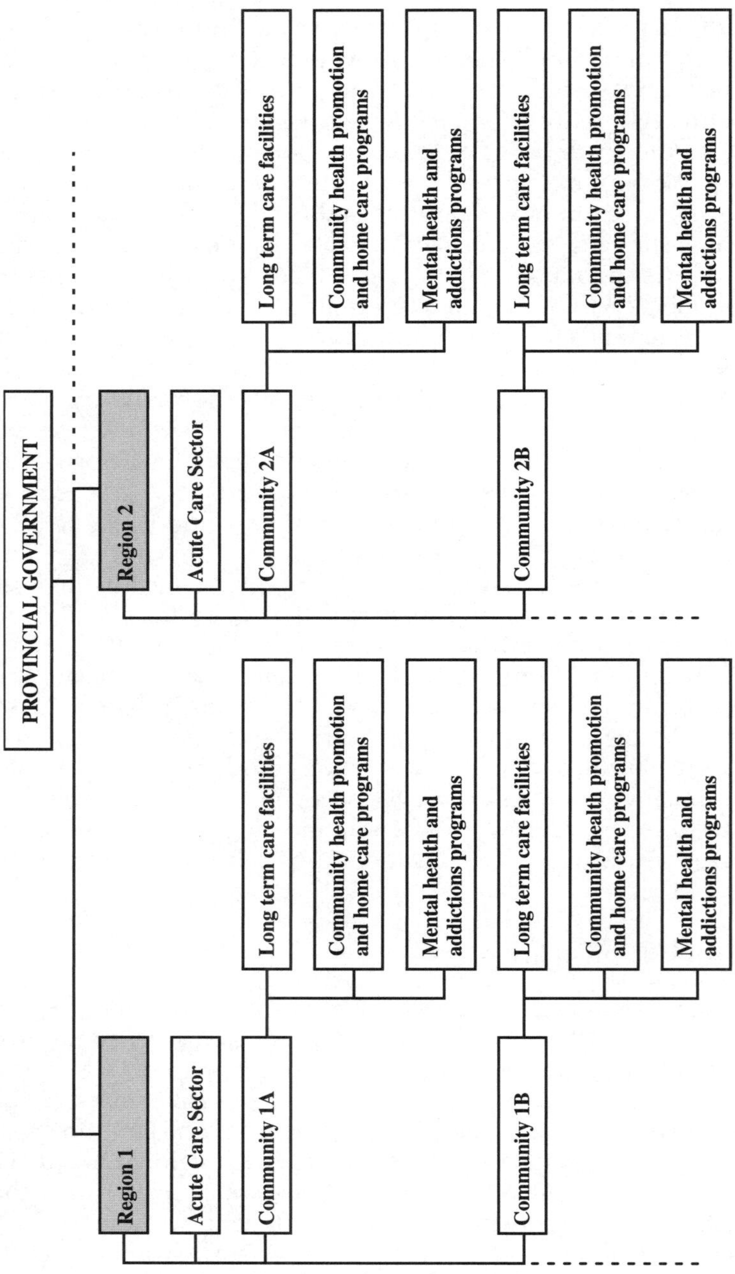

PROVINCIAL GOVERNMENT

Region 1

Acute Care Sector

Community 1A

- Long term care facilities
- Community health promotion and home care programs
- Mental health and addictions programs

Community 1B

- Long term care facilities
- Community health promotion and home care programs
- Mental health and addictions programs

Region 2

Acute Care Sector

Community 2A

- Long term care facilities
- Community health promotion and home care programs
- Mental health and addictions programs

Community 2B

- Long term care facilities
- Community health promotion and home care programs
- Mental health and addictions programs

Figure 6.5
MODEL 5: SINGLE HEALTH AUTHORITY

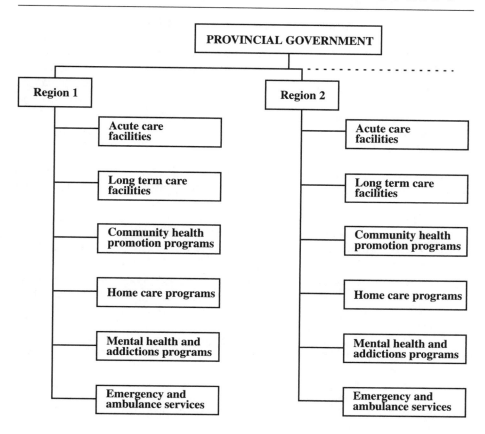

exist. The large regional board receives money from the government, and gives some to the regional hospital board, which has authority over acute-care services on more than one site.

Model 5: Single Regional Health Authority

The fifth type of regional governance is the single regional health authority. This model exists when one regional health board has governance responsibility for a wide range of health-care services, including acute-care and long-term-care facilities, community-based home care, and health promotion services, as well as, in some instances, ambulance, mental-health, and addictions services (see Figure 6.5).

The provinces of Alberta and Saskatchewan have single regional health authorities. Alberta created all seventeen of its regional health authorities at once, in June of 1993. Each authority has jurisdiction over almost all health services delivered in that geographic region, the exceptions at the time of this writing being mental-health and ambulance services. Each health authority is required to have at least one community health council to provide advice on local needs.

The 32 health district boards in Saskatchewan were created in stages, between 1992 and 1997. The transfer of authority from the government also occurred in stages. Although the provincial health budget was not reduced over that time, there were reductions to the acute-care envelope and transfer of monies to community-based services. The new boards had to create health plans in 1993–94 to incorporate these shifts in allocation and support the provincial vision for health system renewal.

Model 6: Single Regional Authority for Human Services

Human services are those that deliver care to individuals in a variety of sectors, including health, social services, housing, and justice. Educational services are not included in this model, although they also serve people directly. (See Figure 6.6).

Prince Edward Island is the only provincial example of this model. Prior to 1997, there was a provincial human services board and five regional boards with governance responsibility for housing, social services, and probation services, in addition to health services from acute-care, long-term, and community sectors. In 1997, the provincial board was dismantled, and the responsibilities of the regional boards were reduced slightly. This province still fits the single human services authority model, for the responsibilities for health, social services, and housing in their jurisdiction have been retained by the regional boards.

MEMBERSHIP

Members of regional health boards can be either appointed by the provincial minister of health or elected by people within a geographic boundary. Most regional health boards across the country have appointed members. Many boards were preceded by appointed planning committees or interim boards that established a foundation for the first governing boards. Appointments are usually made after consultation with local people or after a call for nominations, and confirmed by order-in-council of the provincial cabinet. In October 1995, Saskatchewan became the first and only province with elected members of regional health boards. Eight members of the health district boards are elected by residents of the district, and the remaining four or six members are appointed by the health minister. A few provinces have stated an intention to have elected boards in the future. Other provinces have simply continued to appoint members or have been silent on the issue.

Advantages of appointed boards include greater loyalty to the government's health restructuring goals and greater likelihood that there will be a balanced representation of genders, ethnic minority groups, and ages. The disadvantages include the potential perception that appointments are the

Figure 6.6

MODEL 6: SINGLE HUMAN SERVICES AUTHORITY

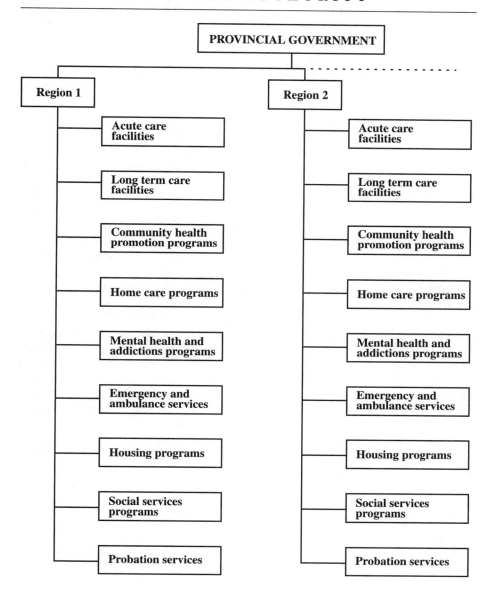

result of government patronage, the possibility that regional and local priorities will be less important than provincial goals, and public concerns regarding board accountability.

Advantages of elected health board members include increased accountability to the citizens of the district, greater likelihood that the board's decisions will reflect the values and interests of the residents, more community involvement in the selection process, and more opportunity for anyone interested in the position to run for the office (Orlikoff & Totten, 1996). Disadvantages include the potential for special-interest groups to field and financially support single-issue candidates. Because elected people would represent geographic areas or specific communities, chances increase that a board might be dominated by people interested in only one issue (Lomas, 1997). In addition, a balanced representation of genders, ethnic minorities, and ages cannot be guaranteed with a wholly elected board, political issues may be more important than the mission of the organization in improving health, and the behaviour of elected members has no restrictions, for the power to remove them rests with the electorate.

The qualifications of people considered eligible to be regional board members is another issue. In Saskatchewan, the only people ineligible for board membership are the chief executive officer and any person reporting to that position, and members of a provincial legislature or of Parliament. Health-care providers and employees of health regions are also permitted to be on boards in British Columbia. In Manitoba and Alberta, the latter two categories are specifically prohibited from board membership. There is a fear that, if health providers or employees are members of the board, they will have undue influence on decisions. As an alternative means of involving these people, volunteer technical advisory committees of health professionals have been established to advise the regional boards in Alberta and Manitoba.

A study was conducted of the sitting members of regional health boards in five provinces during 1995 (Lomas, Veenstra, & Woods, 1997). The response rate was 65 percent, with 514 people completing the survey form. The responding board members, who were all appointed members, "spent 35 hours per month, on average, on work for their board. Members were largely middle-aged, well educated, and well off. Only 36 percent were employed full time. Nine out of ten had previous experience on boards, more often in health care than in social services" (Lomas et al., 1997, p. 513). Although the members considered themselves to be representative of their regions and citizens, their personal characteristics did not match the population of most communities.

RELATIONSHIP BETWEEN BOARDS AND MANAGEMENT

When a new board is established, the relationship with senior administration takes time to develop. Members also need time to orient themselves to their roles and responsibilities, and to the purpose of the board. A regional board must focus on major policy issues because it is impossible to be familiar with all of the detail related to service delivery. Management of organizational activities should be left to the CEO, and the board's role should be to monitor the CEO's effectiveness. The CEO is responsible for ensuring that the board's goals are met and its decisions are carried out.

The most difficult task for a regional health board is deciding priorities among goals, sites or services, and special population groups, and then ensuring that the budget allocations follow those priority decisions. The study of regional health boards carried out by Lomas and colleagues reported:

> The information for decision-making most available to them was information on service costs (68% ...), and utilization (64%); the least available information was that on key informants' opinions (47%), service benefits (37%) and citizens' preferences (28%). Board activity was dominated by setting priorities and assessing needs, secondarily occupied with ensuring the effectiveness and efficiency of services and allocating funds, and least concerned with delivering services and raising revenue. (Lomas et al., 1997, p. 513)

INFLUENCE OF PROVINCIAL POLICIES

Provincial governments have jurisdictional responsibility for health services in Canada. They create the context in which health boards operate through policies and legislation. Boards must stay within those expectations, for the provincial governments are the major funders of health services in Canada. In turn, the provinces must ensure that federal legislation and policies are followed if they wish to retain the federal cash transfers and federal tax points received for health services. Each province has moved at a different pace in legislating health-service restructuring, and each has tackled the aspects in different order.

The basic elements of provincial policy that influence regional health boards are described briefly in this section, with one or two provincial examples.

VISION

A vision is the perception of a future not currently visible. In recent years, visions for the future of health services have been developed in most provinces. Provincial commissions or task forces have studied their respective health services and articulated plans for the future. Provincial governments then either adopted that vision, modified it, or created health councils to define health and establish provincial health goals. In most provinces, these health councils were disbanded as soon as their work was completed, despite recommendations that they continue as watchdogs during restructuring of the health-care system.

The provinces vary in how closely these visions and the restructuring reality are linked. In Alberta, for example, although the Conservative government of Ralph Klein followed the Commission's recommendations for regional health boards, massive budget cuts were imposed without any vision or future care-related goals. By contrast, the New Democratic government of Roy Romanow in Saskatchewan published a series of documents for the new regional health boards that clearly stated why the restructuring was necessary, what the future system would be like, and in which ways it would be better than the old health-care system (Saskatchewan Health, 1992).

If the provincial government does not articulate a vision for the future, regional health boards vary enormously in their goals and priorities, and provide inconsistent levels and types of health-care services. When a vision exists, the regional health boards have clearer guidelines for both long- and short-term decisions. Consistency of service delivery across the province is much more likely where there is an overall provincial vision, for goals and philosophies of those boards will be more similar.

INFORMATION SYSTEMS

Provincial policies and priorities related to information systems are extremely important for health services, because almost all of the infrastructure costs for new systems are borne by the province. The commitment of provincial governments to evaluation of health-system changes is shown by decisions made to invest or not to invest in a provincial health information system. The ability of regional health boards to fulfill their legislated mandate of assessing health needs and monitoring the effectiveness of programs will be determined by the provincial priority given to health information system design and funding.

Technology has begun to change the way information is gathered and used in all fields. In health care, the most radical transformation also includes how care is provided. The transmission of X rays and other diagnostic data over telephone lines has begun, and will increasingly make expert services more accessible for clients and family physicians in rural areas. Most provinces are currently assessing their health information needs, the linkages required, and the type of infrastructure required to support an integrated provincial health-care information and delivery system.

Baseline data on the health of provincial populations does not exist in most provinces, so the impact of changes to the health-care system on health status of people cannot be determined. Health departments and ministries must decide which information is important if an integrated health-care information system is to be centralized to improve access to client health information. Every organization collected its own health information in the past. Clearly, policies on confidentiality of records must be developed. Provincial databases on drug use, service utilization, and physician services have all developed separately, but they need to be linked for evaluation of system efficiency. Some health-promotion activities take more than a decade to show results, so health-system effectiveness may be proven only if data from education and social services and justice are linked to the health data.

Some provinces have established research centres that evaluate health policy and study health-care utilization patterns. Examples include the Health Services Utilization and Research Commission in Saskatchewan, the Centre for Health Economics and Policy Analysis in Ontario, and the Manitoba Centre for Health Policy and Evaluation. These units play an increasingly important role in obtaining the information to support decision-making by both regional and provincial bodies.

FUNDING

Methods of funding health-care organizations determine how services are provided. Most provincial governments used to base funding of both acute-care and long-term-care facilities on numbers of occupied beds. That funding policy encouraged indiscriminate use of those beds. Clients were admitted to acute care on Friday, given a weekend pass, and told to go home until Monday. The bed was "occupied" and the hospital made money, for no meal or housekeeping or care costs were incurred on the weekend.

Provincial health departments used to approve budgets for health organizations in detail, line by line. More recently, hospitals have been funded on global budgets, although the previous year's utilization statistics are still used as a basis for the allocation. This system allows hospitals some freedom to move money between departments and support innovation. Unfortunately, many of these funding policies still compensated hospitals only for the provision of acute care, severely limiting ventures in outpatient, day-program, or community-outreach services.

Many people were admitted permanently to long-term-care facilities without even trying community support services in their homes first. These facilities may have been funded according to the classification of the "bed" as light or heavy care, regardless of the needs of the person who filled the bed. People requiring very light care were therefore often admitted to keep staff workloads at a reasonable level. If the province funded facilities on a line-by-line basis, flexibility across departments was discouraged. If budgets were global, more freedom occurred in programming during the year. (See also Chapter 22.) Funding policies tied to the total number of beds still severely limited the ability of a long-term facility to offer day programs or community outreach services for seniors and the disabled.

Most provinces now fund both hospitals and long-term-care facilities according to the Resource Intensity Weighting of client needs in addition to utilization data. The specificity and accuracy of this measure is not good, but it provides some recognition of the costs of high-need clients for staff resources.

In Saskatchewan, the province began using a "needs-based" funding formula for the health districts in April 1995. (See also Chapter 4.) This formula bases funding on the population of a district, but is adjusted according to several variables specific to health-care sectors (Saskatchewan

Health, 1994). In acute care, for example, a higher number of elderly people and women of childbearing age in the community will mean an increase in the funding allocation, because these groups require more care. In the long-term-care institutional envelope, more money is given when there are greater numbers of single women over the age of 65 years, or of young disabled people; these groups have higher rates of admissions. In the home care sector, the formula is richer for those districts with sparse populations over greater distances, to compensate for the increased costs of providing service. At the time of this writing, health-promotion services were soon to become part of the formula. Even though the model is more population-based than needs-based, this funding policy has given district health boards freedom to allocate resources to areas of greatest need within each sector. There has also been a "one-way-valve" policy in place since 1992; this permits movement of money from institutional sectors to community programs, but forbids transfers from the community side to prop up the retention of institutional beds in acute or long-term care. Successive provincial budgets and policies have supported the provincial goals of reducing institutional services and enhancing community services.

PHYSICIANS

The influence of physicians is powerful, for they are essential to the delivery of effective health services, but they exist outside the system, often in independent businesses. Because physicians are the primary gatekeepers to the health-care system, they generate many of the costs. They control admission to hospital, use of drugs, and use of surgical, laboratory, and some therapy services. Most provinces have a human resource plan in place in an attempt to control the supply of physicians, particularly specialists, who generate high costs to the health-care system.

All provinces have retained the responsibility for physician payment, even where regional boards have been established for as long as five years. The most common method is fee payment for particular services. Physician earnings under the government health insurance plans take about 16 to 18 percent of the provincial health budget. Provincial medical associations bargain with provincial governments for changes to fee schedules.

Provinces vary in their use of alternative methods for paying physicians. In some, nearly all doctors are paid on a fee-for-service basis. In Saskatchewan, nearly 20 percent of doctors receive some alternative method of payment in addition to fee-for-service, including a combination of individual- or group-practice contract payments, salary, and per-capita reimbursement. (See Chapter 4 for further discussion of this subject.)

Regional boards are often preoccupied with physician-related issues, because so many of the health services offered in the region are dependent on the availability and co-operation of physicians. Co-ordination of efforts and development of policies on recruitment, retention, and compensation must occur at the provincial level to be fair to all parts of the province. Physician-payment policies may be created in an attempt to keep doctors content or to retain medical services in remote areas. Quebec has influenced physician distribution by paying less than the negotiated fee schedule to urban doctors, and more than the fee schedule to rural doctors, when both are doing the same procedure. Saskatchewan has provided a one-time $25,000 incentive to doctors who establish practices in rural communities.

Other regional board policies have an enormous influence on physician practice, however, because health facilities and operating rooms are required as a base for many doctors to provide care. Surgeons, cancer specialists, and pathologists, for example, all practice primarily in larger regional facilities. Many decisions are made by regional boards, including acute-care bed closures, summer bed reductions or "slowdowns," the renovation of facilities, new equipment purchases, even the quantity of artificial hips or cataract lenses available per year. If physicians are not included in these decisions, the antagonism about changes to their practice patterns may be communicated to both patients and the media. Provincial and regional health board policies regarding physician payment and practices have a tremendous influence on the delivery of health services, and physicians are absolutely essential to health-care delivery. For health-care restructuring to work effectively, good relationships must be nurtured.

UNIONS

Health-care worker unions are another major factor that must be considered in the restructuring of health services. These unions are powerful, particularly if they are organized provincially or federally. Their mandate is to protect jobs and benefits for their members, so any change to the health-care system is mistrusted. Provincial policies for change affect union negotiations, union jurisdiction, and union involvement. Because approximately 80 percent of health-system operating costs are salaries, a provincial decision not to fund a provincially negotiated contract increase has an enormous effect on regional health boards. The money for contract increases must then be found in existing budgets, and expenses reduced in other departments.

Regional board decisions frequently have implications for employees or unions. Any decisions to consolidate services on fewer sites mean staff positions move to another site and people may have new job descriptions. Any decision to reduce acute-care or long-term-care beds means that jobs disappear, in both care provision and in support services such as housekeeping and laundry. A regional health board decision to offer a new service or program creates new staff positions, but the board has to decide whether to offer the new program directly through its own employees or to contract it out.

Because each site or health-service agency used to have its own board of directors, there were hundreds of employers in the health-care system. Since the advent of regional health boards and amalgamations, the number of employers has been reduced. Unfortunately, union locals have traditionally been site- or program-based, and often the same category of worker has been represented by two or more different unions within the same region.

To complicate matters, sometimes locals of the same union were so separate that a member from one site would not have access to jobs at a different site, or if access was possible, seniority would not be recognized at the new site. If two different unions or if a union and a non-union site were involved, the seniority of a staff member transferred to a different site to do the same work would never be recognized. These jurisdictional problems have created difficulties for regional boards who want to move programs, consolidate services, and have staff with the same skills relieve one another on different sites. Some boards and union locals have been able to negotiate letters of understanding, which enable some of these system changes to benefit both management and workers. Long-term flexibility for both management and worker, however, rests entirely with provincial government policy.

In Saskatchewan, the Dorsey Commission developed solutions to the jurisdictional issues in health care, and the major unions supported the process, even though it was likely that some would lose membership. The recommendations, passed by the provincial cabinet in January 1997, establish that there will be only three categories of workers; nurses, other licensed health workers, and health workers who do not need professional licenses to work (e.g., maintenance workers and office clerks). The first two categories will bargain provincial-wide as two unions. The non-professional category will negotiate as district locals with each district health board; the union affiliation will be the same within a district, but may be different across districts. Existing contracts will be honoured. As these current contracts end, management and union negotiations will work to establish equity in wages and benefits for members of the remaining unions. The process will take at least three years to implement. Then, for each health district, there will be only three union categories of workers, and all workers doing the same job in the same district will be in the same union.

Union jurisdiction will continue to be a problem in all provinces where a provincial solution to the multiplicity of health-care unions and union locals is not adopted.

HEALTH BOARDS AND FIRST-LEVEL MANAGERS

The role of first-level managers is to focus on the delivery of services from a particular unit, program, or health centre. They have responsibilities for direction and supervision of staff; quality of services delivered to patients and clients; hiring and firing of staff; budgeting; and professional-development activities. The relationship to the health board is usually indirect. Only in a small health agency would a first-level manager's report go directly to a board; in larger institutions, it would be channeled through one or more administrators. Only when issues are common across several parts of an agency would they be of importance to the board.

Figure 6.7

COMMUNICATION FLOW BETWEEN
BOARDS AND NURSE MANAGERS

Strategic directions	Board	>>>	Nurse Manager
Monitoring	Board	<<<	Nurse Manager
Linkages to community	Board	←→	Nurse Manager

In a policy governance model, the board role includes establishing the mission and goals of the organization, monitoring their achievement, maintaining linkages with stakeholders, and developing and reviewing policy (Carver, 1990). Establishing strategic directions for the organization includes framing the mission and goals and articulating values and vision. Monitoring the application of those values and achievement of those goals is an important part of the board's accountability to the public and to the Minister of Health. The process of maintaining linkages with both internal and external stakeholders brings the board full circle, using the broadly based information obtained through those linkages to re-evaluate strategic directions. The direction for information flow and type of information is different for each of the three responsibilities: strategic directions, monitoring, and maintaining linkages (see Figure 6.7).

With respect to strategic directions, the communications flow is from board to managers. Managers are expected to review all activities of their units or programs in the light of the values, vision, goals and mission statements articulated by the board, as well as to interpret them to the staff.

In the case of monitoring, the flow of communication is from management to the board once the board has indicated the type of information it needs. The best example is the budget, because the board will want to know how money has been spent, and whether it was spent in accordance with the values and goals of the board. Boards are also keenly interested in outcome data. The effect of the care provided on client health is the most important aspect to monitor, but also the most difficult to demonstrate.

And finally, in relation to linkages with external and internal stakeholders, communication between board and managers flows both ways. External stakeholders include the general public, physicians, professional associations, the provincial government, and other provider organizations. Communication with internal stakeholders usually occurs through the chief executive officer. Mechanisms must be in place to ensure that dialogue and feedback is maintained between board and all stakeholders in relation to values, vision, goals, the budget, and organizational activities.

CONCLUSION

A major purpose of regionalization was to reorient the health-care system away from costly institutional care. From 1992 to 1997 in most provinces, little change was evident in budgets for long-term care and community sectors, particularly in health promotion and mental health services. Boards need to give physicians, acute-care staff, and the public time to adjust. Within ten years from the beginnings of health reform, however, boards should be able to say proudly that the budget allocations are no longer based only on historical funding patterns. Priorities for budgets and service delivery should be driven by the goals of the board and needs of the community.

SUMMARY

- The board of directors governs an organization and establishes what services will be offered to whom at what cost. Management exists to accomplish those activities.
- A board of directors distributes the responsibility for decisions related to the organization across a variety of different individuals.
- The role of the board is to make decisions on the strategic direction of the organization, to monitor activities of both management and the board itself, to establish and maintain linkages with stakeholders, and to develop and review policies to guide itself and the organization.
- The traditional structure of governance in health care consists of many boards for site- or service-specific organizations.
- Most provinces have now established regional health boards; these have responsibility for the delivery of all acute-care, long-term-care, ambulance, home-care, mental-health, substance-abuse, and community-health services offered in the region. The major difference between the various models of regional health-care governance is the number of organizations that receive funding and power directly from the provincial government.
- Provincial governments have jurisdictional responsibility for health services and create the context in which health boards operate through policies and legislation.
- The relationship between health boards and first-level management is generally indirect. The board informs the organization of its strategic directions, people within the organization report activities so the board can monitor success, and there is two-way communication about linkages with other community providers.

FURTHER READINGS
AND RESOURCES

Health and Welfare Canada (1993). *Planning for health: Toward informed decision-making*. Ottawa: Health and Welfare Canada.

Lomas, J., Veenstra, G., & Woods, J. (1997). Devolving authority for health care in Canada's provinces: 3. Motivations, attitudes and approaches of board members. *Canadian Medical Association Journal, 156* (5), 669–676.

Rachlis, M. and Kushner, C. (1994). *Strong medicine: How to save Canada's health care system.* Toronto: HarperCollins.

Zander, A. (1993). *Making boards effective: The dynamics of non-profit governing boards.* San Francisco: Jossey-Bass.

REFERENCES

Carver, J. (1990). *Boards that make a difference.* San Francisco: Jossey-Bass.

De Wolf, G.D., Gregg, R.J., Harris, B.P., & Scargill, M.H. (Eds.). (1997). *Gage Canadian dictionary.* Vancouver: Gage Educational Publishing.

Health and Welfare Canada. (1993). *Planning for health: Toward informed decision-making.* Ottawa: Health and Welfare Canada.

Lomas, J. (1997). Devolving authority for health care in Canada's provinces: 4. Emerging issues and trends. *Canadian Medical Association Journal, 156*(6), 817–823.

Lomas, J., Veenstra, G., & Woods, J. (1997). Devolving authority for health care in Canada's provinces: 2. Backgrounds, resources and activities of board members. *Canadian Medical Association Journal, 156*(4), 513–520.

Lomas, J., Woods, J., & Veenstra, G. (1997). Devolving authority for health care in Canada's provinces: 1. An introduction to the issues. *Canadian Medical Association Journal, 156*(3), 371–377.

Orlikoff, J.E., & Totten, M.K. (1996). *The future of health care governance: Redesigning boards for a new era.* Chicago: American Hospital Publishing.

Pineault, R., Lamarche, P.A., Champagne, F., Contandriopoulos, A-P., and Denis, J-L. (1993). The reform of the Quebec health care system: Potential for innovation? *Journal of Public Health Policy, 14*(2), 198–219.

Saskatchewan Health. (1992). *A Saskatchewan vision for health: A framework for change.* Regina: Saskatchewan Health.

Saskatchewan Health. (1994). *Introduction of needs-based allocation of resources to Saskatchewan district health boards for 1994–1995.* Regina: Saskatchewan Health.

Wagner, P. S. (1996). Quality management challenges in Canadian health care. In J. Schmele (Ed.), *Quality management in nursing and health care.* Toronto: Delmar Publishers.

Chapter 7

▼▼▼▼▼▼▼▼▼▼▼▼▼

Restructuring Health Agencies: From Hierarchies to Programs

Susan VanDeVelde-Coke

KEY OBJECTIVES

In this chapter, you will learn:

- A definition of program management.
- Characteristics that distinguish a traditional centralized professional bureaucracy from program management.
- Macro—and micro—factors that have influenced institutions to implement program management.
- Issues that should be considered during and after the implementation of program management.
- Suggestions to assist senior and junior managers during implementation.
- Implications of program management for nurse managers.

INTRODUCTION

Hospitals, including both community hospitals and tertiary care institutions, traditionally have been organized according to professional disciplines and functional support departments.

Mintzberg (1989) has described this type of structure as a professional bureaucracy. Characteristically, professional bureaucracies are complex environments where professionals function in a relatively autonomous manner, controlled more by the performance standards of their parent professions than by the rules and regulations of the institutions where they work. Professionals by nature tend to establish their own goals and objectives, often making it difficult for hospital administration to develop and implement corporate priorities.

With the rapid expansion of medical knowledge and technology in recent years, the tendency for professional groups has been to become more specialized, or sub-specialized, in order to maintain high levels of expertise in a more focused domain of their disciplines. Mintzberg used the term "pigeonholing" to describe this process, such as the grouping of physicians into specialties (e.g., medicine, surgery, obstetrics) and even further into sub-specialties (e.g., cardiology, nephrology, gastroenterology), all within the broader discipline of internal medicine.

Ironically, as health-care professionals have become more specialized, they have also developed a greater dependence on health-care administrators to provide and co-ordinate the wide range of essential support services (e.g., maintenance, housekeeping, dietary, and financial services) on which they have come to rely. The persisting autonomy of professional groups, however, continues to make the administration of these complex organizations difficult. As a result, hospitals have had more difficulty than many other types of service industries in the business world when they try to implement new approaches, such as automation and quality-assurance programs. The reluctance of professionals to co-operate, the tendency toward pigeonholing, and the complexities of administration all make it difficult for health-care organizations to adapt to changing environments (Mintzberg, 1989).

In an effort to overcome these problems, some professional bureaucracies have attempted to implement a matrix approach to management. (Kolodny, 1979). In a matrix management structure, professionals may be assigned to a specific program or project made up of a multidisciplinary team, each member of which often has special skills or expertise. The team as a whole assumes responsibility for the successful management of the program or project, with each member contributing according to his or her expertise and ability. At the same time, the professionals continue to report through traditional, discipline-specific departments. While this dual reporting approach does help to resolve many of the problems associated with professional bureaucracies, matrix management structures in large complex organizations tend to be costly, can be confusing if lines of responsibility are not clearly defined, and are difficult to co-ordinate (Leatt, Shortell, & Kimberly, 1988). In addition, matrix structures are not well-suited to large support services such as housekeeping, medical records, and dietary; these services and their standards must be maintained throughout the institution and across programs and projects. As a result, many hospitals are now turning to program management as a potential strategy for improving efficiency in a changing environment.

PROGRAM MANAGEMENT: A DEFINITION

Program management is a type of management structure that is being adopted increasingly by health-care organizations, including hospitals ranging from small community facilities to large tertiary-care centres. Within this type of management structure, hospital services are grouped into programs. Definitions may vary but, in general, a program refers to a group of patients or clients who have like needs, and who are usually cared for by groups of physicians, nurses, and other health-care providers who have a special interest and expertise in caring for this population. Frequently, programs in hospitals are grouped by medical specialty (e.g., surgical, medical, pediatric, mental-health programs) or by the types of services provided (e.g., ambulatory care, emergency services, community-care programs). Programs may be further categorized by specific diagnoses or diagnostic groups (e.g., cardiac services, oncology clinics) (Leatt, Lemieux-Charles, & Aird, 1994).

Large programs like surgical services may set up sub-teams (e.g., an orthopedic rehabilitation sub-team) responsible for the day-to-day care of a limited group of patients within the larger surgical program. Each sub-team is also responsible for establishing standards of service and performance, and for developing care maps, while remaining accountable to the central program management team for key management decisions such as resource utilization and budgets. Linking patient-care services in this way to a designated group of health-care providers makes it much easier for managers to link costs to a specific volume and mix of services, as well as to monitor the impact of the expenditures on patient-care outcomes. At the same time, program management not only encourages health-care providers to develop innovative new approaches to patient care, but also makes them more accountable for resource utilization.

Figure 7.1 illustrates a traditional professional bureaucracy in which professionals are divided and centralized into groups representing their profession. Support services are also centralized and organized in a hierarchical fashion. Within this traditional structure, co-ordination of professionals is difficult as each vice-president is responsible primarily for a professional "stovepipe."

Figure 7.2 illustrates a program management structure. Program management organizations will show wide variations in integration of clinical and functional services. Most program management structures include physicians, nurses, and some allied health professionals within the program. Some hospitals have developed a new category of employee often referred to as a multi-skilled worker (a combination of nursing assistants, housekeepers, and unit clerks) (Ellis & Closson, 1994). Multi-skilled workers usually are assigned to specific programs. Most institutions continue to separate and centralize corporate services, such as financial management, strategic planning, human resources, and information systems, from specific programs, although in a pure program management model, these functions too would be decentralized. In summary, program management shifts the focus to patient-care services and outcomes, rather than to traditional discipline-specific hierarchies.

Program management has, in turn, altered the professional bureaucracy into a hybrid model that combines many aspects of the traditional hospital management structure with matrix management.

Figure 7.1

A TRADITIONAL, DIVISIONAL
DESIGN OF A HOSPITAL

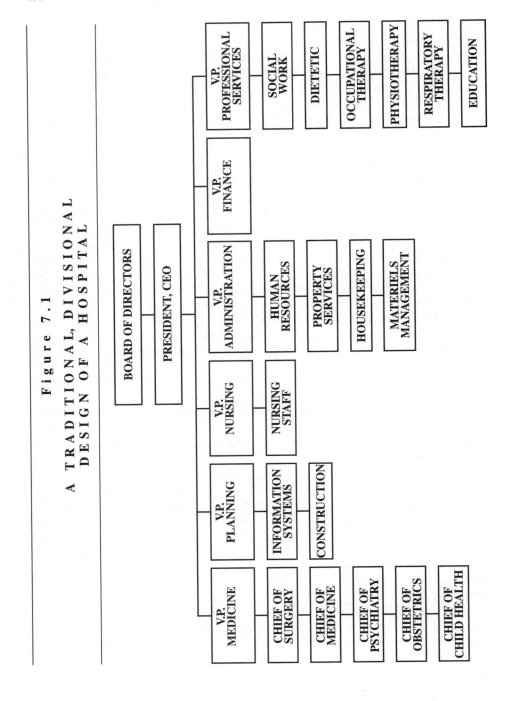

Figure 7.2
PROGRAM MANAGEMENT STRUCTURE

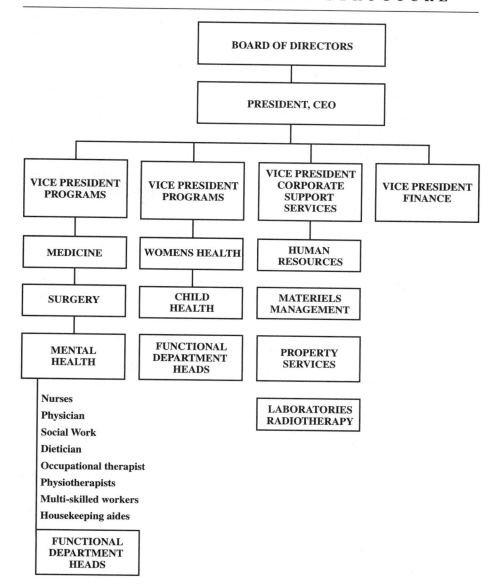

PROGRAM MANAGEMENT: MACRO LEVEL

Unprecedented changes in the health-care system in recent years have compelled institutions to look for new management structures that allow them to respond more rapidly to a changing environment. Bryan (1996) notes that these environmental forces are affected by several factors, such as:

- A commitment to the health-care system. Despite increasing financial constraints, the Canadian public wants its health-care system preserved, while expecting health-care providers to use existing resources more effectively and efficiently.
- Demographic changes. At the same time, demographic changes in the Canadian population are significantly altering the health-care needs of society. These demographic changes include the rapid growth of the elderly population, high immigration rates, and a growing awareness of under-served minority groups such as the aboriginal population. (See also Chapter 2.)
- Well-informed clients. The public in general is becoming better informed about health care and the health-care system. More than ever before, people are insisting on having more input and control over health-care decisions, both in relation to their own use and to the health-care system as a whole.
- Alternative approaches to health and health care. Complementary and alternative therapies are becoming more widely accepted. Consumers now expect more choices.
- Outcome evaluations. Health-care planners are stressing the need to base resource-allocation decisions on outcome evaluations of therapeutic and diagnostic interventions.

For many health-care institutions, program management, which links health-care resources to specific services or activities, appears to be the most logical strategy for responding to these environmental forces. However, although many working examples of program management have been described in the literature or can be observed directly in the Canadian health-care system, few institutions have proactively defined the benefits they wished to achieve through these changes or have evaluated the impact of program management on their performance. Evaluation literature on program management is scant. Nevertheless, most institutions that have introduced program management would not return to a traditional structure (Lemieux-Charles, Leatt, & Aird, 1994).

PROGRAM MANAGEMENT: MICRO LEVEL

At the institutional level, the most influential forces promoting a shift toward program management in hospitals relate primarily to more effective monitoring of health-care expenditures and the need for improved decision making (Ellis & Closson, 1994; Harber, 1994; Leatt, Lemieux-Charles, & Aird, 1994).

Specifically, monitoring of health-care expenditures should include:

- The costs incurred by the institution for groups of patients served by diagnoses, medical specialty, or age group.
- The need to relate patient-care outcomes to the amount of resources allocated to specific patient-care services.
- The best way, in the face of ongoing budget cuts, to determine reallocation of limited resources to patient care services.

Improved decision making should include:

- Ways to promote and facilitate the work of multidisciplinary teams by allocating resources to programs rather than to health-care professionals organized according to discipline.
- A shift of management decisions to front-line managers and staff, especially if some management layers are eliminated in response to budget cuts.
- Reduction of traditional dependency on individual leaders, including the CEO, for day-to-day operations.
- Demonstrations to accreditation bodies and other regulatory agencies that patient care is being provided by multidisciplinary teams capable of dealing directly with management issues without relying on an administrative hierarchy.

PLANNING A CONVERSION TO PROGRAM MANAGEMENT

By its very nature, the introduction of program management into a complex institution such as a hospital does not simply mean re-arranging the organizational chart. It also requires a major change in the attitudes, values, and management practices of the personnel. The adoption of program management is as much a process as an outcome.

In studying major innovative changes in large complex institutions, Cockerill and Barnsley (1997) noted that different organizations use different strategies or approaches for implementation. Some organizations adopt a rational approach based on a clear understanding of the innovation. They proceed by persuading the individual members of the organization about the advantages of the innovation, and then make a formal decision to implement the change. Supported by executive leadership, the innovation is implemented until the change has been institutionalized into the organization (Rogers, 1995).

In contrast, other organizations facing comparable pressures for change may adopt new organizational structures that have been successful for their peers or competitors without any apparent analysis or insight (Abrahamson & Rosenkopf, 1993). This bandwagon or fad approach is simply a form of imitation.

Finally, some organizations adopt strategies for change that resemble a natural selection process. Their implementation strategies do not follow a structural sequence. Rather, the organization initiates a change process and then responds to problems in implementation as they arise. Responses to problems are based on the personal experience and problem-solving abilities of managers and on the adoption, as necessary, of successful solutions developed by other organizations for similar situations (Kaluzny & Hernandez, 1988). For this type of strategy to work effectively, however, the organization must have sufficient internal flexibility to allow for experimentation in responding to problems as they arise.

Whatever the organization's reasons for choosing to implement program management or the strategy adopted for the implementation, senior executives must address a number of practical issues, including the number and types of programs to be included in the new organization, governance strategies for the programs, and ways the organization will deal with the diminished authority or elimination of the traditional professional departments.

DEFINING THE NUMBER AND TYPES OF PROGRAMS

Senior executives and professionals throughout the institution are usually responsible for defining the type and scope of programs and their accompanying structure. Influence from stakeholders will be intense throughout the process and should be solicited to obtain consensus. Complete agreement about what constitutes a "program" is unlikely, although there will probably be more consensus about the most pertinent and logical groupings of patients than about governance within the program itself. Input from the various stakeholders should be sought by senior executives and a number of iterations should be expected before a final decision is made about the number and types of programs.

LEADERSHIP WITHIN THE PROGRAM

Some program management structures are based on the premise that only one person will be in charge of a program, while others have worked with co-directors (Leatt, Lemieux-Charles, & Aird, 1994). The "one director" approach frequently results in a physician becoming head of the program. A co-director approach usually results in a nurse and a physician leading the team, and often a third person will represent the other professional or support members of the team.

The co-director or multiple director approach is more consistent with a multidisciplinary approach to program management and may result in improved co-operation among team members. The directors of the team must decide who will be responsible for specific management activities (e.g., chairing meetings, preparing budgets, financial information, hiring). Some programs may rotate the chair of the program team over a set period of time. The concept of "equal responsibility" for the program must be clearly defined to help ensure that one director does not dominate the team. If domination or an imbalance occurs, team members must be able to state their concerns, to re-establish ground rules, and to redefine the specific responsibilities of each co-director on an operation basis, so that administrative authority remains balanced. An imbalance of this nature is not always easy to correct.

EFFECT OF DELETION OF PROFESSIONAL DEPARTMENTS

In a traditional hospital structure, professionals such as nurses, nutritionists, therapists, and physicians are assigned to relatively autonomous discipline-specific departments that direct and supervise their practice within the institution. Under program management, these departments are either eliminated or altered to de-emphasize professional autonomy and to stress the importance of a multidisciplinary team approach to management. Professionals may view the loss of their departments as a loss of identity for their particular profession within the institution. Senior executives must handle this situation carefully, taking time to meet with the professional groups to define clearly and delineate each group's role within the program management teams.

In addition, separate mechanisms must be set up to manage professional issues, including clinical practice guidelines and standards. "Councils" for the specific professions are suggested as a way to address concerns of those professions and still maintain an emphasis on program management as the main operational structure. Some institutions will continue to maintain a medical advisory council, a nursing council, or an interdisciplinary professional practice council. It is unusual to see the medical advisory council amalgamated into a multidisciplinary professional council, although some hospitals have been successful in doing so. Whatever the mechanism adopted by the institution, it is essential that the professional groups be involved in setting up these councils or alternative structures and in defining their terms of reference. It will take time for professionals to acknowledge and trust the councils as an appropriate alternative forum to replace their traditional professional departments.

Program management may also create unique problems when the number of professionals in a given discipline is limited. For example, occupational therapists working in a hospital may be assigned to a wide range of programs. Given the limited number of practitioners, they may not be able to attend and participate actively in all related team meetings (Monaghan, Alton, & Wojtak, 1994). The structure therefore creates potential conflicts for those individuals between providing patient-care services and participating in management.

IMPLEMENTATION OF PROGRAM MANAGEMENT

Implementing program management within a health-care organization can be a monumental undertaking. If successful, it will result in a major change not only to the administrative structure of the institution but also to its decision-making processes and management culture. For implementation to be carried out successfully while still maintaining the day-to-day operation of the organization, a number of critical roles and procedures within the institution must be preserved and supported by senior management.

SUPPORT AND CORPORATE SERVICES DEPARTMENTS

Even when program management is introduced, support and corporate services (e.g., matériels management, human resources, finance, and planning) usually maintain their traditional structures and are not assigned to individual programs. They remain essential, however, to helping individual programs achieve their goals. With the emphasis shifted onto programs rather than support services, these departments may be overlooked in the aftermath of corporate restructuring. As a result, senior management may need to intervene to ensure that effective links of communication are established and maintained between the newly established programs and those essential support services.

SENIOR MANAGEMENT

The role of executive staff, including the CEO and more particularly the corporate vice-president, will tend to change substantially once program management is introduced. As programs evolve within the organization, these individuals will tend to take on increasing autonomy for day-to-day activities, including resource utilization. At the same time, however, there will be an increasing need to co-ordinate activities across individual programs, to ensure that corporate and not just program-specific goals and objectives are met, and to ensure the continued maintenance of standards across the institution. These duties require effective strategic planning, strong corporate policies and procedures, and efficient control of resource allocation and expenditure across the institution, all supported by effective information systems (Harber, 1994). In general, the corporate vice-president will be charged with ensuring that these kinds of essential infrastructures are in place. However, as programs continue to evolve and become more autonomous, the total number of vice-presidents required within the organization will likely decrease.

PHYSICIANS

Physician involvement with and commitment to program management is essential. Usually, sub-teams are established that will be responsible for groups of specialized patients (e.g., an orthopedic surgical sub-team or a re-habilitation sub-team). Physician involvement is needed at all levels of pro-gram management to co-ordinate these types of activities. In order to facilitate this type of participation, team-building and information sessions should be held at a time when physicians can attend; this often requires scheduling sessions to take place after routine working hours. Some insti-tutions have provided stipends for physicians who commit a significant portion of their time to program management, although this practice is not always possible (Lemieux-Charles et al., 1994).

INFORMATION TECHNOLOGY

To function effectively, program management requires information systems and data to support the decision-making program. Institutions that are planning to implement program management should ensure that they can provide the required statistics about the volume and mix of patient-care services, and that these data can be re-configured to correspond to defined programs. Similarly, programs will need access to related quality assurance information such as morbidity and mortality rates, average duration of stay, infection rates, and rates of recidivism, all grouped around defined pro-grams. Programs also will require access to related financial information broken down by program, often involving the creation of new cost centres. Direct costs for a given program usually can be identified without diffi-culty, but indirect costs also need to be determined and included within the statistical packages. Senior managers, therefore, need to anticipate all the information that will be required when they consider a change to program management, and should ensure that the required data is readily available at implementation.

SCHEDULE OF IMPLEMENTATION

Many institutions opt to carry out a limited application or pilot project using program management before implementing it throughout the organi-zation. Experience has shown, however, that these initial limited applica-tions generally are not helpful to the organization. Interim structures or pilot projects often lead to confusion about the specific roles and responsi-bilities of the new program structure versus the traditional, pre-existing management structures. As a result, institutions that intend to introduce program management are generally encouraged to proceed with full imple-mentation across the entire organization (Ellis & Closson, 1994; Harber, 1994; Monaghan et al., 1994).

According to a study of hospitals where program management has been implemented effectively (Lemieux-Charles et al., 1994), keys to success include:

- A set of values, principles, and objectives guiding the change.
- A strong commitment to change within the institution.
- A clear understanding of the effort involved.
- A willingness to commit resources to implement the change.

ONGOING ISSUES

A number of issues continue to confront those using program management, including communications, definitions of authority, and quality assurance. These will be discussed briefly.

COMMUNICATION MECHANISMS THROUGHOUT THE INSTITUTION

All institutions that have successfully established program management report that communication with staff throughout the process is critical. Not all staff members will be involved in the decision to proceed to program management, but managers who are involved in its implementation must expect questions about why program management is being introduced, and must be prepared to answer them. In addition, resistance, particularly from physician groups, should be anticipated as hospital personnel are re-grouped into teams. A commitment to teamwork is essential, as is education about team function and team building. Many organizations institute formal teaching sessions on team building to facilitate interaction among different professionals.

Most program management teams or sub-teams have worked together informally in the past, but often they have not interacted formally as a management group developing financial plans, goals, or objectives for the program, nor have they shared any other management responsibilities. As a result, the group of health-care providers brought together as a management team may not have any previous experience or knowledge about how to function as one. One of the most common errors in the initiation of program management is the assumption that management teams will be able to function effectively without appropriate education or training. In addition to training program management teams about financial reporting, budget development, strategic planning, and development of program goals and objectives, senior executives should be prepared to provide financial support for team-building sessions. Teams will also require education or training and information about business aspects of the program, including policies and procedures related to human resources and financial management.

It is recommended that ongoing, regular communication mechanisms be instituted throughout the organization when the program management process is started. Individual programs will tend to become involved and insular as they concentrate on specific issues. Other departments not directly involved in the programs may express concerns about isolation and lack of communication. Corporate newsletters and regular, open employee forums about the program and hospital activities are essential to help achieve a flow of information throughout the institution.

DEFINING PROGRAM AUTHORITY

The policies and procedures of an organization should be consistent not only with its structure but also with the way that organization functions.

Program management is based on the principle that decision making should be delegated, whenever possible, to the front-line health-care providers through their program teams. To function effectively, however, program teams must be given some degree of authority, including budgetary authority, commensurate with the responsibilities they are expected to assume.

In implemented management structure, therefore, senior executives must develop clear guidelines defining the authority of program teams, including the extent of their authority concerning capital-equipment purchases, allocation and re-allocation of resources to specific services, and human resource management (e.g., hiring and firing of personnel within the program).

QUALITY ASSURANCE PROCEDURES

Statistics on the volume and mix of services provided, patient-outcome measures, and resource utilization are all essential elements for developing program management in health-care institutions. Once implemented, these elements must be incorporated into a concurrent formal evaluation process, as described in quality-improvement systems, in order for program management to continue to function effectively.

Individual program team members often have already participated in audits or other quality-assurance activities. The team must then decide what specific information is pertinent to monitoring the quality of the program and, in turn, to improving its performance. The Canadian Council on Health Service Accreditation guidelines provides an excellent outline that can help team members develop a quality assurance or quality improvement process specific to the needs of the program.

However, clinical practice standards for specific health-care professions (e.g., physicians, nurses, physiotherapists) must be considered throughout the health-care institution and cannot, therefore, be monitored effectively by program management teams. As a result, health-care institutions implementing program management have found that they must still retain directors, such as chief medical and chief nursing officers, for the major professional groups responsible for establishing and maintaining clinical practice standards in each profession, often with the assistance of a discipline-specific professional council.

A NEW SET OF "STOVEPIPES"

In traditional management structures, institutions are divided into hierarchical professional and support departments. As seen in Figure 7.1, traditional departments were organized under a series of vice-presidents, typically a vice-president medicine, vice-president nursing or patient services, vice-president operations, and a vice-president research/planning. Under this structure, professionals formed discipline-specific hierarchies, with policies, procedures, and standards of practice that were easily understood by the individuals within the hierarchy since they all shared similar professional training and experience. These structure have been described as "stovepipes" or "silos."

Program management, by design, dismantles traditional hierarchies. Under program management, each team is theoretically responsible for the total operation of its program, including strategic planning and resource management. However, problems may still develop when a program incurs a deficit or wants to expand its services. Under a traditional structure, a vice-president nursing could transfer personnel and other resources from surgical units to medical or obstetrical units, as required, to meet the needs of the institution. Under program management, however, if one program requires expanded nursing resources, it often must seek them from other programs within the institution. Any significant re-allocation of resources, therefore, tends to become a potential source of conflict.

The vice-presidents, or, in some cases, the CEO in charge of a group of programs, may choose to transfer funds from one program to another. It is rare, however, that the programs themselves will be willing or able to transfer resources among themselves, unless criteria have already been established to determine how the transfer should occur. Most programs will tend to become protective of their own resources, and tend to focus primarily on ways to enhance their own efficiencies to expand or improve their services (MacLeod, 1994). Considerable energy is required to work in a multidisciplinary structure. There is usually little time or sympathy to understand and appreciate the concerns of other programs. Mintzberg (1989) describes co-ordination and innovation as the biggest challenges in a traditional professional bureaucracy. Although the potential for innovation may improve with program management because of its multidisciplinary and autonomous nature, co-ordination of activities across programs within the overall strategic plan for the institution remains a major challenge for senior executives.

Distributing resources fairly throughout the institution is the mandate of senior executives. With the implementation of program management, programs usually receive the same resources that had been previously allocated to the area. Programs that had too few resources prior to implementation often find it increasingly difficult to compete for resources from other programs once the structure is in place. Programs tend to "lock-in" to their own resources, and generally will resist any effort to transfer personnel, funds, equipment, or space to other programs, regardless of the apparent need. The CEO, vice-presidents, and program teams therefore must force the challenge of developing mechanisms to redistribute resources among programs or to allocate reductions fairly when budget cuts are introduced.

Suggestions that have been developed by existing program management teams for this process include:

1. Sharing program information among the programs. This information should include activity and workload statistics, budgeted resources, actual resource utilization, waiting lists, and other information that will help educate the program teams about each other.

2. Developing objective criteria, with input from program teams, for moving resources from one program to another to cope with challenges such as:

    a. Gaps in services (e.g., insufficient occupational therapy services in a program). There may be valid arguments for moving resources from one program to another because of long waiting lists or clearly documented shortages.

    b. Changes in technology requiring a shift in resources from one segment to another (e.g., from inpatient wards to ambulatory care).

    c. Mechanisms to distribute capital resources across the institution. Programs and support departments must first rank their own capital-resource requests, and then meet to defend or re-prioritize a list of capital purchases over the coming fiscal year. Physical plant priorities must be considered in conjunction with the program priorities.

    d. New services being considered by a program. New services must be consistent with the mission and strategic direction of the institution.

REGIONALIZATION AND THE FUTURE OF PROGRAM MANAGEMENT

Most provinces across Canada have instituted some form of regionalization in an effort to improve the delivery of health-care services and reduce costs (see Chapters 4 and 6). Programs, particularly those based in academic centres, will be affected by these changes. Frequently, programs in academic or tertiary-care centres become the fulcrum for change for the rest of the region. From a regional perspective, a surgical program includes not only the academic institution but also the community hospitals, ambulatory-care centres, and other community agencies. With the introduction of regionalization, governance of programs then becomes a regional issue. The strategic plan for a program must include the whole region, with multiple partners. Program teams in one institution may be dismantled, rearranged, or added from other hospitals or the community. The role of CEOs and vice-presidents tends to be altered or, possibly, eliminated when regionalization forces changes to governance structures for all the health-care institutions in the region. The overall impact of regionalization on program management remains to be seen, but it likely will be profound. Box 7.1 illustrates one example of a large organization moving to a program management model.

IMPLICATIONS FOR NURSE MANAGERS

Many nurses view program management as threatening. (Flynn, 1991) However, the implementation and operation of program management is fairly straightforward for nurse managers. Nurse managers have global and practical

Box 7.1

CASE EXAMPLE: FROM ADMINISTRATIVE HIERARCHY TO PROGRAM MANAGEMENT

This case example illustrates the experience of a large tertiary-care centre that changed from a traditional administrative hierarchy to program management. As is frequently seen in today's health-care environment, many other changes occurred within the institution at the same time that the management reorganization was implemented, illustrating a vital point: Major management changes rarely, if ever, occur in a vacuum.

Budget Reduction Exercise

The Health Sciences Centre was created through the amalgamation of four separate hospitals, all located close to one another geographically. The centre employs close to 5,000 staff, excluding physicians, and has an operating budget of approximately $250 million per year. In the early 1990s, the provincial government reduced the centre's budget by more than $30 million over a three-year period. A massive budget exercise was undertaken with the assistance of an external consulting agency, whose mandate was to facilitate and educate the staff on how to re-engineer most front-line jobs within the institution. To improve efficiency, more than 700 staff members were directly involved in multiple team exercises to investigate how to streamline, to eliminate procedures, to remove redundant positions, to delete layers of management, and to improve administrative relationships within the organization.

The budget-reduction project took approximately one year and resulted in recommendations for $19 million in savings in the operating budget. The majority of participating teams believed they had achieved as much efficiency and cost savings as possible. There was considerable burnout as a result of the process. Some teams were ridden with guilt because they had recommended the introduction of multi-skilled workers, which would lead to

the elimination of jobs. In some cases, elimination of entire job classifications (e.g., Licensed Practical Nurses) was recommended. Overall, however, this multidisciplinary approach involving front-line health-care providers appealed to hospital personnel to such an extent that many reported to senior executives they did not want to go back to the traditional departmental administrative structure that had existed before the restructuring project.

The Move Towards Program Management

The project also forced the institution to re-examine the structure and organization of its senior executive staff. The president became convinced that the organization should move to program management. Coupled with informal feedback from staff members calling for the maintenance of a team approach, the executive staff decided to proceed with the change. To initiate the process, senior executives held a series of meetings and retreats to plan a new structure, with ongoing feedback from the department heads within each existing portfolio. Final decisions about the content of each new portfolio, however, remained with the president. At the end of the process, seven programs were identified: surgery; medicine and rehabilitation; women's health; children's health; mental health; dialysis; and adult ambulatory care. These programs fit well with the geography and physical plant of the centre, since the Women's Hospital, Children's Hospital, Provincial Psychiatric Centre, and Rehabilitation Hospital are all separate physical structures, and are responsible for defined provincial or regional programs.

Support departments, such as matériels management, laboratories, dietary, and information systems, were distributed evenly across the patient-care portfolios, with each department reporting to one of the area presidents.

Professional departments, such as nursing, occupational therapy, and physiotherapy, were dissolved, and professional staff were assigned to the patient-care programs. Each profession, (e.g., occupational therapy, physiotherapy) except nursing and medicine, maintained a "discipline" director responsible for maintaining the professional and clinical practice standards of that profession. One vice-president was appointed as spokesperson for nursing and nursing standards. A second vice-president, who was a physician, served in the same role for the physicians, although the senior executive made a conscious decision to eliminate the formal positions of chief nursing officer and chief medical officer. The Medical Advisory Committee continued as the vehicle for medical professional issues. Two other new professional councils were established, one for nursing and one for all other allied health-care professionals.

The new structure was announced six months before implementation. A number of individuals, departments, and professional groups lobbied for changes in the structure, resulting in some minor changes. Overall, however, the new structure was maintained from the original announcement. Each program had two, or sometimes three, co-directors representing medicine and nursing, with an allied health-care professional when appropriate.

During the six-month period prior to implementation, job descriptions for program directors, discipline directors, and a number of other positions were completed. Considerable work was also required to finish up the cost-saving restructuring exercise and establish time frames for implementing the recommendations. Downsizing, the introduction of multi-skilled workers, and other recommended changes to achieve cost savings as well as introduce the new management structure continued to cause considerable disruption throughout the institution over the next year.

Implementation

The new structure was implemented as planned. During the aftermath, a number of major events took place that greatly influenced the implementation of the new management structure, including team building, elimination of management positions, accreditation, and strategic planning and evaluation.

Team Building

Budget reductions, implementation of program management, and continuous uncertainty about the direction of provincial health care left the whole organization in turmoil. As is seen in the literature, staff who experience this amount of change in addition to other related emotional trauma from layoffs, position deletions, or loss of structure are unable to focus on their immediate jobs, much less continue to bring forth the creativity required for future planning. As a result, members of the senior executive brought in a second consulting group to analyze the situation and to develop a plan that would help managers and staff re-focus.

A major exercise was undertaken to help managers learn how to work productively in teams, manage conflict situations, define and understand decision-making modalities, run meetings more effectively, and gain greater insight into the ways they, as individuals, worked in teams. As part of this exercise, each manager spent three days working in teams doing highly structured problem-solving exercises; these required active, often physical, participation. The exercise left the managers re-focused and energized.

Four separate multidisciplinary teams were set up to continue the work of restructuring and team building. Each team was instructed to concentrate on one of the following tasks:

- Educating managers and staff about team building;
- Developing an ongoing, centre wide communication strategy;
- Defining the responsibility and authority of each program and of senior management;
- Developing a set of management principles and ethics for the new organization. These included a code of conduct, a performance appraisal system, and a set of values to help all staff members behave and practice in a manner

that would demonstrate respect for each other and their team members.

The four teams were made up of personnel drawn from all different levels and departments within the institution. Each team reported directly to executive staff and regularly provided reports on its progress. Funding for these plans was approved by the senior executive. Ongoing efforts to educate the remaining staff about team building, decision making, conflict resolution, and a code of conduct proved to be the most costly component of this process with an anticipated three-year time frame for completion.

The values and governance teams completed their work within six months, but it was decided that the communication and education teams should become permanent entities and report regularly to the executive about their progress.

Accreditation

The Canadian Council for Health Services Accreditation surveyed the centre less than a year after program management was first implemented. This review process created considerable anxiety throughout the organization. Although all teams were functioning effectively, not all sub-teams had been firmly established by the time the survey team arrived.

In addition, many allied health-care professionals felt they did not have adequate representation within the new management structure, and that this put standards of practice at risk. However, the strongly positive accreditation review supported the initiatives to establish program management and gave the institution the needed feedback and encouragement to complete the process.

Strategic Planning Process/ Evaluation of Program Management

Each program was required to develop a strategic plan, working in collaboration with a Strategic Planning Committee set up by the centre's board. Approximately six months after the accreditation review, all programs reported progress on their strategic plans. Despite continuing financial constraints and political uncertainties at the ministerial level, each program had been able to accomplish most of the goals it had defined two years previously.

The last task for each team was to develop evaluation tools and to assess the performance and accomplishments of its program. The most common problems experienced by all programs in developing effective evaluation tools were:

- The lack of or inability to obtain data specific to the needs of the program to assess its performance.
- Incomplete information for case costing. Although some data were available on direct costs, information on indirect costs was rarely available.
- Team members often had limited knowledge and experience in developing operating and capital budgets, which led, in turn, to the inefficient operation of programs.
- Most team members were attempting to improve their knowledge not only about management techniques and finance but also about evaluation methods and the ways other programs functioned. Many teams went through a "storming" stage within their own group before moving on to a productive relationship. In addition, a new set of "stove-pipes" tended to emerge in the teams, with little sharing of resources. Effective collaboration among programs did not begin to develop until much later in the process.

knowledge of how professional and support departments work together. Using this knowledge to facilitate program management is a fairly easy transition. Nurse managers soon discover that other members of the team rely on their knowledge and expertise not only to co-ordinate daily management of programs, but also for strategic planning.

Nurses still make up the largest single group of professionals within the hospital, and are the only professionals invariably present 24 hours a day, seven days a week. It is essential, therefore, that there is a voice for the nursing profession at the senior executive level, either as a vice-president or as chief nursing officer. The principles for a professional practice environment established by the Canadian Nurses Association (see Haines, 1993, p. 22) are helpful for any nursing department implementing program management. If these principles are followed, the nursing profession should have little difficulty in participating in program management.

CONCLUSION

Participation in team-building exercises, helping to educate teams, listening to the concerns of the other professionals, establishing clear job descriptions, and developing criteria for measuring outcomes are all key roles for nurse managers. Most nurse managers will find that program management enhances and illuminates more clearly for other professionals the essential role that nurse managers fill in the operation of their institution.

SUMMARY

- The decision to implement program management is often the result of a combination of a logical rational process and a bandwagon approach as defined by Cockerill and Barnsley (1994). In Box 7.1 a case example is presented in which the senior executives were influenced by the experience of employees working as teams to achieve objectives in a budget-reduction exercise, as well as by positive experiences reported by comparable centres that had already implemented program management.
- The co-director approach may create difficulties at first, but will help establish equality among professionals. In the example, the position descriptions for program directors were similar, whether the director was a nurse or a physician. The directors, therefore, were obliged to define who would be responsible for each of the operations of the program based on that individual's ability and experience.
- Monitoring is essential, once professional departments are eliminated, to assure professionals that standards of practice are being maintained across the institution.
- Lack of information, technology, and evaluation tools will slow the work of the programs until databases are established.
- Team building is time consuming, at times frustrating, and potentially explosive but it is essential to the implementation of program management, as is ongoing communication throughout the institution. In the case study, the establishment of corporate values and a code of conduct for the institution proved to be an essential part of the process.
- Despite reorganization, new "stovepipes" tend to develop. Criteria and administrative mechanisms are required to allow the shift of resources across programs as needed, in order to meet corporate goals.

FURTHER READINGS AND RESOURCES

Armstrong-Stassen, M., Cameron, S.J., & Horsburgh M.E. (1996). The impact of organizational downsizing on the job satisfaction of nurses. *Canadian Journal of Nursing Administration, 9*(4), 8–32.

Isaak, S., & McCutcheon, D., (1997), Organizational restructuring in health care: A successful approach. *Healthcare Management Forum, 10*(3), 34–41.

O'Malley, J., Cummings, S., & Serpico, D. (1991). Pragmatic strategies for product-line management. *Nursing Administration Quarterly, 15*(2), 9–5.

Read, N., & Gehrs, M. (1997). Innovative service redesign and resource reallocation: Responding to political realities, mental health reform and community mental health needs. *Canadian Journal of Nursing Administration, 10*(4), 7–22.

Rook, M., & Shulman, K.I. (1996). Revolutionary versus evolutionary change: The experience of a university hospital department of psychiatry. *Healthcare Management Forum, 9*(4), 53–55.

REFERENCES

Abrahamson, E., & Rosenkopf, L. (1993). Institutional and competitive bandwagons: Using mathematical modeling as a tool to explore innovation diffusion. *Academy of Management Review, 18*(3), 487–517.

Bryan, L. (1996). *A design for the future of health care.* Toronto: Key Porter.

Cockerill, R., & Barnsley, J. (1997). Innovation theory and its applicability to our understanding of the diffusion of new management practices in health care organizations. *Healthcare Management Forum, 10*(1), 35–38.

Ellis, P.H., & Closson, T. (1994). Realigning around the patient: The application of restructuring and process re-engineering at Sunnybrook Health Science Centre. In P. Leatt, C. Lemieux-Charles, & C. Aird (Eds.), *Program Management and Beyond: Management Innovations in Ontario Hospitals* (pp. 55–65). Ottawa: Canadian College of Health Service Executives.

Flynn, M. K. (1991) Product-line management: Threat or opportunity for nursing. *Nursing Administration Quarterly, 15*(2), 9–15.

Haines, J. (1993). *Leading in a time of change: The challenge for the nursing profession. A discussion paper.* Ottawa: Canadian Nurses Association.

Harber, B.W. (1994). Program management at Peel Memorial Hospital: Advancing our patient care focus. In P. Leatt, L. Lemieux-Charles & C. Aird (Eds.), *Program management and beyond: Management innovations in Ontario hospitals* (pp. 17–28). Ottawa: Canadian College of Health Service Executives.

Kaluzny, A. D., & Hernandez, S. R. (1988). Organizational Change and Innovation. In S. M. Shortell & A.D. Kaluzny (Eds.), *Health care management* (pp. 379–417). New York: John Wiley & Sons.

Kolodny, H. F. (1979). Evolution to a matrix organization. *Academy of Management Review*. Vol. 4 [#4], 543–553.

Leatt, P. Lemieux-Charles, L., & Aird, C. (1994). Program management: Introduction and overview. In P. Leatt, L. Lemieux-Charles & C. Aird (Eds.), *Program management and beyond: Management innovations in Ontario hospitals* (pp. 1–10). Ottawa: Canadian College of Health Service Executives.

Leatt, P., Shortell, S.M., & Kimberley, J.R. (1988). Organizational Design. In S.M. Shortell & A.D. Kaluzny (Eds.), *Health care management* (pp. 307–343). New York: John Wiley & Sons.

Lemieux-Charles, L., Leatt, P., & Aird, C. (1994). Lessons learned and future directions: Translating a vision into reality. In P. Leatt, L. Lemieux—Charles & C. Aird (Eds.), *Program management and beyond: Management innovations in Ontario hospitals* (pp.85–89). Ottawa: Canadian College of Health Service Executives.

MacLeod, W.B. (1994). Program management at Women's College Hospital. In P. Leatt, L. Lemieux-Charles, & C. Aird (Eds.), *Program management and beyond: Management innovations in Ontario hospitals* (pp. 11–15). Ottawa: Canadian College of Health Service Executives.

Mintzberg, H. (1989). *Mintzberg on management: Inside our strange world of organization*. New York: The Free Press.

Monaghan, B.J., Alton, L., & Wojtak, A. (1994). Program management at West Park Hospital. In P. Leatt, L. Lemieux-Charles, & C. Aird (Eds.), *Program management and beyond: Management innovations in Ontario hospitals* (pp. 43–54). Ottawa: Canadian College of Health Service Executives.

Rogers, E.M. (1995). Lessons for guidelines from the diffusion of innovations. *Journal of Quality Improvement, 21*(7), 324–328.

Chapter 8

▼▼▼▼▼▼▼▼▼▼▼▼▼

Work Process Redesign and Nurses' Work

Bonnie L. Lendrum

KEY OBJECTIVES

In this chapter, you will learn:

- How the work of health care professionals has become disconnected from the whole process of patient and family care.
- How work process redesign offers a method of reconnecting healthcare professionals to the process of care.
- How to differentiate surface change in health care from fundamental change.
- Critical steps to be considered when embarking on work process redesign.

INTRODUCTION

The design of nurses' work has traditionally been viewed in terms of relationships. Those relationships have been to the patient (primary nursing), to other nurses (team nursing), to the geographic distribution of the patients (modular nursing), and to the division of work involved in patient care (functional nursing) (Lendrum, 1994; McPhail, 1991). Over the years, each of the traditional designs has been touted for its benefits to patients and to nurses. There have been no conclusive studies, however, that show one design consistently produces more or better patient outcomes, or more or greater efficiencies, than another does.

The respective designs have generated enthusiastic supporters over the years. Considerable time, money, and effort have been spent to introduce one model or another to health care organizations. There is, however, no body of substantive evidence that can support one design over the other. Selection of a model for care delivery, or an approach to organizing work, may best be determined by a host of factors such as length of stay, acuity versus chronicity, staffing levels, and skill mix—but that research also has not yet been done.

This absence of compelling evidence for the design of nurses' work has left nurses poorly situated at a time of fiscal constraint. Consumer expectations of quality and spiralling healthcare costs have forced health-care organizations to examine the outcomes of the care they provide, as well as the methods for its provision. New verbs such as restructure, re-engineer, and redesign have become part of our vocabulary. Throughout North America, the work of health care is currently being examined by applying a work redesign framework.

This chapter will introduce the reader to work process redesign: its origins and theory, its goals, its fit with organizational structure, and its methods (redesign, evaluation plan, and implementation). A final note will address political realties of current redesign work.

ORIGINS AND THEORY OF WORK PROCESS REDESIGN

Work process redesign has its origins in the quality improvement literature that emerged just after World War II (1939-1945). However, methods associated with quality improvement pre-date the industrial revolution. The work of artisans is a wonderful illustration of quality-improvement methods. Artisans attended to complete processes from the time a customer communicated his needs and wishes for a product, through purchase of materials, construction of the work and, finally, to delivery of the product. Apprentices were trained to assist with components or steps in the process and ultimately learned to perform the whole process to the satisfaction of the artisan, measured against the artisan's standard for quality. That standard would have been one that assured customer satisfaction and, therefore, an ongoing source of livelihood for the artisan. Positive opinion came directly to the artisan through referrals and more commissions. Negative feedback came by way of requests to repair or rework the product. The net result of cumulative negative feedback would be the loss of a livelihood.

The industrial revolution separated artisans from their customers and removed them from a view of the entire process. With mass production came the need to separate work. New types of work were created, such as order acquisition, raw materials purchasing, manufacturing, work inspection, and product distribution. Scientific management (Taylor, 1912) further divided the labour into smaller units of work, with the result that workers became one step in the production of goods rather than managers of the whole production process. Mathematical measures were introduced as surrogates (e.g., number of defects per 1000 pieces) for the original artisan's measure of satisfaction (or standards).

In the post-industrial revolution, consumers continue to provide feedback to the entire production process through their buying patterns and return of unsatisfactory goods. But just as workers have become distanced from the process of production, so too have consumers. An unhappy consumer can complain to the store where a purchase was made and perhaps receive an apology and a replacement product. However, that complaint may not be heard by the product manufacturer whose business may ultimately suffer. The separation of workers from the process of production can ultimately lead to loss of market share and job loss. When the views of workers and their participation in the process becomes limited to the components of work immediately before and after their own, they no longer contribute value for people who use the product or service. Hammer (1996) says "value-adding work is easy to identify. It consists of all the activities that create the goods and services that customers want.... Value-adding work can rarely be eliminated from a process, although it can be improved" (p.33).

Health care organizations today are analogous to the post-industrial revolution model of manufacturing and distribution. Individual artisans (professionals) no longer directly influence the process of care, and in some instances have lost sight of the whole process of care. Work-design strategies such as primary nursing and case management are well intended efforts to help the professional influence the whole process, and the introduction of roles such as clinical nurse specialist have provided a larger scope of practice. However, the roles and the work designs fail because organizations have not been structured to emphasize the central processes of providing health services. Primary nursing, case management, and clinical nurse specialist roles do not usually have structural nor operational authority, and even when well performed by experts they may fail to systematically and consistently improve care. Individual complaints may be heard respectfully and addressed at the point of care. Some patients may even have the clinical specialist or the case manager accompany them through the process, but the system or processes underlying these complaints may not be changed. The goal of work process redesign is to reconnect health-care professionals and ancillary workers to the process of care, and thereby to the quality of care experienced by patients.

Nurses can take pride in their history, which is marked by continual efforts to increase the quality of care for patients. Primary nursing and case management are two recent examples of work designs that increase both the co-ordination and continuity of care, while reducing the number of health workers involved in the patient's care. The patient's experience, however, extends beyond the nursing unit, and beyond the hospital. Beyond those walls, a primary nurse has little influence, and a case manager has only slightly more. The reality for nurses is that their daily frustrations do not rest with the patients but with the way the systems around them function. Work process redesign offers a means for nurses to increase their patients' quality of care and their own quality of work life.

THE GOAL OF WORK PROCESS REDESIGN

Work process redesign figuratively turns an organization on its side to examine and reconstruct how it works. That means examining how care and service delivery cut across departments, and what is accomplished along the way. Work process redesign addresses more than the incremental improvement of tasks; it examines the changes that may be required in the whole process of care to improve service and create value for the client.

What does creating value for patients and their families mean? Patients and families can tell us about value—and have done so in an articulate, impassioned manner in *Through the Patient's Eyes* (Gerteis, Edgman-Levitan, Daley, & Delbanco, 1993). When value has been created, they express pleasure that tests are done quickly, accurately, and comfortably, and done only once. Patients and families express relief that staff took time to understand their worries and explain the steps they would come across in diagnosis or recovery. They comment on competency of staff they met and on the system itself, how all the pieces fit together. They feel cared for, respected, and treated as partners in their care. They are proud to live in a community where care of this quality is available and accessible to them. What patients and families are describing is the value that has been added to their illness experience. They describe not only quality care, but a series of processes that weave together to create a seamless experience with no loose threads and no holes.

An examination of the diagnostic process provides an illustration of how work process design can leave patients and families with powerful impressions of receiving quality care. The diagnostic process is a useful exemplar because it intersects other processes and engages a range of professional and support staff. The diagnostic process begins when a sick person sees a physician and is assessed for the unexplained and rapid onset of symptoms. An example might be an instance of apparent renal failure. The physician orders a series of investigations to be done in hospital and the person is admitted to a nursing unit by a nurse and then interacts with a number of different staff from different departments as different investigations are conducted over time. The physician receives and reviews the reports, keeps the patient informed, and finally communicates the diagnosis to the patient. From the patient's point of view, the system has worked flawlessly if his or her experience is as described below:

- The time from booking the admission to the time of admission is short.
- Tests are explained in a manner that addresses the patient's worries and respects the fact that he or she is a partner in the care.
- The patient is asked to fast for a period of time prior to investigations and finds this reasonable.
- Transport to and from the diagnostic areas is achieved in comfort.
- Investigations are performed by staff who are knowledgeable and efficient with their techniques, and also seem to care about the patient's comfort and dignity.
- The nurse greets the patient, inquires about the investigation, and brings medication to relieve discomfort arising from the investigation.
- The next meal arrives as expected.
- The nurse returns to talk with the patient about the tests being conducted the next day.

- The doctor arrives later that afternoon and informs the patient of the first batch of test results.

In this instance, the patient has connected with the visible parts of the process and found them acceptable. Behind the curtains are other, invisible parts of the process, or the machines and moving parts that construct the tapestry of care: booking of the diagnostic tests to match with acceptable levels of fasting; cancelling of one meal tray and restarting of the next one; matching of the correct patient's name to the correct diagnostic test; preparation, transport, and administration of medication necessary to a successful test; preparation of the room where the test will be conducted; preparation and sterilization of the equipment necessary for the investigation; performance of the right investigation on the right person; correct labelling of specimens procured from the investigation; transport of specimens to the lab; examination of specimens; matching of the specimens to the pathology report; and, finally, return of the report to the patient's chart.

The visible and the invisible components of the process are all parts of a larger overall process. In this example, the diagnostic process is intersected by the admission process (e.g., booking of the bed and assignment of the bed on the day of admission), by sub-processes of the care process (e.g., interaction with the nurse for assessment and teaching; interaction of the nurse and patient with the medication system), and sub-processes of the facilities management process (i.e., arrival of the meal tray; transport to and from tests). The diagnostic process itself is a complex one and it requires interaction of staff from different departments with the patient, and associated pieces of paper or electronic files.

There are many instances in which one person or department "hands off" successive parts of the process to another and, with them, many opportunities for the process to break down. If the admission is delayed, so too is the diagnosis, and the patient is left with uncertainty about the illness. Delays in "paperwork" can result in a delay in communicating the diagnosis to the patient. If the paperwork is lost, the patient will be retested and subjected to unnecessary discomfort. At the same time, retesting doubles the cost to the health-care system and delays the testing of the next patient in line. If the patient's tray has not been cancelled and the patient, not understanding the fasting requirements, eats breakfast, then the test is delayed another day. Again, inefficiencies are experienced in staffing and supplies, and the next patient waiting to come to hospital experiences delays. For a compelling account of how hospitals have incrementally built in inefficiency and a failure to respond to the client, read Lathrop (1993).

Processes that do not weave together tightly do not add value to the patient's experience. Rather, the patient may be left with uncertainty about the nature of the illness and may experience unnecessary physical discomfort. The physician, the patient, and the primary nurse may complain about booking delays, but the absence of someone in charge of the diagnostic process—the *process owner,* to use a phrase coined by Hammer and Champy (1993)—means that nothing is changed. If the patient is left feeling chilly, exposed, and uncomfortable during transport and throughout investigations, the physician, the patient, and the primary nurse may complain. But if no single individual feels responsible for the diagnostic process or has the authority to deal with processes, nothing is likely to change. If the paperwork is lost and the patient is retested, the physician, the patient, and the primary nurse may complain, but, again, the absence of someone in charge of the diagnostic process will be an obstacle to its improvement.

Ignoring the manner in which processes cut across departments can amount to tacit approval of inefficiency, substandard responsiveness, and poor communication, as well as of lack of courtesy, respect, and caring. Failure to attend to whole processes can become a way of preserving system incompetence.

FIT OF WORK REDESIGN TO ORGANIZATIONAL STRUCTURE

Restructuring an organization is no guarantee that work processes will be redesigned. The objective of work process redesign is to develop a system where a program or service is provided in the best possible way to give the client the desired outcome with the least possible degree of harm (Clark, Cudmore, Hammons, et al., 1995).

To accomplish this objective, restructuring is often the first wave of an organization's attempt to improve consumer satisfaction and manage costs. It becomes visible within and beyond the organization as the organization's partners and stakeholders engage in strategic planning. Ultimately, care units are grouped differently, new titles are applied to the groupings, and the organizational chart is redrawn. Restructuring may mean the loss of traditional departments of nursing, surgery, and medicine. These may be replaced with new labels, such as women's health program or adult-specialty services program. Nursing and other health professional groups may be entirely devolved to these programs.

The changes that result from restructuring may seem large, and when a professional department has been lost the changes may be demoralizing. If such restructuring has the effect of reorienting the managers in the organization to take a holistic view of its processes, and to work together as a team, the initial steps of restructuring can lead to a deeper level of change. Front-line workers are affected by restructuring when reporting relationships are changed or when colleagues lose positions through job reassignment or job deletion. Re-engineering or work process redesign involves and requires a deep level of change that will also have a dramatic impact on the work of the front-line worker. When it is conducted well, it can improve quality of care, the fiscal bottom line, and quality of work life.

METHODS EMPLOYED IN WORK PROCESS REDESIGN

Initiating work process redesign involves a large-scale organizational change. It requires a dedicated team to lead the process and mobilize the work force. By the time an organization has committed to work process redesign, consultants have likely been engaged to introduce the change effort. They may continue to be involved as guides or coaches until the change effort is well underway. An internal team of project-seconded employees may be put in place to assist with the redesign effort.

The methods used to examine work processes stem from the early 1900s and have been described in the quality-improvement literature. Lewin's work on force-field analysis would have been an early example of the methods used to examine change and social forces. While the methods of redesign are the same as the methods of quality improvement, the approach is different. Quality improvement leads to incremental changes in work processes over time, whereas work process redesign is undertaken with the objective of making radical changes to processes throughout the organization. The gains made from redesign then need to be sustained or advanced by using the tools and methods of quality improvement. For an informative and entertaining introduction to quality improvement the reader is referred to Townsend and Gebhardt (1992). Boulerice's (1994) chapter in the first edition of this text provides a summary of the trend towards quality improvement. Greater depth is provided in the following readings: Gaucher and Coffey (1993); Berwick, Godfrey, and Roessner (1990); and Early (1989).

The remainder of this chapter will help the reader gain an understanding of the approaches and methods employed throughout process redesign. This description is not intended to serve as a guide to help the reader undertake work redesign. Readers interested in such primers would be well advised to read Hammer and Champy (1993) and Hammer (1996) and to talk with colleagues who have participated in a work process redesign project.

PLANNING THE REDESIGN

Work process redesign begins with understanding a process from the perspective of its customers and its providers. This understanding involves more than analysis of the process; it also requires that the redesigners learn about their clients' goals. These goals can be numerous and complex. Referring again to the examples of the diagnostic process, a primary nurse and an internist may say that they want fast accurate reports from investigations. They would also want their patients treated with care and respect, and informed about the process of the investigation. They may specify that pre-test preparations should cause as little patient discomfort as possible (e.g., tests that require fasting are done first thing in the morning). The unit clerk, in addition to managing the work load on the inpatient unit, would want a friendly reception when calling for a booking, and would want patients cared for in a manner that would minimize discomfort and make efficient use of the patient's time. The patient would want to be investigated by caring competent staff who perform efficiently while keeping him informed and comfortable. The patient would also want to know the results as soon as possible. The patient's family members would want to have a comfortable place to sit or stand during the investigation, and would want to be included as partners in the care. The receptionist in the diagnostic area would want to reduce the time from patient arrival to investigation, and from end of investigation to transport back to the unit. The investigation team would want a patient who had been correctly medicated and had the site prepared and who had received an explanation that would assure an understanding of the procedure about to be done.

This example illustrates the multitude of goals held by clients and stakeholders. It shows that redesign cannot be done in one marathon re-design session by a manager in an office, nor can it be done as a paper-and-pen exercise by staff members from a single work area. Rovin (1991, Chapter 1) have suggested that typical planning methods do not work. Planning for redesign involves teamwork, and requires that various stakeholders and clients, with their different goals and perspectives, be brought together to create a new process. Ackoff (1981) suggests a model entitled "interactive planning." This model engages the people who will use the products of the change in the planning of the change. Interactive planning is creative in that the goal is not to fix a problem or to pull out several million dollars; the goal is to have participants identify and achieve what they desire (Rovin, 1991). Interactive planning is a values-driven process based upon systems thinking. One of its by-products is a new culture.

Redesign unleashes creativity by moving people out of their pre-existing frameworks. Starting with the end in mind, the redesign process works backward from that future ideal to the present. Preconceived notions of steps that must be taken, or who does what task, will fall by the wayside. The end-point is clear and desirable, and it is recognized that there are many ways of achieving the goal. The work of interactive planning is to achieve the goal in the best way possible for the clients.

Quality improvement (QI) methods have proven a useful way of unleashing creativity. A *focus group* conducted by a skilled facilitator is one means of gaining an understanding of client and stakeholder perspectives about the process. That understanding may include what is valued and what is not; what is essential and what is not; what works and what does not. Focus groups can act as the initial unfreezing step in the process of change.

Brainstorming is a method that gives individuals permission to move outside their pre-existing frameworks. It results in the building of bigger and better ideas. A prompt for brainstorming may be to imagine that the hospital has been swallowed up by an earthquake and no longer exists. The redesign team has the opportunity to build new processes for a hospital about to be constructed. If mental boundaries still need to be loosened, the redesigners could be urged to think of the process as something completely different, such as a car. How would the engine sound? What would it look like from the outside? Or feel like on the inside?

Flow diagrams are an essential quality-improvement tool used by interactive planners, who diagram existing process as well as different ways of achieving goals of a redesigned process. The selection of the best process will likely be the one that reduces the number of steps and hand-offs, and the duplications and wait times, as well as the time it takes to get from beginning to end (sometimes referred to as the cycle time or turn-around time).

Other tools used in the redesign process are *Cause and Effect Fishbone Diagrams, Force Field Analysis,* and *Interrelationship Digraphs.* The reader interested in more information about these tools is advised to become familiar with materials published by the Juran Institute (see Early, 1989).

As a work redesign project is planned, an evaluation plan is also developed. Establishing an evaluation plan at the beginning allows planners to know what their milestones will be, what their trip wires will look like, and what data will be collected and analyzed by whom along the way. The evaluation is such an important piece of work process redesign that it needs to be addressed more fully.

PLANNING THE EVALUATION

It is a sad reality that organizations planning for change do not often include planning for evaluation. Managers and clinicians build evaluation into their research proposals, but do not transfer that practice to planning and evaluation of organizational change. One hears bizarre statements such as "We will evaluate when we finish," or "I will evaluate when I have solved all the problems." Failure to plan for evaluation at the time of planning for change eliminates the opportunity to learn from the process of the change. If clinicians were to evaluate only at the *end* of a patient's stay in hospital, they would miss many opportunities to provide appropriate clinical intervention along the way. Documenting performance to goals at the end of a patient's stay means not capturing whether that goal was achieved at day two, day four, or the last day of stay. These analogies hold true for organizational change and evaluation.

It makes good sense to plan the evaluation at the same time as the redesign. Markers of success can be determined, early warning signs of problems can be anticipated, and preventative steps taken. Measurement of indicators along with the associated data collection, analysis, and communication of results can be assigned.

Evaluation of organizational change is best done formatively—that is, as the change happens, not just at the end. Evaluating organizational change is not like conducting a randomized, controlled trial. The change happens in the course of people's daily work lives, and so the purpose of the evaluation is to inform the management of the process of change.

Declarative cause-and-effect statements cannot be made, but it is possible to comment on progress toward the desired end.

Planning of the evaluation means working with pen, paper, flip chart, and black board to begin making the evaluation plans visible. People planning the evaluation should be the same people who are designing and implementing the change. Why? These people are the "implementation planners" (Rovin, 1991). They are designing a process with which they will have to work on a daily basis. The problems will be theirs to identify and to resolve; the successes will be theirs to celebrate. Evaluation is not something to be handed off to another group who may be more expert at counting and calculating means. "Anyone who can follow a recipe, understand sports statistics, or read a map can use measurement on the job" (Townsend & Gebhardt, 1992, p. 209).

Although expert consultation may be sought along the way, and even for an extended period of time, the people involved with the change need to acquire the evaluation skills. This way, evaluation can be done not just during the introduction of change and but also at the end of change, and will continue indefinitely. Once the change process has become normal practice, staff will evaluate to determine whether the gains they made in redesign have held over time. When there is an opportunity in the future to reduce redundancies, shorten turn-around time, or increase throughput, the staff will evaluate again. Evaluation should occur at a predetermined frequency that provides staff with information for practice. If data are being "warehoused"—that is, collected, reported, but not acted on—staff need to question whether the data are needed. Staff ownership of evaluation is essential to accountability (Porter-O'Grady, 1996).

There is more than one way to evaluate change. Two approaches are presented here. The common feature to both approaches is a thorough understanding of the goal of the change, the purpose of the change, and the anticipated outcomes. Box 8.1 illustrates an approach that works well for process changes. The questions come from a work book that was designed to help staff develop evaluation plans step by step. The links between designing a new process and its evaluation are evident. If the design has been done thoroughly, the first four questions are already answered.

A second approach is to develop a program logic model (see Rush & Ogbourne, 1991 for a full discussion) with an evaluation matrix. The program-evaluation approach is useful when the change involves more than one process with multiple intersections (e.g., a change that includes new workers and new processes). The logic model requires that the set of activities in the program be identified, along with their respective implementation objectives, outputs, and short-term and long-term objectives. Once the model is complete, the evaluation matrix is developed. The matrix includes: objectives, questions, strategies for answering questions, tools for collecting data, data sources, analysis plan, and the communication plan. The toughest part of the matrix is determining answerable questions and then selecting the critical questions to answer. It will not be possible to answer all the questions; the reality for most implementation planners is that

Box 8.1

QUESTIONS TO GUIDE EVALUATION OF WORK PROCESS REDESIGN

Planning the evaluation: defining the action plan

What will the process accomplish?

- What is the aim of this process?
- Who will be the clients (suppliers, patients, providers, recipients) of this process?
- What are the features of this process that will be most important to its different clients?
- How will the new process work/flow? Create a diagram of this process.
- What are the other projects that could impact on the evaluation of this project?
- What are the other projects that could be affected by the evaluation of this project?
- What are the products, services, and information that will be produced as a result of the new process?
- What information is required for you to evaluate this change? What are the sources of the information? Is that information available to you?
- What changes or parts of the process carry the greatest risk to quality of care, quality of worklife, or to savings?

As we change the process, how will we know if it is an improvement?

- How will we recognize our success? (What will we see?) (If we could graph the change, what would be on the vertical axis and what would be on the horizontal axis?)
- What might be most important to measure relative to the output of this process?
- How will we track progress?
- What will be learned from the information harvested from this measurement?

- What may happen that we have not anticipated? What can we do to rapidly identify such an occurrence? Is there an early warning system?

What will be done, when, how, and by whom?

- Who will be most responsible for evaluating the change?
- When will the data be collected?
- How often will the data be collected?
- For how long will the data be collected?
- Where will the data be collected?
- Who will collect the data?
- Will data entry be immediate or delayed (by how long)? Will data entry be manual or automated? Who will be responsible for performing the data entry function?
- Who do we need to communicate progress to within the implementation unit and beyond the implementation unit?
- What resources (people, paper, tools, etc.) will we require?

What might we encounter while we are doing the pilot?

- What will help our team's evaluation? How can we capitalize on that help?
- What will hinder the evaluation? How can we overcome the hindrance?
- How will we collect information on things we did not anticipate happening?
- How will we know the plan was actually followed?
- How will we give recognition and celebrate progress?
- How will our team maintain the positive factors?
- How will our team minimize the negative factors?

Source: J. McIntosh and B. L. Lendrum, *A Workbook to Guide the Evaluation of Re-engineering Ideas* (Hamilton, ON: Chedoke-McMaster Hospitals, 1996). Reprinted with permission.

evaluation needs to be conducted in the course of daily work. A good screen to use in selecting questions that must be answered is to ask "Which questions address issues of high risk, high volume, or high cost?"

Just as the redesign group will want to test their idea for a redesigned process with other stakeholders in the hospital and community, they should also validate their evaluation plan. It is important to obtain a range of perspectives. It is useful to pay close attention to committed supporters and to nay-sayers. Nay-sayers will point out why the redesign will not work and will state why the evaluation plan has no merit. Criticisms like these are better attended to at the outset. Sceptics should also be included when the evaluation is planned. They may say that data sources are being missed, and that when the analysis is done the evidence will not be strong enough to demonstrate the usefulness of going ahead with the change. Considering a range of perspectives will help in the construction of a strong evaluation plan.

IMPLEMENTING THE PLAN

Planning is the operative word with redesign activities. Once the redesign and the evaluation have been planned, the implementation of the redesign project must also be planned. QI tools that help the implementation planning process include *activity network diagrams, flowcharts, gantt charts, matrix diagrams, tree diagrams*, and *process-decision program charts*. Planning the re-design, evaluation, and implementation are much more complex activities then actually implementing the plan. If the planning of all three phases has been thorough, the implementation should go well. However, there will always be events that were not anticipated. In planning the evaluation, the implementation planners should try to predict unanticipated events and determine ahead of time how they will be addressed.

Organizational redesign has little meaning for most people in the organization until it begins to affect their work life (Bridges, 1991). Implementation planners need to be aware of the transitions that will affect staff. They can anticipate experiences that staff will have, and suggest ways of responding to that experience in a timely and caring manner.

Communicating results of a redesign project throughout implementation is an important means of keeping stakeholders informed of progress toward goals. The communication has both an informational and a motivational purpose. Celebrations or acknowledgements at various milestones are a way of recognizing contributions toward the change. Once the goals of the change have been met, implementation planners will want to have a plan in place for maintaining the positive factors and minimizing the negative factors. The planners are then entering into their own continuous-quality improvement cycle, which spins off from the radical changes of redesign.

POLITICAL REALITIES OF CURRENT REDESIGN

Unlike the United States, where redesign is being done for competitive advantage in a market-driven healthcare system, redesign in Canada is being done to reduce the percentage of provincial budget dollars allocated to health care. Redesign features in the United States, such as multi-skilling of professionals and introduction of unlicensed assistive personnel, are a consequence of nursing shortages. In Canada, some of the same redesign features are being introduced to reduce salary costs, and others may be necessary as an anticipated nursing shortage materializes.

Redesign tends to be viewed with a different lens depending on the driving forces. Healthcare reform has long been needed in Canada. When the changes are viewed through a lens of budget cutting and job loss, however, health-care professionals worry about patient safety and their own futures. Reframing the changes as opportunities to begin health-care reform and create a more comprehensive, co-ordinated system might help professionals embrace the opportunities provided by redesign projects.

Opportunities that could emerge are:

1. **Creation of true interdisciplinary teams.** In such teams, each member's frame of reference is understood and valued by other team members, and the shared skill-set is much larger than that which currently exists in specialized practice silos (see Schweikhart and Smith-Daniels, 1996, for a discussion about the "focussed" team). The patient and family would ideally experience fewer hand-offs to others and greater co-ordination and continuity of care. Recent work on employee attitudes has resulted in recognition of interpersonal relationships as a motivational factor of the work environment (Rantz, Scott, & Porter, 1996). The implication for health care is that employees motivated by their interpersonal relationships will work on issues and problem-solving as a collective team and be predisposed to work with other teams.

   Team work across organizational boundaries would break down walls and could accomplish good for patients and for the health-care system. The shift would be one of emphasis and attention. Hospital care, because it is a sporadic event for most of the population, would play a supporting role to the community. Salaried primary-care providers working in health-service organizations would co-ordinate the team function across the system of care. Practice guidelines adopted by regional health authorities could be the tool for communicating timelines and performance expectations from the team of professionals. Hospital consultants would find themselves serving two sets of clients, the patient and family, and the primary-care providers. Communication with both sets of clients would be an important vehicle for continuity of care.

2. **A seamless system of care.** Patients want their health care to be co-ordinated and integrated and they want to experience continuity with

their transitions (Gerteis, Edgman-Levitan, Daley, & Delbanco, 1993). Care providers are often as frustrated as patients by the system's disrespect for patients and by their own productivity losses. Care management and case management offer partial solutions to co-ordination, integration, and continuity. A full solution would mean examining the process of care within and beyond the hospital, reducing redundancies, wait times, and hand-offs while increasing communication, efficiency, and caring.

3. **Development and assignment of assistive personnel to enhance patient care.** The work of nurses has always included work that could be done by people other than nurses (Davis, 1982). In the current budget-cutting climate, new workers who do non-nursing work may not be welcome. Reframing their introduction as a means of enhancing the patient experience is positive and worthwhile. New roles may combine the work of several different job classifications (Marshall, 1995; Pischke-Winn & Minnick, 1996; Trerise & Lemieux-Charles, 1996) and thereby reduce human-resource system redundancies and costs. When the new role results in a decentralization of support services, hand-offs to other workers are reduced, as are wait times. From the patient's perspective, the number of interactions with different service providers is reduced. When scheduling of the new role matches the peaks and valleys of service demands on a unit, or program, clients may be better served, and professional staff better supported.

As a new role for assistive personnel (sometimes called multi-skilled workers) is introduced, it is important to align the responsibilities of the new role with the knowledge, skills, and abilities required to perform the role. If clinical judgement is required, a clinician should perform the function. Introduction of new workers will require changes in ways existing workers conduct their work. Training sessions on communication, teamwork, delegation, and work-flow analysis may be helpful. The arrival of new workers can create opportunities to engage in team renewal. The articles by Pischke-Winn and Minnick (1996) and by Trerise and Lemieux-Charles (1996) provide useful summaries of lessons that have been learned when introducing multi-skilled workers.

CONCLUSION

Redesign is hard work intended to improve quality and increase efficiency. It may lead to the loss of existing jobs as new and fewer jobs are created. It will mean, at the outset, the disintegration of familiar work patterns and social relationships. Although healthcare professionals may value the outcomes of work process redesign for their patients, they may, while participating in a redesign project, feel like victims of a social experiment. An evaluation of the early days of change in one organization (Lendrum & Hastie, 1997) revealed that staff quality of work life had changed. People struggling with the change expressed concern about the persistent threat of losing jobs, about seeing colleagues lose jobs, and about the stresses associated with working with colleagues who were similarly worried. Others were glad to experience the growth in their new jobs, and thought their clinical skills would be used more effectively and clients served much better.

SUMMARY

- Work process redesign is a fundamental change in the way work is organized and carried out. It often takes place with, or following, organizational restructuring. However, redesign changes are not immediately visible to the public. Unlike restructuring initiatives, process redesign changes are not generally the subject of press releases. However, patients or clients who experience care in organizations where processes have been redesigned recognize the benefits and improvements if redesign efforts have been successful.
- Work process redesign provides a framework within which intentional communication occurs to inform process performers about how well clients' goals are being met. In health organizations, front-line nursing managers will sit with front-line service managers to review performance that is measured, reported, and acted upon. "Process owners" will be responsible for connecting with their peers to examine quality of care and service at the points where various processes intersect.
- Work process redesign has the potential to enable primary nurses and case managers to influence the process of care beyond the walls of the unit, and across organizational boundaries. Their concerns can be directed to their front-line manager, who will have a legitimate forum to raise and resolve work process issues.

ACKNOWLEDGEMENT

Grateful acknowledgement is extended to colleagues who critiqued the manuscript for this chapter: Lorine Besel, Nancy Carter, Stephanie MacArthur, Shelley Marshall, Janis North, and Jan Park Dorsay.

FURTHER READINGS AND RESOURCES

Borzo, G. (1992) Patient-focused hospitals reporting good results. *Strategic Management, 10*(8), 17–24.

O'Malley, J., & Llorente, B. (1990). Back to the future: Redesigning the workplace. *Nursing Management, 21*(10), 46–48.

Weber, D.O. (1991). Six models of patient-focused care. *Health Care Forum Journal, 34*(4), 23–31.

REFERENCES

Ackoff, R. L. (1981). *Creating the corporate future.* New York: John Wiley & Sons.

Berwick, D.M., Godfrey, A.B., & Roessner, J. (1990). *Curing health care: New strategies for quality improvement.* San Francisco: Jossey-Bass.

Bridges, W. (1991). *Managing transitions: Making the most of change.* Reading, MA: Addison-Wesley.

Boulerice, M. (1994). Quality Management: From QA to TQM. In J. M. Hibberd & M.E. Kyle (Eds.), *Nursing management in Canada* (pp. 250–269). Toronto: W.B. Saunders.

Clark, L., Cudmore, J., Hammons, D., Holt, A., Hunt, M., McIntosh, J., & Watts, J. (1995). *Quality improvement: Ensuring care and service for the clients of CMH.* Hamilton, ON: Chedoke-McMaster Hospitals.

Davis, K. (1982) Non-nursing functions: Our readers respond. *American Journal of Nursing, 82* (12), 1857–1860.

Early, J.F. (Ed.) (1989). *Quality improvement tools.* Wilton, CT: Juran Institute.

Gaucher, E.J., & Coffey, R.J. (1993). *Total quality in health care: From theory to practice.* San Francisco: Jossey-Bass.

Gerteis, M., Edgman-Levitan, S., Daley, J., & Delbanco, T.L. (1993). *Through the patient's eyes: Understanding and promoting patient-centred care.* San Francisco: Jossey-Bass.

Hammer, M., & Champy, J. (1993). *Reengineering the corporation: A manifesto for business revolution.* New York: Harper Business.

Hammer, M. (1996). *Beyond reengineering.* New York: Harper Business.

Lathrop, J.P. (1993). *Restructuring health care: The patient focused paradigm.* San Francisco: Jossey-Bass.

Lendrum, B. L. & Hastie, J. (1997). *Summary of the qualitative analysis of the early days reports from the first roll-out units.* Hamilton, ON: Hamilton Health Sciences Corporation.

Lendrum, B.L. (1994). Organization of patient care. In J. M. Hibberd & M. E. Kyle (Eds.), *Nursing management in Canada* (pp. 312–330). Toronto: W.B. Saunders.

Marshall, K. (1995). Multi-skilling—Re-engineering work process. *Health Management Forum, 8* (2), 32–36.

McIntosh, J., & Lendrum, B. L. (1996). *A workbook to guide the evaluation of re-engineering ideas.* Hamilton, ON: Chedoke-McMaster Hospitals.

McPhail, J. (1991). Organization for nursing care: Primary nursing, traditional approaches, or both? In J. Kerr & J. McPhail (Eds.), *Canadian nursing issues and perspectives* (2nd ed.) (pp. 179–188). Toronto: McGraw-Hill Ryerson.

Pischke-Winn, K., & Minnick, A. (1996). Lessons learned from introducing a multitask environmental worker program. *Journal of Nursing Administration, 26* (6), 31–38.

Porter-O'Grady, T. (1996). The seven basic rules for successful redesign. *Journal of Nursing Administration, 26* (1), 46–53.

Rantz, M.J., Scott, J., & Porter, R. (1996). Employee motivation: New perspectives of the age-old challenge of work motivation. *Nursing Forum, 31* (3), 29–36.

Rovin S., (1991). The process of planning. In S. Rovin & L. Ginsberg (Eds.), *Managing hospitals: Lessons from the Johnson & Johnson-Wharton Fellows program in management for nurses* (pp. 3–38). San Francisco: Jossey-Bass.

Rush, B., & Ogbourne, A. (1991). Program logic models: Expanding their role and structure for program planning and evaluation. *The Canadian Journal of Program Evaluation, 6* (2), 95–106.

Schweikhart, S., & Smith Daniels, V. (1996). Reengineering the work of caregivers: Role redefinition, team structures, and organization redesign. *Hospital & Health Services Administration, 41* (1), 19–36.

Taylor, F.W. (1912). *The principles of scientific management.* New York: Harpers.

Townsend, P.L., & Gebhardt, J.E. (1992). *Quality in action: 93 lessons in leadership, participation, and measurement.* Toronto: John Wiley & Sons.

Trerise, B., & Lemieux-Charles, L. (1996). An assessment of the introduction of a multi-skilled worker into an acute care setting. *Health Management Forum, 9* (3), 43–48.

Chapter 9

▼▼▼▼▼▼▼▼▼▼▼▼▼▼

Service Integration and Case Management

JANE E. SMITH AND DONNA LYNN SMITH

KEY OBJECTIVES

In this chapter, you will learn:

- Ways in which organizational factors, professional boundaries and a variety of funding mechanisms can contribute to fragmentation and lack of integration among health services.
- Why clients with complex, long-term needs are particularly susceptible to the problems arising from fragmented delivery systems.
- Some of the issues involved in defining case management and why a client-centred definition is desirable.
- Factors that influence the way case management services are designed and implemented.
- Some of the elements of a case manager's role and some reasons why the role may differ from one setting to another.
- Similarities and differences between the nursing process and the process of case management.
- Similarities and differences between the traditional role of a first-line manager and a case manager.
- About the evolution of case management and its current importance within the Canadian health system.

INTRODUCTION

People who need health and human services are often faced with a bewildering array of service providers and arrangements. They must often find the services they need through a process of trial and error, in a system where such services are delivered in many different programs, provided by different health professionals, and funded or paid for in a variety of ways. The more complex a person's health or social problems become, the more difficult it may be for them to obtain access to services or to move from one service, provider, or location to another. Vulnerable client groups are particularly susceptible to the problems arising from fragmented service-delivery systems and multiple payors. Gaps and duplications in the service-delivery system and in the care of individuals and their families can be a source of inefficiency, added costs, and sometimes of mistakes. One goal of health reform is to achieve better integration of services and to assure that people are directed to the right care provider or service at the right time, and in the location or service setting most appropriate to their needs.

Case management is a process and a professional service that can help to achieve the goal of more integrated and cost-effective care. The role, skills, and organizational base of the case manager are best determined by the needs and characteristics of various client groups whose needs are sufficiently complex to warrant case management services. In this chapter, case management is introduced from a historical perspective and is also examined in current contexts, so that leaders and managers in the health system can assess its appropriateness and potential benefit for the client groups they serve.

WHAT IS CASE MANAGEMENT?

The term "case management" arose in an earlier era, and today the term itself presents some problems. One client reminded health professionals that it is care that needs managing, not clients, by stating, "We're not cases and you're not managers" (Everett & Nelson, 1992, p. 60). In response to this concern, many health professionals and organizations now describe case management in a more client-centred way, preferring terms such as "care co-ordination," "service co-ordination," and "care management." The generic term "case management" is used in this chapter because it continues to provide a convenient entry point to the professional literature on the subject.

DEFINING CASE MANAGEMENT

Case management is a generic term with multiple definitions. It has been said that "Case management ... derives its definition in large part from the nature and needs of a system whose component parts it will be co-ordinating and integrating ... it must be a creature of its environment, tuned to the specific characteristics and needs of its host system"(Beatrice, 1981, p. 124). For example, Austin (1993) defines case management as "an intervention whereby a human-service professional arranges and monitors an optimum package of long-term care services" (p. 452). In a slightly different vein, the American Public Welfare Association describes it as the "brokering and co-ordination of the multiple social health, education, and employment services necessary to promote self-sufficiency and strengthen family life" (cited in Pearlmutter & Johnson, 1996, p. 179). The Case Management Society of America (1994) describes case management as "a collaborative process which assesses, plans, implements, co-ordinates, monitors and evaluates options and services to meet an individual's health needs through communications and available resources to promote quality cost-effective outcomes" (p. 60). Intagliata (1982) states that case management is "a process or method for ensuring that consumers are provided with whatever services they need in a co-ordinated, effective and efficient manner" (p. 657). Geron and Chassler (1994) define case management as "a service that links and co-ordinates assistance from both paid providers and unpaid help from family and friends to enable consumers with chronic functional and/or cognitive limitations to obtain the highest level of independence consistent with their capacity and their preference for care" (p. v). While these definitions have commonalities, they also illustrate some differences in perspective.

In this chapter case management is defined as a professional service that attempts to prevent people from "falling through the cracks" of health and human service systems. It is a process intended to facilitate access to services, and includes assessment, planning, co-ordination, delivery, and monitoring of the services that are provided to individuals and families. By assuring that these services are appropriate and accountable, case managers contribute to positive health outcomes and cost-effectiveness in the service-delivery system. The degree of integration in any health and human services system can be improved if increased continuity of attention is provided to clients and families as they make their way across the boundaries that separate programs, service settings, care providers and geographic locations where services are provided. Ideally, a single case manager would assist a client or family throughout an entire episode of illness, or through the many transitions that must be navigated by people who require support over long periods of time because of chronic illness or disability.

ORIGINS OF CASE MANAGEMENT

Many disciplines have contributed to the evolution of case management practice. At the turn of the century, nurses implemented public health programs and visiting nurse services, and Lillian Ward established the Henry Street Settlement for individuals requiring home care. Family physicians also arranged and co-ordinated services for patients requiring care, and in the 1940s, the American worker's compensation board inaugurated a more formal approach to medical case management (Henderson & Collard, 1988). Community-based social work can be traced back to groups of ministers in the 1830s, charity boards in the late nineteenth century, and settlement houses in the early twentieth century (Austin & McClelland, 1996).

In the mid-1970s, the term "case management" began to be used in North America to refer to a formal process through which professionals responded to the needs of the mentally ill, the aged, and other groups for whom services were fragmented or unavailable. De-institutionalization of the mentally ill in the 1950s had resulted in the discharge of these clients into communities that were unprepared to meet their needs. Problems escalated as these clients attempted to access a network of services that was highly complex, fragmented, duplicative, and uncoordinated (Intagliata, 1982). At the same time, long-term care for the elderly in nursing homes was becoming too expensive for the aged population, whose numbers were rapidly growing, and community-based models were developed to address this issue (Austin, 1996). In the late 1970s, the role of case manager was usually filled by social workers, who were working with the mentally ill and the aged in the community.

By the mid-1980s, case management had become prominent in hospital-based systems in the United States as one approach to containing the escalating costs of high-tech health care. A nursing case management model at the New England Medical Centre Hospitals (NEMCH) in the early 1980s is generally credited with inaugurating the practice of case management by nurses in acute-care settings. This model incorporated critical paths (Zander, 1988) and became a prototype for many subsequent hospital-based case management initiatives, including one at the Toronto Hospital (Lamb, Deber, Naylor, & Hastings, 1991).

Case management continues to be used to co-ordinate services for people with mental health needs and the elderly living in the community, as well as other client populations with complex health and rehabilitation needs. The role has expanded into home care and other human-service settings, such as worker's compensation, child welfare programs, and the justice system. More recently, persons with AIDS; people with substance-abuse problems; victims of spinal-cord, brain, and other traumatic injuries; and children with developmental disabilities have also received case management services.

There are powerful financial incentives to control costs by restricting access to high-cost services, and to improve hospital-utilization management by achieving early discharge. For these reasons, the benefits of case management have received increasing recognition from insurance companies as well as health-care institutions.

CORE COMPONENTS

Although today numerous definitions of case management exist, there is widespread agreement about the core activities in the case management process. These are:

1. **Targeting:**   Case management services begin by identifying, or targeting, individuals who need case management services. Clients are usually people with complex, long-term needs, requiring a variety of services over an extended period of time. Not all clients require case management services and case management can be expensive. Therefore, targeting case management services to those clients most likely to benefit from them is particularly important.

2. **Assessment:**   Assessment requirements vary among organizations, and can include measurement of the physical, cognitive, psychosocial,

functional, and financial status, as well as the caregiver support system. An in-depth assessment provides the information necessary to determine needs and service priorities. When an interdisciplinary team is involved, assessments can become repetitive and sometimes exhausting for clients. The goal should be to develop an integrated, interdisciplinary assessment in which information needed by all participating disciplines is gathered only once to create a cumulative data base that is specific to each client.

3. **Care planning:**   Information gathered in the assessment phase is formulated into a multidisciplinary care plan that indicates how each of the identified needs will be met. A working knowledge of services and resources is required at this stage.

4. **Implementation:**   At this stage, formal and informal providers are contacted to arrange needed services. The case manager authorizes services, allocates resources, and co-ordinates service delivery.

5. **Monitoring:**   Monitoring ensures that services are achieving the agreed-upon goals and are available as required by the client. This is particularly important in case management, as clients are usually dependent on services over long periods of time. Ongoing contact with the client enables the case manager to respond quickly, as needs and priorities change.

6. **Reassessment:**   A client's needs for case management services change over time. During the reassessment process the case manager determines what services are still needed, and makes any necessary changes to the care plan in consultation with those receiving and providing services.

The nature of case management is shaped by: each client's needs and circumstances; the availability of resources in the community; the worker to client ratio; the system of case management; the education and background of case managers; the budgets of service agencies; and organizational structure. Ideally, the case manager will work proactively with each client and/or family to develop a realistic and attainable service plan. The core activities of case management can be adapted in response to differences among client groups, organizational changes, environmental influences, and fiscal requirements.

THE ROLE OF THE CASE MANAGER

The case manager in today's health system requires wide-angled lenses if he or she is to serve as an effective link between the client and the service-delivery system. Role descriptions for case managers vary considerably because the objectives, goals, and mission of an organization are taken into account as the case management process and role are defined. The goal of case management in an integrated system is to provide the client with continuity, consistency, and co-ordination of care across service settings and boundaries, to assist the client with daily coping skills, and to advocate for resources that are unavailable in the community.

At present, hospital-based case management and community-based case management are the two main areas of practice, and although both have some common goals, there are also some differences in the approaches used. These two management areas have the following features in common:

- promoting interdisciplinary practice among health professionals;
- ensuring that all participating care providers co-ordinate and collaborate in their efforts to meet the goals of the care plan as efficiently as possible;
- promoting quality care for the client; and
- ensuring the appropriate and efficient use of resources and services.

Hospital and community-based case management often differ in the following respects:

- **The duration of care.**   Hospital-based case management has usually been limited to co-ordination of services during the episode of care or immediately afterward. Care plans developed for clients with complex needs in the community must often provide for case management and certain other services to continue for a longer period and, sometimes, indefinitely.
- **The standardization of care.**   The overall plan of care in hospital-based case management (which is sometimes called a care map or a clinical pathway) is standardized from pre-admission to discharge, although it may sometimes be individualized to reflect some preferences of individual physicians or the programmatic interests of some service providers. Case management plans for community care are usually developed individually after in-depth assessments, and the goals, objectives and service plan are more likely to be developed with the involvement of the client and family.

The degree of integration within hospital- or community-based case management systems may vary considerably. From the client's perspective, a high degree of integration within either of these two sectors is desirable, and the integration of hospital and community services with each other is even more important.

The role of a case manager encompasses wide and diverse responsibilities. Some of these are summarized in Box 9.1.

A case manager's actual activities "are shaped ultimately by the constraints of the environment within which they work, not by their formal job descriptions" (Intagliata, 1982, p. 670). Today case managers come from a variety of professional backgrounds including nursing, social work, rehabilitation therapies, and medicine. In many instances, family members or informal caregivers act as case managers without the support of a case management service.

QUALIFICATIONS AND EDUCATION FOR THE ROLE OF CASE MANAGER

Comprehensive case management practice requires professionals with the knowledge and skills to work with clients who have complex needs,

---

Box 9.1
ROLES AND RESPONSIBILITIES
OF A CASE MANAGER

---

1. **Clinical Expert** provides in-depth assessment, care planning, and consultation regarding the client's needs and issues

2. **Facilitator** eases the client's interaction with the system

3. **Liaison** brings services/resources to the client/family level

4. **Supporter** promotes the client's confidence in becoming the "insider expert" (Lamb & Stempel, 1994) of his or her own care

5. **Educator** provides information so that the client/family can make informed decisions

6. **Researcher** identifies areas of concern and initiates research to aid in the development of evidence-based practice

7. **Negotiator** intercedes and/or brings problems to the attention of others so that change can be initiated

8. **Monitor** ensures that the client and services are doing what they have agreed to do, and identifies problems, gaps, and/or necessary changes at an early stage

9. **Advocate** provides support and/or assists the client to identify goals and objectives that ensure a client-driven plan of care

10. **Manager** develops care plans that are creative and innovative

---

within existing bureaucratic and organizational service systems. Kanter (1989), for example, recognized the need for case managers to have generic interdisciplinary training augmented by years of continuing education and clinical supervision. All members of an interdisciplinary team contribute their expertise to enhance the appropriateness, quality, and co-ordination of services provided.

As the importance of the case manager role becomes more widely recognized, educational requirements are changing. Many case managers have acquired the specialized knowledge and skills they require through a combination of on-the-job experience and in-service education provided by their organizations. More recently, structured continuing-education and certificate programs in case management have been established.

It is becoming increasingly obvious that the specialized knowledge and skills required by case managers should be built upon a foundation of professional education in a health or human-service discipline. Many organizations and health agencies now require, as prerequisites for the case management role, a minimum standard of a baccalaureate degree and relevant clinical experience with the client group to be served. Cronin & Maklebust (1989) describe a project at the Detroit Medical Centre in which BScN-prepared nurses piloted the role of case manager. It was found that although the nurses reported an increase in the quality of care provided and increased job satisfaction, they felt ill-prepared to collaborate and delegate with their level of educational preparation. The next project in this setting was successfully initiated with Master's-prepared nurses.

Authors of the most recent literature on case management believe that practitioners with advanced skills, such as Clinical Nurse Specialists or professionals prepared at the Master's level, are best qualified to be case managers. Educational institutions are now developing case management education at the graduate level. For example, the University of San Francisco has recently implemented a Master's program that focusses on the case management needs of older people (Haw, 1995).

MODELS OF CASE MANAGEMENT

The rapid growth in popularity of case management has resulted in a profusion of models and frameworks of case management practice. In their classic discussion, Applebaum and Austin (1990) identified three types of models that are differentiated from one another by the way the roles of case managers are structured. In "brokerage" models, case managers serve as links between consumers and the system, making referrals and allocating services but not providing or monitoring care, and not allocating funds. These models are widely used with insurance and private practices. Case managers in "service management" models are fiscally responsible for the care plans they develop, although they may not provide services directly to the client. In "managed care" models, a major focus for case managers is to keep costs below a capitated payment. Providers are pre-paid a specific amount and are at risk for any excess costs. More recently, a "generalist model," in which one case manager performs a majority of case management activities, has been described by Roberts-DeGennaro (1993).

Case management models can also be differentiated from one another in terms of the settings or programs out of which they have developed. Desimone (1988) described seven types of case management models. "Social case management," geared to a relatively healthy population, is a multidisciplinary approach used to delay hospitalization by emphasizing long-term community care services. In "primary care case management," the physician has traditionally assumed the role of gate-keeper to services. The "medical/social" model focuses on the long-term client, co-ordinating health and social resources, both formal and informal, in the community. "Health Maintenance Organization" (HMO) models co-ordinate a limited number of services to treat an episode of illness. "Independent (private) case management" services have evolved to meet the needs of clients outside the publicly funded systems of care. "Insurance case management," usually a pre-paid service, includes an incentive to manage costs of service. "In-house case management" refers to models developed by internal or intra-facility settings within an institution or organization.

Distinctions can also be made between case management models that involve working within specific program settings, and those that are intended to bridge many settings. More and Mandell (1997) have used the term "internal case management" to describe models in which a case manager is employed within a single health-care organization or facility, such as an acute-care hospital, a rehabilitation program, or a home-care program. In contrast, "external case management" takes place outside the health-care network. External case managers may work for insurance companies, worker's compensation programs, and private companies. Cohen and Cesta (1997) classified models of case management as "within the walls" (tertiary-care settings such as acute-care hospitals) and "beyond the walls" (primary-care settings such as community/home care). Numerous examples in the literature illustrate how core activities of care may be applied in a variety of settings.

In the past decade, the nursing profession has become actively involved in the development of models for case management. Pelletier and Blouin (1990) define nursing case management as "a system of patient care which strategically positions nursing and recognizes the key role nursing plays in the allocation of resources, consumer perceptions and the overall profitability of health-care organizations" (p. 55). Lamb (1992) identifies three categories of nursing case management models: hospital-based models; hospital-to-community models; and community-based models.

The nursing literature provides a number of examples of programs with a nursing case management focus, and several of these are included in the reference list for this chapter (Brett & Tonges, 1990; Gibson, Martin, Johnson, Blue & Miller, 1994; Olivas, Del Togno-Armanasco, Erickson, & Harter, 1989; Ethridge & Lamb, 1989). Such publications indicate a growing recognition of the role case management can play in the integration of nursing care with other services across more than one setting.

CASE MANAGEMENT AND NURSING

Some authors have drawn parallels between case management and the nursing process. Both involve the application of knowledge and skills in a systematic approach to assessing and managing clients' health needs. While the two processes have these and some other elements in common, it is important to recognize that the process of planning for, obtaining, co-ordinating, and monitoring services provided in a succession of settings, by more than one agency, and through more than one funding avenue, is a vastly more complex function than that of developing care plans for one or more individuals within a single unit, program or agency.

In a number of contemporary textbooks on nursing administration, case management is presented as a way of organizing or assigning nurses' work. It is described in conjunction with other care-delivery models such as functional, team, and primary nursing (Lendrum 1994), and the progression from primary nursing to case management is often depicted as a logical evolutionary step. Case management is touted, as other care delivery models have been in the past, as a way of enabling nurses to achieve their full potential as professionals.

Case management may indeed provide a convenient approach to the organization or assignment of nurses' work, and some of the precepts of primary nursing can certainly be applied to case management. However, it is important to note that there are some crucial differences between the organization of nursing work and the process of case management. For example, in hospital-based primary nursing the primary nurse's accountability usually extends only to the point of the client's discharge from that unit. If the client is transferred to another area in the same hospital, a new primary nurse would normally be assigned, thus breaking the continuity of care. A primary nurse based in a hospital-care unit is not typically expected or empowered to remain involved with the client after discharge.

Those involved in home-care programs are often assumed to be more aware of the need for co-ordination and continuity of care than those employed in hospitals, and many home-care professionals take pride in incorporating a case management model. When examined closely, however, home-care and hospital-based case management may prove to be more similar than different. The work of home-care nurses is not necessarily structured so that they can act as primary nurses or case managers for their clients. In home-care programs, the case management function is often limited to planning care and co-ordinating and monitoring personnel from a single agency, or to co-ordinating services provided by health professionals, or to gate-keeping and resource management. The actual care received in the home by a single individual or family may be delivered by several different workers, disciplines and agencies, and the overall provision of care may, therefore, be as task-oriented and fragmented as that provided in hospitals.

Fragmentation in the health and human services system is taken for granted to such an extent that if discharge or other service arrangements fail, professionals have not traditionally been held accountable, or expected to take responsibility for preventing or rectifying problems outside of their own program setting. Ironically, while it is assumed that professionals working within one setting cannot be held responsible for assuring continuity of care when clients move to other settings, it is also assumed that clients and their families can navigate the system on their own without the benefit of "insider" knowledge!

One of the central differences between the role of a nurse in primary nursing and the role of a case manager is a difference in perspective, in which the emphasis shifts from a single episode of illness in one setting to the co-ordination of services over the entire episode of illness and/or disability (Smith & Smith, 1997). Case management can be viewed as an enlargement of the role of primary nurse to include a broader range of assessment, care planning, and other skills. Nursing has an historic tradition of providing and co-ordinating highly skilled care, 24 hours a day, in many settings. Therefore, nurses are often seen as particularly suited for case management roles. Professional experience in settings where primary nursing or some other accountability-oriented model of care delivery has been implemented, and in settings where interdisciplinary teamwork has been valued and required, provides nurses with a strong foundation upon which to build the additional skills required to practice in a case management role within an integrated service-delivery system.

CASE MANAGEMENT AND TRADITIONAL MANAGEMENT ROLES

Generally speaking, when roles are designated as "managerial," it is because they incorporate responsibility for the hiring, supervision, and discipline or termination of employees, as well as either shared or direct accountability for the expenditure and management of financial resources. Managerial work is also distinguished from other types of work in terms of the amount of discretionary decision-making, personal initiative, and problem-solving that is expected.

Case management involves responsibility for individual clients and groups of clients, but it also usually includes responsibilities at the level of programs, organizations, or service-delivery systems. A case management role that focusses on gate-keeping, care planning, or clinical activities may require superior organizational skills, but may not be designated as a management position if it does not entail responsibility for supervising staff or managing a budget. However, it has already been noted that the effectiveness with which gate-keeping and utilization management functions are carried out will have a direct effect on expenditures. Some case management roles incorporate responsibility for obtaining, training, supervising, and evaluating the workers who will deliver direct services, whereas others may involve only authorization and payment for direct services provided by collaborating agencies. When case managers are accountable for managing human and financial resources, using skills that would not normally be needed by professionals acting in a clinical capacity, their jobs may be defined as managerial.

When case managers function in situations where there is a high level of ambiguity and uncertainty, the decision-making dilemmas they face in locating and mobilizing services for clients with complex needs may be as complex as those faced by managers in more conventional roles. The noted organizational theorist, Charles Perrow, has used the term "unanalysable search" to describe the requirement for high level discretionary decision-making in some professional roles (Perrow, 1970, p 83). There is clearly a high requirement for personal initiative, high-level communications skills—including the ability to influence others—and discretionary decision-making in case management roles, where many boundaries must be crossed in the process of locating, co-ordinating, and monitoring services provided by many different disciplines and workers from a variety of programs, organizations, and geographic locations. Clinical Nurse Specialists and other professionals whose highly specialized knowledge and skills equip them for boundary spanning and discretionary decision making often have their positions classified within the management stream of the organizations in which they work. Case management roles may also be defined as advanced practice managerial positions, for this reason.

Grisham, White, & Miller (1983) distinguished among case management models by depicting their placement on a continuum, depending on the level of authority and responsibility of the case manager. They suggested that case management services are not present when each health professional controls some of the resources, and is independently responsible for the services he or she provides. The intensity of case management service changes as authority and responsibility for total client care and financial resources increases. Clearly, case management roles vary in complexity and other dimensions. Therefore, the extent to which a case manager's role has elements in common with more traditional managerial roles depends upon the authority, accountability, and discretionary decision making expected of a case manager within a particular organizational context.

Managers at various levels in the health and human services system may find it helpful to their understanding of the role of a case manager to compare it with other specialist roles that cut across functional or departmental boundaries to accomplish defined tasks. As work redesign efforts (such as those described in Chapter 8 of this book) are undertaken by health and human service organizations, it may become more common to design roles in which case managers are empowered to act as client-centred advocates, facilitating the transitions that clients make across the boundaries within or between disciplines, departments, programs and service settings.

CASE MANAGEMENT IN THE CANADIAN HEALTH SYSTEM

Since the introduction of the Hospital and Diagnostic Services Act in 1957 and the National Medicare Insurance Act in 1966, Canada has had a "single payer" for hospital and physician services through its universal health insurance system. In the Canadian health system the availability of universal public insurance coverage of hospital and medical services has created incentives for overuse of the acute-care sector of the health system. Not surprisingly, Canada lagged behind Scandinavian countries and Britain in developing and funding such services as home care, community mental health, and community-based home and family support services.

In the last two decades, chronic mental and physical illnesses have been more widely recognized and effectively treated, and the Canadian population has aged. These developments have created a need for services not provided by doctors or in hospitals. In response to this growing need, a variety of services have been developed under the auspices of religious and voluntary groups, community organizations and other not-for-profit organizations, as well as by businesses that market health and personal-care services. Some agencies provide their services free of charge; others charge fees based on clients' ability to pay; while others require full payment, either directly or via private insurance plans. The more vulnerable people are, or the more complex their health or social problems, the more likely they are to need these community-based services. The problems created by a scarcity of these community services, and the economic benefit of using such services where appropriate in place of higher cost, medically oriented care, have been well documented (Angus, Auer, & Cloutier, 1995).

Case management services in Canada were first widely utilized in the area of mental health. Goering and colleagues conducted a number of studies of mentally ill clients in a community-outreach program in Toronto, Ontario. They found that, although the rate of hospitalization did not change, clients in the program had higher occupational functioning (Goering, Wasylenki, Farkas, Lancee, & Ballantyne, 1988a), improved role performance (Goering, Farkas, Wasylenki, Lancee, & Ballantyne, 1988b), and decreased gender differences in social skills, supportive networks, and housing conditions (Goering, Wasylenki, St. Onge, Paduchak, & Lancee, 1992).

In an intensive case management program in the Waterloo region of Ontario, Nelson, Sadler, and Cragg (1995) found differences in the hospitalization rates of clients who had received case management services. The study associated these rates with the ratio of clients to case managers, program philosophy, and the availability of hospital beds.

Mercier and Racine (1995) surveyed 25 homeless women with substance-abuse problems in Montreal to determine the frequency, type, nature, and location of the contacts that case managers had with these women. They found that developing and maintaining a significant relationship with the clients constituted a major part of the case manager's work. A high staff-to-client ratio was necessary to respond adequately to the multiple needs of homeless people. This conclusion is supported by Pyke, Clark and Walters (1991), who suggest three themes in providing case management services to clients with long-term mental illness: (a) the relationship between the case manager and the client is essential; (b) the case manager must respect the client's values and choices; and (c) the case manager must keep in mind that he or she has a number of clients—including not only the client, but also the client's informal and formal networks. When seventeen nurses practising case management in publicly supported community-based agencies across Canada were interviewed, they placed high value on nurse-client relationships (Rheaume, Frisch, Smith, & Kennedy, 1994).

In the past two decades, case management services have expanded into other areas of health and human services, as the shift to community care continues. Most health regions in Canada will be forced to provide services that were once provided within institutions at lower cost in community settings. Given the diverse demographics in Canada, case managers will require advanced educational programs to prepare them with the knowledge, skills, and cultural competency necessary for this complex role.

The trends toward program management and work redesign in Canadian hospitals has been motivated to a large degree by the need to improve utilization management and reduce costs. All provinces have taken measures to restrict health spending, and these have curtailed the availability of hospital services and created financial incentives for hospitals to screen and restrict admissions, shorten lengths of stay, and discharge clients to their homes or community services even when they still have extensive health-care needs. This means that clients will assume many of the costs of the services, drugs, and supplies that were formerly provided to them without charge in or by hospitals. One outcome of these trends has already been that the number and variety of non-insured services available has increased, particularly those provided by the for-profit sector. These contextual developments help to explain why the need for case management services in Canada is now greater than ever before.

MOVING TOWARD INTEGRATED SERVICES

Clients with complex needs require continuity of attention, and unnecessary costs can often be avoided if case management services are provided. To achieve service integration, or what is often wistfully referred to as a "seamless system," it is desirable that a single case manager (or a case management team) works on behalf of clients and their families to assess their needs on an ongoing basis, and to assist them to obtain, plan, co-ordinate, and monitor services for as long as they are needed, irrespective of the client's location within the system. When this is not possible, incentives and procedural mechanisms to improve the accountability of one service provider or program for what happens in the next program or care setting can help to make incremental improvements in the continuity or care and integration of services. The case examples at the end of this chapter in Box 9.2 illustrate recent initiatives for improving the integration of services.

CONCLUSION

Although research about case management has mainly been focused on cost savings, early indications also indicate other positive outcome measures. Health care becomes more cost-effective as duplication and mistakes in services are reduced. Proactive care leads to early intervention and prevention of costly complications. As clients become more confident in a responsive, proactive community-based care system, hospital utilization is reduced. Increased client confidence can, in turn, lead to a reduction in family burnout and stronger, longer lasting, informal networks. This can result in decreased usage of the health-care system by family members as they experience decreased physical and emotional symptoms of burnout (Smith & Smith, 1997).

SUMMARY

- Clients with complex, long-term needs are particularly susceptible to the problems arising from fragmented delivery systems.

Box 9.2
CASE EXAMPLES: CURRENT INITIATIVES FOR IMPROVING THE INTEGRATION OF SERVICES

1. Development of a Care Map for Transurethral Resection of the Prostate

This article describes the development of a care map that was designed to deliver a continuum of care between hospital and community services in Edmonton, Alberta. The development and implementation of this care map required extensive collaboration, planning and evaluation by members of many professions from a variety of different program and service settings. (Raiwet, C., Halliwell, G., Andruski, L., & Wilson, D. (1997) Care maps across the continuum. *The Canadian Nurse* 93(1), 26-30.

2. Integrating Care for Clients From the Westview Health Region Who Have Joint Replacement Surgery

The Westview Health Region serves a number of communities extending from the municipal boundaries of the City of Edmonton to Jasper, Alberta. Area team leaders located in the various communities in the region are responsible for managing and co-ordinating the client-care services in their respective communities. These area team leaders report to a regional director of health services.

Any client from the region who requires joint replacement surgery is referred to one of two tertiary-care hospitals in Edmonton. A care co-ordination process and a care map are developed to assure that integrated service is provided to these clients. The intake co-ordinator of the Westview Home Care Program monitors the wait-list of clients for joint replacement surgery, and makes contact with the

clients to begin gathering the information needed to plan their care. When surgery has been booked, the client attends a pre-admission clinic and a data base from which to develop a discharge plan and follow-up care is completed.

The Westview Home Care Program monitors the client's post-operative progress in hospital, and facilitates transfer arrangements, rehabilitation services, home care and any other services that may be required. The goal of the program is to prevent any complications or to deal with them promptly, and to return clients to active living as soon as possible. (Personal communication from Barbara Rocchio, RN, MEd, Director of Health Services, Westview Regional Health Authority.)

3. Case Management by the Co-ordinated Assessment Unit in Saskatoon, Saskatchewan

Saskatoon District Health is the regional governing authority for all health services in the City of Saskatoon. The corporate structure has been designed to support increased integration of services for groups of clients who have similar needs. All services are provided through twelve care groups, eight of which receive case management services provided by the Co-ordinated Assessment Unit (CAU).

The case management services provided by the CAU are offered independently of various programs such as acute care, continuing care or home care. Case managers in the CAU are responsible for arranging services for clients in the various care groups as they move from one program, service provider, or site to another, and back again. In some cases (for example, with many of the clients within the surgery-care group), involvement by the case manager is time-limited by the client's needs. For other care groups, such as continuing care and geriatrics, palliative care, or rehabilitation whose clients include people with brain injuries, the case manager's involvement will be ongoing and may include providing continuity of attention over a period of months or years as the needs of client and family change.

The CAU calls upon a variety of services including home care (both professional services and personal or homemaking services), community day programs, social work, physiotherapy, occupational therapy, and various housing, community-support and private services. Waiting lists for special care homes and continuing-care facilities are managed by the CAU.

Case managers in the CAU share responsibility for resource allocation and utilization with the managers of programs that provide services. (Personal communication from Sue Mellrose, the registered social worker who is the manager of the CAU. She works with a team of three assistant managers, one of whom is a registered nurse, one a physiotherapist, and one a social worker.)

4. The Comprehensive Home Option of Integrated Care for the Elderly (CHOICE™)

This program was established in 1995 to provide integrated care for seniors in Edmonton, Alberta. There are two program sites; one is owned and operated by the Capital Care Group (a publicly owned multi-site provider of continuing-care services), and the other by the Good Samaritan Society (a voluntary continuing-care provider).

Modelled on the Program for All-Inclusive Care (known as PACE) in the United States, CHOICE offers a systematic and integrated approach to meeting the health and social needs of older people who may otherwise be eligible for admission to a continuing-care facility. The goal is to maintain frail older persons in their own homes for as long as possible within the bounds of medical, social, and economic feasibility. Participants are usually functionally or medically frail; have chronic mental illness, or are in various stages of dementia. Care is provided by a multidisciplinary team using a case management approach. The core program elements include: a day health centre; health clinic; home support; transportation; and sub-acute care beds. Medical services are provided by a salaried physician who becomes responsible for clients' medical needs when they are admitted to the program.

Admission to the CHOICE program is through the Regional Single Point of Entry for Continuing Care Services. Clients are accepted for a trial admission following an interdisciplinary team conference. During the trial admission, assessments are conducted in the core service areas of social work, medicine, physical therapy, occupational therapy, nutrition, home support, recreational therapy, and pharmacy. The interdisciplinary team then meets to discuss the assessment results and make the admission decision.

Once a participant is admitted, an interdisciplinary care plan is developed. All team members are responsible for implementing the plan and contributing to the achievement of the established goals. If a participant requires services beyond those offered directly through the program, staff of the CHOICE program will organize access to these services. Discharge from the program is infrequent, as one of the objectives of the program is to maintain participants in the program for as long as possible by altering services as required. In this innovative program the core elements of case management are vital to the achievement of objectives for individual clients and for the program. (The information for this case example was provided by the Continuing Care and Public Health Division of the Capital Health Authority, which is responsible for the program.)

- Case management is a process and a professional service that can help achieve the goal of integrated and cost-effective care.
- There are a number of common elements to the case management process; however, the way they are applied is dependent upon a number of factors including the client group being served, the goals of care, the program setting, the way the case management role is structured, and the organizational characteristics.
- Many authors have compared the nursing process and primary nursing to the process of case management and, while there are certain similarities, there are also important differences.
- The case manager serves as a link between the client and the delivery system, providing the client with continuity, consistency, and coordination of care across service settings and boundaries.
- The availability of universal public insurance coverage in the Canadian health system has created incentives for overuse of the acute-care sector of the health system. At the same time chronic mental and physical illnesses have been more widely recognized and effectively treated, and the Canadian population has aged. These developments have created a need for community and home health services to supplement those provided by doctors and hospitals.
- The development of community and home health services and their integration with services provided by doctors and hospitals will be a key factor is ensuring the financial viability of the Canadian health system.
- The extent to which the case management role is "managerial" in nature depends upon the degree of authority, accountability, and discretionary decision-making expected of a case manager within a particular organizational context.

FURTHER READINGS AND RESOURCES

Callwood, J. (1986). *Twelve weeks in spring*. Toronto: Key Porter. When case management services are not provided through the formal system, family members and friends often become case managers. This book describes a situation in which a group of individuals in Toronto, many of them strangers to each other, came together to help a dying friend remain in her home during the last three months of her life.

More, P.K., & Mandell, S. (1997). *Nursing case management: An evolving practice*. New York: McGraw-Hill. This introductory text describes the role of the nurse case manager in the institutional setting, the community, and the insurance field. The authors describe key components of case management and skills required by case managers.

Pyke, J. (1996). Case management and mental health services. *The Canadian Nurse* 92(7), 31-35. In this article the author, a case management consultant in Toronto, provides a review of case management services for mental health clients in Canada, and suggests criteria that can be used to assess whether case management is appropriate within a particular organizational context.

REFERENCES

Angus, D. E., Auer, L., Cloutier, J.E., Albett, T. *Sustainable health care for Canada: Synthesis report.*(1995) University of Ottawa Economics Project. Ottawa: Renouf.

Applebaum, R.A., & Austin, C.D. (1990). *Long-term care case management: Design and evaluation.* New York: Springer.

Austin, C.D. (1996). Aging and long-term care. In C. D. Austin, & R. W. McClelland (Eds), *Perspectives on case management practice* (pp. 73–98). Milwaukee, WI: Families International.

Austin, C. D. (1993). Families in society. *The Journal of Contemporary Human Services,* 451–459.

Austin, C. D., & McClelland, R. W. (1996). Introduction: Case management—everybody's doing it. In C. D. Austin & R. W. McClelland (Eds.), *Perspectives on case management practice* (pp. 1–16). Milwaukee, WI: Families International Inc.

Beatrice, D. F. (1981). Case management: A policy option for long-term care. In J. J. Callahan, & S. S. Wallack (Eds), *Reforming the long-term-care system* (pp. 121–161). Toronto: Lexington.

Brett, J. L., & Tonges, M. C. (1990). Restructured patient care delivery: Evaluation of the ProACT model. *Nursing Economics,* 8 (1), 36–44.

Case Management Society of America. (1994). CMSA proposes standards of practice. *The Case Manager,* 5(1), 59–71.

Cohen, E. L., & Cesta, T. G. (1997). *Nursing case management: From concept to evaluation* (2 ed). St. Louis, MO: Mosby.

Cronin, C. J., & Maklebust, J. (1989). Case-managed care: Capitalizing on the CNS. *Nursing Management,* 20(3), 38–47.

Desimone, B. S. (1988). The case for case management. *Continuing Care,* 22–23.

Ethridge, P., & Lamb, G. S. (1989). Professional nursing case management improves quality, access and costs. *Nursing Management,* 20(3), 30–35.

Everett, B., & Nelson, A. (1992). We're not cases and you're not managers: An account of a client-professional partnership developed in response to the "borderline" diagnosis. *Psychosocial Rehabilitation Journal,* 15(4), 49–60.

Geron, S. M., & Chassler, D. (1994). The quest for uniform guidelines for long-term care case management practice. *Journal of Case Management,* 3(3), 91–97.

Gibson, S. J., Martin, S. M., Johnson, M. B., Blue, R., & Miller, D. S. (1994). CNS-directed case management: cost and quality in harmony. *Journal of Nursing Administration,* 24(6), 45–51.

Goering, P. N., Farkas, M., Wasylenki, D. A., Lancee, W. J., & Ballantyne, R. (1988b). Improved functioning for case management clients. *Psychosocial Rehabilitation Journal,* 12(1), 2–17.

Goering, P. N., Wasylenki, D. A., Farkas, M., Lancee, W. J., & Ballantyne, R. (1988a). What difference does case management make? *Hospital and Community Psychiatry,* 39(3), 272–276.

Goering, P., Wasylenki, D., St. Onge, M., Paduchak, D., & Lancee, W. (1992). Gender differences of a case management program for the homeless. *Hospital and Community Psychiatry ,* 43(2), 160–165.

Grisham, M., White, M., & Miller, L. S. (1983). Case management as a problem solving strategy. *Pride Journal of Long Term Home Health Care, 2*(4), 21–28.

Haw, M. A. (1995). State-of-the-art education for case management in long-term care. *Journal of Case Management 4*(3), 85–94.

Henderson, M. G., & Collard, A. (1988). Measuring quality in medical case management programs. *Quality Review Bulletin, 33–39.*

Intagliata, J. (1982). Improving the quality of community care for the chronically mentally disabled: The role of case management. *Schizophrenia Bulletin, 8*(4), 655–674.

Kanter, J. (1989). Clinical case management: Definition, principles, components. Hospital and *Community Psychiatry, 40*(4), 361–368.

Lamb, G. S. (1992). Conceptual and methodological issues in nurse case management research. *Advances in Nursing Sciences, 15*(2), 16–24.

Lamb, M., Deber, R., Naylor, C. D., & Hastings, J.E. (1991). Managed care in Canada: *The Toronto Hospital's proposed comprehensive health organization.* Ottawa: Canadian Hospital Association Press.

Lendrum, B. L. (1994). Organization of patient care. In J. M. Hibberd & M. E. Kyle (Eds), *Nursing management in Canada* (pp. 312–330). Toronto: W. B. Saunders.

Mercier, C., & Racine, G. (1995). Case management with homeless women: A descriptive study. *Community Mental Health Journal, 31*(1), 25–37.

More, P. K., & Mandell, S. (1997). *Nursing case management.* New York: McGraw-Hill.

Nelson, G., Sadler, C., & Cragg, S. M. (1995). Changes in rates of hospitalization and cost savings for psychiatric consumers participating in a case management program. *Psychosocial Rehabilitation Journal 18*(3), 25–37.

Olivas, G. S., Del Togno-Armanasco, V., Erickson, J. R., & Harter, S. (1989). Case management—A bottom-line care delivery model. Part I: The concept. *Journal of Nursing Administration, 19*(11), 16–20.

Pearlmutter, S., & Johnson, R. (1996). Case management in the public welfare system. In C. D. Austin & R. W. McClelland (Eds), *Perspectives on case management practice* (pp. 175–202). Milwaukee: Families International.

Pelletier, M. G., & Blouin, A. S. (1990). Case study: Case management; Success in a community hospital. *Definition, 5*(3), 55–56.

Perrow, C. (1970). *Organizational analysis: A sociological view.* Belmont, CA: Wadsworth.

Pyke, J., Clark, S., & Walters, J. (1991). Case management. *The Canadian Nurse 87*(1), 22–25.

Raiwet, C., Halliwell, G., Andruski, L., & Wilson, D. (1997). Care maps across the continuum. *The Canadian Nurse 93*(1), 26–30.

Rheaume, A., Frisch, S., Smith, A., & Kennedy, C. (1994). Case management and nursing practice. *Journal of Nursing Administration, 24*(3), 30–36.

Roberts-DeGennaro, M. (1993). Generalist model of case management practice. *Journal of Case Management, 2*(3), 106–111.

Smith, J. E., & Smith, D. L. (1997, February). *Achieving evidence-based case management nursing practice.* Paper presented at the Canadian Association of University Schools of Nursing Conference, Edmonton, Alberta.

Zander, K. (1988). Managing care within acute care settings: Design and implementation via nursing case management. *Health Care Supervisor 6*(2), 27–43.

Chapter 10

▼▼▼▼▼▼▼▼▼▼▼▼▼▼▼▼▼

Leading and Participating in Workgroups and Teams

Dorothy M. Wylie and Donna Lynn Smith

KEY OBJECTIVES

In this chapter, you will learn:

- The importance of teamwork in health organizations.
- Similarities and differences between workgroups and teams.
- Some key features of group structure and process that provide a background for understanding workgroups and teams.
- Various roles that may be assumed by members of groups or teams.
- Some models of group development.
- Special characteristics and challenges of health-care teams.
- Some reasons why teams don't work.
- Characteristics of effective teams.
- Factors to be considered when building and leading a group or team.
- Why organizational support for teamwork is important.

INTRODUCTION

As is true in most other disciplines, there is increasing recognition in the health-care field today of the added value that effective teamwork can bring to organizations and their clients. An aging population and the increasing number of persons with chronic illnesses has created a growing demand for a blend of health services that can meet medical, nursing, rehabilitative, psychosocial, and recreational needs. No single discipline has the expertise and capability to provide the entire range of necessary services, and inter-disciplinary teams are now considered essential in the provision of more integrated care. There is a growing interest in understanding how teams work, and how obstacles to effective team performance can be overcome. The ability to influence groups of people to work cohesively and productively together as part of a team is now seen as a skill that is nearly indispensable for leaders and managers at all levels and in all fields.

Health-care settings are complex environments in which a variety of services must be provided to clients with multiple and diverse health-care needs. There is almost always a need for those who provide health services to communicate and co-operate with others, and to co-ordinate their efforts. They may work together as staff members in a unit or program, they may be part of an interdisciplinary team that brings together expertise to provide service to a defined group of clients, or they may come together to accomplish a specific task or to carry out a project.

As discussed in Chapter 9 of this book, significant risks and costs are associated with the gaps, duplication, and lack of co-ordination that have characterized the health system in recent years. Although there are many obstacles to effective teamwork in health organizations, developing more effective workgroups and teams in health-care settings is more than a challenge: it is a necessity.

This necessity is increasingly acknowledged by such initiatives as the new standards recently established by the Canadian Council of Health Services Accreditation (CCHSA, 1995). In the past, health-care organizations have been assessed on how well each department or profession met standards that had been developed by professionals in their own fields. The emerging approach is one in which accreditors interview teams of professionals who care for particular client groups, thereby assessing the performance of the workgroup or team, rather than that of individual disciplines or departments. The development of interdisciplinary standards and leadership approaches within health organizations are other current examples that indicate that administrators in health-care organizations have become aware of the importance of effective teamwork, and are working to achieve it (Beverley, Dobson, Atkinson, & Caldwell, 1997; Young, Ang, & Findlay, 1997).

GROUP DYNAMICS AND STRUCTURE

Group dynamics was defined by Luft (1970) as the "study of individuals interacting in small groups" (p. 1). An understanding of basic concepts about the way small groups work is the starting point for effective group and team leadership and participation.

A "group" consists of two or more people who come together, or who are brought together, to achieve a purpose through communication and interaction. Individuals usually belong to several groups, whether in the home, workplace, or classroom, or as members of associations or clubs. Many groups are formed for the purpose of accomplishing a task, but people often voluntarily join groups to meet their own needs for affiliation, self-esteem, or recognition. Groups may be needed to accomplish organizational goals in the workplace, but they can also meet personal needs of group members.

A group is a social system with its own boundaries, structure, and culture. The structure and culture of a group can become so firmly established that it can be extremely difficult to change the ways the group has developed for doing business (Dimock, 1987). Group membership tends to become inclusive for the members and exclusive for those who are not members. Non-members may be viewed as outsiders or may see themselves that way. In fact, it may be easier to start a new group than to get an existing group to change behaviours. Many changes in organizational structure come about because it is assumed that groups of people cannot, or will not, change the way they work.

The size of a group can be a significant factor in its effectiveness. Group interaction tends to decrease as the number of persons in the group increases (Zander, 1986). As a result, persons who belong to large groups are often less satisfied with membership in the group as there is less opportunity for participation and interaction. In large groups with limited interaction, a group member may feel anonymous. This can result in a lack of co-operation or commitment.

GROUP TASKS AND NORMS

Tasks, interaction, and self-orientation are the three basic functions that affect the group process (Boshear & Albrecht, 1977).

Task behaviours achieve the goals of the group and can be called the work of the group. They include such things as gathering facts, developing goals, sharing information, clarifying issues, or reaching consensus in problem-solving.

Interaction activities are the processes that determine how the group performs. They include communicating, expressing feelings, attempting to resolve disagreements, and establishing the norms of behaviour for the group.

Self-oriented behaviours are those behaviours that the group members use to meet their individual needs. These may not always be useful to the achievement of group goals or to positive interaction. For example, members may dwell on personal concerns and issues, waste time, dominate the discussion, have side conversations with others, not listen, or continually interrupt.

The functions of task, interaction, and self-orientation can be carried out directly or indirectly. Direct activities are open, and group members share the reasons for their behaviour with the group. Open communication, including the sharing of personal needs and wishes by group members, can often lead to resolution of interpersonal issues. Sometimes, however, undisclosed intentions or motivations of group members may be reflected in "hidden agendas."

Individuals who are attempting to pursue a hidden agenda within a group may do so by undermining projects, making hidden agreements with other members, promoting personal needs above others, and suppressing or avoiding interpersonal issues. Hidden agendas may arise around the group task, group leadership, or the individual member. Groups may work well at the surface level, when the hidden agenda is resting or has been settled, but at times of crisis, unresolved hidden agendas may give rise to an increase in indirect activities within the group. All groups have both surface agendas and hidden agendas and work at both at the same time (Bradford, 1978).

Groups often establish norms of behaviour early in their development. Norms are the expectations of the group about how their members will behave in the achievement of the task. Norms may be formalized into written statements of procedure or may be informal and unexpressed. Regardless of their format, norms can strongly influence an individual's behaviour in a group. When groups demand strict adherence to group norms, there is a high degree of conformity and cohesiveness. In some situations this is positive; in others, it may not be constructive and can lead to "groupthink". This term was coined by Janis (1983) and is defined as an extreme occurrence in which poor group decisions result from a limited exploration of various alternative solutions to problems.

ROLES OF GROUP MEMBERS

Fourteen roles that group members carry out to achieve the functions of the group were described by Dimock (1985). These roles are summarized in Table 10.1. The task roles and the group building and maintenance roles contain eleven functions, all of which are essential to development of the group. The self-orientation role is carried out through three individual functions. Group roles can be assessed through group observation and keeping a record of the roles each member plays.

MODELS OF GROUP DEVELOPMENT

Many different models of group development have been described (Bales, 1950; Bion, 1961; Schutz, 1958; Tuckman, 1965; Tuckman & Jensen, 1977; Jones, 1974; Lacoursiere, 1974). Although the terminology differs with the model, each portrays the task and interpersonal behaviours within a group as it moves through various stages. Sometimes groups become bogged down in the early stages of development and cannot achieve the stage of interdependence where roles and functions are shared among group members.

One five-stage model of group development (Tuckman, 1965; Tuckman & Jensen, 1977) describes the first stage, *forming*, as a time of orientation when members seek guidance from the leader, and direction on rules and functions. During this phase, they also determine their commitment to the group. The second stage, *storming*, is characterized by competition and conflict with resistance to other members' roles and ideas. Members experience discomfort in this stage; some become passive and others vocal and hostile. During the third stage, *norming*, a sense of cohesion starts to develop. Team members buy into the group as trust and open communication emerge. There can be a sense of energy and creativity during this phase. When the fourth stage, *performing*, is reached, the group operates interdependently, and its goals and roles are clear yet flexible. Members are more confident, morale is good, and productivity related to task is high. At the fifth stage, *adjourning*, the task has been completed and the relationships that have de-

Table 10.1
ROLES OF GROUP MEMBERS

Task Functions

1. **Defines problems.** Group problem is defined; overall purpose of group is defined.
2. **Seeks information.** Requests factual information about group problem, methods to be used, or clarifies a suggestion.
3. **Gives information.** Offers facts or general information about group problem, methods to be used, or clarifies a suggestion.
4. **Seeks opinions.** Asks for the opinions of others relevant to discussion.
5. **Gives opinions.** States beliefs or opinions relevant to discussion.
6. **Tests feasibility.** Questions reality, checks practicality of suggested solutions.

Group-Building and Maintenance Functions

7. **Coordinating.** A recent statement is clarified and related to another statement in such a way as to bring them together. Proposed alternatives are reviewed.
8. **Mediating/harmonizing.** Interceding in disputes or disagreements and attempting to reconcile them. Highlights similarities in views.
9. **Orienting/facilitating.** Keeps group on track, points out deviations from agreed upon procedures or from direction of group discussion. Helping group progress along, proposing other procedures to make group more effective.
10. **Supporting/encouraging.** Expressing approval of anothers' suggestion, praising others' ideas, being warm and responsive to ideas of others.
11. **Following.** Going along with the movement of the group, accepting ideas of others, expressing agreement.

Individual Functions

12. **Blocking.** Interfering with the progress of the group by arguing, resisting, or disagreeing beyond reason, or by coming back to same "dead" issue later.
13. **Out of field.** Withdrawing from discussion, daydreaming, doing something else, whispering to others, leaving room, etc.
14. **Digressing.** Getting off the subject, leading discussion in some personally oriented direction, or making a brief statement into a long, nebulous speech.

Source: Reproduced from Hedley G. Dimock, *How to Observe Your Group* (2nd ed.) (Guelph, ON: University of Guelph, 1985). Reprinted with permission

veloped may be given up. A similar model described by Lacoursiere (1974; 1980) categorized the developmental stages as orientation, dissatisfaction, production and termination.

Figure 10.1 illustrates how groups move through the task and interpersonal dimensions in four stages (Jones,1974). In stage one, as they are becoming oriented to the task, group members are dependent on the leader for guidance and direction. At stage two, members begin to organize their own approaches to the task, and conflict may develop among members as

Figure 10.1
FOUR STAGES OF GROUP DEVELOPMENT

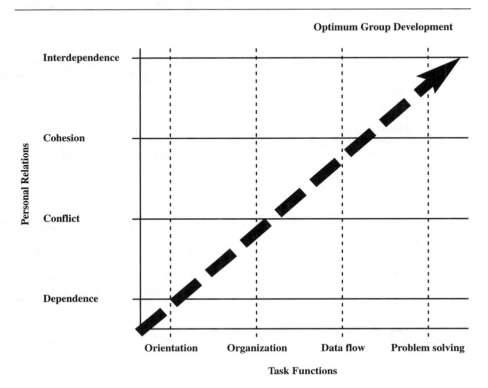

Source: Reprinted from J.W. Pfeiffer (Ed.), *Theories and Models in Applied Behavioral Science*
(Vol. 2) (San Diego: Pfeiffer & Company, 1991), p. 100. Used with permission.

differing ideas, methods, and behaviours begin to surface. In stage three, as
some level of trust begins to emerge and members get to know each other
better, there is movement toward group cohesion. Information begins to
flow as members share perceptions, feelings, and ideas at the task level as
well as the personal level. In stage four, interdependence is evident as members begin to feel more comfortable in working together, can openly share
and communicate, and can work toward a higher level of problem solving.

All groups do not necessarily progress through a predictable or "normal" development process, and not all individuals contribute equally to the
groups in which they participate. Slavin (1992) pointed out that since
group products are the reflection of pooled—rather than individual—learning and accomplishment, achievement can be difficult to assess. Individual
responsibility can be diffused because the group, rather than the individual
members of it, is held accountable for the product or outcome. The term
"free-rider effect" has been used to describe the situation in which a group
member reduces individual effort by taking advantage of the efforts of

others (Kerr & Bruun, 1981, 1983). Alternatively, some group members may reduce their individual efforts if they perceive that others in the group are "free riding" by contributing less than they are able, or less than other members of the group. This has been termed the "sucker effect" (Kerr & Bruun, 1983). These behaviours fall within a broader category of behaviour that has been described as "social loafing" (Hertz-Lazarowitz, Kirkus, & Miller, 1992; Latane, 1986). This term refers to reduction of effort and performance in situations in which a group shares a single goal and individual contributions toward it cannot be readily monitored. Losses of effort attributable to social loafing have been observed in small groups, but increase with the potential for an individual to be "lost in the crowd."

Regardless of the model chosen to illustrate group development, specific elements must be in place for groups to be effective. The goals of the group need to be clear and will need to be clarified from time to time to keep the group on track. The necessary group roles and functions must be carried out to maintain the life of the group. Every group member has a responsibility to see that functions are fulfilled. Open, two-way communication is essential and should provide opportunities for members to express perceptions and feelings as well as ideas. Positive norms need to be established to create a climate of trust and to allow for participation by each member of the group. There should be opportunities for leadership of the group to be shared among the members, and for leadership to alternate according to the skill requirements needed, the functions to be fulfilled, and the abilities of the group members.

WORKGROUPS AND TEAMS: SIMILARITIES AND DIFFERENCES

It is often assumed that any group of people who work together are—or will inevitably become—a team, but this is not the case. Often groups working together remain simply "workgroups." Most organizations are composed of numerous workgroups, and these depend heavily on the ability of managers to provide leadership, so that they can function in a cohesive and collaborative manner to meet the goals of the unit, program, and organization. It is neither necessary nor inevitable that workgroups develop into teams; on the other hand, most teams will first function as effective working groups.

The differences between workgroups and teams have been demonstrated in research conducted by Katzenbach and Smith (1993). Workgroups have a strong, clearly focused leader; the group's purpose fits with the broader organizational mission; individual members are accountable for individual work products or outcomes; work is delegated, decisions are made, and meetings run efficiently. These authors state that "the best working groups come together to share information, perspectives, and insights; to make decisions that help each person to do his or her job better; and to reinforce individual performance standards. But the focus is always on individual accountability." (p. 112).

Larson & LaFasto (1989) defined teams as consisting of two or more people with specific performance objectives or goals to be achieved. Teamwork or co-ordination of activity between or among members is required for the attainment of the objectives or goals. In teams, leadership roles are shared and there is both individual and mutual accountability. The team has a specific purpose and produces work products or outcomes that are the result of collective efforts; and the performance of the team is assessed on the basis of these collective accomplishments. The focus on group goals and the satisfaction of achieving them creates a direction, momentum, and commitment that goes beyond that seen in workgroups. Senior management provides teams with a mandate and a "performance challenge," but teams act independently and flexibly in establishing their own specific goals and work plans in response to demands or opportunities presented to them.

Workgroups and teams also differ in their composition. The membership of a workgroup may be determined by various factors including past recruitment decisions and shift schedules, or may automatically extend to include all personnel in a unit or program. On teams, in contrast, where the right mix of technical and functional expertise, interpersonal skills, and problem-solving and decision-making abilities is critical, team members are selected for their skills and skill potential. Support for team efforts from higher levels of management is a critical factor in team success and enables the team to develop a form of discipline that includes both clear rules of behaviour and commitment to collective goal achievement.

A majority of the "high performance" teams that were studied by Katzenbach and Smith had no more than ten members. Such teams frequently have fun together, and develop an energy of their own. They are not necessarily better than workgroups in every situation—which is fortunate, because highly effective teams are relatively rare. However, when such teams do emerge, they are a valuable organizational resource.

CREATING EFFECTIVE TEAMS AND WORKGROUPS

Whether the goal is to develop more effective workgroups or high performance teams, training is a key factor. Anderson (1993) cites a number of authorities including Edward Deming, the founder of the quality improvement paradigm that gained prominence in the 1980s, who believes that training in team processes and process improvement needs to be supplemented by training for self-improvement. Training to develop communications skills, and related skills for chairing and participating in meetings, resolving conflict, and problem solving, benefits both the organization and the individual.

Blanchard (1991) emphasizes that a group's overall level of productivity and morale are shaped by specific behaviours that can be performed by any member of the group. The two key behaviours are *giving direction* and *giving support*. Giving direction is accomplished in three ways:

1. by creating structure through the use of tools like agendas, and role and task descriptions;
2. by controlling, through the use of scheduling and time-management tools; and
3. by supervision, including the identification of areas of activity where the group needs assistance in order to reach its goals.

Giving support includes:

1. praising constructive contributions;
2. listening to various points of view; and
3. facilitating participation so that all members of the group develop an appreciation for each other's contributions, and experience a growing sense of commitment to one another and to the goals of the unit, program or organization.

WORKGROUPS AND TEAMS IN HEALTH CARE

Workgroups and teams in health-care settings must address and overcome certain challenges and difficulties that are specific to the health-care environment if they are to function effectively. These challenges affect both intradisciplinary and interdisciplinary workgroups and teams.

Intradisciplinary teams, composed of members of the same profession, have been common in health organizations for many years. Physicians who work together in a practice or specialty area frequently do so as a team, and in teaching hospitals such teams often include medical students at various stages of their training. In the early 1950s, the concept of team nursing began to be promoted in order to provide care more efficiently and effectively to groups of patients during severe nursing shortages. More recently, the advantages of team building within nursing organizations have been advocated as a means of sharing leadership and optimizing accountability (Jacobsen-Webb, 1985).

Interdisciplinary teams were defined many years ago as "a functioning unit, composed of individuals with varied and specialized training, who coordinate their activities to provide services to a client or group of clients" (Ducanis & Golin, 1979, p. 3). The first intentional efforts to establish health-care teams were seen in community and mental health, child-development, and rehabilitation centres. Today interdisciplinary teams exist in both community and hospital settings, and many include nurses, physicians, social workers, rehabilitation therapists, recreation therapists, respiratory therapists, dieticians, pastoral-care professionals, and volunteers. Although the concept of interdisciplinary teams has been in place for many years, studies to examine the effectiveness and outcomes of the team approach are relatively recent and few.

THE CHALLENGE OF TEAMWORK IN HEALTH CARE

Although there is broad agreement that teamwork is necessary in health-care settings, a number of problems associated with interdisciplinary teamwork in health care have been identified in the literature (Anderson, 1993; Baggs & Schmitt, 1997; Baggs, Ryan, Phelps, Richeson, & Johnson, 1992; Briggs, 1991; Chavigny, 1988; Deber & Leatt, 1986; Ducanis & Golin, 1979; Fagin, 1992; Fried & Leatt, 1986; Fried, Leatt, Deber, & Wilson, 1988; Temkin-Greener, 1983). These problems include: lack of clarity of roles, confusion over accountability, leadership issues, lack of clearly defined mutual goals, poor communication skills combined with inadequate problem-solving skills and inadequate decision-making methods, infringement of the disciplinary boundaries, and lack of conflict-management skills. The group-development models provide some insights into how these problems can prevent teams from functioning effectively. Many of these weaknesses in team function arise from lack of group-process skills and poor team management in health-care situations.

Ducanis and Golin (1979) use a team system model (Figure 10.2) to explore the various and complex dimensions of health-team interaction. The health team is conceptualized as an open system incorporating a feedback loop. This feedback loop provides information that will influence and change goals and activities.

Three components affect the goals, activities and outcomes of a team. These are the professional team members, the client, and the organizational setting or context.

PROFESSIONAL TEAM MEMBERS

The professionals who come together to make up an interdisciplinary team have each been educated and socialized into the professional norms and standards unique to their particular discipline. Historically in health care, rigid boundaries have existed around professional disciplines, and members are likely to carry personal perceptions of their own profession and of other professions. Distorted perceptions of others' roles, overlapping of roles, status issues, and varying points of view all contribute to interprofessional conflict and can lead to a poorly functioning team.

Traditional stereotypes colour interactions between professionals and can be illustrated by the "doctor-nurse game" described by Stein in 1967 (Stein, Watts, & Howell, 1990). The relationships between doctors and nurses have traditionally appeared to be those of superiors and subordinates. Open disagreement between the two players was to be avoided at all costs. In communication and consultation, the nurse assumed a passive manner and made recommendations in a way that made these recommendations appear to have been initiated by the physician rather than the nurse. Nurses who work in contemporary health organizations are better educated and more assertive than their earlier counterparts; they seek

F i g u r e   1 0 . 2

T H E   T E A M   S Y S T E M   M O D E L

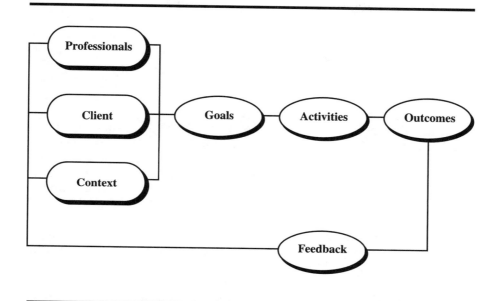

Source: From A. J. Ducanis and A. K. Golin, *The Interdisciplinary Health Care Team: A Handbook* (Germantown, MD: Aspen Systems, 1979).

greater autonomy, and expect to have more equal relationships with physicians. The former hierarchical arrangements are beginning to crumble and dissolve—but at a rather slow pace. (Stein, Watts, and Howell, 1990; Ornstein, 1990).

Other barriers that contribute to tensions between nurses and physicians include: the frequent inability of nurses to describe their roles and scope of practice, differences in education levels, sex-role stereotyping and gender differences, social differences, and a tendency among nurses to accord status to "hands-on" activities rather than intellectual activities (Fagin, 1992). These barriers are not unique to nurse-physician relationships. The same types of issues are played out between and among the other professional groups that make up interdisciplinary teams.

In a study of multidisciplinary renal teams across Canada and in Michigan, Deber and Leatt (1986) contrasted descriptions by health-care team members of their ideal roles in decision making with their perceptions of their actual roles. The teams consisted of nephrologists, physicians, surgeons, nurses, social workers, dietitians, and technicians. The findings showed that the nephrologists took leadership roles on the teams and assumed the major responsibility and accountability for clinical decision making. Team members from other disciplines submitted to the dominant profession, medicine. Nevertheless, the ideal of a collaborative multidisciplinary renal team with equal representation and equal decision making powers was maintained by the members.

Where there are differences between perceptions of the ideal role and the actual role, role conflict and role ambiguity can occur. Role deprivation occurs when the person who occupies a role cannot behave as he or she thinks appropriate. Nurses have expressed feelings of role deprivation in numerous job-satisfaction surveys; burnout, frustration, and high turnover have been some of the results. Lack of role clarity among the group members contributes to dysfunction in health-care teams.

Status differences among the professions often fuel issues that relate to leadership of the team. Physicians have traditionally assumed the leadership role because they are considered to be legally responsible for the patient. However, they often lack the interpersonal and leadership skills necessary to the development of team cohesion, which is required to meet the needs of the patient and to facilitate the effective functioning of the team.

Specific training for collaborative health teamwork is now becoming a priority (Casto, et al.,1994). For example, at the University of Alberta, over the past five years, several hundred senior undergraduate students from the disciplines of pharmacy, rehabilitation medicine, nursing, medicine, dentistry, and physical education have elected to take an interdisciplinary course (IntD 410) that is designed to promote an appreciation for the contributions of each health discipline and to develop skills in collaborative problem solving. A self-directed team of faculty from all participating disciplines leads the course, assisted by tutors from health agencies in the community.

THE CLIENT

Traditionally, the client has not been seen as part of the interdisciplinary team, but as consumers have become more knowledgeable, they have made it clear that they wish to be actively involved in decisions affecting their own health. Today, clients and their families or significant others (often called informal caregivers) are being acknowledged and included as members of the health-care team. One psychologist has described how family and friends can supplement the work of professionals in the creation of a team that works with both the "outer environment" of the patient or client, as well as with that person's "mindfulness" and use of self: "I've seen teams of helpers bring the principles of basic attendance into assisting childbirth, elder-care, and attending the injured, ill and dying. Sometimes these teams have been only loosely knit together; other times they have been well organized and have had team leaders" (Wegela, 1996, p.198). The evolution and relationships within a team like this is described in detail in Callwood's account (1986) of how a group of acquaintances in the city of Toronto were drawn together out their concern for an older friend who was dying. Although most had not previously known each other, they became a team to achieve the common purpose of providing palliative care for their friend in her home until she died.

Recent changes in the structure of the health system have resulted in the need for informal caregivers (a majority of whom are women) to provide many health services to family members in their homes. These structural changes have increased both the level of responsibility and the costs that are borne by families; for example, when intravenous drugs were administered in hospital, professionals were responsible for their administration and the drugs were provided to patients at no charge to them. Many intravenous medications are now administered at home by family members, and in some provinces, the costs of these drugs are now an expense to the patient and family. It is not surprising that families and informal caregivers now expect to be included in the planning, decision making, and evaluation of the health-care they receive and often help to provide.

When patients and families were occasionally included in care conferences in the past, their roles were often passive, and the team objective was usually to obtain their co-operation for a plan that had already been developed by the professional team. Not surprisingly, the experience of "being conferenced" was an intimidating one for patients, whether or not they were present!

In many sectors of the health system today, public advocates are appointed to represent patients or clients who feel that their needs and interests are not being recognized by health professionals and health-care organizations. Teams of health professionals must become more proactive in developing the values and skills required to include the patient and informal caregivers as equal partners in planning their care. This need is also being recognized at the level of the health system, where members of client groups and other stakeholders are increasingly represented on the boards responsible for health-system planning and governance.

While efforts are being made to increase patient involvement in health-care teams, it is worth noting that Spitzer and Roberts (1980) raised several questions about whether people are better off being cared for by teams at all. They asked: Do teams further depersonalize medical care? Do patients prefer health teams? Do they have a choice? Ducanis and Golin (1979) pointed out that the relationship between client and individual professional becomes diluted in the team approach. There is an impact on both the patient and the professional. Clients may experience less structure and support with the group approach, and feel the loss of the one-to-one relationship. There is also the possibility that the client may receive conflicting information from various team members. Some patients and families may feel intimidated by the size and professional composition of the group and, therefore, not see the process as helpful or supportive to them. Little study of client satisfaction with interdisciplinary teams has been carried out, and studies are needed to provide a basis for continuous improvement by health teams.

THE CONTEXT

An organization can be seen as a social system built on a mission statement and based on a philosophy or set of values. Each is, therefore, somewhat unique and displays its own culture and climate. Teams are developed within that particular culture to achieve the goals and objectives set by the organization to achieve its mission.

Superimposed on the specific character and culture of any health-care organization today is the reality of rising costs and increasingly restrained resources. Hospitals are abandoning traditional hierarchical structures and functional departments, and are moving to more decentralized organizational approaches. Program management is emerging with organizational structures that focus on clinical programs (such as rehabilitation services, cardiovascular services, women's and children's health). A clinical and administrative team is set up to manage the programs and build on the concept of the interdisciplinary team. The result of the breakdown of functional departments such as nursing, pharmacy, and social work is a further blurring of roles and boundaries among disciplines. Where functional departments remain in place, the individual team member assumes a dual-reporting relationship in which he or she is accountable to both the program head and to the discipline head. This can lead to conflicting values and goals. Each program has its own goals and objectives which may or may not be synonymous with those of the total organization. Working in these newer organizational structures places even greater pressure on the health-care team and reinforces the need for each member to become proficient in group-membership skills to ensure efficient and effective performance.

Organizational structures that support teamwork are taking some time to develop. Hackman (1990) points out that groups cannot flourish where members have multiple tasks to perform, where staff assignments continually shift or group membership changes, and where organizational rewards are based on the individual rather than the team. Under these conditions, issues about quality of service arise, and tension develops about how to work effectively and efficiently within limited time constraints.

Health-care teams associated with teaching hospitals face particular challenges because these settings often include learners who "rotate" in and out of teams. These learners may not yet have acquired group skills, and the development of their clinical expertise may also be in the early stages. They may be more likely than some permanent members of the group, however, to see issues and situations from a client's perspective, and it is incumbent upon the leaders and permanent members of the team to find ways of including and maximizing the contributions of students.

Another context-related problem faced by interdisciplinary health teams in recent years has been the impact of personnel changes that are the result of layoffs and "bumping"—particularly of nurses, but also of some other professionals. In many health organizations, the number of permanent full-time and part-time positions has decreased while the number of casual or "call-in" workers has increased, so that the organization can reduce costs associated with employee benefits. Ironically, this has happened at a time when teamwork has been recognized as of critical importance, and the elimination of permanent positions to save benefit costs in the short term may well prove to be a false economy. Clearly, a constantly changing membership in workgroups and teams is not conducive to group development or the development of the high levels of cohesiveness and commitment that are necessary for high team productivity.

LEADING AND DEVELOPING WORKGROUPS AND TEAMS

Managers at all levels of health organizations must assume greater responsibility for effective leadership of workgroups and teams, and nurse managers have multiple roles in this regard. First and foremost, they lead working groups of staff in particular nursing units or programs. At this level, workgroups are responsible for many outcomes including meeting the health needs of clients and assuring client and family satisfaction with the care being provided. Staff satisfaction often results when working groups and teams accomplish this work effectively. In addition, the nurse manager and the unit or program staff may participate in one or more interdisciplinary teams, or serve on various inter- and intra-disciplinary committees, task forces or project teams of the kind described in Chapter 24. The nurse manager may take a leadership role in some cases, a membership role in others. It is therefore critical that nurse managers know how to work effectively in team settings.

Varney (1989) believes that managers must not only know what constitutes effective teamwork, but that they must also develop the abilities to observe, diagnose, and problem-solve to promote effectiveness. The nurse manager needs to know the abilities and readiness of team members to take on the responsibility of the tasks they have been assigned, and must be able to adjust his or her leadership style to fit the situation. As groups become empowered and self-managed, the nurse manager needs to know when to step aside and support the group in other ways.

GROUP LEADERSHIP

Studies have shown that leadership styles can range from an autocratic, authoritarian style to a democratic, more participative style. The situational leadership model (Hersey & Blanchard, 1982) provides a framework that is widely applicable to a variety of group situations. It presents the idea that leadership style needs to vary according to the situation and the readiness of group members (or "followers") to undertake the task. Within this framework, leadership style is described as the behaviour pattern of an individual, as perceived by others, when that person is attempting to influence a group.

A leader's own perception of his or her behaviour (self-perception) may be very different from that of the group members. Leadership style is determined by the combination of two factors—task behaviours and relationship behaviours. Task behaviours (sometimes called "initiating structure") are defined as the extent to which the leader organizes the group, and establishes the channels of communication and the ways of getting the task done. Relationship behaviours (sometimes described as "consideration") are behaviours that facilitate relationships between the leader and the group members, open up communication, and provide socio-emotional support. The effectiveness of the leadership style is determined by the appropriateness of that style to the environment where it takes place.

The Situational Leadership Model® shown in Figure 10.3 illustrates how the behaviour of a leader in relation to group members is based on the interaction of three factors: (1) the amount of guidance and direction a leader gives; (2) the amount of socio-emotional support a leader provides; (3) the readiness of a group to perform a task.

The model depicts the style of leadership on a bell-shaped curve passing through four quadrants relating to the task and relationships behaviours of the leader. The concept of readiness is portrayed on a continuum of low readiness (R1) to high readiness (R4). The Situational Leadership theory suggests that there is no one best style to influence group members. Rather, leaders should choose a leadership style that takes the readiness of group members into account. That level is determined by the ability and willingness of people to take responsibility for their own behaviours in relation to a specific task or function. The definitions for readiness levels as indicated by the abbreviation R1 to R4 are described as follows:

R1. Unable and unwilling or insecure
R2. Unable but willing and confident
R3. Able but unwilling or insecure
R4. Able/competent and willing/confident

Four styles of leadership are indicated by abbreviations S1 to S4 and are described as follows:

S1- Telling. This high-task and low-relationship style is used where group members exhibit low readiness. This is a directive style for group members who are insecure or inexperienced in their task or function. It is well suited to group members described as R1, above.
S2- Selling. This high-task and high-relationship style is used with group members with low to moderate readiness. This style provides for directive behaviour accompanied by supportive behaviour to give encouragement and reinforce the willingness of group members. It is well suited to groups whose members are classified as R2, above, who are willing but not able (or confident) to take responsibility for their skills.
S3- Participating. This low-task and high-relationship style is used when working with people who display moderate to high readiness, but who are unwilling to perform (R3, above). These group members may be

Figure 10.3
THE SITUATIONAL LEADERSHIP MODEL® *

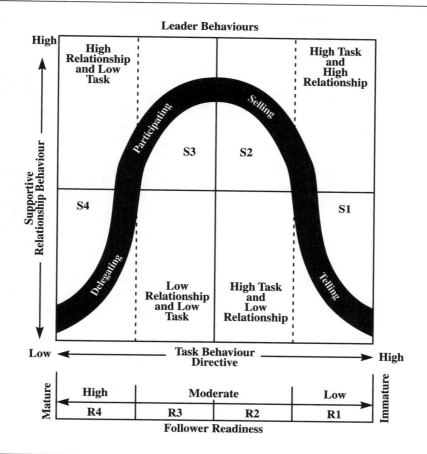

Source: Abstracted from P. Hersey & K. Blanchard, Situational Leadership® handout (San Diego University) (San Diego: Leadership Studies Inc., 1988). Used with permission of Leadership Studies Inc., Escondido, CA.

*Situational Leadership® is a registered trademark of the Center for Leadership Studies. All rights reserved.

competent at the task but unwilling to participate due to lack of confidence (insecurity). A supportive, non-directive style is used to give positive reinforcement and to facilitate the use of group members' individual abilities.

S4- **Delegating.** This low-task and low-relationship style is used where group members are at a high level of readiness and are able and willing to take responsibility for their own efforts (R4, above).

Both the readiness level of individuals and the readiness level of the group as a whole can be considered in this model. Groups that come together frequently and interact to achieve tasks can reach a high level of readiness in their group behaviour. The leader may then choose to deal with the group as a whole with an approach that matches its readiness level. However, the leader also understands that there are differing levels of readiness among the individuals who make up the group, and uses a variety of different styles when interacting with individual members.

Building on this notion, Dimock (1987) suggests that the appropriate leadership style is determined by the group members and the situation. He advises group leaders to start groups off with a structured and directive approach. At the same time, the leader should assess the abilities of the group members and then slowly move along the continuum to a more facilitative coaching style according to member readiness.

In contemporary organizations it is now taken for granted that leaders at all levels must have the skills and willingness to provide leadership to groups and teams. However, recent research (Katzenbach & Smith, 1993) has demonstrated that a specific performance challenge that is clear and compelling to all team members can be as important as the team leader in determining the performance of a team. As a result, all employees—not only those in the most senior organizational ranks—must now be prepared to be willing, able, and constructive participants in groups and teams.

Workgroups or teams are sometimes brought together precisely because the diverse perspectives and skills of their members are needed to accomplish a task or carry out a project. When participants possess high levels of skill, readiness, and a shared commitment to the task at hand, there is often a natural sharing of task leadership among group members, as well as consideration and support. Some organizations provide specific in-service training to employees to assist them in developing skills of group leadership and followership. When such skills are present throughout an organization, when employees are highly motivated, and when time is available to enable groups to plan, co-ordinate, and carry out their activities successfully, a culture of "self-directed" or "leaderless" teams may evolve.

ORGANIZATIONAL SUPPORT FOR TEAMS AND TEAMWORK

There is a growing consensus that significant changes in the culture of organizations are required to support the development of effective teams (Wellins, Byham, & Dixon, 1994, p. 308; Zenger et al., 1994, p 24; see also Lendrum, Chapter 8 of this book). In traditional organizations, work has been determined and planned by managers who were the custodians of information. These people made most organizational decisions and led working groups or teams where they existed. Employees, for the most part, had narrowly-defined roles or skill sets, and when training opportunities were made available they tended to focus on upgrading technical skills. When support staff or specialized skills were needed, they were usually provided by staff specialists imported from outside the working group. Rewards were based on individual performance and there were hazards associated with risk-taking.

In team-centred organizations, by contrast, managers and team members jointly define goals and tasks. Where positions and roles are seen to need broader knowledge, training in interpersonal and administrative skill areas supplements technical knowledge. "Cross-training," in which workers learn skills and roles additional to those associated with their own positions, was once viewed as inefficient, but is now widely advocated. Support staff and skills as well as leadership skills are now often incorporated into teams rather than being provided from a central source. The importance of effective collaboration within workgroups and teams suggests the need for health organizations to review their philosophies, reward systems, supervisory practices, and organizational support systems to assure that they contribute to the development of effective teamwork.

CONCLUSION

The study of groups has a long history, but as Paul S. Goodman & Associates (1986) observed, knowledge specific to designing and maintaining effective workgroups in organizations has not been consolidated and systematically applied. Regardless of the particular task or purpose of the group or team, Hackman (1990) suggests there are three main dimensions to group effectiveness: productivity, the process of the work, and personal well-being of the members. In terms of productivity, the results of the group's work need to conform to a standard of quality, quantity, and timeliness for the client; in other words, clients must be satisfied with the results. The process of doing the work should contribute to the members' satisfaction with the way they interact and achieve the purpose of the group. A relationship is established whereby members enjoy the work and want to continue to work together. Individual group members want to feel they personally have grown and developed throughout the process and have had learning opportunities that contribute to their well-being.

Since groups are social systems they will behave according to the climate they have created. Therefore, those who develop workgroups or teams need to focus on creating conditions that will support their work and enhance their productivity. Building a climate of trust in which risk-taking is encouraged and rewarded is often a precondition of group and team productivity. Trust occurs in an organizational culture that is characterized by honesty and integrity, openness and willingness to share and receive information, consistency of responses and behaviour, and respect that includes treating each other with fairness and dignity (Larson & LaFasto, 1989). Recent research suggests that another critical factor in the development and maintenance of trust in a group over time is that of working together to achieve real results (Katzenbach & Smith, 1993).

SUMMARY

- Health-service organizations now recognize the necessity for members and leaders in all health disciplines to be able to work effectively together in the interests of the client.
- The characteristics of professional roles, accompanied by traditional hierarchical relationships among professions, can produce conflict and dysfunction in workgroups and teams in health-care settings. This can interfere with meeting client needs and achieving organizational goals. Health-care managers must learn ways to address these obstacles in order to make groups function more effectively.
- Groups and teams develop a shared history and life of their own, as demonstrated in the various models of group development. Knowledge about stages of group development and awareness of strategies to shape the course of group development are vital strengths for health-system leaders today and in the future.
- Group or team members can assume various roles and the best approach to leading a group is one that takes into account the maturity and motivation of group members.
- The skills involved in assuming, sharing, and delegating leadership within groups or teams are of critical importance. These skills will become increasingly indispensable as the complexities of client care and organizational life dictate the need for groups and teams to form, perform, and disband quickly and effectively according to needs and circumstances.
- Workgroups and teams in health-care organizations face some unique and complex challenges. Gaps, duplication, and a lack of co-ordination in providing service are some consequences delaying or failing to overcome these challenges. Other consequences may be mistakes or unnecessary costs.
- Progressive health organizations are now developing management approaches, training programs, and organizational supports to facilitate effective teamwork.
- The ability to contribute to groups and teams as a participant or group member is now an essential professional skill that can be improved upon throughout one's career.

FURTHER READINGS AND RESOURCES

Katzenbach, J. R. & Smith, D. K. (1993). *The wisdom of teams*. Boston: Harvard Business School Press. The authors have conducted research with large numbers of teams in business, voluntary, and public organizations. They describe the differences between teams and workgroups and discuss factors involved in improving the performance of teams. An abridged version of the original book (without bibliographical references and index), published by Harper Business (1994), contains a question-and-answer guide that contrasts the commonly assumed answers to questions about teams with the research findings of the authors.

Chaleff, Ira (1995). *The courageous follower: Standing up to and for our leaders*. San Francisco: Berrett-Koehler. The author of this book is a consultant to leading industries and governments. He points out that a follower is not necessarily a subordinate, but shares with the leader a common responsibility for the organization's purpose and its stakeholders. The practical and values-based approach outlined in this book challenges individuals to assume responsibility for sharing leadership, supporting leaders, and where necessary, challenging them.

Zenger, J.H., Musselwhite, E., Hurson, K, & Perrin, C. (1994). *Leading teams: Mastering the new role*. New York: Irwin. The authors of this book have had varied careers in business education, as corporate executives, and as leaders of teams. They link the need for high-level team performance to the widely acknowledged need for organizations to move from being internally driven to customer driven, to move from a focus on process to a focus on function, and to move from a management-centred approach to greater employee involvement. Practical approaches for developing teams are presented. The final section of the book is a series of "profiles in team leadership" that are excerpts from research interviews. These provide insight into the thinking, as well as the skills, of effective team leaders.

Douglass, M. & Douglass, N. (1992). *Time management for teams*. New York: Amacom. This publication of the American Management Association reflects the new organizational reality in which teams assume responsibility for their own leadership and productivity. It includes practical suggestions and worksheets to assist groups in managing their time, as well as sections on making meetings productive, managing "the boss," and teaming up with support staff.

REFERENCES

Anderson, L. K. (1993). Teams: Group process, success, and barriers. *Journal of Nursing Administration, 23*(9), 15–19.

Baggs, J. G., Ryan, S. A., Phelps, C. E., Richeson, J. F., & Johnson, J. (1992). The association between interdisciplinary collaboration and patient outcomes. *Heart & Lung, 21*(1), 18–24.

Baggs, J. G., & Schmitt, M. H. (1997). Nurses' and resident physicians' perceptions of the process of collaboration in an MICU. *Research in Nursing and Health, 20*, 71–80.

Bales, R. F. (1950). *Interaction process analysis: A method for the study of small groups*. Reading, MA: Addison-Wesley.

Beverley, L., Dobson, D., Atkinson, M., & Caldwell, L. (1997). Development and evaluation of interdisciplinary team standards of patient care. *Healthcare Management Forum, 10*(4), 35–39.

Bion, R. W. (1961). *Experiences in groups*. New York: Basic Books.

Blanchard, K. (1991, February). Get your group to perform like a team. *Inside Guide,* 12, 13, 16.

Boshear, W. C., & Albrecht, K. G. (1977). *Understanding people: Models and concepts.* San Diego: University Associates.

Bradford, L. P. (1978). *Group development* (2nd ed.). San Diego: University Associates.

Briggs, M. H. (1991). Team development: Decision-making for early intervention. *Infant-Toddler Intervention: The Transdisciplinary Journal, 1*(1), 1–9.

Callwood, J. (1986). *Twelve weeks in spring.* Toronto: Key Porter.

Canadian Council of Health Services Accreditation. (1995). Ottawa: CCHSA.

Casto, R., Julia, M., Platt, L., Harbaugh, G., Waugaman, W., Thompson, A., Jost, T., Bope, E., Williams, T., & Lee, D. (1994). *Interprofessional care and collaborative practice.* Pacific Grove, CA: Cole.

Chavigny, K. H. (1988). Coalition building between medicine and nursing. *Nursing Economics, 6*(4), 179–184.

Deber, R., & Leatt, P. (1986). The multidisciplinary renal team: Who makes the decisions? *Health Matrix, 4*(3), 3–9.

Dimock, H. G. (1985). *How to observe your group* (2nd ed.). Guelph, ON: University of Guelph.

Dimock, H. G. (1987). *Groups: Leadership and group development* (rev. ed.). San Diego: University Associates.

Ducanis, A. J., & Golin, A. K. (1979). *The interdisciplinary health care team: A handbook.* Germantown, MD: Aspen Systems.

Fagin, C. M. (1992). Collaboration between nurses & physicians: No longer a choice. *Nursing & Health Care, 13*(7), 354–363.

Fried, B. J., & Leatt, P. (1986). Role perceptions among occupational groups in an ambulatory care setting. *Human Relations, 39*(12), 1155–1173.

Fried, B. J., Leatt, P., Deber, R., & Wilson, E. (1988). Multidisciplinary teams in health care: Lessons from oncology and renal teams. *Healthcare Management Forum, 1*(4), 28–34.

Goodman, P. S. & Associates (1986). *Designing effective workgroups.* San Francisco: Jossey-Bass.

Hackman, J. R. (1990). *Groups that work (and those that don't): Creating conditions for effective teamwork.* San Francisco: Jossey-Bass.

Hersey, P., & Blanchard, K. (1982). *Management of organizational behaviour: Utilizing human resources* (4th ed.). Englewood Cliffs, NJ: Prentice-Hall.

Hertz-Lazarowitz, R., Kirkus, V., & Miller, N., (1992). Implications of current research on cooperative interaction for classroom application. In: R. Hertz-Lazarowitz & N. Miller (Eds.) *Interaction in cooperative groups* (pp.253–280). Melbourne: Cambridge University Press.

Jacobsen-Webb, M.-L. (1985). Team building: Key to executive success. *The Journal of Nursing Administration, 15*(2), 16–21.

Janis, I. L. (1983). *Groupthink* (2nd ed.). Boston: Houghton Mifflin.

Jones, J. E. (1974). A model of group development. In J. W. Pfeiffer (Ed.). (1991). *Theories and models in applied behavioral science* (Vol. 2). San Diego: University Associates.

Katzenbach, J. H., & Smith, D. K. (1993, March-April). The discipline of teams. *Harvard Business Review,* 111–120.

Kerr, N. L., & Bruun, S. E. (1983). Dispensability of member effort and group motivation losses: Free-rider effects. *Journal of Personality and Social Psychology.* 44(1) 78–94.

Kerr, N. L., & Bruun, S. E. (1981). Rinbgelmann revisited: alternative explanations for the social loafing effect. *Personality and Social Psychology Bulletin, 7,* 224–231.

Lacoursiere, R. B. (1974). A group method to facilitate learning during the stages of psychiatric affiliation. *International Journal of Group Psychotherapy, 24,* 342–351.

Lacoursiere, R. B. (1980). *The life cycle of groups: Group development stage theory.* New York: Human Science Press.

Larson, C. E., & LaFasto, F. (1989). *Teamwork: What must go right/what can go wrong.* Newbury Park, CA: Sage.

Latane, B. (1986). Responsibility and effort in organizations. In P. S. Goodman & Associates (Eds.), *Designing effective workgroups* (pp. 277–304). San Francisco: Jossey-Bass.

Luft, J. (1970). *Group processes: An introduction to group dynamics* (2nd ed.). Palo Alto, CA: Mayfield.

Ornstein, H. J. (1990). Collaborative practice between Ontario nurses and physicians: Is it possible? *Canadian Journal of Nursing Administration, 3*(4), 10–14.

Schutz, W. (1958). *Firo: A three dimensional theory of interpersonal behavior.* New York: Holt, Rinehart and Winston.

Slavin, R. E. (1992). When and why does cooperative learning increase achievement: theoretical and empirical perspectives. In R. Hertz-Lazarowitz and R. Miller (Eds.) *Interaction in cooperative groups* (pp.145–173). Melbourne: Cambridge University Press.

Spitzer, W. O., & Roberts, R. F. (1980). Twelve questions about teams in health services. *Journal of Community Health, 6*(1), 1–5.

Stein, L. I., Watts, D. T., & Howell, T. (1990). The doctor-nurse game revisited. *The New England Journal of Medicine, 322*(8), 546–549.

Temkin-Greener, H. (1983). Interprofessional perspectives on teamwork in health care: A case study. *Milbank Memorial Fund Quarterly, 61*(4), 641–658.

Tuckman, B. W. (1965). Developmental sequence in small groups. *Psychological Bulletin, 63*(6), 384–399.

Tuckman, B. W., & Jensen, M. A. (1977). Stages of small group development revisited. *Group & Organization Studies, 2*(4), 419–427.

Varney, G. H. (1989). *Building productive teams.* San Francisco: Jossey-Bass.

Wegela, K. K. (1996). *How to be a help instead of a nuisance.* Boston: Shambhala Publications.

Wellins, R., Byham, W., & Dixon, G. (1994). *Inside teams: How 20 world-class organizations are winning through teamwork.* San Francisco: Jossey-Bass.

Young, J. M., Ang, R., & Findlay, T. (1997). Interdisciplinary professional practice leadership within a program model: BC rehab's experience. *Healthcare Management Forum, 10*(4), 48–50.

Zander, A. (1986). *Making groups effective.* San Francisco: Jossey-Bass.

Zenger, J., Musselwhite, E., Hurson, K, & Perrin, C. (1994). *Leading teams: Mastering the new role.* New York: Irwin Professional Publishing

Chapter 11

▼▼▼▼▼▼▼▼▼▼▼▼▼▼▼

Community Health Centres: Innovation in Health Management and Delivery

JOHN CHURCH AND STEPHANIE LAWRENCE

KEY OBJECTIVES

In this chapter, you will learn:

- Historical and political contexts within which community health centres operate.
- What constitutes a community health centre model.
- Current community health centre developments in Canada.
- Benefits of community health centres.
- Unique characteristics of a community health centre model.
- Opportunities for managers offered by the community health centre model.

INTRODUCTION

Traditionally, delivery of health-care services in Canada has been organized to accommodate the needs of the medical profession. Introduction of universal health insurance in Canada during the late 1960s entrenched this bias in the delivery, organization, and financing of primary health services. Physicians continue to deliver health services with a distinct bio-medical focus in hospitals, in individual practices, and sometimes in group practice. Physicians have largely determined the nature and scope of health-care services with relatively little input from the communities they serve.

Despite this reality, Canada is the home of significant innovation in the organization and delivery of primary health-care services. Of particular note is what is generically referred to as the community health centre (CHC). For purposes of this chapter, a CHC is "a non-profit health corporation or association, controlled by an elected community board of directors" (Church, 1994, p. 2). Community health centres provide a range of health and social services including, but not limited to, "clinical diagnostic, therapeutic, and preventive services to regular, special care, and transient patients as well as participatory health promotion to a defined geographic or demographic community" (Birch, Lomas, Rachlis, & Abelson, 1990, p. 1). These services are provided through a broad interdisciplinary team of health and social-service professionals and allied workers on a non-fee-for-service basis, including, but not limited to, nurses, doctors, chiropodists, nutritionists, and social workers (Birch et al., 1990; Hastings, 1972; Ontario Ministry of Health, 1993). The definition chosen for this chapter, then, excludes other forms of primary health services delivery such as "nurse-centred" or "physician-centred" models because these other models are by definition centred on a particular provider (Abelson & Hutchinson, 1994).

In the North American context, the CHC model has been most closely associated with the efforts of community activists, public-health workers, and medical activists to ensure that the poor and other disadvantaged populations receive adequate primary health and social services. Unfortunately, because of the threat that the CHC model poses to their central economic and power position in heath-care delivery systems, established medical interests have often viewed these activities through an ideological prism. CHCs have also been associated with the preventive paradigm of health care because they emphasize a broader range of services than conventional medical practice. As a result of these political characteristics and the incongruence in service delivery patterns and focus, CHCs have been somewhat out of place in conventional North American health-care systems. However, they have become an increasingly attractive option for health-care policy makers because their frameworks emphasize determinants of health, and they have the ability to provide services in lower-cost community settings.

The purpose of this chapter is to discuss the CHC as an organizational model that offers health-sector managers and providers significant opportunities for innovation in management of programs and delivery of services. This discussion will include a description of the model, an overview of the historical context of CHCs, the adaptation of the model in various jurisdictions, research on outcomes associated with CHCs, a profile of a CHC to indicate the uniqueness of the model, and implications for managers. Particular emphasis is placed on the Canadian experience.

THE MODEL

The CHC model offers a means for integrating and co-ordinating health and social services at the community level. The CHC is a non-profit health corporation or association controlled by an elected community board of directors. Development of CHCs is initiated by representatives of community groups, defined either by geography or population. Early community involvement is designed to encourage ownership. Objectives of CHCs include:

- Improving access to appropriate primary-care services.
- Fostering the empowerment of the individual and the community in health and health-services delivery.
- Developing co-ordinated primary health and social services that make the most appropriate and efficient use of service providers and re- sources.
- Promoting health and preventing illness.
- Promoting an interdisciplinary or team approach to meeting health and social needs.

The range of services provided by CHCs might include, but is not limited to:

- Primary health services: treatment, promotion/education, mental health, prevention, dental, dietary, placement, and co-ordination services.
- Social services: information and referral, crisis and emergency services, counselling services, legal services, and community services (food banks, day-care centres, and recreational services).

Funding for CHCs is provided through a variety of mechanisms, including global budgeting, program budgeting, and capitation. Within these organizational funding arrangements, health providers are usually paid through capitation, salary, or sessional arrangements.

HISTORICAL CONTEXT

The CHC model has long been a fixture in the international health-care organizational landscape. A quick scan of the literature indicates that CHCs can be found throughout Europe, North America, and Australia. For the purpose of this chapter, the focus will be on the application of CHCs in the English-speaking democracies, specifically the United Kingdom, the United States, and Canada.

CHCs IN THE UNITED KINGDOM

In the United Kingdom, the CHC model was first articulated in 1920 by the Committee on the Future Provision of Medical and Allied Services (Dawson Committee). The Dawson Committee envisioned two types of health centres: one to provide primary care services through medical gen- eral practices; the other to provide more specialized services. Local author- ities controlling specifically-delineated administrative areas would administer these services. The recommendations of the committee were not adopted, but the Labour Party, Trade Union Congress, and Socialist Medical Associ- ation became advocates for the development of health centres, although there was considerable disagreement over size and function (Hall, Land, Parker, & Webb, 1975).

During the 1930s and early 1940s, the medical profession debated the prospects of a national health system including health centres. The major concern of the medical profession, because of its inherent distrust of local authorities and a desire to maintain control over clinical discretion, was the question of ownership and administration of the centres and their specific focus. However, the medical profession remained generally supportive of the health centre concept as a means of promoting less isolation among general practitioners (Hall et al., 1975).

Recognizing the concerns of the medical profession, the government initially promoted the health centres on an experimental basis, and de-emphasized the ideas of placing physicians on salary and making them subject to control by administrators. However, election of the Labour Party in 1945 revived the idea of a national network of health centres controlled by local authorities as part of the creation of a National Health Service. Section 21 of the National Health Service Act of 1946 required local health authorities to provide, equip, and maintain health centres to deliver a broad spectrum of related health and social services in an integrated fashion. Despite this shift, the immediate post-war period in Britain was characterized by a shortage of public resources. Health centres had to compete with other government priorities, such as the building of roads and schools. The mandatory requirement for local authorities to submit plans for health centres was quickly dropped (Hall et al., 1975).

Between 1945 and 1965, development of health centres became the prerogative of local health authorities. During this period, some 52 "experimental" health centres were developed. In response to growing support for the development of the health centres at the local level, the national government once again began to support the idea in the mid-1960s. This success, characterized by consensus between local health authorities and individual physicians, came about largely through recognition that some sort of common facility for delivering primary care was needed. Doctors could not afford to shoulder the costs of overhead and capital associated with private practice, and the retention rate of physicians in under-served areas was a problem. The government response included: development of standard guidelines for centre development; systematic evaluation; and sponsorship of an annual conference for health centres. Between 1972 and 1981, the number of health centres expanded from 200 to 950. By the early 1980s, approximately 27 percent of general practitioners operated from health centres as part of interdisciplinary teams that included district nurses and health visitors (Allen, 1984).

CHCs IN THE UNITED STATES

In the United States, the CHC model began to emerge following World War I (1914–1918). During the early 1920s, Herman Biggs, the New York State Health Commissioner, developed a plan to establish a network of health centres to provide an integrated set of preventive, diagnostic, and curative services for rural and urban workers. The state medical society was central in preventing this plan from being implemented. However, several experimental health centres were established in New York City by volunteer social agencies. These initial experiments served as the precursor of a federal neighbourhood health-centre program, part of the War on Poverty initiatives of the 1960s. The explicit intent of the federal initiative was to provide broadly defined health services to under-served populations using a framework that emphasized determinants of health. As had earlier been the case in New York State, the federal initiative set off a running battle between the activists, federal bureaucrats and legislators who promoted health centres, and those who opposed them—including the vested medical interests and their bureaucratic and political supporters (Sardell, 1988).

From the initial 150 neighbourhood health centres developed in the United States between 1965 and 1971, nearly 800 additional centres were in operation by 1980. Currently, there are approximately 1,600 clinics providing services to roughly six million people. Neighbourhood health centres are the main source of health care for under-served populations (Freeman, Kiecolt, & Allen, 1982; Health Resources and Services Administration, 1997).

CHCs IN CANADA

In Canada, CHCs have developed sporadically across the country, due both to the nature of constitutional arrangements and to opposition from organized medicine. The first CHC in Canada was developed by the United Steel Workers of America in Sault Ste. Marie in 1958 to provide comprehensive primary medical care to union members. Because this centre operated before government-funded health insurance was introduced, funding came from monthly premiums paid through the union. An elected board of directors contracted for the provision of services with a group of physicians. The method of payment was salary. Ironically, the introduction of government-funded, universal medical care in 1968 posed a serious challenge to the CHC experiment in the Sault, precisely because the government-funded plan enshrined in legislation the fee-for-service model of medical practice (Lomas, 1985).

CHC development in Saskatchewan took a different course. In 1961, the government of that province announced that it intended to introduce universal, compulsory health insurance. This was not surprising, given that Saskatchewan—which had elected the first social democratic government in Canadian history—had introduced universal hospital insurance ten years earlier. The medical profession responded by striking for 23 days. In response to this withdrawal of services, a number of organizations representing affected communities approached the government to support the establishment of CHCs (Naylor, 1986).

While the provincial government and the medical profession continued to haggle over the details of the new health insurance plan, the public began to mobilize to develop community clinics along the lines of a CHC model. By the end of the strike, CHCs had been established in five municipalities, with an additional ten in the process of being developed. The clinics were viewed as a threat by the striking physicians and ultimately became a bargaining chip in the resolution of the dispute. An amendment to the proposed medical care insurance legislation dealt specifically with the issue of lay-controlled clinics and their relationship to physicians (Young, 1975). In the aftermath of the doctors' strike, a total of eight clinics were developed including one in Regina, one in Saskatoon and one in Prince Albert (Badgley & Wolfe, 1967).

When the federal government began to introduce national health insurance legislation in the 1960s, it responded to concerns about the potential cost explosion by establishing a task force. One section of the report of the Task Force on the Costs of Health Services in Canada, which confirmed the worst suspicions about cost escalation, recommended programs for CHC construction. These would be supported by federal and provincial governments, and would house public, mental, and voluntary health personnel, including physicians, to provide appropriate diagnostic services.

A spin-off of this committee was a task force to investigate the potential of the CHC model to re-orient the health-care system from the expensive acute hospital-centred model of delivery to a "people-centred" preventive approach. The report referred to experiences in both the U.S. and Canada and indicated that the CHC model could reduce hospital admissions by between 15 and 50 percent. The report recommended establishment of CHCs with integrated and co-ordinated decentralized (regional) health-care systems within provinces. Despite this recommendation, no nationally co-ordinated plan to develop CHCs was implemented. Provincial medical and hospital associations opposed such an approach (Hastings, 1972; Hastings & Vayda, 1986).

Although no action was taken on a national basis, several provinces moved to introduce CHCs. Quebec took the most systematic approach, opting in 1970 to establish a network of community health and social service centres as part of overall health-care reforms. The network of Centres locaux de services communautaires (CLSCs) is spread over the entire province. Quebec also introduced regional health councils to plan the delivery of health-care services on a regional basis. In an attempt to counter the government efforts to establish CLSCs, organized medicine developed a substantially larger number of physician-sponsored polyclinics across the province.

Unlike Quebec, Ontario chose to move incrementally, developing a small number of centres on an "experimental" basis. This approach resulted in the emergence of two primary care models: a CHC model characterized by community boards and a range of integrated diagnostic and health promotion services; and the health service organization (HSO), essentially a physician group-practice employing a capitation method of payment. In essence, by incorporating an option favourable to physicians into its CHC initiative, the Ontario government has avoided the level of negative response from the medical profession encountered in other Canadian jurisdictions (Church, 1994).

During the late 1980s, there was renewed concern by the provincial and federal governments about increasing levels of expenditures on health care.

Table 11.1

COMMUNITY HEALTH CENTRES IN CANADIAN PROVINCES

Province	Number of Centres
Newfoundland	3
Nova Scotia	7
New Brunswick	1
Prince Edward Island	0
Quebec	161
Ontario	56
Saskatchewan	5
Manitoba	13
Alberta	3
British Columbia	9

In response to this, most provinces introduced a regional health-care system of some kind. Most provinces also moved to introduce some form of CHC on an experimental basis. Table 11.1 provides a breakdown of the number of CHCs in Canada, by province.

APPLICATION BY CANADIAN PROVINCE

British Columbia began developing CHCs during the 1970s. Although commitment from successive provincial governments with ideological differences has vacillated, 13 centres were operating by 1997. Provincial efforts in the mid-1990s to reform the health-care system have placed a renewed emphasis on the development of CHCs as a single point of access for a range of health services that will "encourage community participation, and provide integrated, client-centred services at the local level" (Community Health Centres, B.C., 1993, pp. 1–3).

Alberta has developed three CHCs since the 1970s. The three centres emphasize provision of primary health and related social and community services to under-served and disadvantaged urban populations. The centres provide a range of primary care medical services, referral services, mental-health and public-health care, health promotion and prevention, community nursing outreach services, well-baby clinics, and counselling, as well as social services. Funding is provided by the provincial ministry of health through a variety of arrangements, including an annual grant based on the number of physicians and a negotiated rate for the specific number of patient visits per month (*Sessional payment manual*, 1993).

As discussed earlier, Saskatchewan has had a long history with CHCs. By the mid-1990s, there were three varieties of CHCs in operation: community clinics, community health and social centres, and wellness centres. Each of these variations reflects changing government preferences over time. However, only five clinics fit the definition of CHC adopted for this chapter (*A guide to community health centres*, 1994). Community clinics were developed during the height of the provincial doctor's strike in 1961. Essentially, they are non-profit co-operatives in which physicians are salaried; these equate with the basic CHC model.

Manitoba has developed seven urban and three rural CHCs. The rural CHCs are being integrated into community health resource networks through which a continuum of primary, secondary, and tertiary care will be co-ordinated. In urban areas, these networks are referred to as neighbourhood health resource networks. Additionally, three CHCs are being developed to deliver provincial programs for AIDS, occupational health, and women's health, and one CHC is being developed to address aboriginal health issues.

Ontario has approximately 56 CHCs, serving the poor, seniors, women, and multicultural and aboriginal populations. In 1992, CHCs served approximately 100,000 residents and employed about 100 of the province's 18,000 licensed physicians (0.5%). CHCs in Ontario most closely resemble the general model. They provide services in primary care, health promotion, health prevention, community development, chiropody, dental care, social services, and legal aid. The mix of services varies according to the needs of the client populations (Abelson & Hutchinson, 1994).

Quebec's community health and social centres (its CLSCs) were introduced during the 1970s to provide "basic health and social services with a community orientation" (Bozzini, 1988, p. 349). CLSCs provide a range of primary health, diagnostic, prevention, integrated health and social services, community organizing, mental-health care, and programs for special-needs populations. While the government has been attempting to standardize the range of services provided through CLSCs, in some rural areas, where hospital services are not available, CLSCs also provide emergency health services (Bozzini, 1988). What differentiates Quebec from other provinces is that the 161 CLSCs serve the entire geographic area of the province and make services available to 90 percent of the population. In addition, CLSCs are formally and informally linked to other organizations in a fashion unequalled in other provinces.

New Brunswick has developed one pilot CHC in McAdam to determine the feasibility of delivering primary health care in rural areas of the province. The centre provides primary medical care, health promotion, disease prevention, rehabilitation therapy, and emergency observation services. Unique to this approach is that nurses are legally allowed to assess, treat, and discharge certain types of ailment.

Nova Scotia has seven CHCs that provide varying levels of primary medical and social service, health promotion and disease prevention. The provincial government does not recognize CHCs and, therefore, their major source of funding is from fee-for-service payments for services rendered by physicians.

Newfoundland is pilot testing one CHC and two integrated service delivery models involving acute, chronic, and primary care. The CHC is

governed by a community advisory board and includes salaried family practitioners, community health nurses, and social work intervention services.
The community advisory board provides advice to a locally elected health
council.

THE RESEARCH CONTEXT ON COMMUNITY HEALTH CENTRES

Since the mid-1960s, governments in Canada have been interested in CHCs
for a variety of reasons—including their ability to increase access to services for under-served populations, their increased emphasis on health
promotion and health prevention, and their potential to provide cost-
effective services. An increasing focus on the cost aspect of health-service
delivery has increased government interest in the potential cost savings of
the CHC model; however, wholesale adoption of the model has not occurred in Canada for ideological reasons, and because the evaluation of
CHCs has been plagued by methodological problems.

Since the mid-1980s, a variety of literature reviews have been done on
community-based health services models. These reviews encompass studies examining the cost, quality, and outcomes of the CHC model in the
international and Canadian context. For example, a critical appraisal of the
research on the performance of health service organizations (HSOs) identified eight commonly held assumptions about HSOs when compared to fee-
for-service practice. These included: lower hospital utilization rates;
comparable use of ambulatory care; greater patient loads for physicians;
employment of more ancillary health personnel; higher quality care; structures that facilitate more preventive services; physicians who believe that
the method of payment favours the delivery of more preventive services;
and less patient satisfaction with their care. In examining the evidence in
the literature about these assumptions, the authors concluded that, with
the exception of hospital utilization and personnel substitution, the level of
supportive evidence was not high. This conclusion is attributed to lack of
methodologically rigorous or consistent studies of the performance or outcomes of the CHC model (Birch et al.,1990).

A more recent appraisal of primary care models by Abelson and Hutchison
(1994) contradicts findings of the earlier reviews. These authors suggest
that the evidence to support lower hospital utilization or overall costs when
compared to cost for fee-for-service models is weak. But, despite the apparent lack of rigorous and consistent evidence about the cost effectiveness
of CHCs, a closer look at some of the international and Canadian
literature indicates the potential of CHCs to fulfil the requirements of current government thinking on health policy (Abelson & Hutchison, 1994).

A review of the evaluative literature on neighbourhood health centres
in the U.S. concluded that, in general, health centres have succeeded in
"delivering good comprehensive care, including preventive services

and health supervision through a team approach ... at a reasonable cost" (Seacat, 1977, p. 168). A discussion of the results of two surveys on neighbourhood health centres in the U.S. suggests that access to ambulatory care for low-income and minority populations is enhanced; utilization of hospital ambulatory care is reduced; and patients have measurably lower hospital utilization rates when compared to hospital outpatient populations (Freeman, Kiecolt, & Allen, 1982). An impact assessment of the federally funded CHC program in the U.S. suggests that CHCs have had a significant impact on the infant mortality rate among certain target populations (Goldman & Grossman, 1988).

In the European setting, studies of CHCs in Finland, the Netherlands, and Sweden suggest that CHCs provide comparable quality of care to fee-for-service methods. Health centres in which services are delivered by "small teams consisting of a GP, two nurses, and an assigned social worker" are most successful in terms of responsiveness to population needs, collaboration among health-care providers, service integration and co-ordination, methods of reimbursement, and financial management and accountability practices (Abelson & Hutchison, 1995, p. 26).

Studies of CHCs in Canada are perhaps most intriguing. A study of four CHCs matched to four fee-for-service practices in Saskatchewan indicated that hospital costs were 23 percent lower for the Prince Albert CHC and 30 percent lower for the Saskatoon CHC, and that overall costs were 13 and 17 percent lower for the Prince Albert and Saskatoon CHCs respectively. This significant cost difference was attributed to lower admission rates and fewer prescriptions (Birch et al., 1990). Studies of CLSCs in Quebec indicate that patients are likely to receive a higher quality of care in the treatment of certain ailments, and that they are likely to receive more appropriate prevention services than care provided in other practice settings (Battista & Spitzer, 1983; Renaud, Beauchemin, Lalonde, Poirier, & Berthiaune, 1980). Additional research has suggested that physicians practising in CLSCs may do so because of already internalized values and preferences, which favour preventive activities and quality time with patients. The chosen medical education pathway (e.g., family medicine) may influence these attitudes. Age and gender also affect practice patterns, with young female physicians on salary being more likely to engage in cancer-detection activities and prevention activities, and to encourage patient involvement in treatment. The CHC context may act to reinforce this predisposition (Pineault, Maheux, Lambert, Beland, & Levesque, 1991). Box 11.1 illustrates the operation of a community health centre.

IMPLICATIONS FOR MANAGERS

As the above case example indicates, CHCs offer unique opportunities for innovation in management and service delivery. Community health centres are smaller in scale, have a flatter administrative structure, embrace a determinants-of-health framework, and are more organic in nature than more traditional health-care organizations, such as hospitals. Philosophically, they are committed to redressing the traditional power imbalance

Box 11.1
THE SANDY HILL COMMUNITY HEALTH CENTRE: A CASE EXAMPLE

The neighbourhood of Sandy Hill, in Ottawa, encompasses a relatively heterogeneous population of over 20,000 residents. The Sandy Hill Community Health Centre developed as an initiative of the Sandy Hill Community Development Corporation. The Corporation was originally created in 1973 as a non-profit organization to address issues related to public housing and neighbourhood land-use planning. The mandate of the Corporation allowed it to develop the CHC between 1973 and 1975 (Church, 1994).

Human Resource Management

Like other CHCs, the organization of Sandy Hill allows for a variety of different relationships among staff, clients, board members, management, and community. For example, an individual can be at once a client of the centre, a member of the board, and a member of the community at large; this puts that individual in the unique position of being both client and policy maker. Such arrangements have the potential to strengthen accountability linkages to the service community.

At the root of accountability is the distribution of power among the various stakeholders associated with community health centres. Given the history of CHCs (described above), management and board members are extremely cognizant of maintaining an equitable balance of power. One way in which CHC management tries to keep the power balance in check is by fostering open and mutually supportive relationships with staff.

Sandy Hill has developed a set of management values that emphasize reciprocal communications between management and staff. This is reflected both in the approach to personnel appraisal and to policy and program development. The performance development process created by Sandy Hill looks at factors such as how staff meet the needs of clients, relationships among team members, and what staff contribute to the centre. All staff are encouraged to participate in staff appraisals, but a minimum of four per appraisal is required. The staff member being evaluated is a fully participating member of the evaluation team. Both the staff member being evaluated and the manager choose one member of the evaluation team. The result of this open process is a strengthening of individual members and their teams through group self-appraisal. Staff describe the experience as energizing, affirming, and empowering.

One of the most notable characteristics of CHC management is the ability to react quickly to identified community needs. This can mean anything from developing a new program to completely shifting the approach of an existing program. The role of CHCs is to adapt to the changing needs of their clients and the communities they serve, not to impose their own views and solutions. This management philosophy is reflected in the organization and operation of providers.

Flexible Programming

At the level of operational decision making, staff are organized into service-delivery teams. Recently, the centre's health and social services teams collaborated to develop an innovative strategy to deal with the issue of teen pregnancy. Previously, the centre had focussed its efforts on promoting birth control and preventing teen pregnancy. This meant that other issues such as prenatal care, nutrition, and child-rearing practices were not being addressed. To broaden the focus of their efforts, the staff and management partnered with several outside agencies, including the Youth Services Bureau. The new strategy provides teens with a range of information and services relating to pregnancy and parenting, including a drop-in program that provides food and medical services for expectant mothers. While management continues to emphasize that the policy of the centre is to discourage and prevent teen pregnancy, it prefers to ensure that all teens are equipped to make informed choices about pregnancy and to receive proper care during and after the pregnancy.

Sandy Hill has also developed innovative programming through its community outreach team. Recently, this team identified a need among street people for some sort of new mechanism for networking. The need arose from the increasing number of street people who were getting clean, sober, and properly housed through the work of the outreach team. To address this need, a wood-working program was established to allow street people to learn carpentry skills and to network in a productive, safe, and supportive environment. The program is run through a partnership with another community agency, and is self-funded.

Holistic Care

Community health centres are well known for their "determinants of health" approach to service delivery. This is reflected in the interdisciplinary configuration of providers and the holistic approach to programming. Sandy Hill and other CHCs are in a position not only to help clients find the services and resources they need, but also to advocate on their behalf. For example, Mary, a 25-year-old woman who moved to Sandy Hill, was a stay-at-home mother with two toddlers. Shortly after arriving in Sandy Hill, Mary was involved in a serious car accident. After several surgical operations and repeated stays in the hospital, she was left with mobility problems and chronic pain, for which she began taking prescription painkillers. Mary had increasing difficulties coping with her personal responsibilities for the household and children, and her relationship with her husband began to deteriorate. The pain resulting from her injuries was not getting better. Not sure where to turn, Mary took the advice of a neighbour and contacted the Sandy Hill CHC to seek help with her ongoing problems.

Mary's first contact with Sandy Hill was through the medical service component. With the help of a physician, she was able to identify a problem with prescription drugs. Her physician connected her with the social services and addiction assessment components of the CHC. During the course of counselling, Mary revealed that she was in an abusive marriage and had also suffered abuse as a child. It was at this point that Mary decided to leave her husband and take the children with her. She was assisted with this transition by the social services intake/crisis worker; the worker helped Mary to find shelter for herself and her children until affordable housing was located.

Mary continued to work with the team of providers at Sandy Hill to deal with her complex health problems. She began physiotherapy and developed a strategy for coping with the pain without prescription drugs through alternative therapies (acupuncture, homeopathy, biofeedback, and visualisation). She also received massage therapy through referral to an outside agency. During this time, Mary also continued with regular visits to her nurse and, occasionally, to her physician.

Over time, Mary has rebuilt her life with the assistance of Sandy Hill. Unable to return to full-time employment because of her injury, she turned to the CHC for information and direction on income support, housing, and other social agencies that assist in obtaining employment. Although she has continued with counselling, the frequency of sessions has decreased over time. She is now part of a support group and is a volunteer at the centre.

Although at one point Mary felt her life was not worth living, she now has a very different outlook for herself, her family, and her future. Her physical health has improved significantly. Her children are growing up in a secure and happy environment. She has remarried and is now part of a blended family. Finally, she actively volunteers in the community as an organizer and advocate for the low-income population.

between service providers and lay individuals, and to facilitating community empowerment. These attributes are reflected in the accountability relationships between all health providers (including physicians) to the board of directors, the accountability of the board to the community, and the variety of opportunities for community participation in the development and delivery of programs. A caveat here is that, as the organization grows, the emphasis on organic participation by both clients and staff may be displaced by an institutional culture.

The interdisciplinary team approach to the delivery of services requires physicians to function as equal partners in interdisciplinary teams. This approach is fundamental to the CHC setting. In at least one case, this has resulted in experimenting with a partnership between a physician and nurse practitioner "that is based on mutual respect for the other's experience, knowledge and skills" (Birenbaum, 1994, p. 77). The manager must be flexible enough to allow experimentation with a range of non-traditional interdisciplinary arrangements.

Commitment to a framework that emphasizes the determinants of health results in the development of many partnerships and relationships by CHCs. Intersectoral relationships with existing agencies, and relationships with new or fledgling community groups, increase the potential to address a wide range of health issues that go beyond health care to engage in community development.

Managers operating in this environment need to be creative, flexible, adaptable, responsive, and visionary. Unlike managers in larger organizations, who tend to be more specialized, CHC managers must be adept at facilitating co-operation among a wide range of stakeholders, including federal and provincial funding agencies, providers who come from diverse professional backgrounds, community board members, clients, and local agency partners.

CONCLUSION

Community health centres have been a part of the health-care landscape for a long time. Their development has been characterized by an association with left-wing politics, and tends to be viewed by the medical profession as a threat to their central economic position in the health-care marketplace. However, when considered objectively and without reference to their ideological origins, it is obvious that CHCs offer an innovative means of delivering integrated and co-ordinated primary health and social services through interdisciplinary teams. While research to date has not provided conclusive evidence of the benefits of the model, there is growing evidence that CHCs provide greater access to appropriate primary care for the populations they serve. There is also some evidence to suggest that CHCs provide services in a cost-effective manner when compared to other methods of service delivery. In addition, CHCs have in some cases demonstrated an ability to achieve better clinical and population health outcomes for the prevention or treatment of certain ailments.

As governments are moving to reform the health-care system to deliver services in a more cost-effective and responsive manner, CHCs are becoming an increasingly attractive policy option. The extent to which CHCs will offer opportunities for new managers in the future will be determined largely by the degree to which provincial and regional governments adopt the CHC model as a vehicle for reforming the health-care system. However, the community-based, interdisciplinary nature of CHCs can also be expected to influence more traditional models in the future.

If they are to survive and thrive, CHCs will also have to adapt to the changing environment in health care. The introduction of regional governance and administrative structures for health care in most jurisdictions of Canada is proving a double-edged sword for some community health centres. On the one hand, regional structures and a broadened policy mandate are bringing the rest of the health-care system more in line with the broad philosophical approach of the CHC movement. On the other hand, individual CHCs, which have operated largely as highly autonomous community-based organizations accountable to local communities, are now faced with the prospect of surrendering some or all of their autonomy through integration into regional systems. Past experience has suggested that where CHCs are integrated with hospitals, the hospital culture dominates the new organizational form (Begin, 1977).

If CHCs are to play a significant role in the future health-care system, governments would be wise to invest in systematic research about the potential of CHCs to provide cost-effective services that contribute to improvements in the health of the population. This will involve establishing pilot projects across Canada and conducting rigorous and comparative evaluations of the benefits of the CHC model in different population settings. Community and consumer support for CHCs and their ability to integrate a variety of health and community services in a low cost, easily accessible setting can be expected to increase support for this innovative model.

SUMMARY

- Community health centres are non-profit agencies, controlled by elected boards, which deliver a range of primary health and social services through broad interdisciplinary teams.
- Community health centres have not been viewed favourably by the medical profession because of the threat the model poses to the dominant position of physicians in health care.
- Currently, most provincial governments are considering community health centres as mechanisms for reforming primary care.
- While the information on community health centres is incomplete and flawed, CHCs have demonstrated the capacity to achieve cost savings while allowing their communities to achieve improvements in health outcomes.

- Both the philosophical underpinnings and organizational design of community health centres offer unique opportunities for managers to develop innovative strategies for human-resource and program management, and for service delivery.

ACKNOWLEDGEMENTS

The authors wish to thank Jean-Marc Dupont, Sue McMurray, Denise Albrecht, Jeanette Edwards, Carole Dilworth, Bonny Hoyt-Hallet, Carole Anne Duffy and Brenda Fitzgerald for providing input on various aspects of the chapter.

FURTHER READINGS AND RESOURCES

ARA Consulting Group. (1992). *Evaluability assessment of Ontario's Community Health Centre Program*. Final Report. An assessment of the potential to evaluate the CHC Program in Ontario conducted by the ARA consulting group for the Ontario Ministry of Health.

Ginzberg, E., & Ostow, M. (1985). The community health center: Current status and future directions. *Journal of Health Politics, Policy and Law, 10*(2), 245–267. A descriptive assessment of the Robert Wood Johnson Foundation's Municipal Health Services Program.

Pong, R., Saunders, L. D., Church, W.J.B., Wanke, M.I., & Cappon, P. (1995). Health human resources in community-based health care: A review of the literature. *Building a Stronger Foundation: A Framework for Planning and Evaluating Community-Based Health Services in Canada*, Component 1. Ottawa: Health Promotion and Programs Branch, Health Canada. A systematic review of the literature conducted for the Federal/Provincial Advisory Committee on Health Human Resources on health human resources in community-based settings, including policy recommendations.

Weiner, J. (1988). Primary care delivery in the United States and four northwest European countries: Comparing the "corporatized" with the "socialized." *The Milbank Quarterly, 65*(3), 426–461. A descriptive comparison of primary care delivery models in the United States, Sweden, Finland, Denmark, and the United Kingdom.

Wanke, M.I., Saunders, L.D., Pong, R., & Church, W.J.B. (1995). *Building a stronger foundation: A framework for planning and evaluating community-based health services in Canada*. Ottawa: Health Promotion and Programs Branch, Health Canada. A discussion of issues relating to community-based health delivery, and the presentation of a framework for evaluating community-based models, prepared for the Federal/Provincial Advisory Committee on Health Human Resources.

REFERENCES

Abelson, J., & Hutchison, B. (1994). *Primary health care delivery models: A review of the international literature.* McMaster University Centre for Health Economics and Policy Analysis Working Paper 94–15, September, 1994.

Allen, D. (1984). Health services in England. In Marshall W. Raffel (Ed.), *Comparative health systems: Descriptive analyses of fourteen systems* (pp. 197–257). University Park, PA: Pennsylvania State.

Badgley, R., & Wolfe, S. (1967). *Doctors' strike: Medical care and conflict in Saskatchewan.* Toronto: Macmillan.

Battista, R., & Spitzer, W. (1983). Adult cancer prevention in primary care: Contrast among primary care practice settings in Quebec. *American Journal of Public Health.* 73 (8), 1040–1041.

Begin, C. (1977). Can the HCs and CLSCs co-exist? *Mental health in Canada, 5*(4), 11–15.

Birch, S., Lomas, J., Rachlis, M., & Abelson, J. (1990). *HSO performance: A critical appraisal of current research.* Centre for Health Economics and Policy Working Paper Series #90–1, January, 1990.

Birenbaum, R. (1994). Nurse practitioners and physicians: Competition or collaboration? *Canadian Medical Association Journal, 151*(1), 76–78.

Bozzini, L. (1988). Local community services centres (CLSCs) in Quebec: Description, evaluation, perspectives. *Journal of Public Health Policy, 9*(3), 346–375.

Church, W.J.B. (1994). *Health politics and structural interests: The development of community health centres in Ontario.* Unpublished doctoral dissertation, London, ON: University of Western Ontario.

Church, W. J. B., Saunders, L. D., Wanke, M. I., & Pong, R. (1995). Organizational models in community-based health care: A review of the literature. *Building a stronger foundation: A framework for planning and evaluating community-based health services in Canada, Component 2.* Ottawa: Health Promotion and Programs Branch, Health Canada.

Community health centres. (1993). Victoria: British Columbia Ministry of Health.

Community health centres: A picture of health (1993). Toronto: Ontario Ministry of Health.

Freeman, H.E., Kiecolt, K.J., & Allen II, H.M. (1982). Community health centers: An initiative of enduring utility. *Milbank Memorial Quarterly, 60*(2), 245–267.

Goldman, F., & Grossman, M. (1988). The impact of public health policy: The case of community health centers. *Eastern Economic Journal, 14*(1), 63–72.

A guide to community health centres in Saskatchewan. (1994). Regina, SK: Saskatchewan Ministry of Health.

Hall, P., Land, L., Parker, R., &. Webb, A. (1975). Change, choice and conflict. In P. Hall, L. Land, R. Parker, & A. Webb (Eds.), *Social policy* (pp. 277–310). London: Heinemann.

Hastings, J. E. F. (1972). *The community health centre in Canada: Report of the Community Health Centre Project to the Conference of Health Ministers.* Ottawa: Queen's Printer.

Hastings, J. E. F., & Vayda, E. (1986). Health services organization and delivery: Promise and reality. In R. G. Evans & G. L. Stoddart (Eds). *Medicare at maturity: Achievements, lessons, challenges* (pp. 337–384). Calgary, AB: University of Calgary Press.

Health Resources and Services Administration, Bureau of Primary Health Care Supported Health Centers. (1997). *Community health center program* [On-line] Available: http://158.72.85.159/chc/chc1.htm.

Lomas, J. (1985). *First and foremost in community health centres: The Centre at Sault Ste. Marie and the CHC alternative.* Toronto: University of Toronto Press.

Naylor, D. (1986). *Private practice, public payment.* Kingston, ON: McGill-Queen's University Press.

Pineault, R., Maheux, B., Lambert, J., Beland, F., & Levesque, A. (1991). Characteristics of physicians practising in alternative primary care settings: A Quebec study of local community service centre physicians. *International Journal of Health Services, 21*(1), 49–58.

Renaud, M., Beauchemin, J., Lalonde, C., Poirier, H., & Berthiaune, S. (1980). Practice settings and prescribing profiles: The simulation of tension headaches to general practitioners working in different practice settings in the Montreal area. *American Journal of Public Health, 70* (10), 1068–1073.

Sardell, A. (1988). *The U.S. experiment in social medicine: The community health center program*, 1965–1986. Pittsburgh, PA.: University of Pittsburgh.

Seacat, M. S. (1977). Neighborhood health centers: A decade of experience. *Journal of Community Health, 3*(2), 156–170.

Sessional payment manual. (1993). Edmonton, AB: Alberta Ministry of Health.

Young, T. K. (1975). Lay-professional conflict in a Canadian community health centre: A case report. *Medical Care, 13* (11), 897–904.

Chapter 12

▼▼▼▼▼▼▼▼▼▼▼▼▼▼▼▼▼▼▼

Work Force Issues

SONIA ACORN, ELAINE M. BAXTER, AND JANET WALKER

KEY OBJECTIVES

In this chapter, you will learn:

- How demographic, social, and economic trends shape the nursing work force and its needs.
- Implications of contemporary issues related to individual problems and cultural issues.
- The nurse manager's role in shaping the work environment.

INTRODUCTION

Changing trends in the Canadian social, economic, and health environments are also changing the work force and the ways first-line nurse managers provide leadership. Effective leadership depends on knowing about and using current trends and issues within a framework of progressive management practices. A first-line manager is in a key position to shape the work environment so that quality care can be delivered.

In this chapter, key demographic, social, economic, and health-care trends that are shaping the profile of today's and tomorrow's work force are identified. Current challenges that are coming to the forefront of attention for first-line managers are addressed. These challenges include such topics as: incorporating human rights practices, understanding the needs of a multiculturally diverse staff, managing stresses and strains within the modern workplace, and facilitating quality care. Implications—both theoretical and practical—for first-line managers are provided throughout.

BACKGROUND TRENDS

Historical background on the development of the Canadian health-care system and on political, social, and economic forces was provided in

Chapter 1. Information on ways to retrieve and use basic demographic and epidemiological information was provided in Chapter 2. In order to be effective, front-line managers must be familiar with the demographics of the work force, and gain an appreciation for the ways in which the working population is affected by social values and attitudes. Health-care managers must also understand the implications of a changing health-care environment on issues relating to the workplace.

WORK FORCE DEMOGRAPHICS

Changes in population structures or demographics help form basic characteristics of the nursing work force. In an earlier edition of this text, significant trends for Canada and Canada's nurses were documented. National trends that were shared by nurses included an aging population and the increase in cultural diversity. Specific to the nursing work force, significant trends included high and stable employment rates and a continuing increase in part-time employment (Acorn & Walker, 1994). The latest demographic information reflects a continuation in these trends. For example, 55 percent of employed nurses in Canada are age 40 years or older and 37 percent are age 45 years or older. Employment rates remain high, at 88.7 percent, and part-time employment continues to grow. Forty percent of hospital nurses and 48 percent of home care and community nurses are now working part time (Statistics Canada, 1996).

A growing number of men practise nursing and their employment characteristics are set out in editions of *Health Reports* prepared by Statistics Canada (1996). In 1985, male nurses in Canada represented 2.4 percent of the total nursing work force; by 1995, this figure grew to 3.8 percent (or approximately 10,000 nurses). Half of these nurses are in the province of Quebec and occupy 7.9 percent of that province's nursing population. For other provinces and territories, the percentage of male nurses ranges between one and three percent. Like their female counterparts, just over half of Canada's male nurses are employed in general hospitals. The part-time employment rate for male nurses (23%) is roughly half that for female nurses, but double that of male workers in general. Nurses of both genders significantly exceed the part-time employment rates of the overall work force. In Canada, 11 percent of men and 28 percent of women are employed on a part-time basis.

Nurses make up 47 percent of all workers employed in Canadian health care (OECD, 1995). The nurse group is made up predominantly of women. These two facts, together with available demographic and statistical information, have significant implications. Take the aging trend, for example. By the year 2005, nearly 40 percent of working nurses will be 55 years of age or older. Given the growing preference for early retirement among all Canadians, and the physically demanding nature of most nursing jobs, Canada could see more than one-third of its nursing work force disappear. Added to this are indications that adequate replacements are not coming. Student enrollments in nursing are generally smaller; women are choosing professions other than nursing, and enrollments in nursing education are falling (Ross, 1996).

With respect to participation rates in employment, Butlin (1995) reports that the participation rate of women in the workplace is at a stand-still. This ends a multi-decade trend of growth, and analysts are continuing to evaluate possible reasons. Other labour statistics reflect increased amounts of work time lost for personal and family reasons. This trend, most evident in the health-care and social-services sector, is attributed to the high percentage of women in these fields and their responsibilities in balancing work and family life (Akyeampong, 1995).

VALUES

Both attitudes and values fashion the expectations and behaviours of the work force. Drawing on ten years of data (1981-1991) and a world-wide survey of advanced industrialized countries, Nevitte (1996) reports on the changing values of Canadian people on topics that range from politics to the family and the workplace. In all spheres, Canadians reveal their declining deference to authority. There is less confidence in both government and non-government institutions. There is significant support for social movements, such as human rights, and an appreciation for individual rights and relationships. Value for egalitarian relationships is highly rated by both men and women, particularly spousal relationships. Parent-child relationships are undergoing transition towards a less hierarchical form.

In the workplace, motivation to work is driven by needs for self-actualization and there are expectations for greater participation and decision making. Detailed analysis reveals that these two significant workplace values are positively linked to age and education. The younger and more educated the individual, the greater the need for personal achievement and participation in the workplace. However, these shifting workplace values are present in all advanced industrialized countries, and Nevitte suggests that a new work ethic is emerging—one that relies on such work values as responsibility, achievement, engagement, and initiative. Incorporated in this study is a comparison between values of new Canadians and Canadians born in Canada. On 20 of the 24 values measured, findings show that new Canadians are no different than those who are Canadian by birth; however, four significant differences are noted. Within political orientations, new Canadians report a greater interest in politics and tend to be more cosmopolitan. In the workplace (part of economic orientations), new Canadians register less deference to authority and exhibit a greater preference for participation in decision making. Within social orientations (e.g., social intolerance, family relations), new Canadians register no differences.

HEALTH CARE

While detailed discussions about Canada's health-care system are available in other parts of this book (see especially Chapters 1 and 4), it may be helpful to examine this topic briefly here for the purpose of identifying some key trends relevant to work force issues. The state of a health-care system generates the environment in which the work force functions.

In Canada, health care is increasingly viewed as too costly and in need of reform. In a survey of health-care systems among industrialized countries and a review of the Canadian system in particular, McArthur, Ramsay, and Walker (1996) make several points related to economics. First, health care is a government responsibility, and the health-care sector is the largest single employer in Canada. Because Canada's population is aging, this economic sector is expected to continue to expand. Second, health-care costs are the largest and fastest-growing part of provincial government budgets. Third, given Canada's current debt level, the ability to pay for future health care, as it is presently organized, is doubtful.

In 1993, Health and Welfare Canada (1993) produced a summary of literature on emerging trends related to organization and delivery of health-care services. Six significant trends were identified:

1. decentralization or regionalization;
2. shift in resources to community-based health care;
3. creation of partnerships across health-care sectors;
4. role redefinition among health-care providers;
5. increased consumer participation; and
6. increased use of alternative medicine.

For the health-care system in general, the picture is one of transition. Driven by growing need, declining dollars, and changing public preferences, a transformation is being seen in the number and nature of services provided, where and how those services are provided, and by whom the services are provided.

TREND INFORMATION AND MANAGERS

Knowledge of pertinent trends is essential for effective management and human resource planning. Drawing on such information, managers can anticipate the various impacts in their areas of responsibility. Further, managers can be in a position to develop plans either to enhance or to mitigate the expected effects of the trends.

HEALTH-CARE SYSTEM TRENDS AND THE MANAGER

It is important for a manager to be attuned to the changing state of the health-care system for at least two reasons. First, it shapes the political environment within which the manager gathers resources and achieves particular results. One example is the expected partnerships across the various health-care sectors. The manager who includes such partnerships in planning and resource-sharing will achieve more effective results. Another example of the political environment relates to shrinking budgets. The need for innovation is pressing, and a manager who seeks more creative and cost-effective processes and who encourages such creativity among staff will advance the efficiency of health care.

Second, the changing state of the health-care system shapes the immediate work environment and relationship with staff. With all parts of the system in flux, feelings of fear and insecurity can be expected. For example, all provider roles are coming under intense scrutiny. Today's manager must work with staff to carefully analyze the needs and preferences of the population for whom the service is provided and to match those needs with the appropriate skills. If any resulting staffing changes are experienced as negative, the manager is in a valuable position to mitigate the situation with both personal and professional support.

NURSING WORK FORCE TRENDS AND THE MANAGER

Managers need to be familiar with the characteristics, behaviours, and preferences that are present or emerging among nurses as a group. Trends in demographics, employment characteristics, and values provide a manager with a generic profile of the nursing work force, as summarized in Box 12.1. Such a profile assists managers in planning recruitment strategies and developing positive, effective workplaces.

Implications arising from the profile of the nursing work force relate to a manager's working style. The manager who best fits with working nurses of today and tomorrow is a manager who is energized at the prospect of shared decision making, enjoys mentoring each member of the group, and is sensitive and responsive to the many and varied individual needs of staff. On the practical level, the manager will be focussing on how aspects of the workplace and work atmosphere could be altered to address employee needs, yet maintain or enhance quality of care. The issue of part-time work is one example. On the one hand, part-time work allows women to more effectively balance their home and work responsibilities. On the other hand, part-time work too often means a break in continuity of care, a breakdown in communications, and a weak connection between worker and workgroup. A good manager can involve staff in developing innovative ways to achieve the former without the latter. By acting in concert with people's needs, values, and preferences, managers increase not only the quality of work life but also the quality of care.

WORK FORCE ISSUES WITH IMPLICATIONS FOR FIRST-LINE MANAGERS

As the new millennium approaches, several issues have special implications for first-line nurse managers. Among these are human rights issues,

---

Box 12.1
NURSING WORK FORCE PROFILE

Demographics

Most Nurses are women.

The average age is 40 years and rising. Cultural diversity is rich and prominent.

Interests and Desires

Professional growth and development at work is an important consideration.

Participation in workplace issues and projects is valued.

More part-time work is sought to address personal and lifestyle issues.

Expectations

Employee involvement is solicited for all decisions affecting the work or the worker.

Work itself will meet personal achievement needs.

Individual rights, needs, and preferences are acknowledged, respected, and addressed.

Cultural beliefs and behaviours are identified, valued, and integrated into the daily work.

Practical Needs

Work schedules are increasingly more flexible and creative.

Personal, family, and eldercare responsibilities necessitate more time away from work.

---

including those related to discrimination and sexual harassment. Demographic changes and increasing multicultural awareness mean that managers must be cognizant of cultural diversity in situations involving both staff and clients. As well, managers must be aware of increasing stresses and strains that affect workers and clients alike.

HUMAN RIGHTS

Rights of all kinds are receiving increased attention. While the rights of patients were in evidence as early as 1980 (Rozovsky, 1980), the larger matter of human rights, particularly as applied to employees, is only now receiving serious attention. For managers, knowledge of human rights assists in maintaining a neutral and objective approach with all employees. Further, to ensure consistency in the larger context of organizational and societal behaviours and expectations, managers must understand the basics of human rights legislation and its use as a framework for management. Managers do not have to be experts on human rights, but it is important that they know the main purpose of the legislation, understand the various directives or regulations encompassed within each, and are aware of the implications for the management processes. (See also Chapter 3.)

Human rights legislation is both federal and provincial in nature. At the federal level, the *Charter of Rights and Freedoms* became part of the Canadian Constitution with the 1982 amendments. The Charter contains a measure of human rights within the specifications of the fundamental freedoms for all Canadians. The *Canadian Human Rights Act,* passed in 1985 and amended in 1989, addresses employment and services provided by federal organizations, such as chartered banks, national airlines, telephone companies, and band councils or tribal councils (on reserves). This Act is enforced by the Canadian Human Rights Commission. In each province, legislation addresses employment, housing and services (Desjarlais, Tataryn, & Timberg, 1995).

In British Columbia, for example, the Human Rights Code consists of the B.C. *Human Rights Act* (1984) and the *B.C. Human Rights Amendment Act* (1995). Health-care organizations take their direction from this legislation, which prohibits discrimination on the basis of: race, colour, ancestry, or place of origin; political belief; religion; marital or family status; physical or mental disability; sex; sexual orientation; age; and conviction for a criminal or summary offence unrelated to the job. Employers are prohibited from discriminating on any of these grounds with respect to hiring, dismissal, layoffs, promotions, and transfers, or any other term or condition of employment. Further, employees are protected from harassment in the workplace based upon any of the prohibited grounds, and they have recourse through the B.C. Council of Human Rights for any actual or perceived discrimination (Health Employees Association of B.C., 1996; Wills, 1995).

Also at the provincial level, other legislation specifies various guidelines for the employer/employee relationship. In British Columbia, the *Employment Standards Act* (1996):

- provides, for unionized employees, guidelines about minimum standards of wages and terms of employment;
- establishes basic rights for employers and employees;
- promotes fair treatment for employers/employees; and
- establishes ways to resolve disputes.

For example, this Act includes guidelines for hiring, payment of wages, hours of work, overtime, annual vacation, and termination of employment. The unionized employees covered by collective agreements have as a basis the minimum standards set out in the Employment Standards Act. Collective agreements must meet or exceed the minimum standards or the Act applies.

The first-line manager may experience any number of questions related to human rights issues. In most agencies, a department of human resources (often known as the employee relations department) will be able to provide expert advice on matters related to human rights and interpretation of collective agreements. When such a department is not available, a manager must determine where such expertise can be found—either at the provincial employer association level or via legal counsel with particular expertise. The latter are usually involved when a matter is referred as a complaint to the Council of Human Rights.

Four of the more common issues for today's managers are:

1. Allegations of discrimination in the hiring process.
2. Allegations of discrimination in the process of performance appraisal.

3. Situations of real or potential sexual harassment.
4. Dealing with the "duty to accommodate" provisions of collective agreements.

Allegations of Discrimination in the Hiring Process

During the interview process, it is important for a manager to ensure that interview questions address the neutral criteria of job descriptions. For example, the manager may ask if there are any limitations to meeting the work schedule but may not ask a potential employee about day-care arrangements for children, which could be perceived as discriminatory against someone who has children. Some potential employees may have cultural or religious restrictions that limit their availability for work but employers need to be prepared to accommodate these within reason. For example, a nurse applied for a position on a hospital unit but was not prepared to work on Friday evenings because of religious practices. She was not awarded the position as she could not be available for all of the required shifts. A successful appeal was made to the Human Rights Board, and the hospital was directed to accommodate the nurse's restriction by allowing her to switch shifts, or to take a vacation or unpaid leave when the rotation scheduled her for Friday evenings.

Allegations of Discrimination in the Process of Performance Appraisal

Performance appraisal is another area in which a manager must maintain an unbiased approach in both verbal and written evaluations. Even with such an approach, an employee who is not satisfied with his or her performance appraisal could allege that the evaluation was discriminatory, based upon an infringement of human rights. For example, a community health manager evaluating a home-care aide was accused of racial discrimination when in fact she was dealing with the aide's lack of adequate comprehension of English when caring for clients in the home. Several examples of errors made by the aide resulted from not being able to fully understand or accurately implement the written care plan and communicate effectively with the clients. The aide interpreted the manager's examples as evidence that the manager did not want to work with someone of her cultural background. Through the involvement of the union steward, the aide finally came to understand that English language comprehension was the issue, and accepted the need to take remedial language classes.

Situations of Real or Potential Sexual Harassment

In the area of sexual harassment, the most common situation for managers is to find themselves advising and supporting employees. For example, one manager was contacted by a female nurse who was experiencing problems with a male physician. Allegations included inappropriate remarks made in a patient area, telephone calls to the home requesting a date, and an incident of inappropriate touch. In this type of situation, a manager can do much to assist the nurse by acknowledging the stated concerns and providing advice on the process for remedying the situation. Most agencies have a policy for dealing with sexual harassment. Usually it is an in-house process whereby the allegations are fully examined, parties can meet in a safe, facilitated environment, and remedies or a resolution can be reached. Should the employee choose to lodge a complaint with the Human Rights Council, the process becomes more public and more formal. In either case, the employee needs to be supported throughout the process, and the manager must act immediately to implement appropriate procedures as well as take part in the investigation.

Dealing with Duty-to-Accommodate Provisions of Collective Agreements

As the health-care work force ages, more employees are experiencing injuries, illnesses, or conditions that limit their ability to work in areas or shifts previously assigned. Within most collective agreements, a duty-to-accommodate provision requires the employer to make reasonable changes to enable an employee to return to work (e.g., in a different area or on a restricted shift). This involves collaborating with the union steward, the occupational safety and health (OS&H) department, and human resources representatives to develop a planned return to work, with evaluation. Two examples can be used to illustrate situations a manager may face:

1. A nurse who was returning from three years of disability leave had been advised to return to an area that had fewer physical demands than her previous position. The union identified an outpatient area for which the nurse was qualified to work from a knowledge and skill perspective. After a trial period, it was determined that she was able to successfully carry out the work in the outpatient area. Under the duty-to-accommodate provision, the returning nurse was given a position in the new area and the most junior nurse in the outpatient area was "displaced" and moved to another area of the hospital. The manager's role in the situation was to work with the union and the occupational health officer to arrange the trial, then with the staff in the outpatient area to accept the returning nurse who was displacing their colleague. Support for the displaced nurse was also provided to ensure understanding of the situation and to assist with a smooth transition to an appropriate area.

2. Another nurse, returning from nearly two years on long-term disability, was advised to reduce the length of shift and limit the amount of night shift worked. The nurse had formerly worked in a full-time 11.0 hour rotation on a hospital unit. This unit operated with all full-time positions for the 11.0 hour shift and some part-time positions for the 7.5-hour shift. Although the nurse returned to a 7.5-hour part-time position, there were still a number of night shifts in the schedule. The

manager was asked to change the rotation as much as possible and then allow the nurse to trade shifts or take leaves of absence in order to limit the number of night shifts worked.

In summary, managers must be aware of human rights legislation from the perspective of ensuring a fair workplace for employees. It is also necessary to identify resources for consultation on human rights issues. Finally, it is important to be willing to work with union stewards, human resource department staff, and/or occupational safety and health department staff to develop creative solutions when presented by employees with individual challenges. Maintaining an open mind and a sense of fairness is essential in creating an environment conducive to equity and understanding. (See also Chapter 26.)

CULTURAL DIVERSITY

Canada is a diverse and multicultural nation where immigrants from such places as Hong Kong, India, Philippines, China, Sri Lanka, Italy, Germany, and Greece add to the multicultural mosaic of the country.

In 1991, next to English and French, the mother tongues or languages of preference most frequently used by Canadians were: Italian, Chinese (Mandarin and Cantonese), German, Portuguese, Polish, and Ukrainian (Statistics Canada, 1993). Cultural diversity within Canada will continue to grow in the 21st century and the demographics of these population changes will affect the health-care system in at least two ways. First, there is a need for staff to be sensitive to the cultural norms of clients and to possess the skills to provide culturally sensitive care. Second, managers need to provide the leadership required to guide a culturally diverse work force. Whatever the health-care setting, managers and staff must work closely together to create a healthy work environment where diversity is valued and appreciated. Organizations will not be successful in the future unless they value diversity and learn to manage it as a valued resource (Bruhn, Chesney, & Salcido, 1995).

The term "cultural diversity" has many definitions. *Culture* is frequently defined in relation to colour, religion, and country of origin, but may also include the interrelationship of beliefs, values, language, social relationships, modes of dress, politics, law, norms of behaviour, artifacts, technology, dietary practices, and health-care behaviours (Spector, 1991). *Diversity*, according to Hunt (1994), includes not only race and gender, but "age, socioeconomic class, physical differences, educational background, ethnicity, family structure, religion, sexual orientation, and national origin"(p. 27). This broad definition of diversity appears to adequately reflect the reality and composition of today's work force.

Problems of language, communication, racism, lack of education, and managerial inexperience contribute to the complexity of administration within a culturally diverse environment. The literature suggests that language and communications form major barriers for nurses providing care to culturally diverse clients (Burner, Cunningham, & Hattar, 1990; Murphy & Clarke, 1993; Thiederman, 1989). Language differences, interpretation of mannerisms, eye contact, rate of speech, and body-language interpretation can all add to misunderstandings. Even when people speak the same language, effective communication is often hampered when individuals are not acquainted with idiomatic expressions or connotative meanings.

A major communication problem can occur when staff members speak their mother tongue in the presence of clients who do not speak or understand that particular language. "Speaking around" the client in a language foreign to the client is unprofessional and unacceptable. Staff who are tempted to slip into using their mother tongue must remind themselves of the impact this can have on clients. Another communication problem occurs when staff speak a language other than the dominant language of the organization in a group setting. Staff members who do not understand the language that is being spoken often feel excluded and offended, sometimes even annoyed, and suspicious that they may have been the subject of discussion. Managers must set the tone and lead by example to promote a healthy work environment. Managers and staff need to address issues of a culturally diverse environment and set standards for the work unit.

Problems related to racism and discrimination also appear in the literature (Lowenstein & Glanville, 1991, 1995). Findings from an American study of 481 nurse managers, staff nurses, and nursing assistants indicate that "racial conflict and perception of racial discrimination and prejudice continues to exist in the health-care workplace" (Lowenstein & Glanville, 1995, p. 206). The literature suggests that racism also exists in the Canadian health-care system. In another study, nurses employed in Vancouver hospitals were interviewed about their experience of caring for culturally diverse clients (Reimer, 1995). Findings indicate that overt and covert racism is present in health-care organizations. Nurses find these situations difficult to address and need the guidance of managers to help them resolve workplace issues.

The lack of preparation of nurses in transcultural nursing is evident in both the United States and Canada. Leininger (1995) reports that more than 90 percent of hospital staff in the United States have had limited or no preparation in transcultural health care and that the majority can speak and understand only one language. This is reinforced by Guruge and Donner (1996), who write that "Canadian nurses have little knowledge, formal education or strong theory and research to support their care of people of different social and cultural groups" (p. 37), and in a Canadian study by Reimer (1995), who reported a wide variation in the amount of preparation that nurses receive in nursing school relating to the care of culturally diverse clients. Many nurses receive minimal or no preparation in caring for cultural diverse clients.

Education is needed to help staff understand clients' perceptions of their condition, and to enhance their ability to provide culturally sensitive care (Anderson, 1990; Burner, Cunningham, & Hattar, 1990; Martin, Wimberley, & O'Keefe, 1994). Nurses must become skilled in conducting a thorough assessment of the culturally based wishes of clients. At a minimum, the assessment should include the following:

- Where the client was born or, if an immigrant, how long the client has lived in this country;
- Who the client's major support people (family members, friends) are;
- What are the primary and secondary languages, and the speaking and reading abilities;
- What is the client's religion, its importance in daily life, and current practices;
- What are the client's food preferences and prohibitions;
- What health and illness beliefs and practices will affect care;
- Who the client wishes to have included in his or her care.

Educational sessions on cultural diversity assist staff in understanding how culture influences the way people behave and communicate. Managers themselves must become educated about various cultures and ensure the same education programs are available for staff. Managers and staff must identify the education, knowledge, and skills needed within their organizations. As the cultural make-up of clients and staff differs within organizations, education programs must be agency-specific. Organizational diversity training must have the support of the chief executive officer and must focus on issues familiar to the employees (Henderson, 1994). Although content can be provided through lectures, discussion sessions allow opportunities for ideas to be presented and for employees to reflect on the ideas of others. One simple way to promote informal daily learning and discussion is to use a multifaith calendar in the workplace. One such Canadian calendar describes 13 different faiths, including aboriginal spirituality. All significant festivals or days are marked on the calendar and narrative is conveniently offered on the same page (Multifaith Calendar Committee, 1996).

Blank and Slipp (1994) offer managers the following guidelines in supporting cultural diversity:

- Approach each employee as an individual.
- Understand that cultural tendencies such as language, mannerisms, and communication patterns are not necessarily indicators of a worker's performance and capabilities.
- Recognize and confront the issue of discomfort—your own and others'—in dealing with a diverse work force.
- Appreciate and utilize the different perspectives and styles of diverse workers.
- Confront racist, sexist, or other stereotypic or discriminatory behaviour.

Managerial leadership can promote a culturally healthy environment. Managers must monitor the organization to ensure cultural sensitivity, and model professional attitudes and behaviours desired in a culturally diverse staff. Managers set the tone for the organization and hold a firm belief that diversity is an organizational strength. Commitment is needed from senior management within the organization, with the value of cultural diversity being reflected in the mission statement and managers continuously reinforcing the organization's commitment. Fernandez (1991) states that successful managers of the future will recognize, and be willing to hire, people who do not necessarily think and behave as they do (p. 286). People hired should complement the skills and talent that the successful leaders already possess.

STRESSES AND STRAINS

Many factors in today's workplace contribute to stress: diminished financial resources, organizational downsizing, changes in internal organizational design, and increases in technology all add to an already stressful environment. One result of organizational downsizing is an increased span of control of first-line nurse managers. Some first-line nurse managers now report responsibility for up to 175 individual staff (147 full-time equivalents or FTEs) and areas that have up to 230 beds (Acorn & Crawford, 1996). This is accompanied by an increase in responsibilities for staff nurses.

In addition to the work environment, nurses, like the general population, must handle stress associated with daily life. This may include family caregiving commitments, illness and death in the family, and marital or other relationship problems. Cooper and Williams (1994) emphasize the heavy cost, in both human and financial terms, of a stressful environment, and indicate that it is in the best interests of managers to create healthy workplaces. A stressful environment can contribute to employee problems which, if not addressed, can exert a toll on the organization. Special situations of employees that may interfere with performance include chemical dependency, mental-health problems, financial problems, or relationship problems. Employees with significant challenges that go unaddressed can cost the organization in increased absenteeism, work-related accidents, lower productivity, and higher staff turnover (Marquis & Huston, 1996).

Chemical Impairment

The potential for chemical dependency is high in the health professions. Robinson and Spicer (1987) report that members of the nursing profession have a 50 percent greater risk of becoming chemically addicted than members of other professions. Landry (1987) estimates that eight to ten percent of all registered nurses and licensed practical nurses in the United States have either a drug or alcohol dependency. According to Hughes and Smith (1994), alcohol and Demerol are the most commonly used chemicals. The impairment of health professionals takes its toll on both a personal and a professional level. It is imperative, however, to acknowledge that chemical dependency and addiction are treatable illnesses.

There are several areas in which a manager must be skilled in assisting an employee whose practice may be impaired due to substance abuse. These include identifying the problem, intervening, getting the employee into treatment, and assisting the reintegration of the employee back into the work force. Although the profile of the impaired nurse varies, Landry (1987) states that the behavioural changes generally fall into three areas: job performance, personality or behaviour, and attendance. *Job performance changes* may include: illogical or sloppy charting; high frequency medication errors; judgement errors; and complaints from other staff about the quality of the employee's work. *Personality/behaviour changes* may include: increased irritability; mood swings; change in personal grooming; defensiveness when approached about medication or judgement errors; and forgetfulness. *Attendance changes* are evident in increased absences from work, especially on the day prior to or after regularly scheduled off days; consistent lateness; and a noticeable increase in the use of sick time. As the chemical dependency becomes more severe, these symptoms become more pronounced.

Identifying Employees in Difficulty

Nurse managers who observe any or all of these behaviour changes must be careful not to diagnose the observed behaviour as a chemical dependency problem, as the behaviours may be due to other causes. The manager's role is to identify and articulate performance expectations, and to notify the employee when these expectations are not met. Although managers are no doubt concerned about staff on a personal level, the primary responsibility "is to see that the employee becomes functional again and can meet organizational expectations before returning to the unit" (Marquis & Huston, 1996, p. 454).

Resources for Troubled Employees

Managers should call on professional counselling resources when assisting employees with difficulties. Many health-care organizations have internal employee-family assistance programs (EFAPs), which provide counselling services for personal concerns including, but not limited to, stress, burnout, marital problems, mental-health problems, conflict management, legal problems, financial problems, or chemical dependency. The aim of such programs is to prevent, identify, and treat personal problems that affect job performance (Cooper & Williams, 1994).

Many provincial nursing associations offer professional services to assist troubled nurses. The Registered Nurses Association of British Columbia (RNABC), for example, has the Prevention and Resources for Nurses (PRN) program, a confidential service for nurses with chemical dependency or emotional difficulties. The PRN program is based on two approaches: education and consultation. Education programs help nurses and managers understand the impact of chemical dependency on the nursing profession and how they can intervene with a colleague. Education in this area is critical because, according to Marquis and Huston (1996), most nurses "generally lack sensitivity in identifying behaviours and actions that could signify chemical impairment of an employee or colleague" (p. 447). One researcher (Hughes, 1995) found that 61 percent of chief nurse executives indicated they felt unprepared to deal with alcohol- and drug-dependent nurses.

The RNABC's PRN consultation service is confidential, and may be initiated in one of three ways: a nurse recognizes that he or she has a problem; a colleague needs advice on how to help another nurse; a manager calls seeking guidance on how to help a nurse-employee.

The return to work of an employee after treatment for chemical dependency can be tense for both employee and manager. Smith and Hughes (1996) discuss the advantages of a signed return-to-work contract. Such a contract may include: a plan for treatment; practice restrictions (e.g., prohibition from administering narcotics); attendance at a support group for chemically dependent nurses; agreement to perform at professional standards; and participation in random drug screening, if appropriate. The contract can be developed with input from the nurse employee, the manager, the agency's counsellor and, if appropriate, the professional association. Some contracts also contain a section describing what is to happen if the nurse relapses.

SHAPING THE WORK ENVIRONMENT

One of the greatest challenges facing a front-line manager in the late 1990s is shaping a work environment to support quality care or service while in the centre of massive transitions to health care. For example, financial constraints are forcing organizations to change the type of health-care delivery to ever more efficient systems, consumers are demanding more input to the planning of their own health services, and employees are experiencing multiple conflicts from the ever-changing workplace and the pressures of personal and professional life. Sometimes the only stable part of the system is the employer/employee relationship. A good manager can influence this relationship to ensure that quality care is delivered to the patient, client, or consumer group. The provision of quality care and service is the common goal of all health-care providers and offers common ground for effective work relationships.

The manager's role in the modern organization can best be described as a balancing act among various tensions and opposing forces of the work environment. Some of these tensions merit further exploration and include:

- Interdisciplinary versus single-discipline management;
- Integration versus boundaries;
- Structure versus flexibility;
- Personal versus professional life and commitments.

INTERDISCIPLINARY VERSUS NURSING COMMITMENTS

Some managers have difficulties balancing their commitments to nursing with a need for interdisciplinary planning and service delivery. The demands of working closely with other disciplines through program management models, interdisciplinary care planning and documentation, and development of clinical pathways and protocols often leads to concerns about the place and value of nursing. Some of the questions with which a manager must struggle as roles of health-care professionals become increasingly blurred include:

- What is the most critical skill/knowledge for each discipline and how does this contribute to the overall care of the patient/client/resident?
- Which discipline is most capable of providing a particular aspect of care when many of the skills overlap?
- What is the most efficient and effective way of providing care?

The nurse manager's ability to articulate the unique contribution of nursing and the professional standards of practice is critical. The manager can then guide staff toward their role while valuing the knowledge and skills of all disciplines in the delivery of patient care.

INTEGRATION VERSUS BOUNDARIES

Building a care team or unit usually means describing the profile of patients/clients accessing the service, defining the type of care delivered, and identifying admission and discharge criteria for patients/clients. These activities essentially define the boundaries of the environment within which the staff work. However, as the health-care system comes under closer scrutiny, it is clear that the boundaries between parts of the present system create a number of inefficiencies. For example, discharge of a patient from an inpatient psychiatric unit to a mental-health centre in the community requires phone calls, a referral form from the inpatient unit, and an assessment by the mental-health clinician before a decision on acceptance is reached. This may either delay the discharge or leave the discharged patient in limbo in the community while awaiting out-of-hospital treatment.

The need for an integrated, seamless system in which clients simply transfer between and among services with appropriate planning and follow-up will increase efficiency and effectiveness of care delivery in future. However, to make this happen, a manager needs to work closely with counterparts within the system. The manager must also assist staff in understanding other parts of the system so that they can identify information required to ensure a safe transfer pathway. The emergence of community-based case management will help (see also Chapter 9). When the manager promotes such opportunities for professional growth and learning, work values important to employees are achieved.

STRUCTURE VERSUS FLEXIBILITY

Professional nurses are expected to be able to make autonomous decisions about the care they provide. However, this care is delivered within a system where co-operation is essential. For example, while a nurse on a general medical unit may have sole responsibility for five or more patients on day shift, she or he often cannot provide the physical care without assistance from at least one other staff member. Therefore, specific routines for bathing, ambulation, or turn times may be established so the team can function efficiently with another nurse or assistive personnel joining the primary nurse for certain periods of the shift. In this situation, the manager has the opportunity to help staff determine the appropriate balance of structured times and routines for care while allowing flexibility for these routines to change as the patient or staff mix varies. If staff are to provide care in an efficient, effective way, the manager is responsible for identifying the framework for service delivery. A structured approach is required for the complement of staff, rotations, hours of work, roles of the team members, and other such administrative details, but beyond that, the manager can be more flexible in allowing the staff to deliver the care within pre-established care guidelines. Managers and staff must work together to identify what is structured formally and what can be flexible. In this way, individualized care is ensured and staff are empowered in the work environment.

PERSONAL VERSUS PROFESSIONAL COMMITMENTS

Earlier in this chapter, factors creating stress in the work environment were highlighted. Most staff must regularly balance the responsibilities of a fast-paced, demanding profession with the multiple commitments of family and personal life. Successful managers know enough about their employees to understand many of these pressures, and intervene when the balance is tipped. A change of work assignment, time off, or a listening ear will all be required at different times. Because job satisfaction is most threatened by stress (Blegen, 1993), the manager is in a key position to eliminate or minimize workplace stress and facilitate staff satisfaction.

CONCLUSION

The manager's relationship with employees is critical in meeting work force needs and achieving organizational goals. Staff need to know that they are making a difference and that their contribution is valued. The manager has a unique opportunity to open doors to quality care through the exercise of leadership by articulating a vision and creating an environment that promotes personal value, empowerment, and organizational commitment.

In this chapter, the role of the first-line manager has been explored in relation to current work force issues, from human rights and cultural diversity to personal stresses and strains. These have been set within the broader context of Canadian social, economic, and health-care trends. With care and understanding, the first-line manager can shape the future for the work force and for those receiving care.

SUMMARY

- The nursing work force is aging.
- There may be a shortage of nurses in the new century.
- The work force in Canada, like those in other industrialized countries, is expecting more participation and decision making in the workplace.
- Managers need to keep themselves informed on trends, using them to plan and to address the needs of the work force.
- The contemporary workplace exhibits an increase in cultural diversity, human rights issues and stresses and strains.
- Managers need to practice and encourage innovation and to form partnerships across health-care sectors.
- Managers provide the leadership that influences how employees shape the workplace.
- The quality and style of managerial leadership supports professional growth and development of staff and thus the quality of care.

FURTHER READINGS AND RESOURCES

American Nurses Association (1995). *Nursing care report card for acute care.* Washington, DC: American Nurses Association. This study was commissioned by the American Nurses Association to investigate the impact of workforce restructuring and redesign on the safety and quality of patient care. The purpose was to explore the nature and strength of the linkages between nursing care and patient outcomes, and to identify nursing quality indicators. The study revealed the lack of data necessary to measure and track the 21 nursing quality indicators that were identified. Two major findings indicate that mortality rates and patient satisfaction are both related to quality of nursing care as measured by the ratio of registered nurses and all nursing staff.

Kreitzer, M. J., Wright, D., Hamlin, C., Towey, S., Marko, M., & Disch, J. (1997). Creating a healthy work environment in the midst of organizational change and transition. *Journal of Nursing Administration, 27*(6), 35–41. Staff nurses and nurse leaders at the University of Minnesota Hospital and Clinic took the initiative to address what they felt was a stressful environment created by the many changes around them. In this article, the authors describe various strategies employed over a period of several years to develop a healthy work environment. One of the tasks was to identify and agree on what constitutes a healthy work environment, and the behaviours expected of people. They note that the process does not produce results overnight, but requires acknowledgement of current reality, the development of structures to ensure that organizational changes endure, and active leadership.

Sibbald, B. (1998). The future supply of Registered Nurses in Canada. *Canadian Nurse, 94*(1), 22–23. This short report of a recently commissioned study by the Canadian Nurses Association contains a prediction that there will be a shortfall of nurses in Canada of up to 113,000 RNs by the year 2011 unless urgent action is taken. The principal factors include an increasing demand for nurses, but a diminishing supply due to an aging workforce, inadequate retention, and declining enrollments in schools of nursing.

Whitehorn, D., & Nowlan, M. (1997). Towards an aggression-free health care environment. *Canadian Nurse, 93*(3), 24-26. Recent reports of violence in the workplace, especially against nurses, has led to a change in attitude and a determination by nurses to do something about it. This article is an account of one Nova Scotia health agency's initiative to create a safe, aggression-free environment. The process involved the establishment of an active task group, the development of a hospital policy, staff education programs, emergency response procedures, counselling services for victims of aggression, the maintenance of statistics, and periodic evaluation of organizational response.

REFERENCES

Acorn, S., & Crawford, M. (1996). First-line managers: Scope of responsibility in a time of fiscal restraint. *Healthcare Management Forum, 9*(2), 26–30.

Acorn, S., & Walker, J. (1994). Human resources-human management. In J. M. Hibberd & M. E. Kyle (Eds.), *Nursing management in Canada* (pp. 482–500). Toronto: W. B. Saunders.

Akyeampong, E. B. (1995). Missing work. *Perspectives on Labour and Income, 7*(1), 12–16.

Anderson, J. M. (1990). Health care across cultures. *Nursing Outlook, 38*(3), 136–139.

Blank, R., & Slipp, S. (1994). *Voices of diversity.* New York: American Management Association.

Blegen M. A. (1993). Nurses' job satisfaction: A meta-analysis of related variables. *Nursing Research, 42,* 36–41.

Bruhn, J. G., Chesney, A. P., & Salcido, R. (1995). Health and organizational issues in managing a multicultural work force. *Family & Community Health, 18*(2), 1–8.

Burner, O. Y., Cunningham, P., & Hattar, H. S. (1990). Managing a multicultural nurse staff in a multicultural environment. *Journal of Nursing Administration, 20*(6), 30–34.

Butlin, G. (1995). Adult woman's participation rate at a standstill. *Perspectives on Labour and Income, 7*(3), 30–33.

Canadian Charter of Rights and Freedoms, *Constitution Act* (1982), Part 1.

Cooper, C. L., & Williams, S. (1994). *Creating healthy work organizations.* New York: John Wiley & Sons.

Desjarlais, C., Tataryn, J., & Timberg, T. (1995). *Human rights and discrimination. Same sex, same laws: Lesbians, gay men and the law in BC.* Vancouver: Legal Services Society of B.C.

Employment Standards Act (1996). R.S.B.C., C-113

Fernandez, J. P. (1991). *Managing a diverse work force.* Lexington, MA: Lexington Book.

Guruge, S., & Donner, G. (1996). Transcultural nursing in Canada. *The Canadian Nurse, 92*(8), 36–40.

Health and Welfare Canada (1993). *Planning for health: Toward informed decision-making* (Cat. No. H39-266/1993E). Ottawa: Ministry of Supply and Services.

Health Employees Association of B. C. (1996). *What employees should know about human rights law and the duty to accommodate.* Vancouver: Health Employees Association of B. C.

Henderson, G. (1994). *Cultural diversity in the workplace: Issues and strategies.* Westport, CT: Quorum Books.

Hughes, T. L. (1995). Chief nurse executives' responses to chemically dependent nurses. *Nursing Management, 26*(3), 37–40.

Hughes, T. L., & Smith, L. L. (1994). Is your colleague chemically dependent? *American Journal of Nursing, 94*(9), 31–35.

Hunt, P. L. (1994). Leadership in diversity. *Health Progress, 75*(10), 26–29.

Landry, M. (1987). The impaired nurse. *California Nursing Review, 9*(6), 14–18.

Leininger, M. (1995). *Transcultural nursing: Concepts, theories, research & practices* (2nd. ed.). New York: McGraw-Hill.

Lowenstein, A. J., & Glanville C. (1995). Cultural diversity and conflict in the health care workplace. *Nursing Economics, 13*(4), 203–209, 247.

Lowenstein, A. J., & Glanville, C. (1991). Transcultural concepts applied to nursing administration. *Journal of Nursing Administration, 21*(3), 13–14.

Marquis, B. L., & Huston, C. J. (1996). *Leadership roles and management functions in nursing: Theory & application.* Philadelphia, PA: Lippincott.

Martin, K., Wimberley, D., & O'Keefe, K. (1994). Resolving conflict in a multicultural nursing department. *Nursing Management, 25*(1), 49–51.

McArthur, W. R., Ramsay, C., & Walker, M. (1996). *Healthy incentives: Canadian health reform in an international context.* Vancouver: Fraser Institute.

Multifaith Calendar Committee (1996). *The multifaith calendar 1997.* Port Moody, BC: Multifaith Action Society.

Murphy, K., & Clarke, J. M. (1993). Nurses' experiences of caring for ethnic-minority clients. *Journal of Advanced Nursing, 18,* 442–450.

Nevitte, N. (1996). *The decline of deference: Canadian value change in cross-national perspective.* Peterborough, ON: Broadview Press.

Organization for Economic Cooperation and Development (OECD). (1995, May). *OECD health data* (electronic version #3.6). Paris: OECD.

Reimer, S. (1995). *Nurses' descriptions of the experience of caring for culturally diverse clients.* Unpublished Master's thesis, University of British Columbia, Vancouver, BC.

Robinson, M., & Spicer, J. G. (1987). Impaired employee-Confrontation process. In E. M. Lewis & J. G. Spicer (Eds.), *Human resource management handbook* (pp. 217–227). Rockville, MD: Aspen.

Ross, E. (1996). From shortage to oversupply. The nursing work force pendulum. In J. R. Kerr & J. MacPhail (Eds.), *Canadian nursing issues and perspectives* (3rd ed.) (pp. 196–207). St. Louis, MO: Mosby.

Rozovsky, L. E. (1980). *The Canadian patient's book of rights.* Toronto: Doubleday.

Smith, L. L., & Hughes, T. L. (1996). Re-entry: When a chemically dependent colleague returns to work. *American Journal of Nursing, 96*(2), 32–37.

Spector, R. (1991). *Cultural diversity in health care.* New York: Appleton-Century-Crofts.

Statistics Canada. (1993). *Ethnic origin.* Ottawa: Industry, Science and Technology.

Statistics Canada. (1996). Male Registered Nurses, 1995. *Health Reports, 8*(2), 23–26 (Cat. No. 82-003-XPB). Ottawa: Ministry of Industry.

Statistics Canada (1996). *Nursing in Canada 1995* (Cat. No. 83–243). Ottawa: Statistics Canada.

Thiederman, S. (1989). Managing the foreign-born nurse. *Nursing Management, 20*(7), 13.

Wills, A. (1995). *Human rights: The changing landscape: Current issues for employers.* Vancouver: Harris & Company.

PART THREE

Professional Leadership

Chapter 13

▼▼▼▼▼▼▼▼▼▼▼▼▼▼▼▼▼

Contemporary Perspectives on Leadership

Judith M. Hibberd, with Ginette Lemire Rodger

KEY OBJECTIVES

In this chapter, you will learn:

- Common characteristics of effective contemporary leaders.
- The importance of visible leadership in the nursing profession.
- The changing nature of formal nursing leadership in health-care agencies.
- To distinguish between concepts of management and leadership.
- To describe how leadership skills may be exercised at grass roots levels of health agencies.

INTRODUCTION

Few topics in the social sciences have attracted as much commentary, theory, and research as that of leaders and leadership. There is an immense literature on the subject. Introductory management texts such as this one typically contain an overview of theories of leadership, beginning with early attempts to explain the phenomenon with propositions from the great man theory, trait theory, and behavioural theory. These theories had as their focus the individual leader, but gradually the scope of enquiry broadened to include the leaders and their followers, the situations in which leadership occurs, and a host of other considerations. More recently, theories have focussed on the relationship between leaders and followers, emphasizing the "transformational" nature of effective leadership. It is not intended to provide another survey of leadership theory here; however, several excellent references to such surveys are provided at the end of this chapter as supplementary reading (Grohar-Murray & DiCroce, 1997; Marriner-Tomey, 1993; Wylie, 1994). The development of leadership theory is included in the curriculum of all health professionals because the insights it provides can help them to assess their own aptitude for leadership, as well as to understand the goals and behaviour of the leaders they will encounter on a daily basis.

Theoretical approaches to the explanation of leadership have been evolutionary, with each successive school of thought building on the findings of previous schools. From this ever-expanding body of knowledge, there are few hard and fast principles for the new student of leadership to grasp with any degree of certainty. There is no one best way to design an organization, and so it is with leadership—there is no one best style or leadership role. As dozens of factors can have an impact on leaders and their individual styles; making predictions about how a person might perform in a given role or situation would be hazardous to say the least. However, most thinking on the subject recognizes that leadership is contingent upon a variety of major variables including:

- the leader himself or herself;
- the followers and whether they constitute a group;
- the relationships among group members and between the group and the leader;
- the goals and the nature of the tasks to be achieved;
- available resources;
- the setting or situation; and
- the amount of pressure experienced by the group (Perrow, 1973).

The purpose of this chapter is to present some current perspectives on leadership, and to articulate them in the light of changes discussed in the previous section of this book. In the first half of this chapter, Ginette Lemire Rodger provides a macroscopic view of the need for nursing leadership. In the second half, examples of how nurses are providing leadership in the changing health system environment are discussed.

THE LEADERSHIP IMPERATIVE

A recurrent theme both in the popular press and in professional literature has been the search for effective leadership in a particular field, in business, or in government. There has also been a tendency from time to time to proclaim a crisis of leadership. Perrow in 1973 concluded from his overview of the history of organizational theory that in almost every era there had been a burning cry for "good leadership." Twenty years later, the prominent French historian Jean Lacouture was reported to have said, "In the history of the world, I cannot think of a period where there have been so few great [political] leaders" (cited in Walsh, 1993, p.15). At about the same time, a former president of the Canadian Nurses Association said that there had never been a greater need for nursing leadership—leaders who could cut through the ambiguity of the immediate future and offer a vision to their followers (Harrison, 1992).

Now Ginette Lemire Rodger, a Canadian nurse of national and international leadership repute, issues a similar call for leadership. In her

Box 13.1

CALL FOR NURSING LEADERSHIP,
Ginette Lemire Rodger, RN, PhD

This is a call for *nursing* leadership, not just leadership. The nursing profession needs leadership during this unprecedented period of change, not the kind of leadership that is narrow and self-serving, but the kind of leadership that will guide the profession through transitions. During our professional lifetime as nurses, we are fortunate to have lived in an era in which we have dreamed of a reformed health-care system and we have prepared for it. We are now participating in the transformation, and these are some of the reforms we have dreamed of:

- health, not just health care;
- health services in the community, not just in hospital;
- multidisciplinary networks of practitioners, educators, researchers, and managers, not just solo players;
- public participation in shaping the system, not just public consultation;
- intersectoral health, not just health care;
- appropriate technology, not just "high tech";
- ecology, not just environment.

Nurses have also dreamed of a reformed health-care system in which they can contribute to their full potential, and avoid being under-utilized and under-valued. They have dreamed of being able to implement new ways of increasing quality while reducing costs. They have dreamed of direct access to their services by clients who choose to consult them under the basic health care system of this country.

In examining the ways in which nurses have prepared for a reformed health-care system, a colleague and I undertook a retrospective survey of actions taken by universities and professional associations during the years 1985 to 1993 (Lemire Rodger & Gallagher, 1995). We found that during that period, all except one university program had revised its curriculum to include primary health care as a major

component, in anticipation of expected reforms. Seven professional associations had developed, or were modifying, position statements on the role of the nurse in primary health care; five had included primary health concepts in their scope of practice; and all professional nurses' associations were being represented by nurses on various government task forces related to health-care reform. In the past fifteen years, the nursing research agenda has shifted toward increasing knowledge in the areas of cost-effective practice, the impact of the wellness model, the health concept, the benefits of low technology, and self care. Several demonstration projects have been implemented across Canada in which services are provided to highlight the benefits of alternative modes of delivery in a reformed health-care system. Since its beginnings as a profession, nursing has always envisioned and advocated for reforms in the health system of the day. Although we have not foreseen all the events and trends in recent times, nurses have often been at the forefront of efforts to create a more wellness-oriented and client-centred health system.

In the last several years, a major paradigm shift has been underway, approaching like a tornado, although at differing speeds depending on the province we live in. This type of change brings turmoil and creates circumstances that destabilize our most fundamental values and infrastructures. Many nursing leaders are experiencing difficulty in leading the transformation of nursing services within this reforming health-care system. Many are becoming what might be called "generic executives," involved almost entirely in cutting costs or restructuring the health-care system. In all of these changes costs are paramount, and it is tempting for governments and institutions once they have reduced, restructured, redesigned, and met the bottom line, to stop short of real reform. Reduction and redesign without reform are having serious consequences. In many instances, citizens are left with less of the same, although hopefully delivered more efficiently; consumers are abandoned in their homes; professionals lose opportunities for contributing fully to health-care reform; policy makers are replaced in advance of the next round of cutbacks. The route ahead will be challenging for nursing leaders.

Nursing Leaders

The goals for nursing leaders are fairly clear, but the route to be travelled is not as reassuring because it leads into unfamiliar territory. The focus must be on how to reach those goals. According to Vance (1977), the movement, growth, and value of a profession are inextricably tied to its leadership. In the transition to a new paradigm, the discipline of nursing with its knowledge and professional practice requires transformational leadership. This is the kind of leadership that thrives on change and innovation, and empowers by exercising "power 'with' not power 'to' others" (Barker, l990, p. 39). Leaders in nursing practice, education and research must lead within nursing and alongside or parallel to other stakeholders in the new reality, or risk becoming lost and out of touch with their professional roots. The road is not easy and the map not very precise, but how it will be done will most likely determine the future of our ability as a profession to contribute to the new paradigm into the next century.

There are four key characteristics of the kind of leadership that is needed in nursing, and these are vision, knowledge, confidence, and visibility.

Vision

Leaders must be visionary because vision is definitely 'in.' One definition of vision is "the ability to dream [and] translate those dreams into a reality" (Deveraux, 1989, p. 3). Another is that vision is an image of a possible and desirable future—a future that is realistic, attainable, credible, and attractive (Barker, 1990). Visions that have proven to be successful in transforming organizations have several common characteristics:

- They reflect the core purpose of the organization.
- They are feasible yet challenging.
- They have significance that transcends the organization and impacts society as a whole.
- They appeal to the moral values, emotions, and imagination of the people in the profession and the organization.

Because the goal of health system leadership is to get people to invest their talents, knowledge, and skills in health services with a view to the ultimate success of the system, having a vision is vital. These ideas are illustrated in a simple model suggested by Barker (1990):

Vision → Energized Action for Change → Success and Excellence

Vision is essential because it generates the energy necessary to produce the results of action that in turn leads to success. Although the model may seem simple, nurse leaders enrolled in an international nursing leadership training program found vision to be the most difficult skill to master (Deveraux, 1989). Although they felt they had good ideas, few were accustomed to creating detailed plans and crafting strategies to achieve these ideas. Evidently, moving from the idea (i.e., the dream) to the feasibility was the difficult part. As Deveraux (1989) explains: "a vision is a compelling dream, a picture of a different and a better way to achieve the goal of nursing care. Vision began with the mental journey from the known to the unknown; in essence, creating the future from a montage of facts, figures, hopes, dreams, dangers and opportunities. But it uses [not only] the mental process of imagination and intuition but [also] analytical logic" (p. 7).

Table 13.1

OUTCOMES WHEN ANY ONE OF FIVE CHARACTERISTICS FOR MANAGING CHANGE IS MISSING

Vision +	Skills +	Incentives +	Resources +	Action Plan →	Change
	Skills +	Incentives +	Resources +	Action Plan →	Confusion
Vision +		Incentives +	Resources +	Action Plan →	Anxiety
Vision +	Skills +		Resources +	Action Plan →	Gradual Change
Vision +	Skills +	Incentives +		Action Plan →	Frustration
Vision +	Skills +	Incentives +	Resources +		→ False Start

Source: Presented at the Baker Health Congress in Calgary, Alberta, September 19, 1996.

Even if the power of the mind alone is not sufficient to make a vision a reality, it is nevertheless the key element. For example, Bennis and Nanus (1985) suggest that in envisioning, the leader must have:

- Foresight—a sense of the possible future of the organization.
- A world view—an awareness of the impact of new trends in society and health care.
- Hindsight—an appreciation for cultural and traditional roots.
- Depth of sight—an ability to survey internal and external environments.
- Peripheral vision—an awareness of competitors and stakeholders.
- Revision—a willingness to revisit the vision with changes.

Thus, while visions are important assets en route to the next millennium, they should not be confused with brilliant insights. By themselves, brilliant insights are worthless and do not result in achievements. Intelligence, imagination, and knowledge are essential resources, and it is effective use of these resources that creates a vision.

Knowledge

The knowledge base for effective leadership has been the subject of much scrutiny, including an educational agenda that attempts to contend with contemporary megatrends. Paul (1989), for example, identified the megatrends for which leaders of the third wave must be educated, and we need to be mindful of these megatrends if nursing leadership is to guide our profession through this third wave. In educational programming, there is a shift from:

- strategy to structure;
- centralization to decentralization;
- functions to systems;
- hierarchy to horizontal networking;
- hands to brains;
- individuals to teams;
- "soft" culture to "hard" culture (i.e., outcomes);
- laissez-faire to social accountability.

Awareness of these changes is essential to the knowledge bases of all leaders through the contemporary transition. Nursing leaders must concern themselves with how these trends will fashion our service, education, and research agendas into an integrated whole for the nursing profession.

There are many ways in which we can learn from each other during this time of transition; for example, by publishing our experiences and communicating them widely. As we know, change is not controlled, but managed. We can learn from businesses, many of which are managing highly complex changes. Shell Canada, for instance, identified five major elements that must be recognized when managing major changes: vision; knowledge and skill; incentives; resources; and an action plan. A range of unsatisfactory outcomes occurs if any one of these elements is missing. If you lack vision, for example, the other four elements will create nothing but confusion in your organization. The principles presented in Table 13.1 are as relevant to the nursing profession as they are to the business world.

The knowledge agenda for transition to a new paradigm is crucial if nursing is to fulfil its professional mandate. Any divisions among practice, education, and research are artificial because workplaces must of necessity be learning environments, and part of this revolution.

Confidence

Leaders must have confidence if they are to be successful in implementing reform. Using a strategic contingency model (e.g., Stuart, 1986), it is possible to identify three important variables that nurse leaders must keep in mind when bringing about reform. The first is centrality. Traditionally, it has been the role and responsibility of nurses to co-ordinate the services around the delivery of nursing care, and to integrate their work with all other disciplines. Nursing has therefore enjoyed a central role in the delivery of institutional patient care.

The second variable is substitutability. This means that if the nursing profession is viewed only as the co-ordinator of care done by others, it will be a great disservice, because then other workers could easily be substituted for nurses. We have to be mindful of the precise contribution of nurses to health-care delivery. We know through clinical research, for example, that certain nursing interventions for neonatal infants have a direct impact on their future illness pattern, and growth and development. We also know that particular types of nurse-client interaction with cancer patients have physiological and psychological impacts,

making a difference in the reduction of patient stress, and conservation of energy. Moreover, we know that through interdisciplinary collaboration in diabetes education, complications in diabetics can be reduced by as much as 80 percent. When impacts or outcomes such as these can be attributed to nursing interventions, then it becomes clear that knowledge-based nursing interventions are not substitutable. Knowledge of the contribution of nursing is what confident nursing leadership can articulate as the health system undergoes reform.

And finally, the third variable is uncertainty. Nursing needs confident leaders who have self-esteem and are able to live with insecurity. Confident and knowledgeable leaders can articulate and speak out for health services and the contribution that nurses make within the system. Such leaders are able to think critically, consider the options before them as well as the possibilities, and still confront those options that differ from the management vision. For example, if public participation is part of the management model, but the public is only consulted and does not participate, nursing leaders will raise this issue in debate and obtain modification to the management model. Leaders are not paralysed nor do they despair in times of insecurity, nor do they shrink from the constant challenges that lie ahead.

An anecdote contributed by a colleague will serve to illustrate these points. A vice-president of nursing taking part in a major project, in which a traditional organization was being redesigned to incorporate a program model of organization, became concerned not with the ends of the projects, but with the means (i.e., the way in which changes were being implemented). She felt that the changes went against her beliefs with respect to the delivery of nursing services and that she had a duty to resign. She felt she had not adequately represented the nursing profession. My advice to her was that if she resigned, she could do nothing from outside the system, but that if she remained, she would be there to find a way to support the professional practice of nursing despite the changes. The confident leader, then, is armed with a vision of nursing and health services as a clear agenda. This energizes and mobilizes staff in pursuing their goals and dealing with change. The confident leader works with a team of colleagues to pursue the same goals. Functioning under an umbrella of confidence makes the road of daily crises easier to travel, easier to face, and allows the leader to address and overcome vested interests, resistance to change, and quick-fix solutions.

Visibility

The fourth characteristic needed by leaders is visibility. Remaining visible is particularly challenging for nursing leaders, as so many of the redesigning efforts in health services have introduced organizational models that replace existing professional models with management models. The present wave of organizational changes have characteristically eliminated nursing positions at the policy and senior-management levels of health-care agencies. Some administrators, however, want to have nurses as incumbents in newly created positions because of their nursing knowledge and skills in organizing the delivery of patient care, without regard for the knowledge required for other aspects of the position. As a result, nursing becomes invisible and disposable. Moreover, there is little consistency across regional health authorities.

In one Alberta regional health authority (RHA), for example, there are seven senior managers, six of whom are nurses. In the RHA next door, there is not one nurse among the seven senior-management positions. This sort of inconsistency is occurring in the United States and is of concern to leaders there. As Fagin (1996) noted at an invitational conference on executive leadership in major teaching hospitals and academic health centres:

"In examining some written descriptions of these models, one notes that discipline-specific requirements exist only for physicians. Surely nurses exist and participate in some of the leadership roles, but [their] credentials do not appear. This dangerous situation appears to be part of a growing trend and has implications for the profession and for the public. For the profession, by deliberately leaving out the credential of the nursing license, nursing's power, ethic, roles, and future are made as invisible as the most stereotypic view of nursing we all decry. For the public, the potential absence of professional nurses could lead to lower quality of care and in some cases to life-threatening events (p. 32)."

In one Alberta hospital, where all traces of management by discipline-specific leaders were wiped out, efforts are underway to see how a professional practice model might be re-introduced. It seems that the quality of nursing care is going down together with the visibility of nurses. We may think we have worked hard at explaining to policy makers and to other colleagues the precise nature of our contribution to health care. However, in a 1990 opinion survey that examined the public's view of nurses, they were seen as a vital ingredient in helping people recover from illness; however, 79 percent of respondents felt nurses should always consult a doctor before administering care to a patient. While this percentage fell to 65 in a 1995 survey, the results are still revealing. Fifty-nine percent believed that nurses should always follow a doctor's orders without question; 59 percent however, also believed that a physician should respect a nurse's opinion on patient care (Olafson, 1995; Turner, 1990). This is not ancient history, and we need to be mindful of it. The challenge for visible leaders is of course, to help us develop professional practice models that fit in with the characteristics of the third wave.

We need nursing leaders who are proud to be nurses, but who are effective and visible while creating partnerships in the delivery of an integrated health-care service. This can be done, and some of you here at this conference have successfully guided the practice of nursing through these kinds of changes. The design of a new centre of excellence for diabetes education in Alberta is a good example. This project was spearheaded by nurses in collaboration with dieticians and involved 23 partners, including six regional sites for the delivery of diabetes education, seven faculties, two institutes, and two economic development centres in the cities of St. Albert and Edmonton. This was a multi-organizational, intersectoral, and multimedia collaborative effort to design a central network of physical and virtual sites to promote the self-management of diabetes. There are many similar examples, and while change is inevitable, a lot will depend on us to see that appropriate management models are developed to promote the vision of a reformed health-care system.

Conclusion

We need nurse leaders to guide the transition of the nursing profession. When we are in the centre of a tornado, however, it is difficult to see the big picture, so we need to be guided by radar. This "radar" for the nurse as executive consists of knowledge and management skills to adapt to the third wave; professional values and accountability for excellence in nursing practice; education and research; and ability to work in networks that include individual professionals and governments to attain health goals. The people at this conference represent the legitimate leaders of the profession. You have the authority, and the profession is counting on you to lead through this most challenging time of transition. None of us can disappear into the woodwork and ride out the storm.

Our profession has been socialized in a very visible way and, unfortunately, within a rigid infrastructure. It is not appropriate to move the practice environment forward in ways that remove all visible, reliable infrastructures that support our professional practice. It is true that we need to de-stabilize in moving forward with change, but shock treatment should be abandoned. Shock therapy was abandoned in psychiatry because of its lack of effectiveness and the permanent damage it caused to individuals; shock therapy is also inappropriate for the nursing profession. What is needed is facilitation in this journey.

Nursing leaders have been visionaries in the past, working and lobbying for a reformed health-care system that included reform in nursing practice. Nursing leaders have prepared for this latest reform during the past fifteen years, and they are now in the midst of the transition, preparing for its implementation. The transition requires nursing leaders who are visionary, knowledgeable, confident, and visible in helping nursing re-emerge in a third wave version. This then, is a call for nursing leadership.

REFERENCES

Barker, A. M. (1990). *Transformational nursing leadership.* Baltimore, MA: Williams & Wilkins.

Bennis, W., & Nanus, B. (1985). *Leaders: The strategies for taking charge.* New York: Harper & Row.

Deveraux, M. O. (1989). *Leadership development: Key to effectiveness at the policy level.* Paper presented at the conference Nursing leadership: Using research for policy making in primary health care. Yonsei University, Seoul, Korea.

Fagin, C. M. (1996). Executive leadership: Improving nursing practice, education, and research. *Journal of Nursing Administration, 26*(3), 30–37.

Lemire Rodger, G., & Gallagher, S. (1995). The move toward primary health care in Canada. In M. J. Stewart (Ed.). *Community nursing* (pp. 37–58). Toronto: W. B. Saunders.

Olafson, T. (1995). *Public opinion survey: Report to the Alberta Association of Registered Nurses.* Edmonton: Angus Reid Group.

Paul, J. P. (1989) The consequences of Megatrends on business education. *European Management Journal, 7*(3), 284–285.

Stuart, G. W. (1986). An organizational strategy for empowering nursing. *Nursing Economics, 4*(2), 69–73.

Turner, A., Cook, P. & Associates (1990). Public opinion survey: A special report to the AARN Newsletter. *AARN Newsletter, 46*(1), 5–6.

Vance, C. N. (1977). *Group profile of contemporary influentials in American nursing.* Unpublished doctoral dissertation, Teachers College, Columbia University, New York.

Source: Adapted from an address to the National Conference on Nursing Administration, *Our Heritage as Leaders*, Radisson Hotel, Ottawa, October 22, 1996.

inspirational address to an audience of nursing and health-care administrators, she summarized the trends and the issues that face the health-care system as it undergoes the changes that are needed to bring about true reform. In the text of her address, which is reproduced above, she identifies four essential characteristics needed for effective nursing leadership for the current era and beyond: vision, knowledge, confidence, and visibility. These four characteristics provide a framework for observing leadership in action at all levels in the health-care system.

LEADERSHIP AND MANAGEMENT

Repeated calls for leadership in the literature are testimony to the social and psychological need for the presence of leaders in nearly all walks of life, but seldom do such calls bring us closer to clear definitions of this elusive concept. In discussing leadership qualities, authors often try to distinguish leadership from management. Comparing and contrasting the characteristics of these complementary phenomena usually results in a portrait of management as bureaucratic, rigid, and resistant to change, while leadership is painted as visionary, inspirational, innovative, and committed to challenging the status quo. Bennis and Nanus (1985), for example, go to great lengths to describe the static nature of management and the proactive, creative nature of leadership. They argue that managers "do things right" but that leaders "do the right thing," and note that the distinction is crucial even though both are important. "The difference may be summarized as activities of vision and judgement—*effectiveness*—versus activities of mastering routines—*efficiency* (Bennis & Nanus, 1985, p. 21).

While few would argue seriously with this pronouncement, particularly in view of the emphasis now placed on efficiency and effectiveness in the health-care system, it would be most unusual to find an advertisement for a manager of a hospital or community health service that listed "the mastery of routines" as a desirable qualification for the job. Nevertheless, while it may be possible to be a leader without much knowledge of management, it would be unwise to undertake an administrative role without a sound knowledge of management *and* knowledge *and* demonstrated skills as a leader. Indeed, a cursory review of fifty recent advertisements for health administrators and managers revealed "leadership," "interpersonal skills," "creativity," and "flexibility" as the four most frequently sought qualifications.

If management were to focus on controls, supporting the status quo and the bottom line, the very survival of organizations in the turbulent environment of today's health-care system would be in doubt. Mintzberg (1975) recognized leadership as an integral characteristic of effective chief executive officers whom he studied, and his framework of interpersonal, informational, and decisional managerial roles has been extensively employed as a basis for studying management behaviour. Clearly, administrators and managers must be leaders, and must develop their leadership skills.

Drucker (1996), who has spent more than fifty years studying the role of leaders in scores of organizations, also cites leadership as an integral requirement of effective administrators. He categorically rejects the notion of "born leaders," and the notions of "leadership personality," "leadership style," and "leadership traits." Drucker argues that effective leaders have followers who "do the right things," and who get results. Moreover, he argues that leaders are highly visible and set examples, and that leadership has more to do with acceptance of responsibility than with rank, privilege, title or money.

In his foreword to the book *The leader of the future*, Drucker (1996) talks about the typical behaviour of effective leaders he has known and observed. They tend to ask "what needs to be done [and] what can and should I do to make a difference?" (p. xiii). Leaders are guided by the organization's mission and goals, they demand performance, standards, and values from the people they work with, and they are not afraid to hire people who have more strength or greater talents than themselves.

According to Drucker, the distinction between management and leadership is primarily that management involves an obligation to achieve organizational goals, and increasingly those goals must be achieved through prudent use of human, material, and fiscal resources. Leadership, on the other hand, is about relationships with followers and about influencing the process by which they jointly achieve organizational goals while striving for higher levels of quality and effectiveness. It is well to remember that management and leadership skills can both be learned, and that therefore people who aspire to senior positions in health care are likely to be successful if they combine a sound knowledge of management with skills of leadership.

NEW WAYS OF PROVIDING LEADERSHIP

A substantial amount of the literature on leadership is based on studies of large corporations, governments, and manufacturing plants where men generally dominate the executive ranks. Prescriptions for leadership in nursing and health care draw heavily on these sources.

In general, women have not been well represented in strategic leadership roles either in business or in health care. There are disproportionately more women in the rank and file of hospitals, for example, and disproportionately more men represented in senior executive positions. Many observers have noted that hidden barriers prevent women from advancing beyond middle management, at which point they hit a so-called "glass ceiling" (Moss, 1995).

There are many reasons for the shortage of women in politics and other senior, influential societal roles, not the least of which are their socialization as women, lack of educational opportunities and child-rearing responsibilities. Nevertheless, in the "shifting sands" of health-care reform, nurses have had an unprecedented opportunity to move to the top, creating various structures for cracking the glass ceiling (Moss, 1995). Nurses are well situated and well qualified to compete for top administrative positions in health care (Aburdene & Naisbitt, 1992), and there is growing evidence of their successes. For example, Blair (1997) describes the careers of three prominent Canadian nurses, all of whom are currently occupying chief executive officer positions—one in a provincial health information centre, another as CEO of a hospital, and the third as president of a provincial hospital association. All have impressive educational qualifications, experience, and optimistic outlooks, and all are engaged in managing significant changes in their organizations.

Managing change within the new world order is one of the main themes that arises in current discussions about nursing leadership roles. For example, Kerfoot (1996) suggests that change leaders will be highly sought after because of their ability to identify trends, and provide the vision that empowers and reassures people throughout the process of change. Such leaders, according to Porter-O'Grady (1992) "must recognize that the whole culture of the workplace must reflect change as a constant, value it, and incorporate that understanding into the very culture of work"(p.19). The Canadian Nurses Association (CNA) takes the position that a professional practice environment is one that is supported by "a chief executive nurse who provides valued leadership for the discipline"(CNA, 1993, p.22). Underlying these prescriptions in the context of change is the general assumption that if contemporary nursing leaders occupy positions in the formal structure of health agencies, they will be endowed with sufficient power and authority to ensure that change occurs.

In the past, we have usually assumed that "leaders are leaders by virtue of their positions" (Helgesen, 1996). Nurses have looked to their directors of nursing, nurse managers, clinical development nurses, and clinical nurse specialists to take whatever initiatives were needed to address emerging issues in the practice of nursing, and to represent nurses in solving problems that affect their work. They have expected them to serve as role models by setting high standards of professionalism, and to represent them at senior management and board levels.

Nurses expect their leaders to promote a professional practice environment in which nurses participate in decisions at all levels of the organization, help to determine standards of patient care and decide how resources are to be used, take part in quality improvement and continuing education, and support the goals of research. As the CNA notes, quality of care does not just happen, but is the product of environments that support professional nursing practice (Haines, 1993).

The Magnet Hospital study was one of the first of many to demonstrate the linkages among: certain structural aspects of the workplace; well educated and visible directors of nursing; professional practice environments that produce low levels of staff turnover; and high standards of patient care (McClure, Poulin, Sovie, & Wandelt, 1983). More recently, lower Medicare mortality rates have been reported in hospitals that are known for good nursing care (Aiken, Smith, & Lake, 1994).

Regionalization and the trend toward new organizational structures based on programs rather than functional departments, however, have resulted in the elimination of many positions that can be described as discipline-specific (e.g., directors of nursing, physiotherapy, social work). Table 13.2 contains figures from nursing registration forms across Canada, revealing a steady decline between 1988 and 1996 in the numbers of nurses reporting their positions as directors and assistant directors of nursing, nursing supervisors, and head nurses.

Because of their experience and qualifications, many senior managerial nurses have been able to move into what Rodger refers to as "generic executive" roles, for example, positions as patient-care co-ordinators or directors of patient services, who are responsible for a range of disciplines and departments.

Generic administrative roles have become almost totally devoted to what the CNA refers to as the "corporate" dimension of administrative practice (CNA, 1988). This means that the activities and talents of these nurse leaders are directed toward addressing the mission and functions of the corporation as a whole, with little expectation that their professional knowledge of nursing will be applied to the specific issues and problems in nursing services. Nurses can no longer rely on the incumbents of these positions to champion their goals and aspirations as nurses or to serve as a figureheads or spokespersons. As Rodger notes, when nurses have assumed these "generic" roles, their professional background and identity becomes less visible; indeed, the culture of the workplace may encourage disassociation with professional networks and colleagues. While this may represent a dilemma for the individual "generic executive," it is clear that nurses are able to successfully make the transition to broadly based patient care administrative roles. An example of one such leader is presented in Box 13.2.

Major Mimi Fortin was promoted into a generic or non-traditional role in the Canadian Forces where she has responsibility for the entire range of health-care workers, including physicians and dentists. As she says, she has many opportunities to exercise leadership, but she must do it equally for all health-care professionals under her command. She also notes that nurses who assume the role of Detachment Commander tend to be successful because they have a good grasp of the whole range of disciplines, departments,

Table 13.2

NURSE ADMINISTRATORS BY TYPE OF POSITION AND EDUCATIONAL PREPARATION: 1988, 1992 AND 1996

	1988	1992	1996
Director/Assistant	**5,160**	**5,320**	**4,155**
	%	%	%
Diploma	67.8	64.0	56.0
BScN	25.8	29.0	34.7
Master's/PhD	6.4	6.9	9.3
Supervisor/Co-ordinator	**10,834**	**10,443**	**8,579**
	%	%	%
Diploma	77.7	74.5	68.2
BScN	20.6	23.7	29.1
Master's/PhD	1.7	1.7	2.7
Head Nurse	**15,872**	**9,746**	**8,234**
	%	%	%
Diploma	87.1	79.3	70.2
BScN	12.0	19.0	27.1
Master's/PhD	0.9	0.9	2.6
Nurse Administrators: Total	**31,866**	**25,509**	**20,968**

Source: Based on L. Lemieux-Charles and D. Wylie, "Administrative Issues," in A. Baumgart & J. Larsen, (Eds.), *Canadian Nursing Faces the Future* (St. Louis, MO: Mosby, 1992), p. 254; *Registered Nurses Management Data 1992* (Ottawa: Statistics Canada, Centre for Health Information, 1994); Policy, Regulation, and Research Division, Canadian Nurses Association.

laboratories, diagnostic services, and the organization of patient care. Even if their identity as nurses becomes invisible as generic executives, nurses who report to them should consider them influential resources, get to know them, and lobby them for needed services or improvements for patient care. Because they have been nurses in the past, they will understand how patient care is delivered and be familiar with inherent problems and issues. Moreover, they can speak the language of nursing, and like politicians in a democracy, such people have a duty to represent their constituents no matter what their political or occupational backgrounds.

The loss of senior executive roles in nursing has contributed to the loss of momentum in the development of nursing practice models. For example, shared governance organizations designed to decentralize decision-making and promote greater autonomy in professional practice are at risk in the transition from functional to program-oriented organizations. The irony is that there is a much greater need for professional structures to support the development and maintenance of standards of practice within individual disciplines in redesigned organizations.

Box 13.2
PROFILE OF A GENERIC LEADER

Name:	Major Mimi Fortin, BScN, MN
Position:	Edmonton Detachment Commander Canadian Forces Medical Group Headquarters
Reporting to:	Commanding Officer of the Canadian Forces Medical Group Headquarters, Ottawa
Responsible for:	All health care providers or a medical detachment including medicine and dentistry
Aim:	Maintenance of professional skills and competence in order to respond to any military operational mission(s) for deployment as a part of United Nations peacekeeping force and/or humanitarian mission
Main challenge:	To be prepared to leave at any time to set up complete field hospital in foreign country
Unique initiative:	Forging partnership between Canadian Forces and Capital Health Authority to permit military and non-military personnel to work side-by-side. The purpose is to allow maintenance and updating of skills and knowledge of military personnel as new medical technology and treatments are developed
Concept of leadership:	• knowing the military context and nature of work of all disciplines • ability to guide staff in professional advancement in their own disciplines • flexibility to adjust to any situation • establishing contact, networking, knowing resources • drawing on own professional background as nurse and manager • creating initiatives in health service, education, and research

Source: Based on interview with Major M. Fortin, August 29, 1997. Used with permission.

Some tertiary-level teaching hospitals have recognized the importance of visible nursing leadership to the professional identity of nurses, and in some cases have created roles and structures to support nursing practice, education, and research. The position of Chief of Nursing Practice was established at Women's College Hospital, Toronto to report directly to the Board and Chief Executive Officer (Ross, MacDonald, McDermott & Veldhorst, 1996). The role had no line responsibility for such corporate functions such as budgeting and staffing. It was to be a role to which any nurse could have direct access, and which would be advisory to senior management and the Board. Key aspects of the role were to articulate a vision for nursing; enhance the value and image of nursing; act as a practice resource; and advance nursing research and practice. Clearly, it was intended that there be a visible, expert leader of nurses in the hospital with the same kind of stature given historically to chiefs of medical staff. This model of nursing leadership does not seem to have been widely replicated elsewhere in Canada, but has great potential for facilitating the development of working environments that nurture the professional practice of nursing.

As organizations become less hierarchical, more organic in structure and process, and more program oriented, decisions about patient care will increasingly be made by interdisciplinary teams. Knowledge workers such as nurses and other health professions have access to a range of information generated by new technologies and health-care sciences, and they must have sufficient autonomy to use that information in making the best decisions with and for clients and families. In the forum created by interdisciplinary teams, emerging leadership will stem from expertise and competence rather than from rank and position. Helgesen (1996) remarks that: "As the instrumental use of knowledge continues to redefine the nature and purpose of organizations, we will begin to look to those on the front lines for leadership.... And as grass-roots leadership becomes more common, we will begin to recognize as well led [those] organizations that are most adept at nourishing leadership independent of official rank or status" (p.22).

First-line nurse managers and individual nurses are well situated for offering leadership in promoting effective teamwork and team building, by virtue of their broad knowledge of clients' conditions and the services provided by the other team players. The implications for nursing are that nurses can no longer depend on leadership in nursing to come from the traditional hierarchical structures. Such leadership will increasingly need to come from their own initiatives, from coalitions formed with other groups, and from their professional associations and unions.

In some of the larger restructured health agencies, the nurse with the highest visibility is often the president of the local nurses' union. Through legitimate structures established in the collective agreement, most nurses in Canada have access to a professional responsibility committee, or nursing practice committee. Such committees represent a forum for initiating changes in policies, procedures, practices, and standards of care. Although the goals of a local union are primarily to represent nurses with respect to their terms and conditions of employment, there is little to prevent nurses from exercising leadership through these mechanisms. Forming coalitions with other disciplines is another strategy for creating a power base for advancing proposals relative to patient services, programs, or even organizational problems (see Chapter 14 for more discussion on the formation of coalitions).

Perhaps the greatest opportunities for exercising leadership are happening in the community. Although reform is happening more slowly than expected, many initiatives have resulted from the vision of nurses. Such undertakings in primary health-care include the Comox Wellness Centre in British Columbia, and the ongoing efforts to establish midwifery as an insured service in Alberta and other provinces. In Chapter 9, it was noted that many people fall between the cracks of our health-care system, sometimes with tragic results. The story of one such patient is summarized in the case example in Box 13.3.

The example of leadership depicted in Box 13.3 is typical of what Senge (1996) refers to as the internal networker, or community builder in "learning" organizations. He notes that these leaders come from any level in the organization including the grass roots. They are, he says, the "'seed carriers' of the new culture, who can move freely about the organization to find those who are predisposed to bringing about change, help out in organizational experiments, and aid in the diffusion of new learnings" (p.46). Such leadership roles are precarious as they have little formal authority and for this reason, working in concert with local line leaders and executive leaders can maximize their effectiveness.

It seems clear that in the absence of formal positions responsible solely for nursing services, nurses must be prepared to exercise leadership themselves in experimenting with new ways of providing services.

CONCLUSION

As organizations are restructured and work is redesigned, nurses occupying senior, generic management positions are less likely to have sole responsibility for nursing services. However sympathetic the individuals who occupy these positions may be to the delivery of nursing services, their allegiance is likely to be divided among many disciplines, departments, clinics, and diagnostic or environmental services. Where there are discipline-specific positions in nursing such as directors of nursing, these need to be filled by well qualified nurses who are knowledgeable, visionary, confident, and visible, because such people are most likely to support nursing practice standards and promote environments that are conducive to high standards and effective outcomes for clients and patients. Increasingly, nurses will be expected to provide leadership at the grass roots of organizations and in multidisciplinary teams. Not all nurses are interested in assuming leadership roles, but those who are deserve the support and encouragement of their colleagues, their unions, local line managers, and senior executives.

SUMMARY

- Leadership has many definitions; how leadership is exercised depends on multiple factors including: followers and whether they constitute a group; the relationship between leader and followers; the goal; the nature of tasks; the situation; resources; and pressures experienced by the group.
- Management is generally defined in terms of the achievement of organizational goals, and the efficient use of human, fiscal, and material resources.

Box 13.3

THE NEED FOR GRASS ROOTS
LEADERSHIP: A CASE EXAMPLE

A home care clinical nurse specialist in wound and ostomy management received the referral of a new client, an elderly woman who lived with her older brother deep in the country in an area not usually served by home care. The client, who suffered from chronic ulcerative colitis, had just been discharged from hospital with an ileostomy which required attention at least four to six times a day. The nurse also learned from the referral file that the woman was once admitted to a psychiatric unit in a psychotic state.

When the nurse arrived, her new client was in the basement trying to make the washing machine work, but she seemed confused and didn't appear to understand the fundamental components of the appliance. Her brother was out somewhere working on his tractor, and the household was in need of food, supplies, substantial cleaning, and ventilation. There was no telephone. The purpose of the nurse's visit was to teach the client how to manage her ileostomy.

The nurse who made the initial home visit was new to the province and was still learning how to line up services for her clients, including which agencies were responsible for home-care ileostomy supplies. She quickly assembled a team of players to take care of the range of health-care services needed by this client. She also made sure the agencies who had provided uncoordinated care in the past were contacted, in order to discuss the implications of premature termination of services for subsequent patients under their care.

The leadership exhibited by this nurse did not end here. She had observed that the site selected by the surgeon for the stoma was poorly located in a deep abdominal crease, thus complicating the ileostomy care by the client. As a result, she began soliciting support for the notion that preoperative preparation for ileostomy or colostomy should include discussions with client, clinical nurse specialist, and surgeon on the most practical site for the stoma. Not all surgeons welcomed this suggestion, but the nurse began to plan her change strategy, and with vision, knowledge, confidence, and visibility, she felt that she could make a difference in the management of similar cases.

- As regional health authorities restructure their hospitals and community agencies, new opportunities for nurses to exercise leadership arise.
- Functional management positions such as directors of nursing and nursing supervisors have traditionally provided leadership in nursing but these roles are disappearing. New patient care positions require "generic" types of leadership consistent with managerial responsibility for multiple disciplines and departments.
- Health-care system restructure and reform has led to the call for nursing leadership that is visionary, knowledgeable, confident, and visible.
- Managing health-care services today requires formal knowledge and demonstrated skills in both management and leadership.
- Increasingly, nurses will be expected to provide leadership from the grass roots of organizations, in their communities, and within the context of interdisciplinary teams.

FURTHER READINGS AND RESOURCES

Grohar-Murray, M.E., & DiCroce, H.R. (1997). *Leadership and management in nursing* (2nd ed.). Stamford, CT: Appleton & Lange. Chapter Two of this book is devoted to leadership theory. The authors provide a succinct overview of theories of leadership, and include an excellent glossary of key concepts. Case studies illustrating three styles of leadership (democratic, laissez-fair, and autocratic) are provided to promote an understanding of variations in leadership behaviour. The cases would also help students to identify their own potential for leadership, and their own preferences with respect to leadership style.

Marriner-Tomey, A. (1993). *Transformational leadership in nursing.* St. Louis, MO: Mosby-Yearbook. In her preface, the author explains that the purpose of this book is to describe and advocate the philosophy of transformational leadership, to discuss related concepts and research, and to identify strategies and tools for implementation. She expresses the hope that the book will be both inspirational and practical. The book is a collection of contributed papers by various authors applying the notion of transformational leadership to many aspects of management; for example, decision making, shared governance, creating culture, and organizational networking. This would be a useful reference for instructors as well as for students.

Wylie, D.M. (1994). Leadership theory and practice. In J.M. Hibberd & M.E. Kyle (Eds.). *Nursing management in Canada* (pp. 175–190). Toronto: W.B. Saunders. This chapter on leadership in the first edition of *Nursing Management in Canada* will remain relevant for a good many years to come. The author gives a skilful summary of the leading theories of leadership, and provides a useful list of characteristics that distinguish concepts of management from leadership. Theories discussed include: trait, behavioural, contingency, situational, transactional, transformational, and super-leadership. Wylie also reviews research on leadership and discusses the implications for nursing management.

REFERENCES

Aburdene, P., & Naisbitt, J. (1992). *Megatrends for women.* New York: Villard Books.

Aiken, L., Smith, H., & Lake, E. (1994). Lower Medicare mortality among a set of hospitals known for good nursing care. *Medical Care, 32*(8), 771–787.

Bennis, W., & Nanus, B. (1985). *Leaders: The strategies for taking charge.* New York: Harper and Row.

Blair, K. (1997, September). Movers and shakers: The story of three high-profile nurses. *Canadian nursing management supplement.* No. 112, 1–4.

Canadian Nurses Association (1988). *The role of the nurse administration and standards for nursing administrative practice.* Ottawa: Canadian Nurses Association.

Drucker, P.F. (1996). Foreword: Not enough generals were killed. In F. Hesselbein, M. Goldsmith, & R. Beckhard (Eds.). *The leader of the future: New visions, strategies, and practices for the next era* (pp. xi–xv). San Francisco: Jossey-Bass.

Haines, J. (1993). *Leading in a time of change: The challenge for the nursing profession. A discussion paper.* Ottawa: Canadian Nurses Association.

Harrison, F. (1992). Leadership through alliances. *Canadian Nurse, 88*(6), 20–23.

Helgesen, S. (1996). Leading from the grass roots. In F. Hesselbein, M. Goldsmith, & R. Beckhard (Eds.). *The leader of the future: New visions, strategies, and practices for the next era* (pp. 19–24). San Francisco: Jossey-Bass.

Kerfoot, K. (1996). The new nursing leader for the new world order of health care. *Nursing Economics, 14*(4), 239–240.

McClure, M. L., Poulin, M. A., Sovie, M. D., & Wandelt, M. A. (1983). *Magnet hospitals: Attraction and retention of professional nurses.* Kansas City: American Academy of Nursing.

Mintzberg, H. (1975). The manager's job: Folklore and fact. *Harvard Business Review, 53*(4) 49–51.

Moss, M. T., (1995). Developing glass-breaking skills. *Nursing Administration Quarterly, 19*(2), 41–47.

Perrow, C. (1973). The short and glorious history of organizational theory. *Organizational Dynamics, 2*(1), 2–15.

Porter-O'Grady, T. (1992) Transformational leadership in an age of chaos. *Nursing Adminstration Quartery, 17*(1), 17–24

Ross, E., MacDonald, C., McDermott, K., & Veldhorst, G. (1996). The chief of nursing practice: A model for nursing leadership. *Canadian Journal of Nursing Administration, 9*(1), 7–22.

Senge, P. M. (1996). Leading learning organizations: The bold, the powerful, and the invisible. In F. Hesselbein, M. Goldsmith, & R. Beckhard (Eds.). *The leader of the future: New visions, strategies, and practices for the next era* (pp. 41–57). San Francisco: Jossey-Bass.

Walsh, J. (1993). Where have all the leaders gone? *Time,* July 12, 14–19.

Chapter 14

▼▼▼▼▼▼▼▼▼▼▼▼▼▼▼▼

Intraorganizational Politics

GINETTE LEMIRE RODGER

KEY OBJECTIVES

In this chapter, you will learn:

- The importance of change.
- Definitions of concepts such as power, politics, influence, and political action.
- A five-step political process framework that will help nurse managers prepare strategies to accomplish their goals.
- Commonly recognized sources of power available to nurses in health agencies.
- The importance of temporary alliances and coalitions between sub-groups in organizations (e.g., administrators, physicians, nurses, and other health professionals).
- Some challenges for nurses in first-level management positions.

INTRODUCTION

"Intraorganizational politics" is an important concept for nurse managers to understand. It plays a significant role in every aspect of their professional lives. Important questions such as which health goals are pursued, who receives what type of care and when, which health-care programs are maintained or deleted, which resources are allocated to these programs, which organizational models will be implemented and by whom, are all political issues. Intraorganizational politics are directly related to the ultimate goal of nursing—the health of the consumer.

This first section of the chapter provides an introduction to the forces of change and to the definitions central to organizational politics. In the second section, the five steps in a political process framework are described, with examples. The last section highlights challenges faced by first-line nurse managers when they use the political process.

A TIME OF CHANGE

Political knowledge and skills are now needed more than ever by nurse managers, who find themselves facing unprecedented change as the Canadian health-care system is overhauled, and the role and value of nursing and its place in the system are being questioned and modified. This, however, is the nature of change. In 1963, Erikson predicted that the rate of change would continue to accelerate, that humans and institutions would face multiple simultaneous changes, and that limits of human and institutional adaptability were not yet known. That was more than 30 years ago, when it was difficult to conceptualize that reality; today, change is still accelerating and intensifying.

Kurt Lewin (1951), a well known theorist of change, would call the period of change that the Canadian health-care system is experiencing "the moving stage." Change, according to his theory, has three stages: *the unfreezing stage,* a cognitive phase in which the individual is exposed to the idea of the need for change; *the moving stage,* a cognitive redefinition in which the change is planned and initiated; and *the refreezing stage,* in which the change is integrated and stabilized. During the unfreezing and moving phases, the next direction is initiated and movement begins. This is usually a time of insecurity, repositioning, challenges, and no clear answers. However, it is also a time of opportunity. During this time, effective politics can make a great difference in setting the course of action for a project, a department, or an organization.

MANAGERS AND POLITICAL AWARENESS

As Starke and Rempel (1988) observed, "Because politics is so common, managers in all kinds of organizations must understand what it is and why it occurs. They must also learn to cope with its manifestations if they wish to be successful in their careers" (p. 12). Nurse managers must be knowledgeable about politics and related concepts, such as power, influence, and the political process. Theoretical knowledge is important, but not sufficient. Managers must develop abilities and skills in using these concepts if they are to influence decisions to support nursing goals. It is one thing to know about politics and another thing to be political.

DEFINITIONS

The term "intraorganizational" in this chapter means the organization within a health-care agency. "Politics," as used in this chapter, can be defined broadly as "the capacity to influence." Pfeffer (1981) defines organizational politics as the behaviours of individuals as they attempt "to acquire, develop, and use power and other resources to obtain their preferred outcomes in a situation where there is uncertainty ... about choices" (p. 7). Several other definitions are also relevant to this chapter.

Laswell (1936), for example, defined politics as "the study of influence and the influential" (p. 13), and said that to comprehend politics one must look not only at who draws power but also at the relationship that person has with those affected by the actions. The same notion of politics was echoed in the work of Stevens (1980b) as "a process by which one influences the decisions of others and exerts control over situations and events" (p. 208). If politics is defined in terms of influencing and controlling, so is power. Shiflett and McFarland (1978) defined power as "one person's degree of influence over others, to the extent that obedience or conformity are assumed to follow" (p. 19).

It is also important to define the actions that we associate with the concepts of politics and power. "Political action" or "political process" can be defined as a systematic series of actions directed toward influencing others into conformity with a pursued goal. It is interesting to note that the definitions of politics, power, influence, and the political process have similar roots. The mechanism central to politics and power is the process of planned change. The terms planned change and political process are used interchangeably in this chapter.

POLITICAL PROCESS FRAMEWORK

For more than a decade, the Political Process Framework that appears in Box 14.1 has been used to show nurses how to successfully bring about organizational and social change. This framework highlights some elements of intraorganizational politics, and it can serve as a guide for first-line managers who want to use a political process to bring about change. The same five-step process is followed whether a manager wants to bring about a change, guide a change in a different direction, or prevent a change that could be detrimental to client care. A more detailed analysis of the five steps of the process follows.

ESTABLISH GOAL AND OBJECTIVES

Since change is multifaceted and constant, the setting of a definite goal and objectives is an important step in the political process. First of all, there is a need to set priorities among the competing issues. Which issues are essential to be dealt with, and in what way? Some issues play a pivotal role in an organization because they control other secondary or dependent issues. Therefore, dealing with essential issues will, in fact, influence resolution of other issues.

The political process is most effectively exercised when the purpose is clear. The process of clarifying objectives can take time and involve a lot of thought, consultation, and research, depending on the scope of the issue being addressed. One may begin with a general idea of the desirable results—the goal—but there is also a need to refine the objectives, including what needs to be done, when, and where. The changes made by nurses to the Canada Health Act in 1984 provide a well known example. When

---

Box 14.1

POLITICAL PROCESS FRAMEWORK

1. Establish goal and objectives
2. Assess positive and negative factors
   - Social values and trends
   - Key individuals or groups
   - Sources of power
   - Resources
   - Timing
3. Plan the strategy
4. Implement the strategy
5. Evaluate and re-adjust the strategy

---

refining the objectives, nurses had to be as precise as possible in suggesting exactly what words in the legislation would be removed, what words would be added, and when the changes would be proposed at which seating of the House of Commons Committee. The same applies to change on a unit, service, or department. The products of this step are:

1. a clear goal,
2. a lucid set of objectives,
3. a definite target of individual(s) or group(s) to be addressed, and
4. a specific message that conveys the value of the endeavour.

Barbara Stevens (1980a) stresses that unity among those desiring the change is a prerequisite for effectiveness in such endeavours; therefore, this requirement also must be considered in the first step of the Political Process Framework. Stevens urges nurses working towards change to debate their policies (goals and objectives) internally, make decisions, and then present a united front to the public or the organization they are trying to influence.

For example, two important goals for nurse managers to keep in mind in the present Canadian health-care reform, because they are pivotal issues, are: allocation of health-care resources, and the leadership position of nursing in the health-care system. Specific objectives are being developed by some nurse managers to address these issues in their milieu.

Health-Care Resources

Allocation of scarce resources is often the most vital of issues in any organization, and this is reflected in the organization's political struggles or "power plays." Del Bueno (1986) noted that, "in times of economic scarcity, political activity increases as individuals compete for those declining resources. A power holder must not only have control of valued resources, but must be willing to use them to influence others. When power is hoarded it atrophies and blocks achievement" (pp. 125–126).

In an ideal world, nursing care would be as highly valued as other types of care, allocation of resources would be a non-issue because objective data about the effects of such care would guide allocation. However, this is not the way health-care resources are allocated in the real world. In fact, whoever controls resources influences and moulds the delivery of client care and determines who receives what care. For example, the way a hospital allocates its material resources, such as supplies and equipment, usually reflects the power and influence of physicians (Mason & McCarthy, 1985).

There is ample research evidence that nurses can deliver—cost-effectively and well—many health-care services for which they are not now responsible, both in hospitals and in the community (Canadian Nurses Association, 1993b; Denton, Gafni, Spencer, & Stoddart, 1982; Kassakian, Bailey, Rinker, Stewart, & Yates, 1979; Wilkins, 1993). However, despite the need for cost reductions in health care, there have been major road blocks to the introduction of these changes for more than fifteen years because the resources are controlled by stakeholders who favour the medical and hospital models rather than primary health care, public health, and nursing models.

Nursing has responsibility for an important part of the health-care resources and should use this fact as part of a political process. The ability to influence decisions and gain support for the efficient use of health-care resources will be enhanced by developing political alliances within multidisciplinary teams. (This will be discussed further under the heading Sources of Power.)

Leadership Position Of Nursing

The other pivotal issue to be considered in establishing goals and objectives concerns the leadership role nurses must play in a time of transition. Prescott (1993) says that "registered nurses are one of the hospital's most important resources for achieving and maintaining a competitive advantage because they contribute in important ways both to cost savings and to delivering high-quality care" (p. 192). Prescott documented nursing utility and assets by means of outcomes research, such as the impact of nurses on hospital mortality rates, lengths of stay, costs, and morbidity outcomes. She concluded that nursing is an important component of hospital survival under a reformed health-care system.

Several organizational models introduced in the present wave of organizational change eliminate nursing positions at policy and senior management levels (see Chapter 13). Some administrators have hired nurses as incumbents for the new management positions at this level because these managers recognize the need for nurses' knowledge and skills. In most instances, however, the job description does not refer to the nursing knowledge that is needed and, as a consequence, the nursing component becomes invisible and disposable. Would any other industry wipe out its senior production managers or put them in advisory positions to the production line? Of course not!

In light of this disconcerting state of affairs, the Canadian Nurses Association (CNA) (1993a) has reiterated its position that a chief executive nurse, at the senior management level, is essential. As well, CNA has identified key concepts to guide nurse managers in their quest for strong nursing leadership in their agencies. This is a pivotal issue for all nurses and nurse managers.

Allocation of resources and leadership positions are two examples of goals to be attained through intraorganizational politics. Once the goal is set and the objectives clarified, the second important step of the process is an assessment of the positive and negative factors that will help or hinder the attainment of the goal.

ASSESS POSITIVE AND NEGATIVE FACTORS

The political process, or the exercise of power, requires that consideration be given to what will help achieve the objectives and what will impede progress. These elements are what Kurt Lewin (1951) calls "driving forces" and "resisting forces." Each has to be assessed if a nurse manager wishes to develop an effective strategy for change. Driving forces must be used and maximized while the effects of resisting forces should be minimized. When negative factors are encountered, whether related to values or trends in the environment or to key players, resources, or timing, there are ways to deal with them appropriately and thereby increase chances of success. These options include avoiding, minimizing, or confronting. To marshal these options, thus maximizing the positive forces and dealing with the negative forces, nurse managers need to recognize prevailing values and trends within the organization. (See also Chapter 23.)

Values and Trends

Nurse managers need to know and recognize prevailing social values, trends, and beliefs. If reaching a goal means going against these factors, it will be difficult, if not impossible, to accomplish it. Predominant values and trends in an organization are often referred to as the "organization culture." Edgar Schein (1985) defines organizational culture as "a pattern of basic assumptions—invented, discovered, or developed by a given group as it learns to cope with its problems of external adaptation and internal integration—that has worked well enough to be considered valid and, therefore, to be taught to new members as the correct way to perceive, think, and feel in relation to those problems" (p. 9). Each organization has its own culture, but within a large organization, subcultures also develop within specialized groups, departments, or units (Sovie, 1993). As Drucker (1992) notes, culture does not change, behaviour does. Therefore, if a nurse manager wishes to influence decisions, it is vital in intraorganizational politics to analyze the climate, values, and trends of the work environment.

An example of the effect of trends was an attempt to regroup all long-term care patients in one area of an agency; this attempt failed because it was not acceptable, in this organizational culture at the time, to mix the different types of care. The change was successful five years later because values and trends had changed. It was then considered desirable to have the full continuum of care in one agency as an efficient way of utilizing beds and containing costs.

How can a nurse manager assess organizational culture? Fleeger (1993) identifies two types of clues: *explicit clues,* which include formal contracts, written mission statements, policies and procedures, organizational charts, and job descriptions; and *implicit clues,* which include the informal, unwritten rules and expectations (e.g., regarding dress, communications, and behaviours). Both formal and informal clues must be used as indicators of values and trends in the organization.

Key Players

In planning or coping with change, there also is a need to identify which individuals or groups will affect and be affected by the planned change and to evaluate who might support or oppose the goal. These people might be termed the key players in the change process. It is necessary to assess their strengths and identify their particular goals. It may not be possible to identify all the forces for and against the change, but a nurse manager should make an effort to gather as much useful information as possible to plan the nursing strategy.

Key players who support the goal can be considered as a resource for the project, while key players who oppose the goal are likely to create conflict. Unfortunately, many nurses are not skilful at dealing with conflict. The choices are fairly limited when dealing with negative key players: they can be deliberately avoided; their impact can be minimized by identifying the specific area they oppose and trying to convince them either to support the goal or, at least, to be neutral; they can be confronted by developing arguments that demonstrate why the proposed goal is better.

Del Bueno (1986) discusses these interfaces between individuals at different levels or from different departments or with different values. She states that considerable managerial skill and tactics are necessary to resolve such conflicts, and offers suggestions that have a high probability of success. Some of her suggestions include: build your team; choose your second-in-command carefully; establish alliances with superiors as well as with peers; maintain a flexible position and maneuverability; and project an image of status, power, and material success (pp. 127–128).

Sources of Power

What kinds of power will the key individuals or groups use to support or oppose the goal that was set? Does a group have different types of power than an individual? What are some effective strategies to ensure that the nurse manager has the capacity to influence each situation? What are the key variables that affect attainment of power?

There are various ways of describing types of individual power. French and Raven (1959) identify five sources:

- **Legitimate power,** based on authority vested in a role or position that is accepted and recognized by others in the organization, such as a first-line manager position.
- **Reward power,** based on a person's use of positive sanctions such as money, positive evaluation, or other forms of gain.
- **Coercive power,** based on the use of negative sanctions such as threats or punishment.

- **Expert power**, based on valid knowledge or information in a given domain, such as nursing knowledge and skills.
- **Referent power**, based on positive personal appeal to which others respond, often identified as charisma.

Davidhizar (1993) also identifies charisma as a source of power or political strength, and recognizes that charismatic power is an emerging paradigm for modern managers.

Wieland and Ullrich (1976) discuss two derivative forms of power, usually not mentioned in the nursing literature: *associative power,* which comes from an association with others who are perceived as powerful, and *lower participant power,* which those lower in a hierarchy hold over their managers.

Fergusson (1985) also describes a form of associative power, but refers to this as *power through interdependence.*

Similar types of power can be attributed to a group or an organization. In assessing the power of a group, however, the relative or potential influence should be considered by looking at a combination of factors. Versteeg (1979) identifies five factors that need to be considered:

- **Size.** In terms of political power, the number of group members and the percentage they represent of the total organization is an important factor. For example, nurses usually comprise the largest number of professionals in an agency.
- **Information base.** This includes the information possessed by the membership, especially what it knows about the goal and about relevant professional and social issues.
- **Expertise.** This refers to the knowledge base or special expertise the group offers. It is similar in nature to the expert power of individuals.
- **Physical resources.** Time and money provide a group with the ability to participate in the exercise of power.
- **Personal attributes.** Similar to the referent power or charismatic power of individuals, this refers to the personal appeal of the group collectively and of its spokespersons.

What are some tactics that nurse managers can use with these types of power? The power of an individual is relative to that of others in influencing the behaviour of others, or in the context of this discussion, in influencing decisions. For example, in a hospital or a community health centre, a nurse manager has legitimate power due to his or her position. As well, this individual may have various degrees of the other forms of power, such as expertise and charisma.

It is useful for a nurse manager to determine the sources of power of key participants in relation to the objective, and use these to maximum benefit. The nurse manager needs to weigh the relative importance of positional power over expert power. To use the source of power of key individuals and groups to plan the strategy is known as a power strategy.

Several tactics can be used to acquire and maintain the derivative forms of power (i.e., associative power and lower participant power). For associative power, some of the tactics recommended in the literature include forming coalitions, negotiating or making trade-offs, lobbying, presence on key committees, and involvement in social activities. In other words, a nurse manager needs to be at the right place at the right time with the right people.

As an example, forming a coalition (a temporary alliance between individuals or groups with a common goal) can be effective in influencing others into conformity with the goal. Caplow (1969) studied traditional coalitions in organizations and distribution of power among organizational triads. Sills (1976) later discussed Caplow's theory in light of relative power between the three parts of the triad and, in particular, the relationships in a hospital management triad formed by administrator, physician, and nurse.

Even though the size and the complexity of hospitals and the position titles have changed in recent years, the basic mechanisms of the organizational triads are still valid today. Figure 14.1, which is adapted from the work of Caplow, shows the relationship between a hospital administrator (A), the medical director (B), and the senior nurse manager (C). In the triad, one must keep in mind that the positions are imbedded in the status order of the organization represented by the size of the circles. In fact, the power distribution is largely determined by the actual behaviour of the incumbent. Furthermore, socialization of roles in adult life is often the result of primary and secondary socialization.

In this context, using Caplow's theoretical discussions, one sees that hospital administrators often share with physicians their primary socialization as men and their secondary socialization as university-educated. Physicians and nurses share their secondary socialization in the "laying on of hands" and being educated in closed, caste-like professions with specific codes, entrance requirements, and rituals. So, in health care, a coalition between A and B is considered a "conservative coalition" because it respects the primary and secondary socialization. A coalition between A and C is considered an "improper coalition" because it negates the primary and secondary socialization. A coalition between B and C is considered a "revolutionary coalition," a winning coalition that has the potential to dominate the more powerful member of the organizational triad.

This theory can be applied to a debate over the need for bed closures. For example, a conservative coalition would be one in which the administrator, in coalition with physicians, decides what and how many beds to close and presents their recommendation to the board or the executive committee; such a recommendation would be accepted. An improper coalition exists when the administrator, in coalition with nurses, presents a bed-closure plan despite opposition from physicians; such a recommendation also would likely be accepted. However, if an administrator recommended bed closures, but nurses and physicians, in a revolutionary coalition, opposed that recommendation, the administrator, the board, or the executive committee would be hard-pressed to accept the recommendation.

Sills concluded that the system is kept in balance through rapid intermittent coalitions between administrators and physicians or administrators and nurses which, in fact, prevent "revolutionary coalitions" from taking

Figure 14.1

ORGANIZATIONAL TRIAD IN HOSPITAL

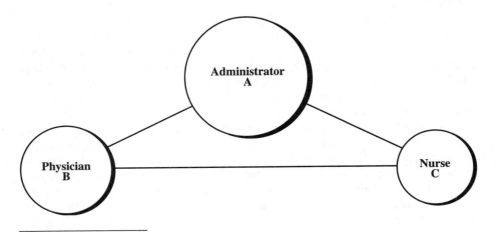

Source: Adapted from T. Caplow, *Two Against One: Coalitions in Triads* (Englewood Cliffs, NJ: Prentice-Hall, 1969) p. 55. Reprinted with permission.

place. An understanding of these patterns can help nurse managers analyze ways in which decision making is carried out in organizations.

On a regular basis, nurses discuss and negotiate issues with other nurses and physicians, but they are not as skilful at influencing interdisciplinary politics or team processes. A political alliance with the multidisciplinary team members is an important asset for nurse managers today. Devereux and Dirschel (1985) offer some guidelines on how to become proficient in the application of interdisciplinary politics:

- Know the situation (e.g., know the patient and problem the team must handle).
- Know the resources available from nursing and, in general, from the institution and/or community.
- Listen to colleagues' concerns and plans for action.
- Emphasize mutuality of goals shared among members of the multidisciplinary team.
- Reinforce what is legal practice of nursing. Work to ensure that all nurses are competent in their areas of practice and be alert to casual encroachment from other disciplines.
- Expand nursing goals to include those of the other disciplines to help build alliances for future interactions.

Nurse managers can also use tactics of lower-participant power. For example, Shiflett and McFarland (1978) noted that a nurse administrator may have power over a hospital administrator through: "1. control of resources upon which the person is dependent; 2. control of the access of others to that person; 3. control of techniques, procedures or knowledge vital to the administrator; and 4. personality attributes such as charm, likeableness, or charisma recognized by the administrator as desirable in subordinates" (p. 20). Shiflett and McFarland also noted that this same type of power can be used by staff members with the first-line manager. One should also remember that derivative forms of power are more uncertain than other forms and that some forms are more likely to be considered legitimate than others, depending on the circumstances.

What are the key variables that affect the attainment of power? Instead of focussing on individual or group sources of power, Hickson, et al, (1971) concentrated on horizontal power, or relationships between groups and sub-units within an organization.

Stuart (1986) also highlighted the importance of interdisciplinary alliances within an organization and referred to this as the strategic-contingencies model:

> Such an approach views intraorganizational conflict and negotiation as ongoing processes with the balance of power to effect change distributed dynamically among the various subunits . . . The division of labor among these subunits is then the source of intraorganizational power, and each subunit's tasks, functioning, and links with the activities of other subunits are crucial power variables. (p. 69)

In Stuart's model, three variables govern a sub-unit's power within the organization (nursing being a sub-unit or a department being a sub-unit): *centrality*—the degree of the sub-unit's interdependence with other sub-units; *substitutability*—the possibility of replacement by others; and *coping with uncertainty*—the ability to handle, through a variety of mechanisms, inevitable but unpredictable occurrences.

In light of these variables, Stuart (1986) recommended four principles to help the nursing profession achieve its goal of quality patient care and control over the practice of nursing:

- Increase connections with other sub-units and maintain the centrality.
- Become irreplaceable.
- Demonstrate nursing assets, as Prescott (1993) does in focussing on the research showing the positive impact of nursing care for clients and for the administration.
- Participate in high-level decision making about goals, resources, and activities desirable for the organization.

Physical Resources and Timing

In addition to assessing trends and values, key players, and sources of power, resources such as time, money and the willingness of individuals to support the project must also be considered. What kinds of people and what mix of each different element will be needed? Will the project require the assistance of consultants, or staff with special skills? Often, the value of the time and energy of the people committed to the goal is underestimated: belief and dedication to a cause is a resource of great value. Any weaknesses identified in the resource area can be compensated for when the strategy is planned. For example, increasing the number of volunteers can offset the shortcoming created by a limited amount of time. If special skills are needed, hiring or enlisting the help of an expert (even a student in that specialty) may be an option.

The timing of an issue is another critical factor. Timing is often so critical that it may be necessary to wait to implement a plan until conditions are more favourable. On the other hand, it may be necessary to be ready to move forward when opportunities present themselves. Favourable and unfavourable times should be identified early in the process and a range of possible deadlines set for the accomplishment of the goal.

PLAN THE STRATEGY

The two first steps—establishing the goal and assessing positive and negative forces—are the stages that require the most time and are the most important. Once these are done, the next step is to plan the strategy. The strategy is the framework within which necessary activities are carried out. It involves an action plan or a defined approach to reaching the goal.

Robbins (1986) has noted that, whereas passion and belief provide the fuel for achieving power, intelligence and logical strategies—in other words, a sound plan—provide the road maps by which success is eventually achieved. Once the goal and objective are clear, and positive and negative factors that will influence change are assessed, it is time to use all that knowledge to develop a strategy.

A viable overall or global strategy may be arrived at by first developing strategies for each individual or group that has been targeted in the first step. At this point, all pieces of the puzzle must be brought together. The choice of activities used in an overall plan should be congruent with the assessment of the positive and negative factors identified in the second step of the process.

IMPLEMENT AND EVALUATE THE STRATEGY

Once the plan is completed, implementation starts. The effectiveness of the tactics selected and the strategy as a whole must be evaluated on an ongoing basis. Some activities or tactics may not be effective and should be replaced by others.

There is always a need to monitor the political process and adapt the strategies in the light of progress and changing conditions. Successful approaches can be duplicated and shared with other groups involved in the political process and unsuccessful approaches can be modified.

CHALLENGES FOR THE MANAGER

Intraorganizational politics and use of the political process is a challenging area. Most studies on the topic, even in the recent literature, identify nurses in general and nursing administrators in particular as ill-prepared and apathetic political spectators (Byers, 1990; Cronkhite, 1991; Small, 1989). In light of the serious consequences of this state of affairs in a time of reform, the situation creates important challenges for the nurse manager.

The first challenge comes from a bias that can be traced back to the Western philosophical view that men are rational thinkers and thus responsible for affairs of the state, while women are emotional and therefore responsible for the affairs of the family—and for the support of men (Lloyd, 1984). Professions that are predominantly female, such as nursing, are affected by these stereotypes. Although much progress has been recorded, these ingrained cultural views explain why such topics as politics and power begin to appear in the nursing literature only in the late 1970s, and why many nurses are still uncomfortable with these concepts in the late 1990s.

The second challenge is to provide positive role models for other nurses by using the political process, encouraging educational programs, and rewarding political participation and behaviour among colleagues.

The third challenge is to provide a climate that encourages nurses to promote unity and consolidate their political power by using the four principles for the attainment of power: increasing connections, becoming irreplaceable, demonstrating nursing assets, and ensuring that nurses participate in high-level decision making (Stuart, 1986).

Knowledge and skills related to intraorganizational politics are essential tools in the arsenal of an effective nurse manager of the new century. Nursing professionals can be part of the solution in restructuring health care, but their involvement depends on a nurse manager's knowledge of intraorganizational politics and on her or his political abilities.

An effective strategy to reach the goal can be planned and implemented through the judicious choice of priorities and the use of a political process drawing on multiple sources of power. These ingredients, plus the determination of all nurse managers, will assure success in influencing decisions that support the goals of nursing.

SUMMARY

- The Canadian health-care system is experiencing the "moving state" as described in Lewin's theory of change. During this time, effective politics can make a great difference in setting the course of a project, department, or organization.
- The Political Process Framework has five steps: establish goal and objectives; assess positive and negative factors related to trends and values, key individuals or groups, sources of power, resources, and timing;

plan a strategy; implement the strategy; and evaluate and readjust the strategy.

- Two pivotal issues for nurse managers in the coming decade are allocation of health-care resources and leadership position of nurses.
- Commonly recognized sources of power include legitimate, reward, coercive, expert, and referent power. Two derivative forms of power are associative power and lower participant power.
- Associative power coalitions are formed among the organizational triad in health care (administrator, physician, and nurse).
- Nurse managers must become proficient in application of essential variables that affect attainment of power (centrality, substitutability, and coping with uncertainty).
- Factors that affect relative or potential influence of a group in an organization include: size, information base, expertise, physical resources, and personal attributes.
- Challenges for first-line nurse managers include the bias in society regarding women and politics, the need for positive role models for nurses, and the creation of a climate that encourage the attainment of power in an organization.
- Knowledge and skills about intraorganizational politics are essential tools in the arsenal of an effective nurse manager.

FURTHER READINGS AND RESOURCES

Canadian Nurses Association. (1993a). *Key concepts for policy statement on the position of the chief executive nurse.* Ottawa: Canadian Nurses Association. The Canadian Nurses Association has identified eleven key concepts for a policy statement on the place of nurses in agencies in order to ensure the quality of nursing care.

Canadian Nurses Association. (1993b). *New directions in health care: Cost effective nursing alternatives.* Ottawa: Canadian Nurses Association. This repository of Canadian studies, which demonstrate cost-effective nursing care, provides good ammunition to persuade other members of the health-care team about the key role of nursing.

Mason, D. J., Talbot, S. W., & Leavitt, J. K. (1993). *Policy and politics for nurses: Action and change in the workplace, government, organizations and community.* Philadelphia: W. B. Saunders. Three units are significant for a first-line manager: a nursing perspective; knowing the process, using the power; and politics in the workplace.

Prescott, P. (1993). Nursing: An important component of hospital survival under a reformed health-care system. *Nursing Economics, 11*(4), 192–199.

This article identifies recent studies that highlight the effectiveness of nursing services in a time of reform.

REFERENCES

Byers, S. R. (1990). *Relationship among staff nurses beliefs, nursing practice and unit ethos.* Unpublished doctoral dissertation, Ohio State University, Colombus. (From CIHNAL 1983–1993, Abstract No. 142524).

Canadian Nurses Association. (1993a). *Key concepts for policy statement on the position of the chief executive nurse.* Ottawa: Canadian Nurses Association.

Canadian Nurses Association. (1993b). *New directions in health care: Cost effective nursing alternatives.* Ottawa: Canadian Nurses Association.

Caplow, T. (1969). *Two against one: Coalitions in triads.* Englewood Cliffs, NJ: PrenticeHall.

Cronkhite, L. M. (1991). *The role of the hospital nurse administrator in a changing health care environment: A study of values and conflicts.* Unpublished doctoral dissertation, University of Wisconsin, Milwaukee. (From CIHNAL 1983–1993, Abstract No. 161175).

Davidhizar, R. (1993). Leading with charisma. *Journal of Advanced Nursing,* 18(4), 675–679.

Del Bueno, D. J. (1986). Power and politics in organizations. *Nursing Outlook,* 34(3), 124–128.

Denton, F. T., Gafni, A., Spencer, B. G., & Stoddart, G. L. (1982). *Potential savings from the adoption of nurse practitioner technology in the Canadian health care system.* (Report #45 - Quantitative Studies in Economics and Population). Hamilton, ON: McMaster University.

Devereux, P. M., & Dirschel, K. M. (1985). Interdisciplinary politics. In D. J. Mason & S. W. Talbot (Eds.), *Political action handbook for nurses* (pp. 240–250). Menlo Park, CA: Addison-Wesley.

Drucker, P. (1992). *Managing for the future: The 1990s and beyond.* New York: Truman Tally Books/Dutton.

Erikson, E. H. (1963). *The challenge of youth.* Garden City, NY: Doubleday.

Fergusson, V. D. (1985). Two perspectives on power. In D. J. Mason & S. W. Talbot (Eds.), *Political action handbook for nurses* (pp. 88–93). Menlo Park, CA: Addison-Wesley.

Fleeger, M. E. (1993). Assessing organizational culture: A planning strategy. *Nursing Management,* 24(2), 39–41.

French, J. R. P., & Raven, B. (1959). The bases of social power. In D. Cartwright (Ed.), *Studies in social power* (pp. 150–167). Ann Arbor, MI: University Press.

Hickson, D., Hinings, C., Lee, C., Schneck, R., & Pennings, J. (1971). A strategic contingencies' theory of organizational power. *Administrative Science Quarterly,* 16(2), 216–229.

Kassakian, M. G., Bailey, L. R., Rinker, M., Stewart, C., & Yates, J. W. (1979). The cost and quality of dying: A comparison of home and hospital. *Nurse Practitioner,* 4(1), 18–23.

Laswell, H. D. (1936). *Politics: Who gets what, when, how.* New York: The World Publishing.

Lewin, K. (1951). *The nature of field theory.* New York: Macmillan.

Lloyd, G. (1984). *The man of reason.* London: Methuen.

Mason, D. J., & McCarthy, A. M. (1985). The politics of patient care. In D. J. Mason & S. W. Talbot (Eds.), *Political action handbook for nurses* (pp. 38–52). Menlo Park, CA: Addison-Wesley.

Pffeffer, J. (1981). *Power in organization.* Boston: Pitman.

Prescott, P. (1993). Nursing: An important component of hospital survival under a re-formed health-care system. *Nursing Economics,* 11(4), 192–199.

Robbins, A. (1986). *Unlimited power.* New York: Simon & Schuster.

Schein, E. (1985). *Organizational culture and leadership: A dynamic view.* San Francisco: Jossey-Bass.

Shiflett, N., & McFarland, D. E. (1978). Power and the nursing administrator. *Journal of Nursing Administration,* 7(3), 19–23.

Sills, G. M. (1976). Nursing, medicine, and hospital administrator. *American Journal of Nursing,* 76(9), 1432–1434.

Small, E. B. (1989). *Factors associated with political participation.* Unpublished doctoral dissertation, North Carolina State University, Chapel Hill. (From CIHNAL 1983–1993, Abstract No. 119031).

Sovie, M. D. (1993). Hospital culture—Why create one? *Nursing Economics,* 11(2), 69–75.

Starke, A., & Rempel, E. (1988). Organizational politics and nursing administration. *Canadian Journal of Nursing Administration,* 1(4), 11–14.

Stevens, B. J. (1980a) Development and use of power in nursing. In National League for Nursing, *Assuring a goal-directed future for nursing* (Publication 52-1814). New York: National League for Nursing.

Stevens, B. J. (1980b). Power and politics for the nurse executive. *Nursing and Health Care,* 1(4), 208–210.

Stevens, B. J. (1982). *Educating the nurse manager: Case studies and group work.* Rockville, MD: Aspen.

Stuart, G. W. (1986). An organizational strategy for empowering nursing. *Nursing Economics,* 4(2), 69–73.

Versteeg, D. F. (1979). The political process: Or the power and glory. *Nursing Dimensions,* 7(2), 20–27.

Wieland, G. F., & Ullrich, R. A. (1976). *Organizations: Behavior, design, and change.* Homewood, IL: Richard D. Irwin.

Wilkins, V. C. (1993). Meeting community needs while conserving healthcare dollars. *Journal of Nursing Administration,* 23(3), 26–28.

CASE STUDY

Nursing staff in the intensive care unit (ICU) and medical/surgical units (MSU) at a local hospital have been upset with each other over co-ordination and communication between their units. Each group feels that the other units are responsible for unnecessary inconvenience and delays.

Complaints of the medical-surgical nurses include:

1. The ICU staff send patients back without warning when they need a bed for a more critical patient.
2. ICU refuses to admit some dying patients from the medical-surgical floors.
3. All patients, even those scheduled ahead of time, seem to come from ICU to the medical-surgical floors at the worst possible time—i.e., midmorning.

Complaints of the ICU nurses include:

1. MSU nurses request admission of every dying patient to intensive care whether or not the patient requires intensive nursing care.

2. New ICU admissions often arrive without warning, so there is no way to inform floors ahead of time when a patient will be transferred to the MSUs.

3. Patients often must be shifted midmorning to accommodate critical surgical cases from the operating rooms.

4. The nursing staff of MSUs refuse to come and pick up patients to be transferred in accordance with the hospital policy. As a result, ICU loses its vitally important skilled help when RNs have to push patients back to the floors.

5. Care on the medical-surgical floors is so poor that physicians tend to use the ICU for patients who could be cared for on the MSUs.

The relevant hospital policy indicates: (a) staff physicians or, in their absence, nurses in charge of units, may make the decision to send a patient to the ICU, or to transfer a patient from ICU to MSU; (b) in general, ICU transfers must be ordered in advance by the physician in charge of the patient's care; (c) in cases of ICU overflow, the ICU nurse-in-charge notifies the MSU when the patient is ready to be transferred; and (d) MSU nursing staff are responsible for transporting patients between units. The policy is broadly stated and offers no further guidelines with respect to its implementation.

Using the ideas presented in this chapter, identify the underlying problems in this case study. Analyze the sources of power available to ICU and MSU nurses. What resources do their nursing staff require to overcome their problems? Are there any potential alliances to be made? Plan appropriate change strategies for ensuring safe and appropriate care of patients.

Source: Based on "Intensive Care Management" in B. J. Stevens, *Educating the Nurse Manager: Case Studies and Group Work* (Rockville, MD: Aspen Systems, 1982), pp. 95-97.

Chapter 15

▼▼▼▼▼▼▼▼▼▼▼▼▼▼▼▼

Structuring and Managing Health Information

Phyllis Giovannetti, Donna Lynn Smith, And Elizabeth Broad

KEY OBJECTIVES

In this chapter, you will learn:

- Why comprehensive health information is critical to the effective management of health organizations and the health system as a whole.
- Definitions of "information technology" and "information management."
- Differences and similarities in the objectives of the management- and clinical-information systems used in health organizations, and some examples of the two types of systems.
- How health information has traditionally been structured, and some limitations of this traditional approach.
- Reasons why information about nursing is not widely available for use in decision making by health organizations or for use in the health system in general.
- About national and international initiatives to structure and manage information about nursing and other health-related matters.
- The importance of a team approach to planning and implementing integrated information systems within health organizations.
- How nursing managers work with information-systems professionals to select, implement, and evaluate information systems for clinical or management purposes.

INTRODUCTION

The impetus for health-care reform at the national and provincial levels is irreversibly altering the landscape of our health-care system. What began in the nineteenth century as a charitable community-based effort to care for the sick and needy has grown into a very large and complex industry. There is now a shift of tremendous magnitude from the traditional view of health care that placed stand-alone acute-care hospitals at the epicentre, towards the development of large, regionally-based systems that are intended to provide for all of the health needs of a given population. Such systems often include networks of merged and affiliated hospitals, as well as community health centres, nursing homes, health-care agencies, pharmacy operations, imaging centres, and various provider groups.

As the health system changes and continues to become more complex, there is increasing emphasis on the need for greater co-ordination and integration. There is a challenge to find new ways of conceptualizing health, and new ways of organizing, delivering, financing, and evaluating health services. These challenges arise from the two fundamental goals of health-care reform in Canada: (a) to improve the individual and collective health status of Canadians, and (b) to ensure effective management and improved performance of the health-care system, with greater emphasis on efficient outputs and effective outcomes. The expectations that data will be linked, quality will be monitored, and costs will be analyzed have been catapulted to the forefront of health-policy directives, and the needs of health professionals for timely, accurate, and easily accessible information at the point of care have become more urgent. These challenges highlight the need for comprehensive integrated health-information systems.

Over the past several decades, information technology has become more convenient to use and more universally available. Its value in supporting management and clinical activities in the health system and in individual health organizations is now widely recognized, although there are great variations among the types and visibility of health-information systems that are being used. Some settings, such as large acute-care hospitals, have introduced a variety of management and clinical applications. Other settings, such as rural hospitals, stand-alone continuing-care centres, and smaller community-health programs may have automated some of their business and accounting processes, but not yet introduced clinical applications. Nurses in all of these settings need timely and useful information.

Hannah (1992) has pointed out that the term "nursing information needs" has a dual meaning. Considered from the perspective of nurses in clinical roles, it includes clinical assessment, the implementation of the nursing process, documentation of clinical observations and care provided, and access to various kinds of reference material within the organization and the nursing discipline. On the other hand, the term also refers to the information needs of organizations as represented by nurse managers, who require information to assist them in managing human resources, in analysing nursing workload as determined by the care requirements of patients in units or programs, in financial management, and in the management of physical resources. Computerized information systems can help to meet all of these needs.

The first part of this chapter is devoted to a discussion of system-level issues, particularly those dealing with how health information is structured. Nurse managers are often involved in the collection, entry and retrieval of health information, and in using and interpreting reports produced by various information systems. They are in a position to observe how health information is structured, and to work with colleagues to maintain the integrity of health information by knowing and correctly using protocols and data definitions. Nurse managers may also participate as implementers and agents of change, as new approaches to the structuring of health information are introduced.

In the latter part of the chapter, information-management issues at the organizational and program levels in health organizations are discussed. The role of the nurse manager in working with information-systems professionals and other colleagues to select, implement, and evaluate information systems is highlighted.

INFORMATION TECHNOLOGY AND INFORMATION MANAGEMENT

"Information technology" refers to the systems (programs and computers) used to manage and process information to support the compilation, analysis and interpretation of large volumes of data. Computer-based systems are the primary information technology and are usually named to indicate the discipline or function they support. For example, nursing-management information systems support nursing administration functions to facilitate the delivery of nursing services. Clinical-nursing information systems and medical information systems support the practices of nursing and medicine respectively.

Information systems may yield three types of content: *data*, *information*, and *knowledge*. According to Blum (1986), *data* refers to discrete entities described objectively without interpretation. *Information* describes data that are interpreted, organized, and structured. *Knowledge* refers to information that has been synthesized so that the interrelationships are identified and formalized.

It is obvious that data does not automatically become information or knowledge. "Information management," including the processes of information-systems planning, is required to structure data so that it becomes useable.

There is now an almost overwhelming array of hardware (the technical and electronic components of information systems); networks (the communication systems linking computers and other devices); and software (the programs or applications that enable information and processes to be operationalized). This contributes to an impression that the hardware and technical aspects of information management are the most important factors to consider in selecting and implementing information systems. This is not the case. Some of the more important factors to consider are:

- What information is needed, when, by whom, and for what purposes?
- How can this information best be structured; in what format should it be collected and displayed; who should collect it; how often should it be updated?

- Who is the custodian of the information? That is, who is responsible for monitoring and maintaining the accuracy and integrity of the databases that will be created as information is collected?
- What information needs to be "on-line" for frequent and interactive use, and what information can be stored for periodic "batch" production and reporting?
- How will the information be retrieved, and by whom?
- How much will the system be relied on when it is functioning normally?
- What regular reports will be produced using the information? What will be required to produce extraordinary reports for special purposes?

The answers to these questions must be known before it is possible to determine whether a particular technical platform or software application will meet the needs it is intended to serve. Every user of a personal computer will appreciate how important it is to be able to structure data being entered in ways that facilitate its convenient and timely retrieval. The catch phrase, "garbage in, garbage out," applies to large data sets and information systems as well as those used by individuals.

OBJECTIVES OF DIFFERENT TYPES OF HEALTH-INFORMATION SYSTEMS

The development and application of information systems to support management activities in health-care organizations pre-dated the development of systems to support clinical activities.

Management and clinical-information systems began for different reasons and to meet different objectives. In the last several years it has been recognized that the two types of systems also have some common objectives. Table 15.1 presents some of the objectives of management information systems. The objectives of clinical information systems and some examples are presented in Table 15.2.

Although they developed at different times and with different objectives, health-management information systems and clinical systems have always had some specific data elements in common. For example, laboratory systems were among the first automated systems to be implemented in hospitals. Data obtained through the analysis of a specimen in the laboratory clearly and directly serves the purpose of clinical decision making. However, a powerful incentive for the development and application of laboratory systems was the emergence of technologies that could substitute automated processes for a significant amount of the repetitive work done by laboratory technologists and other personnel. Before the introduction of automated laboratory processes, an estimated 35 percent of laboratory staff time was spent in transcribing test results so that they could be reported to physicians. A similar development occurred when computer technology was electronically integrated with electrocardiograph (EKG) machines and computer programs written to interpret EKG results. Although controver-

Table 15.1

MANAGEMENT INFORMATION SYSTEMS

Objectives	Examples
• Improve the accuracy and efficiency of statistical record-keeping and reporting. • Make statistical information more widely available for use in management decision making. • Improve resource allocation and management. • Reduce costs by introducing technologies that can automate and/or standardize repetitive annual activities.	• Financial and accounting systems • Inventory control • Payroll/Personnel • Workload-measurement systems • Admission/Transfer/Discharge (ADT) systems for patient registration • Patient-scheduling systems • Staff-scheduling systems

sial at the outset, this application has evolved into an indispensable adjunct to expert discretionary decision making by cardiologists.

More recently, the availability of sophisticated clinical intensive-care monitoring technologies at the bedside has provided clinicians with the ability to simultaneously observe moment-to-moment fluctuations in a number of clinical indicators, and to analyze trends in these indicators for an individual patient over defined periods of time. While the ability to monitor and analyze clinical data has always been available, in the past it was done manually, and often well after the fact. In this case, the introduction of computer technology has improved the ability of clinicians to access, integrate, and interpret many data elements to support decision making. The computer does not substitute for an intensive-care nurse, but enables some clinical monitoring activities to be accomplished more quickly and with greater accuracy. Some of these activities can also be centralized to a remote location by electronic means, thereby increasing the options for nurses' use of their time.

As these examples show, information technologies originally introduced for management purposes are increasingly integrated with clinical processes. It is now widely recognized that aggregate information for management decision making must be "built" from a foundation of client-specific assessment, service events, and outcome indicators. While the clinician may be primarily interested in obtaining faster access to a higher quality of diagnostic or reference information in order to provide optimum care, health-system managers will be interested in identifying what services have been provided, to which clients, by whom, at what cost, and with what outcomes. The same information is needed to satisfy both curiosities.

Although this has not been the case in the past, health-information systems will increasingly be selected and evaluated based on their ability to collect each data element only once; to integrate multiple data elements

Table 15.2

CLINICAL INFORMATION SYSTEMS

Objectives	Examples
• Improve accuracy and efficiency in transmitting and communicating clinical information, including diagnostic results. • Distribute specialized professional information for decision-support to clinical-care providers (e.g., clinic). • Improve the quality of clinical care.	• Nursing (nursing diagnosis, care plans, etc.) • Pharmacy • Dietary • Rehabilitation • Medicine • Social Work • Clinical-care management systems (standard-care plans, care maps, etc.) • On-line compendium of drug information • Clinical practice guidelines

collected at multiple locations and times; and to distribute data optimally to all legitimate users.

STRUCTURING HEALTH-DATA SETS TO CREATE INFORMATION AND KNOWLEDGE

It will likely come as no surprise to the reader to learn that the remarkable Florence Nightingale, over a century ago, was the first to devise a system for gathering minimum uniform health data (Cohen, 1984). Miss Nightingale was interested in a comparative reporting system for London hospitals, including data about admissions, discharges, lengths of stay, recoveries, and deaths. The system was not put into general practice, and over a century later, Miss Nightingale's vision of a uniform data set and comprehensive information for health decision making has still not been achieved.

Most industrialized countries throughout the world collect data at the sites where health services are delivered. This data is then aggregated and summarized to provide a basis for the development of health policies and to provide information on the health of the nation. While some data has been collected at both the provincial and national levels since the beginning of Canada's structured health-care system, it was not until the early 1960s that the concept of a uniform minimum health data set received serious attention. Figure 15.1 illustrates how efforts to structure health information have paralleled technical developments in the field of information-management technology.

As shown in this figure, attempts to structure health information began with the codification of medical diagnoses, which began to be standardized in the 1950s. In the early 1960s, the "discharge abstract" was developed by the Hospital Medical Records Institute (HMRI) to collect clinical information that would serve management purposes in Canada. The HMRI system involves the abstraction, or summary, of medical-records information by technologists following a patient's discharge from hospital. The information listed for each patient includes demographic details, admission and discharge dates, medical diagnoses and procedures, case mix groups, and physician specialities. The data standards and classification methods are consistent for all hospitals, which means that the clinical activity of hospitals in various parts of the country can be compared. The information is used for a variety of purposes including utilization review, strategic planning, comparisons of hospital activities, health work-force planning, cost analysis, support for accreditation, and linkages with other databases. Although the discharge-abstract system has become Canada's most comprehensive and widely used health-care database system, it has been of limited value to nurses.

The HMRI abstract, like most databases, is dependent upon a number of classification systems for the selection of the appropriate codes. For example, medical diagnoses are coded using the International Classification of Diseases (ICD) codes. The ICD developed by the World Health Organization (WHO) is a classification of diseases and other health problems intended to serve a wide variety of needs for mortality and health-care data throughout the world. In the tenth edition of this classification (ICD-10), a new concept was added: the family of disease and health-related classifications. This concept enables nursing diagnoses, which are not disease conditions, to be classified. Currently, the WHO and the International Council of Nurses are working to incorporate nursing diagnoses and other nursing nomenclatures into the ICD.

In addition to disease conditions, costs can be compared and analyzed with data revealed by HMRI abstracts, using a classification scheme known as Case Mix Groups (CMGs). CMGs are derived from data that groups patients according to similarity of clinical characteristics and resource use. In the past decade, considerable research has been conducted to develop CMGs in Canada that are reliable, valid, and sensitive to cost variations.

Another national effort to structure health information was the Management Information Systems (MIS) project. The MIS project was initiated to develop and implement guidelines that would better measure the relationship of input (resources) to output (service activities) by integrating finance-oriented workload and patient-record-keeping systems, and improve the timeliness and comparability of information being collected in Canadian health facilities (McMichael, 1992, p. 184).

A key feature of the MIS project and, indeed, of all efforts to structure information, is the necessity for a common set of data definitions. For example, in the area of work-force costs and reporting, some hospitals might include unit clerks in their tabulation of clinical costs, while others might count them as part of administration. Without agreement as to what items of information are included within particular categories, the problem often described as "comparing apples and oranges" is inevitable. The MIS project

Figure 15.1

INFLUENCE OF TECHNOLOGY DEVELOPMENTS ON THE STRUCTURING OF HEALTH INFORMATION

Key Developments in Information Technology

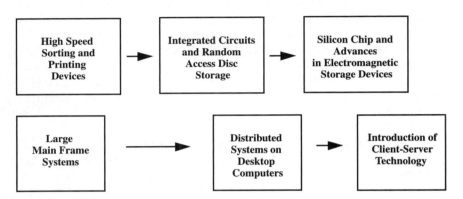

Progress in Structuring Health Information

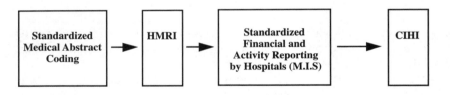

Nursing-Specific Developments

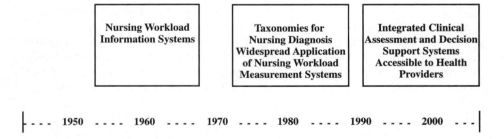

introduced national standards for gathering and processing data and reporting financial and statistical information. Unlike many other systems for
gathering health information, the MIS guidelines contain a category for the

reporting of nursing services as one of the functional areas, or departmental dimensions, within which activities and costs are grouped.

The MIS project was first implemented in hospitals in three pilot sites in different parts of Canada. Over a fifteen-year period, this nationally funded project was diffused to most parts of the country, creating increased awareness of the need for common data standards, and improving the quality of information available for understanding the costs of health care.

CURRENT NATIONAL INITIATIVES IN STRUCTURING HEALTH INFORMATION

The tough economic and fiscal realities facing the Canadian health-care system in the last decades of the century have given rise to new imperatives in the area of health information. A nation-wide consultation and planning process initiated through the National Task Force on Health Information showed that most existing data systems were focused on hospital and medical services. The need for comprehensive information about care in the community and about environmental and occupational health was identified. Existing systems were judged to lack integrity and coherence because they embodied incomparable and inconsistent concepts and definitions. It was recognized that these systems were not adequate for managing the health system as a whole, or for facilitating the assessment of outcomes and effectiveness of various care interventions (Alvarez, 1993). The outcome of the task-force deliberations was the creation of the Canadian Institute for Health Information (CIHI) in 1993.

CIHI is a federally chartered, independent, not-for-profit national organization that is charged with the development and maintenance of a comprehensive and integrated health-information system for Canada. Established by merging the resources of the MIS project and the HMRI, CIHI also assumed functions from the National Health Information Council, the Health Information Division of Health Canada, and some selected health-information resources from Statistics Canada. CIHI analyzes and shares data with health-care facilities, ministries of health, health agencies and organizations, and the private sector. Through these activities, the Institute is responsible for providing accurate and timely information necessary to establish sound health policy, manage the Canadian health system effectively, and create public awareness of factors affecting good health.

CIHI has established databases to provide information in three categories:

1. **Health Human Resources** databases collect information about *who* provides health services in Canada.
2. **Service Events** databases document *what* treatments and interventions are being done.
3. **Health Expenditures** databases track *how much* we spend for health care in Canada.

Currently, a number of health-information data sets exist. These include the CIHI abstract (formerly the HMRI abstract), the Annual Hospital Survey, the Ambulatory Care Costing System, the National Continuing Care Survey, and the National Rehabilitation Survey. Each of these data sets summarizes and aggregates data collected at care-delivery sites. The data are shared at multiple levels—by health-care facilities, health regions, provincial health departments, and nationally—and the health data collected and summarized through this process is used for health planning, evaluation, and policy setting.

In 1996, CIHI established a new program entitled "Partnership for Health Informatics/Telemetrics." The purpose of this program is to bring together professionals from the public and private sectors to adopt and tailor existing international standards for the Canadian health-information environment. The Canadian Nurses Association is a member of the partnership, and is represented in working groups considering such issues as health-information models, security, information exchange, advanced health technologies, and health-identification systems. The establishment of such partnerships is an important step forward, and the initiative to solicit input from all health providers is essential if information systems and health data sets are to be put to optimum use.

The overall goal of informational technology is the provision of data, information, and knowledge to multiple users. The traditional dominance of a medical viewpoint in our health-care system has had major implications for how clinical and administrative information systems and databases have been developed over the last few decades. The original data-collection systems were developed by governmental and private groups, whose members consulted with physicians and their organizations to determine what should be included in the databases. The creation of CIHI, and its potential for a leadership role in ensuring that the goals of health-care reform are achieved, is a positive development for nursing and other non-physician health-care providers whose services have been invisible in the traditional databases.

STRUCTURING INFORMATION ABOUT NURSING INTERVENTIONS AND OUTCOMES

Clark and Lang have succinctly noted that "if we cannot name it, we cannot control it, finance it, research it, teach it, or put it into public policy" (1992, p. 109). Data that reflects the demand for nursing care, the response of nurses to that demand, and the contribution of nurses to the public's health, is generally not available for use in planning, managing, and evaluating the effectiveness of the health system. This may seem surprising, since nurses are the largest group of health-care professionals, and the need for nursing care is the primary reason for most hospital admissions and home-care services. The hospital-discharge abstract, which has for so many years been the basis of the permanent record of hospital activities, contains no information about nursing assessment, goals, interventions or outcomes, and similar deficiencies exist in the data-collection systems of community-health agencies and other sectors of the health-care system. Jacox has outlined the serious ramifications of the "invisibility" of nurses and nursing care in current databases as follows:

- The nursing care received by patients in most health-care settings is not described;

- Much of nursing practice is described as the practice of others, especially physicians;

- The effects of nursing practice on patient outcomes are not described;

- Nursing care within a single setting, or across multiple settings, is not described;

- It is not possible to identify what nurses do so that appropriate reimbursement for nursing services can be calculated;

- It is not possible to tell the difference in patient outcomes and costs when care is delivered by different professional groups (i.e., by physicians or nurses);

- A view of nursing as indistinct from medicine is perpetuated (1995, p. 163).

There are two main reasons why the work of nurses has remained invisible. These are the 1. the lack of a consensual language that describes the practice of nursing, and 2. the fact that data reflecting the practice of nursing are not routinely collected and retained. In view of this, one of the most critical issues for nurses is the need to identify nursing-data elements that should be included in both health-agency information systems and in data sets for the health system as a whole. In order to provide the leadership necessary for this process, nursing leaders and all other nurses must become better informed and more concerned about what data is being collected, summarized, reported, and retained in the various practice settings in which they work. They must also become informed about, and support, provincial and national initiatives to develop a comprehensive set of data elements to describe nursing diagnoses, interventions, and outcomes.

THE DEVELOPMENT OF NURSING DATA SETS

The first efforts toward the development of a minimum data set for nursing began in the United States under the leadership of Dr. Harriet Werley. Cognizant of the fact that patient care is not exclusively physician-directed and that the Uniform Hospital Discharge Data Set (UHDDS), the discharge-abstract system used in the United States, fell short of providing a complete and accurate representation of information related to the operation of hospitals,

Werley and her associates began the job of defining data elements of importance to nursing. They defined Nursing Minimum Data Set (NMDS) as "a minimum set of items of information with uniform definitions and categories concerning the specific dimensions of professional nursing which meets the information needs of multiple data users in the health care system"(Werley, 1988, p. 7).

The benefits of an NMDS, as outlined by Werley, are as follows:

- Access to comparable, minimum nursing-care and resources data at local, regional, national, and international levels.
- Enhanced documentation of nursing care provided.
- Identification of trends related to patient, or client, problems and nursing care provided.
- Impetus to improved costing of nursing services.
- Improved data for quality-assurance evaluations.
- Impetus to further development and refinement of nursing-information systems.
- Comparative research on nursing care, including research on nursing diagnosis, nursing interventions, current status of client problems, and referral for further nursing services.
- Contributions toward advancing nursing as a research-based discipline (Werley, 1988, pp. 427–428).

The NMDS, as conceptualized by nursing leaders in the United States, consists of *nursing-care elements*, *patient-demographic elements,* and *service elements*. The *nursing-care elements* identified were nursing diagnosis, nursing intervention, nursing outcome, and nursing intensity. All of these elements arise from the processes employed by nurses as they plan and provide care in any setting. Most of the *patient-demographic* and *service* elements deemed essential by nurses, with the major exception of a unique nurse-provider identifier, were already contained within the UHDDS and could be accessed through linkages with this data set. In all, sixteen essential data elements were identified for the NMDS.

Standard classification systems are being developed for the nursing-care data elements to aid the collection of uniform, accurate data. These include: the North American Nursing Diagnosis Association (NANDA) taxonomy (NANDA, 1996), The Omaha System: Applications for Community Health Nursing (Martin & Scheet, 1992), The Home Health Care Classification (Saba 1992), the Nursing Interventions Classification (NIC) (Iowa Intervention Project 1996), and Nursing Outcomes Classification (NOC) (Johnson & Maas, 1995).

Canadian nurses have also begun the task of identifying nursing-data elements, and these are beginning to be referred to as Health Information: Nursing Components (HI:NC) to reflect the intention that nursing data be included with other essential health data. A national conference under the auspices of the Canadian Nurses Association (CNA) brought together an international multidisciplinary group of experts and registered nurses from across Canada to deliberate issues related to the development, implementation and evaluation of a nursing minimum data set for use by Canadian nurses (CNA, 1993). The overall purpose of the working conference was to develop a data set to ensure both the availability and accessibility of standardized nursing data. It is intended that HI:NC represent the essential pieces of information concerning the specific dimensions of professional nursing that must be included in federal and provincial compilations of health information.

In the CNA conference proceedings, twenty-one data elements are identified. The proceedings were distributed widely so that nurses in each province could discuss and debate the definitions and decide whether to develop new definitions or to adopt those that have been developed for existing classification schemes for each of the elements. Table 15.3 provides a comparison of the HI:NC with the data set currently in use by CIHI.

The Alberta Association of Registered Nurses (AARN) has been very active in pursuing the aims of the working conference, and its members have developed and endorsed working definitions for the care elements (AARN, 1997, p. 5). These definitions are shown in Box 15.1.

More recently, the CNA, along with its provincial counterparts, has developed a workbook to assist nurses in reaching consensus on HI:NC data elements (Sibbald, 1998). As this edition of *Nursing Management in Canada* goes to press, CIHI is in the process of attaining external review of a newly developed Canadian Classification of Health Interventions (CCI). The main objective of this review, which is being circulated widely among nurses and other health-care professionals in Canada, is to ensure that the proposed classification meets the information needs of multiple users and care providers. Nurses across Canada will study with interest the final CCI interventions list to determine the potential uses of this classification system as an alternative to, for example, the comprehensive nursing intervention classification scheme developed by the Iowa Intervention Project in the United States.

The CCI has several key features that reflect a shift in the development of classification schemes. It is intended to be neutral with respect to service provider and service setting. That is, the same codes are intended to be applicable regardless of whether a physician, nurse or other provider performs an intervention or whether the intervention was done in an operating room, an emergency department, a clinic, or a physician's office. It is expected that information about service providers and service settings would be captured as separate data elements in the client's record, thus overcoming the problem of "invisibility" of nurses and nursing care.

In an effort to recognize the considerable work already completed in developing classification systems for nursing diagnoses, interventions and outcomes, and the urgent need to develop a uniform international language for nurses, the International Council of Nurses (ICN) has begun work on an International Classification of Nursing Practice (ICNP). The ICNP could be used to describe nursing practice and compare nursing data across

Table 15.3

COMPARISON OF CANADIAN INSTITUTE FOR HEALTH INFORMATION (CIHI) AND PROPOSED HEALTH INFORMATION: NURSING COMPONENTS (HI:NC) DATA SETS

CIHI[1]	HI:NC[2]
Care Items	
Medical Diagnosis (most responsible, primary, secondary) Procedures and dates	Client status (Nursing diagnosis) Nursing interventions Client outcomes Nursing intensity
Patient Demographics	
Health card number Date of birth and age Sex Weight (newborn and infants <28 days) Postal Code	Unique lifetime identifier Race and ethnicity Unique geographical location Language Occupation Living arrangments Home environment including physical structure Responsible caregiver upon discharge Functional health status Burden on care provider Education level Literacy level Work environment Lifestyle data (e.g., alcohol and tobacco use) Income level
Service Items	
Prov./Institution # Chart # Most responsible doctor Most responsible consultant Admission date and hour Admission category Admit by ambulance Discharge date and hour Length of stay Institution to alive/death code Responsibility for payment Main patient service	Principal nurse provided Unique nurse identifier

Source: [1]Selected items from Canadian Institute for Health Information, *Abstracting Manual* (Ottawa, ON: CIHI, 1995); [2]Canadian Nurses Association, *Papers from the Nursing Minimum Data Set Conference* (Ottawa, ON: CNA, 1993), pp. 153–54.

> **Box 15.1**
>
> **HEALTH INFORMATION: NURSING COMPONENTS (HI:NC) DEFINITIONS**
>
> **Client status:** A label summarizing a set of indicators that reflects the phenomena for which nurses provide care relative to the health status of clients.
>
> **Nursing interventions:** Purposeful and deliberate health-affecting interventions (independent or collaborative; direct or indirect) based on an assessment of client status and designed to bring about results that benefit clients.
>
> **Nursing intensity:** The amount and type of nursing resources used to provide care.
>
> **Client outcomes:** A client's status at (a) defined point(s) following health-affecting interventions.
>
> Source: Alberta Association of Registered Nurses, *Client Status, Nursing Intervention and Client Outcomes Classification System: A Discussion Paper* (Edmonton, AB: AARN, 1997), p. 5.

clinical populations around the world, and by doing so could support the processes of nursing practice and advance the knowledge necessary for cost-effective delivery of quality nursing care. When developed, it would join the ranks of other well used classification systems such as the International Classification of Diseases (ICD) and the Diagnostic and Statistical Manual of Mental Disorders (DSM).

At this stage in its development the ICNP provides a detailed integration of the principal international classification systems, including those referred to earlier in this chapter relating to nursing diagnoses, interventions and outcomes. In addition, the ICNP provides cross-mapping from the already developed classification systems to ICNP using electronic information systems. In this way nursing data can be compared across practice settings regardless of the particular diagnostic, intervention, and outcome classifications in use.

INFORMATION SYSTEMS IN HEALTH AGENCIES: THE NURSE MANAGER'S ROLE

In the 1970s and early 1980s, it was not uncommon for departmental managers in health organizations to advocate for and implement systems that served their departmental needs. These departmental systems often operated on different hardware and software and were rarely able to communicate with one another or share the same information. Problems of availability, accuracy, and transmission of information from stand-alone systems led to recognition of the need for integrated information systems. Although vendors (companies that sell information technology or software) have often implied that integrated systems are available or can be achieved with minimal effort and cost, this goal has remained elusive (Bilodeau, 1992, pp. 18–20). In the words of the senior nursing officer of Sunnybrook Hospital in Toronto:

> The first time I looked at computer systems to assist us in patient care was in 1975. It is now 1990, and I have yet to see a system fully operating to all of its anticipated objectives anywhere in Canada. What I have seen are bits and pieces of systems, some good and some bad, and many people planning and talking about how much better the health-care world is going to be when these systems are up and operating. Change has not been rapid. I have no reason to believe the next developments will be any more rapid than those over the past 15 years. At least in health care, we are in an automation evolution—not a revolution (Huesing, 1990, p. 27).

In all practice settings, nurse managers play increasingly important roles in the decision to introduce computers and in the selection and implementation of software products. The nurse manager will work with colleagues to define needs or problems in the practice setting that may be amenable to automated solutions. If a problem appears to lend itself to such a solution, then the manager must be prepared to provide more information by means of a detailed "needs analysis." In a needs analysis, the existing practice system is described, usually by developing flow charts or algorithms that break down all major processes into sub-processes, showing their relationships to one another. The current processes are then compared with the processes that might be built into an automated system, so that the impact of the proposed system can be assessed and anticipated. Various approaches to cost analysis are used to develop a "business case" that will illustrate the potential value of the proposed system to the organization and its clients or stakeholders.

Information systems, including not only the technical platforms on which they operate, but also their implementation and maintenance, constitute a major organizational investment. Most large health organizations or health regions now have a chief information officer (CIO) who heads a department of information-systems specialists. The CIO provides professional leadership in the management of the day-to-day operation of information systems, but more importantly, provides guidance in the development of an information structure and strategic direction that will support the organization in achieving its clinical and management goals (Haskell, 1992). Recognizing that a team effort is required to assess information needs and to establish a strategic direction for organization-wide planning, most health organizations now set up a steering committee to coordinate information-systems planning, acquisition, implementation, and evaluation for the organization as a whole. The senior nursing officer of the organization is, or should be, a member of this committee, along with other senior managers in the organization.

PARTICIPATING IN THE ACQUISITION AND IMPLEMENTATION OF AN INFORMATION SYSTEM

The process of acquiring an information system is usually co-ordinated by a staff member of the information-systems department, who acts as a project manager. The project team is made up of people who will use, or be affected by, the system being introduced. Nurses at various levels of the organization will participate in the project team (often called a user group), depending upon the type of system being considered.

A project with significant implications for the organization is not usually initiated unless there is support for it at the senior level (see Chapter 24). This is particularly true for information-systems projects because of their cost and complexity. Therefore, if nurses in an intensive-care unit believe that a patient-monitoring system would assist them in their work, their first task would be to obtain organizational support for the type of in-depth needs assessment that is done before a system is purchased. In this instance, making a case for the benefits of the patient-monitoring system with other clinical professionals who would use or be affected by its introduction would be an important first step. Similarly, if the nurse managers in the organization believe that a staff-scheduling system is needed, it would be to their benefit to enlist the support of the human-resources department at the outset.

Developing and maintaining horizontal relationships with colleagues in the information-systems department can provide nurse managers with insights into the processes through which information-systems projects are initiated in their particular organizations. Where an information-systems steering committee exists, it will usually develop an organization-wide strategic plan for information systems. Within the context of this plan, the committee will review and prioritize all requests to introduce new systems. It will then act as the sponsoring committee for an information-systems project once it has been approved.

Most health organizations require that all major capital assets or consulting services be obtained by means of a formal process that allows vendors or suppliers to compete for the opportunity to supply the product or service. When a decision to acquire an information system has been made, a "request for proposal" (RFP) is usually developed by the organization (sometimes with the assistance of a consulting firm), to describe the needs the information system is intended to meet, and to set forth the technical and functional specifications of the system that is required. A project manager, usually from the information-systems department or a consulting firm, will be responsible for co-ordinating the preparation of this document with the assistance of members of the prospective user group. The intended users have a major role in determining what the functional specifications of the system will be; that is, what the system must be able to do. Once functional requirements are agreed upon, staff members from the information-systems department develop the technical specifications for the proposed system. The RFP is distributed to the vendors who are most likely to be able to supply the type of product and service required, and they have the opportunity to respond with proposals by a specified date.

The user group or project team will play a major role in evaluating the proposals received. The size and cost of the project will determine the number of suppliers who are asked to provide further information and demonstrate their products. Again, at this stage of assessing the capacities of particular products, the user group will be extensively involved.

Some examples of questions that should be considered by nurses and other potential users in a software evaluation are the following:

- How easy is it for novices to use the program?
- Is the program "error-trapping"? In other words, does it stop users from making obvious mistakes?
- Are the messages and reports easy to read and understand?
- Is the system flexible enough to adjust to process changes within the practice setting and organization?
- Is the system interactive with other systems in the organization?
- How are security concerns addressed?

The quality of software documentation is another important aspect that nurses and other users can evaluate. Some examples of questions that might be asked to assess the quality of documentation are:

- Is there a manual with the software? Is it laid out in a logical sequence and understandable enough for inexperienced users?
- Is there a section dealing with common problems?
- Is on-line help available and easy to access?

When the software evaluation and other assessments have taken place, the user group will select the most suitable product and final negotiations about price will take place.

Once a system has been selected, the user group will refocus its attention on planning for and supporting system implementation. It is at this stage that the nurse manager will need to make use of his or her leadership skills to become a champion of the new system and thereby help to motivate staff to accept it, to help design and co-ordinate training opportunities, to identify problems and work with information-systems professionals and others toward their resolution, and to ensure that the system is implemented successfully.

FUTURE DIRECTIONS

Nursing and health informatics are areas of growing importance that have an impact on nurses' clinical, educational, research, and managerial roles. *Informatics* is a term that refers to the combination of computer science and information science as applied, in this case, to the management and processing of nursing and health data (National Center for Nursing Research, 1993). Nurse managers will need to become well informed about these areas. They can do this in a number of ways. Nurses are welcomed as members of the Canadian Association for the Application of Computers in Health, an interdisciplinary national organization for health information-systems professionals. For the last decade there has been a nurse on the board of directors of this organization, and many nurses have been active participants in its Nursing Interest Group. Growing numbers of nurses are developing careers in the area of health informatics. Many are able to do so through opportunistic work experiences, but educational experiences are now becoming available in this area as well. Sibbald (1998) provides information about a number of these opportunities and the potential of nursing informatics to improve the quality of health care in the future.

Today, in Canada, the need to connect large and small health facilities of all kinds in an information network has been accepted. Our geography and relatively small population can reap major benefits from new developments in fibre optics and other forms of communications technology that enable speedy transmission of information and images over long distances. Through developments such as tele-health, clinical and educational expertise can be widely shared to the benefit of clients and care providers from all disciplines and at all levels.

These developments are occurring in parallel with implementation of freedom-of-information and privacy legislation that attempts to address growing concern among consumers that their personal information might be divulged or appropriated without their consent, and given to insurance companies, financial institutions, or other parties. A strong legal precedent has been established with respect to the confidentiality and security of health information and the same rigorous standards will continue to apply as technical advances enable health information to be collected, transmitted, and stored in new ways (Rozovsky & Rozovsky, 1992).

CONCLUSION

The value of structuring health data to reflect interdisciplinary practice across all settings is now being recognized through important national initiatives. Health professionals and managers can expect to see and participate in dramatic developments in the area of health informatics throughout their careers. A forward-looking discussion of how new technologies will support "point-of-service" decision making by health professionals can be found in Parker, Neimeth, & Porter O'Grady (1997). They predict that in the next decade more than 50 percent of capital expenditures for the health system will be devoted to developing a new information infrastructure for health care.

No longer centred on financial management and support to care providers, health-information systems in the future will have the potential to directly benefit clients and their families. Among their other advantages, they will help consumers to become custodians of their own health information, assist them in gaining access to information and services, and equip them and their care providers with knowledge-based systems and best-practice information that will help to improve the overall quality of care.

SUMMARY

- Information technology includes the computers (hardware), networks (communication), and programs (software) used to compile and process health data.
- When data are structured and organized, information can be retrieved and used, and knowledge can be developed. Therefore, it is important to be aware of past, present, and future efforts to structure health data sets.
- Before developing processes and selecting technologies for information processing, it is necessary to know why information is being collected and what it will be used for. Many unnecessary costs can be attributed to a failure to plan for the types and uses of information to be collected and stored in information systems.
- It is now widely recognized that aggregate information for management decision making must be built from a foundation of client-specific data arising from professional assessment, service events, and outcome indicators.
- Although this has not been the case in the past, health-information systems will be selected and evaluated based on their ability to collect each data element only once, to integrate multiple data elements collected at multiple locations and at different times, and to distribute data optimally to all legitimate users.
- Information systems are introduced in health organizations for a variety of reasons. Although management and clinical systems began with different goals, both types of system are now increasingly concerned with collecting information only once and then sharing and integrating it to serve multiple purposes.
- Efforts to structure health information were initially medically oriented, and nursing has been "invisible" in traditional health data sets. This problem is being corrected through current efforts to structure health information in ways that are client-centered and "neutral" as to care provider and setting.
- Most health organizations establish an organization-wide steering committee to carry out strategic planning and to set priorities for information-systems initiatives. Senior nurse managers and/or program managers are usually represented on these committees.
- Nurse managers play important roles in identifying and validating the need for information systems, in documenting current procedures and designing improved procedures to be automated, and in selecting and evaluating systems.

- Skilled first-line leadership is a key variable in the successful implementation of information systems.
- Throughout their careers, clinical nurses and nurse managers can expect to see and be involved in a variety of exciting developments arising from new technological and scientific advances that will make it easier and less expensive to collect and distribute information to multiple users.

FURTHER READINGS AND RESOURCES

American Nurses Association (1994). *Scope of practice for nursing informatics*. Washington, DC: ANA.

American Nurses Association (1995). *Nursing informatics standards of practice*. Washington, DC: ANA.

Ball, M.J., Hannah, K.J., Newbold, S.K., Douglas, J.V. (Eds.) (1995). *Nursing informatics: Where caring and technology meet*. New York: Springer-Verlag.

Canadian Nurses Association (1998). *Nursing and health information: Towards consensus on nursing care elements*. Ottawa, ON: CNA.

Johnson, J.M. (1987). Implementing a computer software system. *Journal of Nursing Administration, 17*(10), 16–21.

McAlindon, M.N., Danz, S.M., & Theodoroff, R.A., (1987). Choosing the hospital information system: A nursing perspective. *Journal of Nursing Administration. 17*(10) 11–15.

Mowry, M. (1992). Computerization and quality. In M. Johnson (Ed.), *Series on Nursing Administration Vol. 3: The delivery of quality care* (pp. 153–171). St. Louis, MO: Mosby.

Ogilvie, M. & Sawyer, E. (Eds.) (1992). *Managing information in Canadian health facilities*. Ottawa, ON: Canadian Hospital Association Press.

REFERENCES

Alberta Association of Registered Nurses (1997). *Client status, nursing intervention and client outcomes classification system: A discussion paper.* Edmonton, AB: AARN.

Alvarez, D. (1993). Health information strategy. In Canadian Nursing Association (Eds.), *Papers from the Nursing Minimum Data Set Conference* (pp.16–20). Ottawa, ON: CNA.

Bilodeau, M. (1992) Information integration: Is it feasible or practical? In M. Ogilvie & E. Sawyer (Eds.), *Managing information in Canadian health care facilities* (pp. 15–30). Ottawa, ON: Canadian Hospital Association Press.

Blum, B.I. (Ed.) (1986). *Clinical information systems.* New York: Springer-Verlag.

Canadian Nurses Association (1993). *Papers from the Nursing Minimum Data Set Conference.* Ottawa, ON: CNA.

Clark, J. & Lang, N. (1992). Nursing's next advance: An international classification for nursing practice. *International Nursing Review, 39*(4), 109–112.

Cohen, I.B. (1984). Florence Nightingale. *Scientific American, 250,* 128–133, 136–137, 144.

Hannah, K. (1992). Nursing management of information. In M. Ogilvie & E. Sawyer (Eds.), *Managing information in Canadian health facilities* (pp. 99–112). Ottawa, ON: Canadian Hospital Association.

Haskell, A. (1992). The role of the chief information officer. In M. Oglivie & E. Sawyer (Eds.). *Managing information in Canadian health care facilities* (pp.69–82). Ottawa, ON: Canadian Hospital Association.

Huesing, S. (1990). Nursing informatics: The nurse administrator's perspective. *Healthcare Computing and Communications Canada, 4*(2), 20–27.

Iowa Intervention Project (1996). *Nursing interventions classification (NIC)* (2nd ed.). St. Louis, MO: Mosby.

Jacox, A. (1995). Practice and policy implications of clinical and administrative databases. In American Nurses Association (Ed.). *Nursing data systems: The emerging framework* (pp. 161–165). Washington, DC: ANA.

Johnson, M. & Maas, M. (1995). Classification of nursing-sensitive patient outcomes. In American Nurses Association (Ed.), *Nursing data systems: The emerging framework* (pp. 177–183). Washington, DC: ANA.

Martin, K.S. & Scheet, N.J. (1992). *The Omaha system: Applications for community health nursing.* Philadelphia, PA: W.B. Saunders.

McMichael, S. (1992). The management information systems project. In: M. Ogilvie & E Sawyer (Eds.), *Managing information in Canadian health facilities* (pp. 183–194). Ottawa, ON: Canadian Hospital Association.

National Center for Nursing Research (l993). *Nursing informatics: Enhancing patient care.* Bethesda, MD: U.S. Department of Health and Human Services.

North American Nursing Diagnosis Association (1996). *NANDA nursing diagnosis: Definitions and classifications.* Philadelphia, PA: NANDA.

Parker, M., Neimeth, L., & Porter-O'Grady, T. (1997). Information management for point-of-service decision making. In T. Porter-O'Grady, M. Hawkins & M. Parker (Eds.). *Whole systems shared governance: Architecture for integration* (pp.257–288). Gaithersburg MD: Aspen.

Rozovsky, L.E. & Rosovsky, F.A. (1992). *Canadian health information: A legal and risk management guide.* Toronto: Butterworths.

Saba, V.K. (1992). The classification of home health care nursing diagnoses and interventions. *Caring, 11* (3), 50–57.

Sibbald, B.J. (1998). Nursing informatics. *The Canadian Nurse, 94*(4), 22–30.

Werley, H.H. (1988). Research Directions. In H.H. Werley & N.M. Lang, (Eds.), *Identification of the nursing minimum data set* (pp. 427–431). New York: Springer.

Werley, H.H. (1988). Introduction to the nursing minimum data set and its development. In H.H. Werley and N.M. Lang (Eds.) *Indentification of the nursing minimum data set* (pp. 1–15). New York: Springer.

Chapter 16

▼▼▼▼▼▼▼▼▼▼▼▼▼▼▼▼▼▼▼▼▼▼

Professional Governance

DONNA ARMANN-HUTTON

KEY OBJECTIVES

In this chapter, you will learn:

- The purpose of professional legislation in regulating professional practice.
- The regulations encompassed in the professional statutes, including: registration requirements for practice; requirements for mandatory continuing education; complaint and disciplinary procedures; and limitations on service.
- The collective and individual responsibilities of the medical staff as described in the medical staff by-laws.
- The committee structure that supports the nursing discipline within a health-care facility.
- The interprofessional relationships that will be required in the health-care organization of the future.

INTRODUCTION

The complex nature of the responsibilities of nurse managers requires them to have not only clinical knowledge and an awareness of the operational processes of the health-care facilities in which they work, but also to be familiar with the legislation that regulates their professional practice and the practice of those with whom they work. Professional governance standards provide security for professionals as well as for patients, and nurse managers are wise to make themselves aware of the implications of these standards.

PROFESSIONAL LEGISLATION AND RIGHT TO TITLE

Professional legislation establishes an exclusive scope of practice for a particular profession only if the public interest is clearly served by doing so, and if the benefit of public protection outweighs the cost. Such legislation grants registered practitioners the exclusive right to use a specific title, so that the public can distinguish between practitioners who are governed by professional legislation (e.g., registered nurses) and those who are not (e.g., therapeutic touch practitioners). Practitioners who are not members of a regulated profession are not permitted to represent themselves as registered. A professional who is registered, therefore, is governed by professional legislation and requirements. This supports the advocacy of competent practice.

PROFESSIONAL SELF-REGULATION

It is important to note that professions such as nursing and medicine are self-regulated. This means that these professionals ensure safe practice by monitoring themselves and their colleagues within the jurisdiction of professional legislation.

The fundamental purpose of professional legislation is to provide regulation in the public interest and in the case of nurses, physicians, and other registered health-care providers, this provides protection to the consumer of health services from practitioners who are incompetent or unethical.

Professional legislation establishes standards, procedures, and controls that regulate professional practice in order to:

- provide a quality, efficient and cost-effective service;
- balance the rights and responsibilities of professionals, service users, and the public; and
- enable service users to exercise informed judgement and freedom of choice regarding professional services (Government of Alberta, 1990, p. 1).

In disciplines such as medicine and nursing, the privileges, responsibilities, and processes of self-governance are delegated to professional associations by government on behalf of the public, by means of professional legislation. The association is thereby made accountable to the public and the government for the performance of its statutory functions.

Regulations encompassed within professional statutes include registration requirements; scope of practice; mandatory continuing education; complaint and disciplinary procedures; and limitations on service. Regulations must be approved by the profession's governing body, the government, and the majority of the profession's membership. By-laws address administrative matters only, and they require approval of the majority of membership (e.g., medical staff by-laws which are specific to a hospital or health authority are approved by the hospital's medical staff and regulating board). These regulations and by-laws outline the processes by which a profession strives to ensure the competence of its members, and also outlines the measures to be taken if standards of competence are not met. The goal of such guidelines is always to serve the best interests of patients and the public.

PUBLIC REPRESENTATION

In order to facilitate public accountability, representation on professional association councils and disciplinary committees by members of the public is required. This helps to ensure that the patient's perspective is voiced, and that an objective "ear" participates in the decision-making process. At present, most professional councils require at least two public representatives.

STANDARDS OF COMPETENCY AND CONDUCT

In order to ensure that licensed practitioners maintain acceptable standards of competency and conduct, the following mechanisms have been implemented by professional organizations:

- **Registration requirements.** In order to practice, professionals must be registered within their province or state. Requirements for registration are established by the professional association and include educational prerequisites.
- **Educational Standards.** Individuals being registered by the professional association must have graduated from institutions that meet specified standards in regard to curriculum and the provision of clinical training.
- **Credential Reciprocity and Portability.** Professional associations have developed processes, including acceptance of national standards (e.g. the Canadian Nurses Association Testing Service), that facilitate interprovincial reciprocity and portability of credentials.
- **Practice Review.** In each association, a professional practice review committee establishes desirable standards of practice and competence and reviews, as appropriate, the practice of registered or licensed practitioners to ensure that they are maintaining acceptable standards. Although professional bodies attempt to monitor their members' competence through these processes, improvements could be made.

A survey of five self-regulating health professions in Canada (Fooks, Rachlis & Kushner, 1990) suggests that current mechanisms for assessing the quality of care provided by practitioners are in an early, unsophisticated stage that focus on identifying poor performance. The authors suggest the development of explicit criteria for standards of patient care (e.g., for the use of caesarian sections or the treatment of deep vein thrombosis). These criteria could be used to guide professional practice and to identify problem areas in relation to individual practitioners. In the continuous-quality-improvement approach, research-based evidence would be used as the basis for standards development and for judgements about appropriateness of care. By establishing patterns of care on research-based evidence, care-mapping processes within managed-care programs could provide multidisciplinary standards for patient care.

The Canadian Council on Health Services Accreditation advocates the use of practice indicators to evaluate care. This body has taken a leadership role in developing standard patient-care indicators for health facilities. Collaboration among professional bodies to establish standards of care is to be encouraged so that resources may be pooled, both across provinces and across professions.

Relying only on a complaints program is seen by many as an insufficient system for assessing the quality of care provided by practitioners, and for protecting the public from incompetence and harm. If the public has to complain after the fact, it is not being fully protected. (Fooks et al., 1990, p. 21).

- **Code of Ethics.** Each profession has established a code of ethics which provides for enforceable standards of practice and conduct, and emphasizes public protection. Ethical responsibilities identify the practitioner as an advocate for the patient, and require that individuals who may compromise a patient's safety be reported.

  In the case study accompanying this chapter, it is the professional code of ethics that would provide guidance to the nurse manager and the reporting nurse in the case of the narcotics theft. In this situation, the nurse's professional responsibility would be to report her colleague to the professional association, giving substantiating evidence for the protection of the patients on the nursing unit.

- **Continuing Education.** Each profession establishes appropriate regulations in relation to requirements for continuing education. Ongoing participation in professional development facilitates currency within the field of practice, thereby assisting in the maintenance of practice competence. Continuing-education credits are required in the medical profession, and pharmacists are also required to attend educational sessions every year in order to be eligible for annual registration. In the near future, Canadian nurses will also require continuing-education credits, as has been the case for many years for their colleagues in other countries.

COMPLAINTS AND DISCIPLINE

Legislation establishes procedures which enable any citizen to make complaints about the conduct of registered or licensed practitioners, and to ensure thorough investigations with appropriate sanctions imposed against those found to be incompetent or unethical. The complaint process serves two purposes. First, it provides the patient with the means to ensure that complaints against an individual professional are investigated, by triggering the professional standards function of the college or association. Secondly, it provides the professional association with the mechanism to become aware of "problem" members so that the regulatory mandate may be carried out.

Mandatory reporting of health professionals by their colleagues is a relatively new requirement that was created in direct response to public concerns regarding professional accountability (Bohnen, 1994, p. 93). At present, if employment is terminated for professional misconduct, incompetence, or incapacity, the employer must file a written report with the registrar of the employee's professional association.

In many situations where a colleague is incompetent, incapacitated (as in alcohol or drug abuse), or has demonstrated misconduct, members are hesitant to lay a complaint with a professional association, in case it is seen as "blowing the whistle." In the interests of public safety, as well as individual professional responsibility, organizations should ensure that policies and procedures clearly describe the reporting and complaint process for staff, and should provide ongoing education regarding individual professional responsibilities. In the first incident described in the case study that accompanies this chapter, for example, the nurse manager should explain the discipline and reporting process as part of a discussion of the staff nurse's professional responsibilities. A clear policy, outlining responsibilities and including recommended procedures, will assist with this process.

ECONOMIC CONSIDERATIONS

In order to avoid conflicts of interest, professional associations that are responsible for both regulatory and collective-bargaining functions on behalf of members are required to ensure that the two functions are structurally and functionally independent of each other. For this reason, most professional associations have a professional arm (e.g., a college of physicians and surgeons) as well as a collective-bargaining association (e.g., a provincial medical association).

THE FUTURE OF PROFESSIONAL REGULATIONS

Professional licensing laws that are developed to protect a title, such as "registered nurse" or "medical doctor," are to a large extent unable to restrict others from practising the profession (Cutshall, 1996). In Alberta and British Columbia, proposals have been submitted that would restrict specific activities included in the Health Professions Act (e.g., Government of Alberta, 1995). In Ontario, legislation already exists to restrict specific acts, particularly those that could involve danger to a patient if improperly executed. Across the country, increasing attention is being paid to assessing ongoing competency and minimum qualifications rather than focusing only on entry credentials. In order to successfully accomplish this, it will be necessary for a common language or a standard of competency to be established.

A greater emphasis on public input and involvement in professional governance is reflected in proposals that would require up to 25 percent of the governing bodies of professional associations to be composed of public representatives. The question then becomes how these representatives could be selected and oriented to their responsibilities, and supported so that their input had maximum benefit.

In the future, professional bodies must go beyond defining practice and protecting the public. They must be directly involved in improving quality of care.

MEDICAL STAFF BY-LAWS

The mechanism in health-care facilities by which physicians operationalize the professional requirements of their discipline is the medical staff by-laws. In most cases, the facility's governing board works directly with the medical advisory committee, as designated in the medical staff by-laws.

Medical staff by-laws establish the collective and individual responsibilities of the medical staff to the health authority. In addition, they establish the medical administrative structure, and provide rules, procedures, and other mechanisms as required by relevant legislation (Capital Regional Health Authority, 1996).

The medical staff by-laws include responsibility for:

1. Ensuring that a high professional standard of care consistent with available resources is rendered to all patients;
2. Providing continuing improvement in educational and professional standards;
3. Ensuring high ethical standards of practice; and
4. Supporting medical student education.

Medical staff by-laws also outline the process for medical-staff appointments, and the specific nature of designated medical privileges that go with the appointments. They define retirement policy, as well as the process for general review of performance including the medical practice outcomes of individual physicians, suspension of privileges, and dispute resolution. In addition, the by-laws define terms of reference for the medical advisory committee (which advises the board on matters related to patient care) as well as the medical staff association (collective bargaining function).

In reference to the second incident described in the case study accompanying this chapter, the nurse manager should consult the relevant medical staff by-laws in regard to the surgeon's credentials. The by-laws will identify the requirements for proof of a surgeon's competence and the procedure for verification, and will also include stipulations for periodic review and updating of the designation of privilege. The nurse manager can share this process with the staff nurse and review the facility's compliance with the procedures outlined.

GOVERNANCE MODELS

In this age of regionalization, mergers, and facility amalgamation, a variety of governance models exist (Dagnone, Goddard, & Wilson, 1994, p. 39, 40) and these have an impact on the development of medical staff by-laws. Professional governance models serve to:

F i g u r e 1 6 . 1

CORPORATE BOARD WITH LOCAL GOVERNING BOARDS

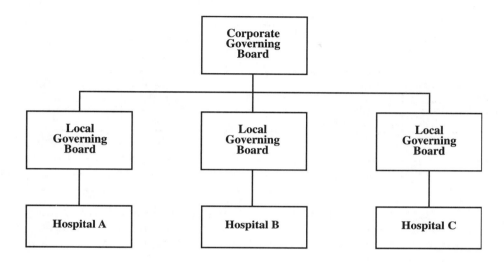

a. provide decision-making procedures with respect to the practice of the discipline;

b. ensure mechanisms are in place to monitor standards of professional practice and the performance of individual practitioners;

c. establish the means for evaluating credentials of individuals applying for positions on the staff;

d. identify the rights, privileges and responsibilities of professionals appointed to the staff; and

e. ensure that the discipline engages in education and research activities.

All models attempt to produce a system in which the board's responsibility to ensure quality of care is balanced with the profession's responsibility to govern itself.

In Figure 16.1, the traditional facility-based governing board has been maintained for each hospital with a corporate structure superimposed. This structure is often problematic as clear role delineation among the various boards is difficult, and medical staff by-laws may not be consistent among the institutions.

In the model illustrated in Figure 16.2, there is recognition of the differences among facilities and the need to provide an advisory structure to provide input to and communication from the board. The difference between this model and the one in Figure 16.1 is that a common set of medical staff by-laws would be established and implemented by the advisory boards.

Figure 16.2

CORPORATE BOARD WITH LOCAL ADVISORY BOARDS

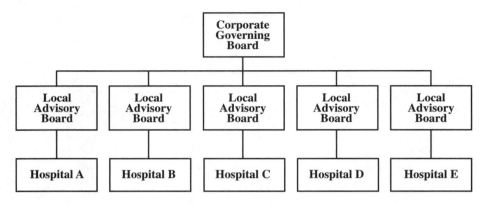

In Figure 16.3, the structure is very flat and does not demonstrate a clear communication process between the respective hospitals and the corporate governing board. In this model, ensuring compliance with medical staff by-laws can be problematic.

Many health facilities are adopting the structure illustrated in Figure 16.2, with representatives from individual hospitals participating on a regional medical council as well as on a facility advisory committee (Dagnone, Goddard & Wilson, 1994).

FACILITY AND MEDICAL COMMITTEES

In organizations which are functioning within a program management structure, medical advisory committees have sometimes been replaced by facility committees with multidisciplinary representation. The by-laws in these organizations describe the purpose of the facility committee as responsible to the board for clinical and scientific practice of the hospital, as well as the professional practice of the treatment team. This committee is further charged with setting standards to monitor and assess patient care (Alberta Cancer Board, 1996).

In addition to the facility committee, a medical committee may be charged with the responsibility for providing advice to the board on appointments, re-appointments, suspensions, terminations, and delineations of privileges of medical staff. In addition, various hospital committees are responsible for providing the advisory body or facility committee with recommendations related to patient care. They include committees responsible for such areas as infection control, medical quality assurance, pharmacy, therapeutics and health records. Each committee has its own terms of reference, and provides for standardization of practice within its designated area. It also ensures that quality-improvement measures are consistently undertaken to improve the standard of care.

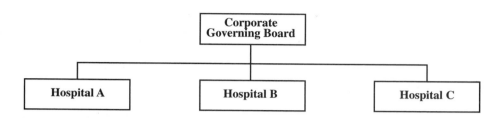

Figure 16.3
CORPORATE MODEL

NURSING GOVERNANCE

In the past, responsibility for nursing practice standards and governance issues in traditional organizations rested primarily with directors of nursing. Although many of these administrators encouraged participation in decision making by their staff nurses, it was a rarity to find nursing organizations with similar degrees of professional autonomy and self-governance as have been established for physicians under medical staff by-laws. A detailed discussion of the various reasons for the lack of professional autonomy traditionally accorded nursing departments in health agencies can be found in Monk's (1994) chapter on nursing (or shared) governance in the first edition of this book. The principal objective of shared governance is to empower nurses "by giving them opportunities to play a significant role in decisions that affect [their practice] and by systematically sharing authority and accountability"(Monk, 1994, p. 199). The term "shared governance" underscores a major difference between the practice of medicine and nursing within health agencies; namely, that physicians are generally given privileges to practice independently within a hospital, while nurses are typically employees of health-agency boards and thus are subject to the constraints of an employment relationship. (See Chapter 26 for details of employment relations.) The focus of shared-governance and nursing-practice models is on clinical nursing practice and the role that staff nurses can play in determining and monitoring professional standards. In such models, individual nurses frequently represent the discipline of nursing on medical and other committees. Additionally, the function of management generally evolves into one of facilitation, integration, and co-ordination of the practice of nursing.

Many of the nursing shared-governance models that began to take shape in the 1980s did not survive the structural changes that took place in the 1990s. (Refer to Chapter 7 for a discussion of these structural changes.) In some cases the introduction of program management had a profound impact on the organization of nursing practice in Canadian health agencies, including the loss of nursing management positions (see Chapter 13).

Under shared-governance models, different types of nursing committees generally existed to support the development and ongoing evaluation of nursing practice standards. These committees included:

- Procedures and policy committees, which establish evidence-based nursing practice based upon current nursing research;
- Nursing practice committees, which review the nursing-practice standards established by both the national and provincial professional bodies as well as specialty bodies for specific areas of practice (e.g., nephrology, oncology, critical care);
- Nursing research committees, which provide support to the improvement of standards and practice; and
- Nursing education committees, which provide educational offerings to staff to promote professional development.

Following the implementation of program management, some of these committees became inter-professional committees comprised of representatives from many disciplines.

INTERPROFESSIONAL RELATIONSHIPS

The process of program management, care mapping, rationalization of resources, outcome measurement, and total quality improvement have set the stage for greater collaboration among physicians and nurses. Both disciplines, indeed all disciplines within the health structure, must be less concerned with protecting their own scopes of practice, and become more concerned with sharing expertise to allow for the most positive patient outcomes possible within available resources. Committee structures created in support of quality improvement are based upon collaborative problem solving and evaluation of improved standards of practice. Organizations are establishing designated committees to address professional issues associated with both disciplines (e.g., joint conference committees); "The vision is, in fact emerging in reality; it involves the effective and efficient provision of appropriate care by a collaborative partnership of physicians, nurses, other caregivers and administrators who live the core values of respect, partnership and continual improvement (Andrews & Wensel, 1992, p. 33)."

CONCLUSION

Professional legislation provides for regulation of professions in the public's interest. Regulations are in place to ensure the provision of competent and ethical health care. In addition to the professional bodies regulated by means of legislation, each employing agency, hospital, health-care institution, or community facility also regulates the operation of its health disciplines with more specific by-laws.

Nurse managers today work within an ever-changing health-care environment. It is their responsibility to be aware of changes to professional legislation governing standards and practice, and of changes to the by-laws and processes that support such legislation. Governance structures exist to protect the practitioner and the client, and to assist professionals in providing guidance to their colleagues.

SUMMARY

- Professional legislation establishes standards, procedures, and controls regulating professional practice.
- Standards of competency and conduct are supported through such mechanisms as registration, the setting of educational standards, credentialling, reciprocity among provinces, practice reviews, enforcement of codes of ethics, and continuing-education requirements.
- Complaints and discipline processes exist to protect the public.
- Medical staff by-laws outline the processes by which the provision of a high standard of patient care is ensured and maintained.
- The provision of appropriate patient care must be accomplished through a collaborative partnership of all health-care professionals.

FURTHER READINGS AND RESOURCES

Porter-O'Grady, T., Hawkins, M., & Parker, M. (1997). *Whole-systems shared governance: Architecture for integration.* Gainesburg, MD: Aspen. The authors discuss a number of areas in which changes to the health system must occur to prepare for future demands. They believe that a new model of service and relationship must emerge and should be designed around the core themes of partnership, equity, accountability, and ownership. This model of whole-system shared governance is necessary because of the increasing importance of teamwork and integration in the delivery of health services. Within this new model, the traditional hierarchy of professional disciplines and organizational levels is replaced by interdisciplinary councils focused on the goals and tasks of patient care, operations, and governance. The vision presented in this book is supported by practical knowledge and examples that illustrate why whole-system shared governance is both a necessary and practical way of refocusing the health system to be more client focused and cost-effective.

REFERENCES

Alberta Cancer Board. (1996). *Medical staff by-laws.* Available from the Corporate Office, Alberta Cancer Board, Edmonton, Alberta.

Andrews, H., & Wensel, R. (1992). Promoting physician-nurse collaboration throughout the organization. *Healthcare Management Forum, 5*(4), 28–33.

Bohnen, L. (1994). *Regulated health professions act: A practical guide.* Aurora, Ontario: Canada Law Book.

Capital Regional Health Authority. (1996). *Medical staff by-laws, draft no. 9.* Available from Dr. R. Wensel, Capital Health Authority, Edmonton, Alberta.

Cutshall, P. (1996). Megatrends in professional regulation: Towards the year 2000. *International Nursing Review, 43*(4), 110–112.

Dagnone, C., Goddard, P., & Wilson, B. (1994). Governance models within multi-institutional systems. *Leadership in Health Services, 3*(4), 36–40.

Fooks K., Rachlis, M., & Kushner, C. (1990). *Assessing concepts of quality of care: Results of a national survey of five self-regulating professionals in Canada.* (CHEPA Working Paper Series No. 90-7, McMaster University). Hamilton, ON: McMaster University.

Monk, M. (1994). Nursing governance. In J.M. Hibberd & M.E. Kyle (Eds.). *Nursing management in Canada* (pp. 191–211). Toronto: W.B. Saunders.

Principles and policies governing professional legislation in Alberta (1990). Alberta Health, Alberta Workforce Planning Branch.

Principles and recommendations for the regulation of health professionals in Alberta: Final Report of the Health Workforce Re-balancing Committee (1995). Alberta Health: Health Workforce Planning Branch.

CASE STUDY

As a newly appointed nurse manager of a large surgical unit and operating room, the following situations have been reported to you by staff nurses on your units:

1. A nurse on the surgical unit is concerned that a colleague is stealing narcotics from the narcotic cupboard and is not providing patients with appropriate pain-control medication. The nurse has observed a change in her colleague's behaviour and is concerned with the safety of the patients under her care. The nurse is uncertain as to her professional responsibilities to report this individual, and of her moral and ethical responsibilities to the patient. She has come to you for advice. What course of action should you take?

2. A nurse on your staff is assisting in the operating room with a physician who has visiting privileges to your institution. The procedure that he is performing is quite complex and she is concerned that his designation of privileges, the description of which is available in your office, may not be current. She wonders what processes are in place to ensure that the information is current, and that this physician has met requirements of the hospital for provision of medical services. What is your role in resolving her concern?

Editor's Note: A catastrophic example of the second incident above is reported by Sibbald (1997). In this article, a group of OR nurses at the Winnipeg Health Sciences Centre Children's Hospital discuss their attempts to draw attention to what they considered to be evidence of a higher-than-expected mortality rate for babies undergoing open-heart surgery. This case illustrates how important it is for all registered and student nurses to understand the communication and goverence structures and the concept of professional accountability discussed in this chapter. It is strongly recommended that readers of this chapter refer to Sibbald's article and consider the following questions:

1. What are the issues and underlying problems in the case?
2. Are there any other actions that these nurses could have taken to make their voices heard?
3. What organizational supports need to be in place to assisst nurses and other health professionals to fulfil their professional responsibilities in relation to such cases?
4. What administrative actions might have prevented the infant deaths?

Chapter 17

▼▼▼▼▼▼▼▼▼▼▼▼▼▼▼

Promoting Evidence-Based Practice

CAROLYN J. PEPLER

KEY OBJECTIVES

In this chapter, you will learn:

- The importance of scientific evidence as a base for decision-making in nursing.
- That research activities include conduct of research, use of other researchers' findings to build practice, and use of rigorous research techniques in daily practice.
- The need for structural support and continuing education to facilitate evidence-based practice in a health-care agency.
- Strategies that nurse managers use to promote research activities.
- The need to be aware of the costs involved in conducting and participating in research, along with the health and economic benefits of evidence-based practice.

INTRODUCTION

Florence Nightingale advocated nursing practice based on nursing research: "And nothing but observation and experience will teach us ways to maintain or to bring back the state of health" (Nightingale, 1859, p. 74). She used detailed observation, measurement, and statistical analysis as the evidence on which to base conclusions about the nursing care during the Crimean War. Since that time, nursing knowledge and research skills have grown considerably, but what constitutes the best available evidence and its use in decision-making is not always clear.

Knowledge may be acquired in many ways, but it is useful to think of conventional wisdom attained by thoughtful analysis of experience, and scientific knowledge gained through research. Both constitute evidence and, in different situations, one or the other will form an appropriate basis for decision making for practice. "The key is for the decision-maker to understand the limitations of the evidence at hand, and the impact and relevance it will have on decision outcomes" (National Forum on Health, 1997, p. 6).

Much of the knowledge in any practice discipline is that of conventional wisdom, but as the knowledge base expands and becomes more complex, it becomes increasingly important to build practice on scientific research. Research is a process of systematic examination of phenomena to increase knowledge of these phenomena, their characteristics, occurrence, and relationships with other variables. The rigour involved in a scientific process provides for a careful examination of variables, reduces bias in data collection and analysis, and allows for critique and testing by clinicians and researchers. Clinicians are able to explain and predict outcomes of their practice and to re-examine practice as new knowledge becomes available.

The Canadian Nurses Association (1990) established three goals for nursing research: to develop nurse researchers, to develop nursing research, and to develop a research reality. A research reality is a world of nursing in which research is part of the substance of practice in all fields. Decisions are based on sound research: decisions that nurses make in relation to their clients and health care; decisions that administrators make in relation to staff and policies; and decisions that educators make in relation to students and learning. The National Forum on Health defines evidence-based decision-making as "the systematic application of the best available evidence to the evaluation of options and to decision-making in clinical, management and policy settings" (National Forum on Health, 1997, p. 6).

To build practice on scientific evidence, four interdependent components are needed: meaningful research questions that are relevant to practice; sound research to answer the questions; knowledgeable nurses with skills in using research findings; and clinical environments open to inquiry and change. Figure 17.1 illustrates the cyclical nature of the relationships among these components.

Advantages of a research base for practice include increased clarity in articulating the role of nursing, improved quality of care, increased cost-effectiveness of health care, and increased nurses' satisfaction. This chapter discusses research activities, nursing department strategies to promote these activities, the role of the nurse manager in developing research-based practice, and the economics of research.

CONDUCT AND UTILIZATION OF RESEARCH IN NURSING

Research activities include those involved in both the conduct and the utilization of research. The conduct of research is the planning and implementation of a research project for the purpose of generating knowledge. The utilization of research has two major components: interpretation and use in practice of other people's research findings, and use of rigorous research methods in practice (Crane, 1989; Horsley, 1985; Stetler, 1994). Research utilization is an integral part of sound clinical, administrative, and educational nursing practice and is essential for quality management.

Figure 17.1
INTERDEPENDENCY OF COMPONENTS FOR RESEARCH-BASED NURSING PRACTICE

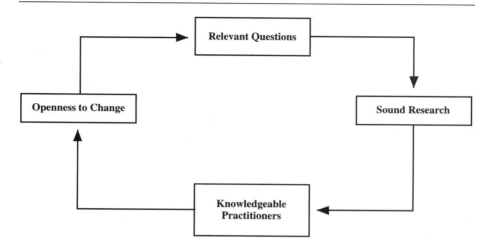

The level and type of nurses' involvement in research activities requires different knowledge and skills, so it is not expected that all nurses will participate in the same ways (Estabrooks, 1997). However, it is possible for all nurses to participate to some extent. For example, nurses from a 42-bed rural hospital in the United States have had an international impact on research utilization through the activities of their research committee and the production of an award-winning videotape on the topic (Horn Video Productions, 1987).

Understanding the value of research is the responsibility of all nurses. Fostering research and its use is the responsibility of all nursing leaders.

MODELS OF NURSING RESEARCH UTILIZATION

There are several models, or frameworks, for the steps needed to use research findings in nursing practice. In their project, the Conduct and Utilization of Research in Nursing (CURN), Horsley and her associates teamed researchers and clinicians, who worked together to critique research reports of tested interventions addressing relevant clinical problems (Horsley, Crane, Crabtree, & Wood, 1983). The findings from the research were transformed into a clinical plan that could be readily understood and implemented. The teams also developed a procedure to test the intervention on a small scale. This process was used in decision making about breastfeeding information in postpartum care (Ashcroft & Kristjanson, 1994).

Information about breast-feeding had been identified by staff nurses as a priority issue, and findings from research literature were used to design an instructional booklet for nurses.

Another process, developed by Stetler and Marram from a clinical perspective, was refined in 1994 (Stetler, 1994). It includes six phases: identification of the problem and preparation, validation of the findings, comparative evaluation, decision-making, translation/application, and evaluation. One advantage of this model is that it allows for cognitive application of findings from descriptive studies. For example, a qualitative study on the impact of cancer pain on the family (Ferrell, Rhiner, Cohen, & Grant, 1991) provides a vivid description of families' perspectives of living with a family member with pain. Nurses can relate the experiences of families in the study to those of clients with whom they work, thereby using a richer knowledge base in their own practice. This is a cognitive application of research findings.

The Stetler/Marram model also identifies symbolic use of research findings, an application that can be extremely useful for nurse managers. This refers to the use of data from the literature or scientific projects for building and supporting an argument. For instance, if a nurse manager has knowledge of the criteria for ideal computerized data management for nursing decisions, grounds for specific computer needs can be stronger.

In 1991, the Registered Nurses Association of British Columbia (RNABC) launched a province-wide program to help nurses understand and use research findings in their practice. The RNABC framework is similar to the Stetler/Marram model, but it also provides direction for decision-makers about when to abandon or continue a project (RNABC, 1991).

Research utilization may progress through several phases. One group of nurses in an immunodeficiency clinic had been using knowledge of social support research cognitively. The nurses knew that people with HIV infection have complex social support networks that influence their ability to cope with their illness. To introduce a more systematic measure of social support to track changes over time, they adapted a sociogram (Maxwell, 1982) and a social support measure (Norbeck, Lindsey, & Carrieri, 1983) for their own clinical use. Clients reported that the measurement process itself helped them become more aware of their resources. The nurses completed a pilot study to test the effects of the measurement process, and are now planning an experimental study. These nurses work in an environment that promotes research activities.

DEPARTMENTAL STRATEGIES TO PROMOTE RESEARCH ACTIVITIES

The paramount requirement for the successful development of evidence-based practice within a department of nursing is a spirit of inquiry and openness to change. Without willingness to question and to challenge rituals and traditions, clinical agencies will not develop practice with a sound scientific base (Walsh & Ford, 1989). In 1992, van Koot and Laverty reported on the process of building policies and procedures on research. Creating a research climate is a key responsibility of the nurse executives (Simms, Price, & Pfoutz, 1987).

The working environment is a major factor supporting or obstructing evidence-based practice. Barriers to research utilization are found in four categories: the setting, the nurse, the research, and the presentation (Funk, Champagne, Wiese, & Tornquist, 1991a) (see Table 17.1). In an American study, Funk and her colleagues (1991b) found that eight of the ten most frequently reported barriers were related to the setting.

Overcoming these barriers requires a commitment to encourage and support nurses' pursuit of questions. This commitment is shown, first of all, in the philosophy and policies of the agency and the nursing department, then in the substantive support of an infrastructure for research, and also in staff development.

AN INFRASTRUCTURE FOR RESEARCH

The infrastructure for research in clinical agencies will depend on resources as well as on philosophy, and can vary from a nursing research committee to a full department. Resources include an administrative structure that fosters research, personnel with research training, access to literature, time, support staff, space, and equipment.

A committee structure is an essential component. Stimulation of ideas and mutual support from a group process is advantageous and, because many different research activities are involved, the workload can then be shared. A nursing research committee can review literature and disseminate findings, facilitate research utilization, provide information about research activities and resources, develop a research agenda, and review proposals for research (Vessey & Campos, 1992). Depending on the size and clinical scope of an agency, research may be best advanced by an agency-wide committee (Henderson & Brouse, 1992), unit-based committees (Hoare & Earenfight, 1986), or thematic interest groups, such as a pain management group (Belair, 1992).

Nurses with research training are those prepared at the graduate level. They may be full-time staff, part-time staff, or available only on consultation. Two positions that have been shown to be effective are the clinical nurse researcher, who is usually prepared at the doctoral level, and the clinical nurse specialist, who has master's preparation. The clinical nurse researcher may conduct research, foster a research climate, provide consultation to nursing staff on research projects, advise administrators on research-based decisions, review research proposals, and co-ordinate a research program. The title and responsibilities vary, but the ability to develop the role and relate to staff nurses and clinical issues is crucial (Knafl, Hagle, Bevis, & Kirchhoff, 1987).

The clinical nurse specialist, whose role is usually directly related to patient care, also contributes to research (Fitch, 1992; Utz & Gleit, 1995). The clinical nurse specialist may conduct research, particularly in team projects,

Table 17.1

BARRIERS TO RESEARCH UTILIZATION, RANKED AND SHOWING TYPE OF BARRIER

Rank Order	Barrier	Type of Barrier
1	The nurse does not feel she/he has enough authority to change patient-care procedures.	Setting
2	There is insufficient time on the job to implement new ideas.	Setting
3	The nurse is unaware of the research.	Nurse
4	Physicians will not co-operate with implementation.	Setting
5	Administration will not allow implementation.	Setting
6	Other staff are not supportive of implementation.	Setting
7	The nurse feels results are not generalizable to own setting.	Setting
8	The facilities are inadequate for implementation.	Setting
9	Statistical analyses are not understandable.	Present*
10	The nurse does not have time to read research.	Setting
11	The nurse is isolated from knowledgeable colleagues with whom to discuss the research.	Nurse
12	The relevant literature is not compiled in one place.	Present
13	Implications for practice are not made clear.	Present
14	The nurse does not feel capable of evaluating the quality of the research.	Nurse
15	Research reports/articles are not readily available.	Present
16	The research has not been replicated.	Research
17	The research is not reported clearly and readably.	Present
18	The research is not relevant to the nurse's practice.	Present
19	The nurse feels the benefits of changing practice will be minimal.	Nurse
20	The nurse sees little benefit for self.	Nurse
21	The nurse is uncertain whether to believe the results of the research.	Research
22	The nurse is unwilling to change/try new ideas.	Nurse
23	The literature reports conflicting results.	Research
24	The research has methodological inadequacies.	Research
25	There is not a documented need to change practice.	Nurse
26	The nurse does not see the value of research for practice.	Nurse
27	Research reports/articles are not published fast enough.	Research
28	The conclusions drawn from the research are not justified.	Research

Present = Presentation

Source: Adapted from Sandra G. Funk, Mary T. Champagne, Ruth A. Wiese and Elizabeth M. Tornquist, "Barriers to Using Research Findings in Practice: The Clinician's Perspective," *Applied Nursing Research, 4*(2), p. 92, by permission.

identify researchable clinical questions, interpret research findings for application in practice, and implement research-based innovations.

If it is not feasible to find agency staff with research training, arrangements can be made with consultants from academic settings or other agencies. Consultants with particular expertise may be sought for specific projects, or a consultant may meet with staff regularly to discuss a variety of clinical questions (Goode, Lovett, Hayes, & Butcher, 1987).

Access to literature may also depend on outside resources, and arrangements with inter-library loan systems may be needed. Other aspects of seeking literature are discussed in relation to the role of the nurse manager, but time to seek consultation or use library resources is essential in any agency with a commitment to evidence-based practice.

Other structural resources such as space, support staff, and equipment demonstrate the commitment of the department of nursing (Fitch, 1992; Pepler, 1988). These not only provide tangible evidence of support, but can greatly enhance the productivity of researchers.

DEMYSTIFYING RESEARCH

Research activities are often perceived by nurses as "something that somebody else does." The idea of research involvement may be threatening for nurses without background preparation, and staff development programs for nurses at all levels will help to demystify research. Whether nurses have had an introductory course in a baccalaureate program or not, knowledge and skills in using research concepts in practice need to be developed.

The nursing department may facilitate nurses' participation in courses outside the agency, or programs may be offered within the department. A series of workshops for different groups of nurses may be expedient for introducing staff to ideas and strategies. It is appropriate to start with managers and senior nurses who will be leaders in an agency-wide program. A course, rather than a workshop, has the advantage of allowing nurses to use the new knowledge over time in their practice between sessions (Pepler, 1992).

Involvement of nursing staff in research activities is a powerful learning process as well (Fitch & Thompson, 1996; Parker, Gordon, & Brannon, 1992). Links with schools of nursing provide an opportunity for students and staff alike to raise relevant questions and gain practical experience in integrating research and practice (Janken, Dufault, & Yeaw, 1988).

THE NURSE MANAGER AS FACILITATOR OF RESEARCH ACTIVITIES

A spirit of inquiry within the nursing department and the structural components of a research commitment will support the nurse manager in efforts to develop research-mindedness in the staff. The manager at the unit level still has a key role in helping staff raise questions, find answers, participate in research, conduct studies, and use findings in practice.

RAISING QUESTIONS

The nurse manager is the pivotal person in creating an environment open to questions. The questions may arise from any source: staff nurses, other nurse managers, senior nursing administrators, or members of other disciplines. The progress from "I wonder if ...." or "How come ...?" to research activities and improved practice can be determined by the initial response of front-line managers. Productive responses come from managers who are at ease with not knowing. Otherwise, the initial response may be "We tried that before," or "We can't because ...." The manager who is secure without an answer will be comfortable in facilitating a search for one.

To find an answer, it is essential to clarify the question. The first question raised is often either vague or too specific. Through clarification, the nurse manager not only can show support, but also can help find an answer by either focussing or expanding the question. For instance, if the question is related to one patient, it may be useful to identify broader characteristics or commonalties across several patients to develop a meaningful question with greater relevancy. If a question is vague or ambiguous, it will be helpful to clarify specific circumstances or particular variables that are of interest.

FINDING VALID ANSWERS

In any research process, the first activity is searching the literature. This takes time. Nurse managers can facilitate the process by providing time to go to accessible libraries and read or bring material to the unit.

Computer searching is a relatively simple process, readily learned, and invaluable in providing a comprehensive search and saving time. It also promotes browsing and stimulates curiosity. On-line searching from the nursing unit is possible in many hospitals. Librarians may be able to send tables of contents from relevant journals to the units, so staff can browse more readily for articles. It is helpful to encourage subscriptions to journals on the unit. While access to a few journals is not sufficient for a comprehensive review, it is useful for keeping up-to-date. The staff might be willing to share a subscription, costs could be negotiated with the administrator, or gifts could be directed toward subscriptions.

Nurse managers can encourage staff to read research reports and think about the value and usability of findings. It is best when reading is triggered by genuine interest in the topic, and it is most effective when a series of articles on the same topic are discussed over time. The issue can be explored in depth, and the similarities and differences in research methods and findings can be examined. A review article is a good beginning because it will give an overall critique and a comprehensive reference list (cf. Atkins, 1991, on children's coping; Clement & Buck, 1996, on weaning from mechanical ventilatory support; Danner, Beck, Heacock, & Modlin, 1993, on working with cognitively impaired elders; Krapohl, 1995, on visiting hours in intensive care units).

In the nursing research literature, there are three broad categories of research reports: descriptive studies of clinical phenomena, client characteristics, or clinical problems; tests of measures or instruments; and experimental studies of nursing interventions. Those in the first category increase the reader's knowledge base and can be extremely useful in working with patients and families in similar circumstances, but these studies do not give directions for care. Those in the second category can be used by clinicians to measure clinical phenomena more accurately. The third category includes reports of interventions which, if found to be effective, can be implemented.

Each research report must be critiqued to determine the potential usability of the information. Nurse managers can help staff read critically by encouraging participation in courses and staff-development programs, and by providing opportunities for discussion with a nurse with a knowledge of research. This may be a staff nurse, the manager, a clinical nurse specialist, or a faculty member. A number of questions need to be asked:

- Is the purpose of the study clearly explained?
- Is other relevant research reviewed adequately?
- Is the study design suitable to answer the research question?
- Is the sample adequate in terms of size, and is it representative?
- Are variables clearly explained, if appropriate?
- Are data-collection methods and measures valid and reliable?
- Are analyses appropriate and sufficiently comprehensive?
- Are findings reported clearly?
- Are findings discussed in relation to the theory and other research?
- Are conclusions and implications for practice derived from valid findings?

All of these questions are important, but the last is critical. It is sometimes problematic for clinicians because the author may make a quantum leap from tentative findings to recommendations for practice. Some knowledge of research terminology, design, and methods is needed.

The nurse manager needs to be supportive and creative when immediate answers are not found. In some situations, the search may be redirected. For example, there is limited literature on family involvement in the care of hospitalized elders, but two related areas from which knowledge can be gained are quite well developed: literature on family involvement in nursing homes, and family participation in the care of hospitalized children. Other times the nurse manager may support the staff in seeking help to conduct a study to find an answer to their question.

PARTICIPATING IN RESEARCH

Answers generated through unit-based research are meaningful to informed nursing staff and usually relevant to their practice. Nurses may help to plan a project, such as discussing the question, methods, and feasibility with a researcher at an early stage. Having input to research design increases nurses' sense of involvement and commitment to the project.

Nurses' participation in an on-going study could include: 1. identifying potential subjects through a designated screening process, 2. asking patients if they are willing to speak to a researcher, 3. carrying out an intervention according to a protocol, 4. obtaining data (such as recording observations or collecting specimens), or 5. participating as a subject.

Nurse managers have many responsibilities related to the unit involvement in research conducted by nurses and other disciplines (see Box 17.1). These include both facilitating participation and limiting involvement as necessary. Both require a high level of awareness of potential projects, a clear understanding of the meaning and ramifications of involvement, and skill in facilitating approved projects. The nurse manager should be knowledgeable about all proposed research, regardless of the researcher's discipline and, if nurses are likely to be involved, the manager should review research projects in detail before they begin. Special responsibilities regarding patients' and staff rights are discussed later.

CONDUCTING A STUDY

Nurses who are planning to conduct a study need the nurse manager's input and support. Research projects conducted by a single individual are rare, so teams and consultation should be encouraged. Few staff nurses have research preparation, but many projects are manageable within normal nursing practice, with consultation and shared workload (Youngkins, 1991).

The nurse manager is a key person to respond to nurses' ideas for projects. It is important to be supportive—but realistic about the demands of research. If the nurse manager does not have the experience or expertise, nurses can be referred to a consultant.

The details of conducting research are beyond the scope of this chapter, but can be found in appropriate textbooks. Similar steps may be used in the process of testing findings from previous studies on a small scale on one unit. This is one stage in the process of using research findings in practice.

USING RESEARCH FINDINGS IN PRACTICE

Although every nurse can be involved in using research findings in practice, it is unrealistic to expect all nurses to lead the way. This is an important component of the nurse manager's role, with support from the nursing department and from prepared staff, such as a clinical nurse specialist or senior staff nurse.

The first step to using research findings is a thorough critique of the research reports to determine the validity of the findings, as outlined above. The next phase, which Stetler (1994) identifies as comparative evaluation, is a careful comparison between the situation reported in the research and

Box 17.1

NURSE MANAGERS' RESPONSIBILITIES RELATED TO UNIT INVOLVEMENT IN PROJECTS CONDUCTED BY OUTSIDE RESEARCHERS

- Identify opportunities for involvement.
- Review proposals for feasibility, including:
    Potential for access to subjects (patients, family, staff)
    On-going projects
    Nursing skills
    Nursing time
    Study time frame and unit activities
- Arrange information sessions for researcher and staff.
- Ensure that staff on all shifts are aware of project.
- Facilitate training sessions for staff if applicable.
- Collaborate with researcher regarding procedures.
- Facilitate access to resources if applicable, e.g., space, records.
- Maintain regular contact with researcher for mutual updates
- Keep staff informed of study progress.
- Arrange for session for researcher to report findings to staff .
- Encourage staff to attend other presentations and read publications on the project.

the particular clinical situation of the reader. At this point, clinical expertise is essential, as is a sound knowledge of the clinical situation. The nurse manager may be the best person to help staff nurses make this assessment. Again, a series of questions is useful to consider:

- What are the similarities and differences between the problem identified in the study and the situation in the unit?
- What are the similarities and differences between the setting in the study and the setting in question?
- What are the similarities and differences between the people (patients, family members, staff) studied and those in the unit?
- How does a possible innovation fit with the philosophy and policies in the agency?
- How feasible is it to carry out the innovation on the unit?
- How feasible is it to use the same measurement techniques to assess the effectiveness of the innovation? If identical measures are not feasible, what alternatives are there?

In the decision-making phase, the nurse manager can help staff decide whether to use the findings cognitively or whether to take action based on the findings (MacGuire, 1990). Even cognitive application does not happen automatically. Suppose a researcher reports on the experience of specific problems or factors related to the well-being of a particular population—for instance, long-term survivors of AIDS (Barroso, 1997), psychiatric patients

(Holdcraft & Williamson, 1991), women whose family members have breast cancer (Chalmers & Thomson, 1996), postpartum mothers (Carty, Bradley & Winslow, 1996), or mothers of hospitalized children (Schepp, 1991). The nurse manager can arrange for a discussion of how the findings relate to the population in the setting and how the new knowledge might influence care.

If action is to be taken, the nurse manager may use the new information as evidence of the need for change. Many groups may resist change (see also Chapter 23) and the stronger the evidence, the more effective the argument. The research findings may prompt the nurse manager and staff to evaluate their own situation. Are they collecting enough information about clients to determine a need for change? What are the actual outcomes of current practice? What are the costs—human and financial—of current practice?

The final decision is whether to use an innovation as a model for a change in practice. It is useful to plan a trial period with a comparison before and after or a control group for whom the innovation is not used. One effective way to conduct a trial is to replicate the original study as closely as possible. Several sources provide clear information on this process (Horsley et al., 1983; Haller, Reynolds, & Horsley, 1979). Also, the original researcher can be consulted.

Once the new information has been in use for a period of time an evaluation of the impact is essential. Assessment of change may be part of a regular review of nursing care or may be specific to the innovation. It is, therefore, important to have accurate data about the situation prior to the change.

PROTECTING PATIENT AND STAFF RIGHTS IN RELATION TO RESEARCH

A nurse manager has a responsibility to protect patient and staff rights in relation to any research. The first step, when the possibility of a research project is known, is to assure that the project has been approved by an appropriate research ethical review board. This is essential, regardless of the researcher's discipline or institutional affiliation. A staff physician, a nurse from a graduate program, a university professor, or a psychologist from a community agency all need approval for research projects. In teaching agencies, there is likely an established procedure, but in any agency the nurse manager is often the first contact researchers make. It is imperative that approval be verified. A nursing administrator or nurse researcher should sit on the review board.

It is also important that nurse managers have an understanding of the research protocol, purpose, procedures, and involvement of patients. If it is medical research or a project that does not involve nursing, the manager may still be called upon to answer questions or refer patients or family members to the researcher. The manager may be the only person who knows what other projects are in process. Patients or staff may need to be protected from "research overload." It may simply be an issue of timing. Data for one study may be collected at one time, and those for another at a different time of the day or day of the week. This may not make a difference to the research, but it can make a big difference to the running of the unit.

If the manager or nursing staff are involved in a screening process for research subjects, the researcher should plan this in advance with the manager. Any screening that is not built into the project can seriously jeopardize the validity of the results.

Nurse managers also need to be involved in the approval process if the study includes any nursing staff participation. Nurses need to be informed participants. They need to know why the study is being done, why specific data are being collected, what the risks and benefits are for patients, and so on. Managers may be doing a balancing act between encouraging and facilitating research on one hand and limiting access to patients or staff on the other.

ECONOMICS OF RESEARCH

As with any other aspect of nursing, there are costs and benefits to nursing research. Knowledge of these economics in general, and in relation to particular studies, will help nurse managers in their research role.

An important distinction needs to be made between research and quality-management activities. Nurse managers are responsible for the quality of care in their jurisdictions, and quality management is addressed elsewhere in this text (see Chapter 19). The activities of identifying problems, collecting data, testing solutions, and analyzing results may be similar, and the long-term goal of both activities is improved nursing practice. However, the purpose of research is to add to the knowledge base, rather than to promote a high quality of care in a specific area. Thurston and Best (1990) discuss methods for integration of the two programs to improve nursing care.

COSTS OF DOING RESEARCH

Nurse managers need to be aware of the indirect costs of participating in research, whether nurses or researchers in other disciplines are conducting the study. Cronenwett (1987) suggests asking several questions related to space, changes in nursing practice, staff involvement and time, patient time, numbers of study patients at one time, and supplies or other costs. Many of these costs should be built into the grant budget.

The primary costs for nursing research involve personnel. In general, nurses do not use expensive equipment or procedures, but many nursing studies are labour-intensive. The same questions need to be considered, whether the study is a large funded project or a small in-house study by nursing staff. It is essential to have time for planning, for data collection, for data analysis, and for writing the report. Pringle (1989) noted that one of the realities of research is that it is a long-term process. Benefits make the costs worthwhile, but it is also well worthwhile to consider outside funding for research.

FUNDING RESOURCES

Obtaining funding is a challenge in this time of restraint and limited resources available for nursing research. However, a truism also pertains: Nurses will not get funding if they do not apply. Federal and provincial government agencies fund research, as do non-governmental organizations, such as the Canadian Heart Foundation or The Arthritis Society. The Canadian Nurses Foundation and some provincial nursing associations have funds for small projects. The Canadian Nurses Association regularly publishes a list of resources for research funding.

Although seeking funds adds to the overall time for research, having deadlines for submission can provide a major stimulus to planning. For nurses unfamiliar with the process, it is essential to get a knowledgeable consultant involved, as grant applications are highly competitive.

ECONOMIC BENEFITS OF NURSING RESEARCH

As health-care costs soar and resources diminish, nursing research has demonstrated that it can make a difference. In broad-based studies of delivery systems, nursing care has been found to offer better care at less cost (Fagin, 1990). Fagin pointed out that nursing programs such as long-term or hospital follow-up home care have been successful in reducing costs "*if they have served as an alternative to other types of care*" (p. 29).

At a more specific level, studies of nursing interventions have shown how costs can be reduced. For example, a program with advanced nurse clinicians in a respiratory intensive care unit reduced ventilator days and chest X-rays in relation to a comparison unit, thereby reducing costs despite new positions (Ahrens & Padwojski, 1990). Brooten and her colleagues (1986) demonstrated that an early-discharge program for very-low-birth-weight infants with counselling and home care by a hospital-based nurse specialist yielded a net saving of US$18,560 per infant. A clinical nurse specialist program for elderly cardiac patients in an acute care setting was effective in reducing the number of readmissions and total days during readmission for patients from the medical units, but not those from the surgical units (Naylor et al., 1994). An analysis of seventeen studies of the use of a saline flush rather than heparin for peripheral intravenous locks showed that saline was safe and could produce annual savings of over US$100,000,000 in American health-care costs (Goode et al., 1991). One team in critical care encourages all staff to identify clinical questions for which the group does a clinical/cost kinetics analysis (White, Bartrug, & Bride, 1995).

It is important for nursing researchers to consider the benefits in patient outcomes in terms of both better health and reduced health-care costs, and it is important for nursing leaders to take advantage of sound research to improve care at a lower cost.

SUMMARY

This chapter focuses on evidence-based nursing practice and the role of nurse managers in developing it.

- Four interdependent components needed for evidence-based nursing practice are meaningful research questions that are relevant to practice; sound research to answer the questions; knowledgeable nurses with skills in using research findings; and clinical environments open to inquiry and change.
- Research activities include the conduct of research, the use of other researchers' findings, and the use of rigorous research techniques in daily practice.
- All nurses can participate in some of these activities with the help of their leaders.
- The working environment constitutes one of the major barriers to the use of research findings and the nurse manager is the key person in creating a climate of openness and inquiry.
- The nursing department can provide structural supports and continuing education to facilitate research-based practice.
- Nurse managers can help staff directly to raise questions, find answers, participate in research, conduct studies and use findings in practice.
- There are costs involved in conducting and participating in research, but benefits for patients and health-care costs are significant. Nurse managers have a particular responsibility to develop nursing practice in their areas that is based on sound economics and sound evidence.

FURTHER READINGS AND RESOURCES

Davies, B., & Logan, J. (1993). *Reading research: A user-friendly guide for nurses and other health professionals.* Ottawa: Canadian Nurses Association. This 22-page pamphlet is a general guide for staff nurses to help them read and understand research literature. It would be a useful guide for nurse managers to have on hand as a reference for staff.

Howell, S. L., Foster, R.L., Hester, N. O., Vojir, C. P., & Miller, K. L. (1996). Evaluating a pediatric pain management research utilization program. *Canadian Journal of Nursing Research, 28*(2) 37-57. This article is a report of how nurses in a teaching hospital developed an educational program for pediatric nurses on state-of-the-art children's pain assessment and management.

Program educators delivered awareness knowledge and "how to" knowledge in five 30-minute classes. The classes were videotaped for nurses who were unable to attend. A Pain Experience History, Pain Observation Scale, and Pain Flow Sheet were developed that incorporated: the child's experience with pain; behavioural assessment; assessment date and time; child and/or parent pain ratings; and nurse's judgement of pain intensity and interventions, including non-pharmacological strategies. Multiple data sources were used to evaluate the outcome and highlight elements of change that were important to the success of the program. Nurses reported that the assessment aids and distraction material for non-pharmacological interventions were the most useful. Six months later, nurses were using the assessment tools more than they had during the three months immediately following the program.

REFERENCES

Ahrens, T. S., & Padwojski, A. (1990). Economic effectiveness of an advanced nurse clinician model. *Nursing Management*, 21(11 Critical Care Management Ed.), 72J, 72N, 72P.

Ashcroft, T., & Kristjanson, L. J. (1994). Research utilization in maternal-child nursing: Application of the CURN model. *Canadian Journal of Nursing Administration*, 7(5), 90–101.

Atkins, F. D. (1991). Children's perspectives of stress and coping: An integrative review. *Issues of Mental Health Nursing*, 12(2), 171–178.

Barroso, J. (1997). Restructuring my life: Becoming a long-term survivor of AIDS. *Qualitative Health Research*,7(1), 57–74.

Belair, J. (1992). Pain management interest group. *Nursing Horizons*, 10(2), 12.

Brooten, D., Kumar, S., Brown, L. P., Butts, P., Finkler, S. A., Bakewell-Sachs, S., Gibbons, A., & Delivoria-Papadopoulos, M. (1986). A randomized clinical trial of early hospital discharge and home follow-up of very-low-birth-weight infants. *New England Journal of Medicine*, 315(15), 934–939.

Canadian Nurses Association. (1990). *Research imperative for nursing in Canada: The next five years 1990–1995*. Ottawa: Canadian Nurses Association.

Carty, E. M., Bradley, C., & Winslow, W. (1996). Women's perceptions of fatigue during pregnancy and postpartum: The impact of length of hospital stay. *Clinical Nursing Research*, 5(1), 67–80.

Chalmers, K., & Thomson, K. (1996). Coming to terms with the risk of breast cancer: Perceptions of women with primary relatives with breast cancer. *Qualitative Health Research*, 6(2), 256–282.

Clement, J. M., & Buck, E. A. (1996). Weaning from mechanical ventilatory support. *Dimensions of Critical Care Nursing*, 15(3), 114–129.

Crane, J. (1989). *Factors associated with the use of research-based knowledge in nursing*. Doctoral dissertation, University of Michigan, Ann Arbor, MI: University Microfilms International.

Cronenwett, L. R. (1987). The indirect costs of nursing research. *Journal of Nursing Administration*, 17(9), 6–8.

Danner, C., Beck, C., Heacock, P., & Modlin, T. (1993). Cognitively impaired elders: Using research findings to improve nursing care. *Journal of Gerontological Nursing*, 19(4), 5–11.

Estabrooks, C. A. (1997). Research utilization in nursing: An examination of formal structure and influencing factors. Unpublished doctoral dissertation. University of Alberta.

Fagin, C. M. (1990). Nursing's value proves itself. *American Journal of Nursing, 90*(10), 17–30.

Ferrell, B. R., Rhiner, M., Cohen, M. Z., & Grant, M. (1991). Pain as a metaphor for illness, Part 1: Impact of cancer pain on family caregivers. *Oncology Nursing Forum, 18*(8), 1303–1309.

Fitch, M. I. (1992). Five years in the life of a nursing research and professional development division. *Canadian Journal of Nursing Administration, 5*(1), 21–27.

Fitch, M. I., & Thompson, L. (1996). Fostering the growth of research-based oncology nursing practice. *Oncology Nursing Forum, 23*(4), 631–637.

Funk, S. G., Champagne, M. T., Wiese, R. A., & Tornquist, E. M. (1991a). BARRIERS: The barriers to research utilization scale. *Applied Nursing Research, 4*(1), 39–45.

Funk, S. G., Champagne, M. T., Wiese, R. A., & Tornquist, E. M. (1991b). Barriers to using findings in practice: The clinician's perspective. *Applied Nursing Research, 4*(2), 90–95.

Goode, C. J., Lovett, M. K., Hayes, J. E., & Butcher, A. L. (1987). Use of research based knowledge in clinical practice. *Journal of Nursing Administration, 17*(12), 11–18.

Goode, C. J., Titler, M., Rakel, B, Ones, D. S., Kleiber, C., Small, S., & Triolo, P. K. (1991). A meta-analysis of effects of heparin flush and saline flush: Quality and cost implications. *Nursing Research, 40*(6), 324–330.

Haller, K. B., Reynolds, M. A., & Horsley, J. A. (1979). Developing research-based innovation protocols: Process, criteria, and issues. *Research in Nursing & Health, 2,* 45–51.

Henderson, A., & Brouse, J. (1992). Development of a research committee in a community hospital. *Canadian Journal of Nursing Research, 5*(2), 17–19.

Hoare, K., & Earenfight, J. (1986). Unit-based research in a service setting. *Journal of Nursing Administration, 16*(4), 35–39.

Holdcraft, C., & Williamson, C. (1991). Assessment of hope in psychiatric and chemically dependent patients. *Applied Nursing Research, 4*(3), 129–134.

Horn Video Productions. (1987). *Using research in clinical nursing practice.* Ida Grove, IA: Horn Video Productions.

Horsley, J. A. (1985). Using research in practice: The current context. *Western Journal of Nursing Research, 7*(1), 135–139.

Horsley, J. A., Crane, J., Crabtree, K., & Wood, D. J. (1983). *Using research to improve nursing practice: A guide.* New York: Grune & Stratton.

Janken, J. K., Dufault, M. A., & Yeaw, E. M. S. (1988). Research round tables: Increasing student/staff nurse awareness of the relevancy of research to practice. *Journal of Professional Nursing, 4*(3), 186–191.

Knafl, K. A., Hagle, M., Bevis, M., & Kirchhoff, K. (1987). Clinical nurse researchers: Strategies for success. *Journal of Nursing Administration, 17*(10), 27–31.

Krapohl, G. L. (1995). Visiting hours in the adult intensive care unit: Using research to develop a system that works. *Dimensions of Critical Care Nursing, 14*(5), 245–258.

MacGuire, J. M. (1990). Putting nursing research findings into practice: Research utilization as an aspect of the management of change. *Journal of Advanced Nursing, 15*(5), 614–620.

Maxwell, M. B. (1982). The use of social networks to help cancer patients maximize support. *Cancer Nursing, 5*(8), 275–281.

National Forum on Health. (1997). Canada health action: Building the legacy. Synthesis reports and papers. Creating a culture of evidence-based decision-making. Ottawa: Health Canada.

Naylor, M., Brooten, D., Jones, R., Lavizzo-Mourey, R., Mezey, M., & Pauly, M. (1994). Comprehensive discharge planning for the hospitalized elderly. *Annals of Internal Medicine,120*(12), 999–1006.

Nightingale, F. (1859). Notes on nursing: What it is and what it is not. London: Harrison.

Norbeck, J. S., Lindsey, A. M., & Carrieri, V. L. (1983). Further development of the Norbeck social support questionnaire: Normative data and validity testing. *Nursing Research, 32,* 4–9

Parker, M. E., Gordon, S. C., & Brannon, P. T. (1992). Involving nursing staff in research: A non-traditional approach. *Journal of Nursing Administration, 22*(4), 58–63.

Pepler, C. J. (1988). The nurse researcher in the clinical setting. In L. Besel & R. Stock, (Eds.), *Benchmarks: A Sourcebook for Canadian Nursing Management.* Toronto: Carswell.

Pepler, C. J. (1992). Fostering change through education. *Canadian Nurse, 88*(1), 25–27.

Pringle, D. (1989). Another twist on the double helix: Research and practice. *Canadian Journal of Nursing Research, 21*(1), 47–60.

Registered Nurses Association of British Columbia. (1991). *Making a difference: From ritual to research-based practice.* Vancouver: RNABC.

Schepp, K. G. (1991). Factors influencing the coping effort of mothers of hospitalized children. *Nursing Research, 40*(1), 42–46, 1991.

Simms, L. M., Price, S. A., & Pfoutz, S. K. (1987). Creating the research climate: A key responsibility for nurse executives. *Nursing Economics, 5*(4), 174–179.

Stetler, C. H. (1994). Refinement of the Stetler/Marram model for application of research findings to practice. *Nursing Outlook, 42*(1), 15–25.

Thurston, N., & Best, M. (1990). Clinical nursing research and quality assurance: Integration for improved patient care. *Canadian Journal of Nursing Administration, 3*(2), 19–23.

Utz, S. W., & Gleit, C. J. (1995). Current developments in research-based interventions: Enhancing and advancing the CNS role. *Clinical Nurse Specialist, 9*(1), 8–11.

van Koot, B., & Laverty, P. (1992). A research foundation for policies and procedures. *Canadian Nurse, 88*(1), 39–41.

Vessey, J. A., & Campos, R. G. (1992). The role of nursing research committees. *Nursing Research, 41*(4), 247–249.

Walsh, M., & Ford, P. (1989). *Nursing rituals: Research and rational action.* Oxford: Heinemann Professional Publishing.

White, S. K., Bartrug, B., & Bride, W. (1995). Supporting nursing innovations in a cost-conscious environment. *Critical Care Nursing Clinics of North America, 7*(2), 399–406.

Youngkins, J. M. (1991). The impact of one staff nurse's research. *MCN, 16,* 133–137.

CASE STUDY

Betty Thorston and Lou Brownlee, registered nurses on a long-term care unit, had frequently discussed the problems associated with assessing pain levels in elderly patients. Other colleagues and staff on the unit had also commented on the difficulties associated with this when a patient approached and asked "Is it time yet for my pain pill?" They took their idea for research to Jordan Maxwell, the nurse manager of their unit, which was part of a large, urban teaching hospital. If you were Jordan:

1. How would you go about assessing whether this was a suitable project for research, and at what level?
2. What steps would you take if you and your nursing staff thought that the topic warranted further investigation?

Chapter 18

▼▼▼▼▼▼▼▼▼▼▼▼▼▼▼▼▼▼▼

Ethical Dimensions of Leadership

JANET L. STORCH

KEY OBJECTIVES

In this chapter, you will learn:

- Common ethical problems of first-level managers.
- The scope of ethical responsibilities in health-care management.
- Common ethical theories and principles applied to health care.
- Recent theoretical thinking in ethics applied to management.
- Ways in which first-level managers can build a moral community.

INTRODUCTION

Increased recognition of the leadership role of first-level managers and the return to greater consideration of everyday ethics in health care, along with the more global issues of biomedical ethics, have paved the way for a broader appreciation of ethics as both a managerial responsibility and as a leadership imperative. There is little doubt that the excursion into moral philosophy and biomedical ethics which began in the 1960s (Pellegrino, 1993) has contributed significantly to enhanced understanding about ethics in health care. Yet, in that process, common understanding of ethical comportment and ethical obligations in relationships between health professionals and their patients/clients, health professionals and their communities, and leaders/managers and health professionals have received uneven and often limited attention.

The purpose of this chapter is to encourage reflection about the ethical dimensions of leading and managing. Although the chapter is geared towards first-level nurse managers, the considerations included are common to non-nursing first-line managers as well. The chapter includes examples of management problems which involve tough moral choices, and require sound ethical decision-making. Principles and theories as approaches to ethical reasoning are reviewed, and their relevance to ethical decision-making in management is elaborated. The chapter concludes with a discussion of ways in which first-level managers can support and reinforce values-based practice.

LEADERSHIP AND ETHICS

Theories of management and leadership have tended to focus on managing people through direction and control. This is true from the classical bureaucratic theories (including time and motion studies) to theories that recognize the human factor in management—including those supporting the notion that leadership in management is contingent upon setting (see Chapter 5). The concept of transformational leadership draws our attention to the reality that people, and particularly health-care professionals, cannot be managed—but they can be led. Transformational leadership is leadership that appeals to higher ideals and moral values, such as humanitarianism, liberty, equality, and justice. It is leadership that commits people to action.

The concept of transformational leadership highlights the manager as a leader who motivates the group of workers by integrating personal and organizational values in such a way as to influence commitment, rather than attempting to motivate through direction and control (Marriner-Tomey, 1993). This requires us to examine the nature and potential of management from entirely new perspectives. It means that almost every action by a manager involves ethical considerations, because attempting to influence the commitment of others means placing one's values squarely before them. It follows that if first-level managers in health care are expected to convey values and influence nurses and other health-care professionals to commit to those values, those managers will require a broadened perspective on the meanings of, and the requirements for, ethical leadership.

Being an ethical leader requires at least three foci of being and doing (Mitchell, 1996). The first is *to be a person of moral character;* the second is *to demonstrate moral behaviour* (i.e. engaging in appropriate moral behaviour and role-modeling moral behaviour); the third is to work *to establish a moral community.* This requires that the leader ask the question, "What am I to do?" and "Why would I choose this course of action over another"? and "How can I enable my staff to be committed to 'right' action?"

ETHICAL PROBLEMS OF THE FIRST-LEVEL MANAGER

The types of ethical problems confronting health-care professionals and their managers fall into three main categories. The first category includes violations of understood ethical commitments—including those stated in codes of ethics or in other sets of rules and guidelines governing ethics, and those generally understood as societal laws or ethical norms. In this category, there is little doubt about the action that should or should not be taken, because a decision to do otherwise would be a 'wrong' choice.

The second type of ethical problem is a dilemma in which a difficult choice must be made between competitive and equally compelling arguments for opposing positions and actions. The third type of ethical problem is one in which health professionals and their managers have little choice except to act, even though that action does not 'seem right,' because there are no better alternatives. This may involve a situation in which individuals are required to act against their sense of rightness because of a course of action has been decided by those in positions of greater authority. This latter type of ethical problem has been labeled a situation of moral distress and ethical distress (CNA, 1997).

Codes of ethics can provide guidance for appropriate actions in dealing with ethical violations. Codes serve as a shared reference point (Kidder, 1995) to clarify for professionals and the public the commitments they should expect. For example, the Canadian Nurses Association Code of Ethics for Registered Nurses (1997) includes seven statements of values with guidance for RNs in fulfilling their major responsibilities in each area. These include values of health and well-being, choice, dignity, confidentiality, fairness, accountability, and practice environments conducive to safe, competent, and ethical practice.

Moral action in situations of ethical dilemma and ethical distress defies easy prescription, as illustrated by the four case examples below. For these situations, some understanding of ethics is important. The cases involving nurse managers described in Box 18.1 will be used to illustrate how ethical theories and principles can be applied to the practice of moral management and ethical leadership.

The case examples shown in Box 18.1 raise the kinds of ethical problems that nurse managers may face at any time. How they deal with these situations depends upon their sensitivity to the fact that their decisions involve ethical choices, and upon their overall ability to deal with ethical issues. Rushforth Kidder (1995), an educational ethicist, emphasizes the importance of "ethical fitness." This seems an apt term to emphasize the importance of preparation for the ethical leadership role the nurse manager must provide.

BEING "ETHICALLY FIT"

To be "ethically fit" is to be mentally engaged in the human activity of ethical reflection and justification. Such fitness requires a certain degree of knowledge and skill in ethical problem-solving. It involves being and becoming a person of good moral character, engaging in ethical conduct, and building a moral community.

In the following section, an overview of the substance of these requirements is provided, with liberal use of references to take the nurse

Box 18.1
MANAGERIAL PROBLEMS INVOLVING ETHICS: FOUR CASE EXAMPLES

The Case of Mary Grace

Mary Grace had been a first-level nurse manager and clinical nurse specialist in gerontology for more than ten years. When the provincial government moved to full-scale regionalization of health services, several hospitals and other health agencies were amalgamated, and a new chief executive officer (CEO) was appointed with a mandate to restructure service delivery in the region. As part of the restructuring, the CEO moved all first-level nurse managers to different portfolios, emphasizing that she wanted their managerial expertise, not their clinical expertise. At the same time, she insisted that the main task of these nurse managers was to stay within budget by restricting admissions, and by planning systems for earlier discharge.

Mary Grace now serves as nurse manager of the cardiac care unit. Nurses on the unit have become increasingly distressed that patients are being discharged too early and without adequate provision for home care. They have begun to question Ms. Grace's leadership and her values, suggesting that her clinical competence (knowledge base) is inadequate for her role which, in their view, includes representing this problem to upper management based upon both sound clinical *and* managerial knowledge. Mary Grace has tried to interpret to her staff the region's fiscal constraints, and the need to preserve funds for future care as well as meeting present care demands. But she is troubled by her staff's conviction that current patients are suffering.

How can Mary Grace help her clients, her staff, and herself? To what degree does senior management face a moral problem in this situation?

The Case of Beth Wallace

Beth Wallace is nurse manager of an adult medical day-care unit that is currently operating as a demonstration project. Upon her return from a two-week vacation, she learns that due to a nursing medication error, a client's recovery has been delayed by approximately a week. Mrs. P., the client, will experience no long-term negative effects. Mrs. P. happens to be the wife of a local newsman who has been highly critical of the hospital's operation of the demonstration unit, alleging that it provides substandard care. Ms. Wallace has checked out all of the newsman's allegations and found them to be without substance. Further, a recent visit from the health agency's accrediting body has commended the unit's operation and its client outcomes.

Mrs. P. and her family have been informed that her setback was due to an unanticipated drug reaction, and Ms. Wallace is informed that they seem satisfied with that explanation. She knows that any adverse publicity for the unit could be damaging at this point. She thinks about the effects on present and future clients should further negative reporting by the newsman lead to closure of the unit. She also thinks about the fact that staff have not told Mrs. P. and her family the real reasons for her setback.

What should Beth Wallace do? Why? What responsibility does senior management have in this situation?

The Case of Diane Wong

Clarence Cook is a 41-year-old registered nurse who recently returned to nursing after a ten-year interim career in the computer industry. During his nursing refresher program, he spent eight weeks in a preceptored learning experience with the home-care division of the regional health authority. The RNs in the division enjoyed having Mr. Cook with them during the eight-week period, particularly because he was able to help them adjust to the division's new computer system. Upon completion of the refresher course, he was invited to apply for a position with the division, and he began work there within a week. Almost immediately, he was required to pick up independent case assignments because of a shortage in staff over the summer.

In early October Diane Wong, the nurse manager, received two complaints from families about the care Mr. Cook was providing, but after a brief discussion with him she concluded that these were matters of misunderstanding, not questionable competence. In mid-November, a homemaker visiting these same clients informed Ms. Wong that the clients had asked that Clarence Cook not be allowed to continue to provide them with nursing care. Further checking by Ms. Wong raised serious questions about Mr. Cook's competence. When she approached him about specific instances of substandard care, he denied all problems and labeled her actions "reverse discrimination."

Diane Wong is concerned about the clients' safety and standard of care, but she is also concerned about being fair to Clarence Cook. She feels responsible for the situation, since she did not provide him with appropriate orientation and supervision. The other RN staff have decided that she is treating Mr. Cook unfairly, and this has created a serious morale problem in the division. (Adapted from Silva, 1990).

What should Diane Wong do? Is this a moral problem?

The Case of Lynda Lightfoot

After a long career as manager of a small nursing home, Lynda Lightfoot has moved to an urban center where she has become a nurse manager in a large, multi-level, long-term-care facility. Ms. Lightfoot's new supervisor tells her that the agency is known for its cost efficiency, and that she is expected to maintain high standards of care while keeping within the budget.

Within two weeks of her arrival, Ms. Lightfoot becomes aware that it is common practice for one staff member to feed four to five patients at a time. She also observes that clients who refuse food when it is first offered, or are slow to eat, are not always fed, and that staff become impatient with residents whose feeding is slowed by bouts of coughing. Lynda Lightfoot discusses her concerns with the residential-care aides, but they seem puzzled. They explain that meal times in the agency have always been handled this way.

Ms. Lightfoot is now concerned not only about the poor standard of nutritional care of the agency's elderly clients, but also about the indifference of the staff who do not see this as any kind of an ethical problem. Compounding her concern is the condition under which she was hired—i.e., that they keep within budget. (Case based upon research of Kayser-Jones, 1997).

Is Lynda Lightfoot's problem an ethical one? Why? What should she do? What responsibility does senior management have in this situation?

manager, or other first-level manager, further along the path towards "ethical fitness."

Being and Becoming a Person of Good Moral Character

The idea of the source of good moral choice as residing in moral character is based upon the theory of virtue ethics. According to the theory of virtue ethics, virtuous persons are persons of moral character who would be expected to choose ethical actions because their deeply held values would direct them to wise and informed ethical deliberation, leading to good

choices. Such values develop during early socialization and can be cultivated throughout a lifetime.

Our understanding of virtue in the Western world originated with
Greek philosophers, particularly Aristotle who emphasized the dispositions
"an agent habitually brings to his acts . . . that make a person good and enable him to do well" (Pellegrino & Thomasma, 1993, p. 5; Aristotle, 1962,
p.38). Virtue ethics has been restored to an important place in ethical decision-making only during the past decade. Particular virtues considered
worthy of respect and emulation include: *trust; compassion; prudence; justice; fortitude; temperance; integrity;* and *self-effacement* (see Box 18.2).

To suggest that the manager and leader must be a person of sound
moral character is to say that it matters a good deal that nurse managers and
other health-care managers are people who intend to do good, who are
good people, and who have a "deep core of ethical values" (Kidder, 1995,
p. 13). Being a professional is to profess to have knowledge which will be
used to benefit others (Hughes, 1963). The combination of nursing knowledge and managerial knowledge creates a powerful potential for good, if the
manager is a virtuous person, that is, a person who has certain moral traits
of character which are embedded in an intention to do good.

Virtues form the basis of the intent to do good which is crucial to making good choices and executing right actions. For example, in the case of
Mary Grace, virtues of trust, compassion, justice, and temperance are required; in the cases of Beth Wallace and Diane Wong, trust, prudence, and
integrity are needed; and in the case of Lynda Lightfoot, there is a demand
for compassion, justice, and fortitude. Understanding the significance of
these virtues to the commitments of the health-care enterprise is critical for
first-level managers.

Most theorists suggest that moral character alone would be insufficient
for moral action, and that knowledge and application of general principles
and theories are also required (Pellegrino & Thomasma, 1993, p. 14–15) to
guide the provision of care and to guide managerial practice.

Ethical Theories And Principles

Because moral virtues (i.e., the disposition to do what is ethically right) are
not sufficient for ethical decision-making, knowledge of theories and principles is considered an essential tool for health professionals and their managers. Such knowledge enables a nurse manager to understand ethical
quandaries of managerial life, and to come to terms with ethical problems
by finding the discourse (the terminology) that helps give meaning to these
situations.

Two main theories derived from moral philosophy have dominated
bioethical thinking. One is the ethic of utility (utilitarianism, or ends-based
thinking) which continues to be employed as strong justification for many
managerial actions in health care. This is increasingly manifest in the current turbulent and fiscally restrained health-care environment. Essentially,
the ethic of utility is based upon the premise that choices of actions can be

Box 18.2
VIRTUES APPLIED TO HEALTH MANAGERS AND PROFESSIONALS

THE FIDELITY TO TRUST involves a relationship with a client of care or a fellow worker (for example, in mutual planning of care) that is characterized by sensitivity to the needs of the other person, but also maintains intellectual honesty and humility.

THE VIRTUE OF COMPASSION is the ability to co-experience the suffering of another person to the extent that one is able to employ one's professional knowledge and competence to attend to that suffering.

THE VIRTUE OF PRUDENCE is the combination of intellectual virtue (theoretical wisdom and understanding) and moral virtue (self-control, beneficence, etc.) that leads to good judgement in dealing with clinical and ethical problems.

THE VIRTUE OF MORAL JUSTICE is the "strict habit of rendering what is due to others" (p. 92) as an extension of the love or charity we should show to others.

THE VIRTUE OF FORTITUDE is the moral courage which makes a person willing to suffer personal harm for the sake of a moral good (for example, advocating for the vulnerable in health care despite a potential risk to one's own status or position).

THE VIRTUE OF TEMPERANCE is the responsible use of power for the good of patients, and the control of excesses in the use of science and technology.

THE VIRTUE OF INTEGRITY is being "predictable about responses to specific situations" (p. 127) and able to integrate all virtues into the whole. It involves wise judgement as to the relative importance of principles, rules and guidelines in reaching a decision to act.

THE VIRTUE OF SELF EFFACEMENT is the ability to accept responsibility for moral malaise, and to seek to restore health/healing practices to be a moral enterprise.

Source: From *The Virtues in Medical Practice* by Edmund D. Pellegrino and David C. Thomasma. Copyright © 1993 by Oxford University Press, Inc. Used by permission of Oxford University Press, Inc.

considered 'good' if those choices lead to good outcomes. Generally, 'good outcomes' are those that lead to the greatest number of people experiencing the greatest good, whether that good is happiness, or access to health care, or general economic good. Jeremy Bentham and John Stuart Mill are regarded as the architects of this approach. In raw form, a utilitarian ethicist might argue that a good outcome for a sizeable number of individuals justifies the ways in which the outcomes are achieved. That is why this theoretical approach is often described as one in which 'the end justifies the means.'

Using 'ends-based thinking' in the case of Mary Grace, a utilitarian would argue that while it is a shame that some patients have to be discharged early and experience some degree of suffering as a result, increased access to the limited service for others justifies the early discharge. In the case of Beth Wallace, the utilitarian argument might be that the deception about the medication should not have occurred but continuity of the unit depends upon public confidence in the unit: because of this assumption, maintaining public confidence outweighs the principle of honesty. In effect, in view of the fact that closure could result from negative media attention, the needs of many elderly patients for the services of the unit outweigh the importance of telling the truth to one patient and her family.

A second main theory of moral philosophy is the ethic of duty (deontological theory, or rule-based thinking). The theory of the ethic of duty is based upon duties or obligations derived from several sources, including theological sources. Secular ethics in our society, however, is mainly derived from the work of Immanuel Kant, a German philosopher who held that obligations or duties should be the basis of moral choices irrespective of the consequences of such actions. Kant (1948) suggested that there ought to be an imperative that one would never act unless he or she believed that such an action should become the rule of conduct for all. In the case of Beth Wallace, therefore, one might hold that individuals have a duty to be honest with one another, regardless of the consequences, because this is a sound general rule for all to follow. Such honesty takes priority over whatever outcomes may result by the revelation of the drug error "cover-up" because of the overbearing importance of honesty. In the case of Mary Grace, an ethic of duty theorist might argue that the duty to alleviate the suffering of individuals in care takes priority over the potential harm that might be caused to others awaiting access to the unit.

In order to provide a more accessible means of ethical decision-making for health-care professionals and managers, bioethics emerged as an applied discipline with theories and principles which were largely developed in the late 1970s and early 1980s. Bioethical principles had been introduced into the mainstream of health-care scholarship and practice mainly through rediscovery of the writings of W.D. Ross (1930) and the work of Tom Beauchamp and James Childress in their popular text, *Principles of Biomedical Ethics* (1994) first published in 1979. The four-principle approach is now quite well known and widely used, the principles being *autonomy, beneficence, non-maleficence* and *justice* (see Box 18.3).

Numerous textbooks of nursing ethics, medical ethics and health-care ethics have employed these principles as a means of enabling health professionals to become "ethically fit" (Kidder, 1995), and thereby to make sound ethical choices. The principles assist in clarifying ethical dilemmas and situations of ethical distress, and serve as a set of counterpoints in ethical decision-making. In the case of Mary Grace, for example, the principle of justice for many must be weighed against the principle of beneficence for a few; in the case of Beth Wallace, the principle of truthfulness as part of beneficence must be weighed against the principle of justice; in the case of Diane Wong, the principle of non-maleficence (i.e., the potential or real harm to clients) must be weighed against the principle of fairness (justice) for the individual employee; and in the case of Lynda Lightfoot the principle of non-maleficence predominates. A good working understanding of these principles assists nurse managers to consider what is at stake when tough choices must be made.

Box 18.3

ETHICAL PRINCIPLES

AUTONOMY: The principle of autonomy is the right to choose for oneself what one believes to be in one's best interests. It is the concept of self-determination, of being in charge of one's person. From this principle of autonomy comes our commitment to respect clients' choices in treatment and their need to make informed choices about matters of life and death. The rights to refuse treatment, to privacy, to truth-telling, and to confidentiality are also duties which evolve from this principle.

BENEFICENCE: The principle of beneficence is the duty to benefit others. A central belief reflected in this principle is the duty or obligation to assist others, to contribute to their welfare, and in doing so, to always act in the best interests of the patient or client.

NON-MALEFICENCE: The principle of non-maleficence is the duty to do no harm and to protect others from harm. Non-maleficence includes minimizing harms that may be necessary in the course of treatment, anticipating harms which may occur, and avoiding harm. Such harms are not restricted to physical harms, but include feelings of helplessness, isolation, and powerlessness, to name just a few of many important considerations for all health professionals.

DISTRIBUTIVE JUSTICE: The principle of distributive justice has as its underlying value that there be fairness based on the equal worth of individuals. While there are several criteria that may be applied to determine fairness, e.g. to each according to worth, to each according to need, to each according to contribution, etc., a value commonly held in Canada is that of equity. Equity is fairness according to need.

Source: From Alberta Association of Registered Nurses, *Ethical Decision-Making for Registered Nurses in Alberta: Guidelines and Recommendations.* (Edmonton, AB: AARN, 1996), pp. 7–8.

Partly in reaction to the fact that these principles appear to be more simple than they are, making them susceptible to misuse, scholars of ethics (among them nurse ethicists) have proposed different approaches to ethical decision-making. Carol Gilligan (1982) criticized principlism as based too solidly in a justice perspective (or rights-based ethic) rather than an ethic of responsibility, which she described as an "ethic of care." Many nurse ethicists, educators and practitioners have found a theory of an ethic of care appealing, in that it is a theory which takes into account the context of care (the setting, the patient's significant others, the patient's history, etc.) as well as the health professional's obligations in relation to the patient and his or her care.

Bergum (1994), a nurse ethicist, has suggested that the "...kind of knowledge needed for ethical care must be constructed in the relationship between professional and patient..." (p. 72). In that relationship, the nurse seeks to understand the patient's experience of disease and illness, and to explore with the patient the meaning of the condition for that individual patient. Bergum has also focused on the development of a theory of "relational ethics" which incorporates principles (a justice-based approach) and an ethic of care (an approach to caring that focuses on context, person, and relationship). Relational ethics involve a commitment to the context and the lived experience of those in situations of health care, and the consideration of principles only in the context of those relationships (Bergum, 1994).

Applying an ethic of care and relational ethics to the case of Diane Wong would focus the nurse manager's attention on the context in which health care is being provided (home care, fiscal restraint, etc.), as well as on the duty of safe care, and the responsibility for fair consideration of the individual nurse (AARN, 1996). In an ethic of responsibility, a nurse manager like Mary Grace, who was forced to consider the duties owed to both present and future clients, might be motivated to involve the staff in identifying important dimensions of care for these patients. She might work with staff to develop a petition (or proposal) to senior management for fair treatment of these patients, documenting evidence of the harms they are experiencing. In the case of Beth Wallace, the nurse manager would attempt to consider all individuals involved—client, family, nurse, and relative—and to seek ways to be faithful to the needs of all, while upholding the fundamental value of honesty.

In view of the foregoing, it bears repeating that nurse managers, in ethical decision-making, must recognize the ease with which it is possible to slide into models of ethical decision-making that are too simple and too comfortable, and which do not always force full clarification and consideration of the ethical dimensions of difficult situations. In some cases the use of principles alone, however helpful they may be, can produce a result that approximates a "medical work-up," or a "nursing process," or some other scientific problem-solving approach. When utilized in these linear thinking models, principles may even obscure the meaning of the ethical dilemma for everyone involved. As one practitioner noted, when we make ethical decisions regarding clients in care, we too frequently take a "snapshot" rather than consider the "mural" of the patient's life (Moss, 1994). Further, broader organizational contexts which may have created situations of ethical distress are too frequently discounted or overlooked. Senior management and governing boards often bear significant responsibility for creating serious ethical problems for front-line managers and their staff: these individuals, too, need to become "ethically fit."

Alternate Approaches To Guide Ethical Decision Making

Over the past decade, numerous models have been proposed for ethical thinking and problem-solving within the health-care literature. Many such models or ethics decision frameworks are principle-based, often utilizing the four principles or some variation of those principles. Silva (1990) offers examples of numerous decision-making models in her stellar text, *Ethical Decision-making in Nursing Administration*, and she provides case studies with step-by-step comments that address the ethical dilemmas inherent in the cases. First-level managers will find her text most helpful.

A relatively neglected resource in health-care ethics has been the work of Rushforth Kidder (1995), whose approach seems particularly applicable to ethical issues facing health-care managers. Kidder emphasizes the reality that ethical dilemmas are normally 'right-versus-right' situations, and urges those who would be ethical to seek some middle ground in such dilemmas whenever possible. He has noted that since a dilemma forces a choice between two "seemingly implacable alternatives," stepping back from the ethical problem and considering it in terms of the four choices below may well uncover a third option. He refers to this type of situation as a "trilemma" (p. 167), and suggests it be examined in the context of the following four choices: *justice* versus *mercy*, *short-term* versus *long-term*, *individual* versus *community*, and *truth* versus *loyalty*.

Kidder also proposes several steps in ethical decision-making, similar to those of health-care ethicists but including some unique features. His step-wise model is roughly as follows:

1. Identify that there is a moral issue (don't brush it aside or mistake it for another sort of issue);
2. Determine the actor (i.e., who is responsible);
3. Gather the relevant facts;
4. Test for 'right-versus-wrong' issues (is there wrongdoing or violation of some duty?);
5. Test for 'right-versus-right' choices (as described in the paragraph above) to bring the issue into focus;
6. Apply resolution principles (ends-based, rule-based, or care-based) "to locate the line of reasoning that seems most relevant and persuasive to the issue at hand" (Kidder, 1995, p.185);
7. Investigate the possibility of a third option (the "trilemma");
8. Make the decision; and
9. Revisit and reflect on the decision (Kidder, 1995, pp. 183-186).

Using Kidder's approach for the case of Lynda Lightfoot, we might conclude early in our decision-making that there is wrongdoing on the part of the staff. While the wrongdoing is probably not deliberate, a group of elderly people is nonetheless being subjected to a poor standard of nutritional care. This violates the moral duty to prevent harm and to avoid discrimination against elderly, vulnerable people. The circumstances call for advocacy to senior administration, including a request that the situation be rectified. In the case of Diane Wong, we might move through Kidder's steps to recognize the importance of providing safe and competent care for clients in home care *and* providing adequate orientation and supervision of new RN staff. Based upon a care-based ethic or a relational ethic, a nurse manager might consider a third option (the middle ground) of providing the RN with the missed orientation and supervision—to clarify expectations and to give him an opportunity to improve his practice, ensuring that evaluation of his performance and client satisfaction is measured in a timely manner. In extending that caring concern to the clients who requested that Clarence Cook not be permitted to continue to provide their care, Diane Wong would ensure that his supervised nursing practice was with different clients.

No one 'fixed' approach to ethical thinking can fit all nurses, or all health professionals. Nurse managers must discover individually the approaches that work best for them, and that enable them to lead in a way that encourages staff to ask questions, to identify issues, and to pursue ethically justifiable choices. Thus, in addition to continued development of moral character, nurse managers need to choose models for ethical decision-making that are meaningful and helpful to them.

Building A Moral Community

The imperative to work towards building a moral community is a third critical element of the leadership role of the nurse manager. In their capacity as individuals who share their vision with a team of workers, transformational leaders can significantly influence moral behaviour within their units or programs and within agencies by way of their example. In fostering a moral community, nurse managers share information and their own interpretation of that information among and between their staff, and demonstrate how ideals can be translated into conduct (Biordi, 1993).

The nurse manager's task of building a moral community with her staff goes beyond obligations to others and incorporates thoughtful reflection about the kind of nursing practice life they consider to be important and worthwhile. Such considerations are critical to choosing what type of a society we want to be, and to become—and these issues are particularly significant in contemporary Canadian health-care settings (Yeo, 1993). Although such reflections may seem remote from the everyday world of the first-line manager, it is through the daily use of moral action, and formal and informal ethical decision-making, that a moral community is ultimately realized.

Within the world of managerial practice there are numerous obstacles to building a moral community. A primary obstacle may be the nurse manager's own understanding and response to the perceived value of the objectivity of management 'science' and of medical 'science.' This matters because the theories of management (or of medicine, health, and healing) determine what we treat as 'facts' (Astley, 1985). There are no 'bare facts'; 'facts' depend upon, and are defined by, the 'theories' of a manager. 'Theories' are comprised of certain terms and specific language, that is, a particular vocabulary. Each of these languages or vocabularies incorporates certain assumptions about values: these values are not normally made explicit.

No where is this more apparent than in the confusing and often misleading vocabulary of health-care management, including nursing management. Through the magic of language, it is possible to diminish the nature of a moral community by redefining client or agency problems. In doing so, meaning can be extracted from client experiences of health and illness, and from the health professional's experience of ethical distress. A common example of this phenomenon is the way in which nursing advocacy for better staffing to ensure safe and competent client care is often reduced by politicians or senior executives to "whining by nurses," or to accusations of "staff protecting their jobs" (see Chapter 5 for a case presentation of this type of situation). For first-level managers caught between opposing positions, exercising "ethical fitness" is a way to remain true to oneself and to one's values in everyday work life.

Nurse managers are cautioned to remember that such commonly used terms as "quality," "total quality management," "clinical practice guidelines" and "evidence-based care" are based on value-laden concepts. Within health agencies these conceptual models can determine what counts as important information for planning and evaluation. Many times, the supposedly objective facts of numbers and statistics are given priority over the more subjective aspects of client care and progress. It is not that any of these concepts are inherently wrong, but in building a moral community they must be understood for what they are: tools to be used by health-care managers, nurse managers, and health professionals. Unfortunately, too often these tools have been misused in practice because they are treated as ends in themselves rather than as means to an end. Unless the tools are appropriately used and take into account consideration of broader issues, such as what patients consider important, they miss the mark (Redman, 1996).

THE NURSE MANAGER AND ETHICAL LEADERSHIP

In the introduction to this chapter, three main dimensions of ethical leadership were noted, namely, being a person of moral character, being a person who engages in moral behaviour, and being someone who builds a moral community. Values are critical to moral leadership. Nurse managers must be clear about the values that are important to them, and recognize that commitment to these values will place demands on them (ICN, 1997, p. 128).

A critical element in ethical leadership is the way in which important values are communicated to staff as a vision of care and service. To gain their commitment and involvement in their work towards those ends, the manager-leader works to establish a culture in which attention to ethics plays a pivotal role. It must be a culture in which staff are encouraged to see ethical problems in the workplace, are "free to challenge standards or practices they consider unethical" (Longest, 1996), are encouraged to keep themselves ethically fit, are supported in agonizing over tough ethical choices, and are supported in addressing ethical concerns.

Such support can be provided through formal structures or by informal means. As long as a climate of openness to ethics and ethical discussion exists on a unit or set of units, questions about ethical practice in specific cases, or application of the Canadian Nurses Association Code of Ethics for Registered Nurses in particular circumstances, can occur as an integral part of the nurses' dialogue in the provision of care. Based upon ethically troublesome and recurring situations with agency-wide implications, nurses can be encouraged to initiate discussion and to draft proposals for agency ethics statements or policies.

Ethics committees can also be an important structure to promote ethical practice. Such committees bring visibility to the priority of ethics in the health agency, and also serve as a useful learning forum for managers and staff. Many health agencies have such committees. Unfortunately, too often nursing staff have been unaware of the existence of these clinical ethics committees and of their work (Storch & Griener, 1992). The nurse manager can do much to raise awareness of ethics committees with staff members, and facilitate their involvement in and use of such committees. The manager can encourage staff to take everyday ethics problems to such committees for consideration.

Some nurses have found themselves intimidated at the prospect of being involved in an agency ethics committee; some are uncomfortable even with the idea of submitting a problem case or issue to such a committee. Yet, these same nurses have often conveyed a deep commitment to ethics, are concerned about ethical practice, and are experiencing ethical distress on a daily basis. Creating formal or informal ethics committees or discussion groups within nursing departments or units, where nurses can share their concerns with colleagues, can be encouraged by nurse managers. Such dialogue can be a way to enhance the level of comfort of staff towards full participation in agency ethics committees and ethics education. If no agency ethics committee exists, the nursing ethics committee or the interdisciplinary ethics committee within a unit may well become the embryo for development of a committee that meets to reflect and consult on ethical problems in the health agency as a whole.

Liberal use of opportunities for ethics education for the nurse manager and staff is yet another way to stimulate reflection and discussion. This approach is particularly important as health regions, health agencies, and units within agencies grapple with such issues as advance treatment directives, research involving patients with dementia, privatizing health programs, and the apparent erosion of standards of confidentiality in occupational health services.

All these types of initiatives not only bring greater visibility to the priority of ethics among staff, but serve as useful forums for mutual learning for managers and staff.

CONCLUSION

Ethical leadership demands that managers be persons of moral character and of moral action, who are intent on building moral communities. They can provide ethical leadership by helping staff to develop a commitment to moral values and to ethical reflection. Tools for "ethical fitness" include knowledge of theories and principles, and a sense of how these can be used to clarify ethical problems and to make good choices. Ethical dilemmas can arise on a daily basis in a health-care setting. It is imperative that nurse managers reflect on the values that are important to them, and that their actions reflect their ethical leadership.

SUMMARY

- Nurse managers manage by leading, not by direction and control.
- Leadership commits staff to action by appealing to higher ideals and moral values.
- Almost every action a manager takes involves ethics.
- The Canadian Nurses Association Code of Ethics for Registered Nurses (1997) offers guidance for nurse managers and nursing staff.
- Being 'ethically fit' means being engaged in ethical reflection and justification.
- Ethical fitness involves being and becoming a person of sound moral character, knowing and applying ethical theories and principles, and building a moral community.
- A person of moral character intends to do good, and has a 'deep core of ethical values' and particular moral traits (or virtues).
- Ends-based thinking, rule-based thinking, and relational-based thinking are three theoretical approaches to ethics, while principles help to illuminate ethical understanding and decision-making.
- Building a moral community involves establishing a culture wherein ethics play a pivotal role.
- Informal ethics discussions, formalized ethics statements or policies, and ethics committees are structures which support a moral community.

FURTHER READINGS AND RESOURCES

Beauchamp, T.L. and Childress, J.F. (1994). *Principles of biomedical ethics.* 4th edition. New York: Oxford University Press. This is a classic text because it provides a comprehensive discussion of the ethical principles of respect for autonomy, beneficence, non-maleficence, and justice, with liberal use of examples to illustrate the application of these principles in health-care practice. Included, as well, is an overview of types of ethical theory, discussion of professional-patient relationships, and attention to virtues and ideals in professional life.

Pellegrino, E.D. and Thomasma, D.C. (1992). *The virtues in medical practice.* New York: Oxford University Press. Virtue theory and the virtues of medicine (appropriate to all health professionals) are given comprehensive treatment in this text. The authors have been able to provide a counter-balancing theory to the principle-based approach, while emphasizing the merits of principles and theories.

Silva, M.C. (1990). *Ethical decision-making in nursing administration.* Norwalk, Conn.: Appleton and Lange. In addition to providing a fine overview of classical ethical theories and principles, Silva offers a wide range of applications for a decision-making model. Included in her text are six case studies which are thoroughly analyzed, plus an additional six ethical dilemmas involving nursing administrators. This is a very useful text for nurse managers and administrators.

Tschudin, V. (1994). *Deciding ethically: A practical approach to nursing challenges.* London: Baillière-Tindall. Although there are numerous fine nursing ethics texts written in North America, this small book authored in the United Kingdom is suggested here because it offers some novel perspectives on ethics. Tschudin provides a practical approach to nursing challenges by covering theories, principles and virtues, with liberal use of illustrations from nursing practice.

REFERENCES

Alberta Association of Registered Nurses (1996). *Ethical decision-making for registered nurses in Alberta: Guidelines and recommendations.* Edmonton: AARN.

Aristotle (1962). *Nicomachean ethics.* (Translated by Martin Ostwald). Englewood Cliffs, NJ: Prentice Hall.

Astley, W. G. (1985). Administrative science as socially constructed truth. *Administrative Science Quarterly, 30,* 497–513.

Beauchamp, T. L. & Childress, J. F. (1994). *Principles of biomedical ethics* (4th ed.). New York: Oxford University Press.

Bergum, V. (1994). Knowledge for ethical care. *Nursing Ethics.* 1(2): 71–79.

Biordi, D. L. (1993). Ethical leadership. In A. Marriner-Tomey (Ed.), *Transformational Leadership in Nursing* (pp. 51–68). St. Louis, MO: Mosby.

Canadian Nurses Association. (1997). *Code of ethics for registered nurses.* Ottawa: Canadian Nurses Association.

Gilligan, C. (1982). *In a different voice.* Cambridge: Harvard University Press.

Hughes, E. C. (1963). Professions. *Daedalus, 92* (Fall), 655–668.

Kant, I. (1948). *Groundwork of the metaphysic of morals.* (Translated and analyzed by H. J. Paton). New York: Harper and Row.

Kayser-Jones, J. (1997). Nutritional care of the elderly: Ethical issues. *Abstracts and Symposia: International Council of Nurses* (p.185). Geneva: ICN.

Kidder, R. M. (1995). *How good people make tough choices.* New York: Fireside.

Longest, B. B. (1996). *Health professionals in management.* Stamford, CN: Appleton and Lange.

Marriner-Tomey, A. (1993). *Transformational leadership in nursing.* St. Louis, MO: Mosby.

Mitchell, C. (1996). *Workshop presentation: Practical bioethics for nurses.* 1996 Bioethics Conference: A Future of Dignity. Hawaii: St. Francis Medical Center.

Moss, A. H. (1994). Narrative ethics: A patient friendly approach to 'doing ethics.' *Network of Ethics Committees Newsletter.* Morgantown, WV: Network.

Pellegrino, E. D. (1993). The metamorphosis of medical ethics. *Journal of the American Medical Association, 269* (9), 1158–1162.

Pellegrino, E. D. & Thomasma, D. C. (1993). *The virtues in medical practice.* New York: Oxford University Press.

Redman, B. K. (1996). Ethical issues in the development and use of guidelines for clinical practice. *The Journal of Clinical Ethics.* 7(3): 251–256.

Ross, W. D. (1930). *The right and the good.* Indianapolis, IN: Hackett.

Silva, M. C. (1990). *Ethical decision-making in nursing administration.* Norwalk, CT.: Appleton and Lange.

Storch, J. L. & Griener, G.G. (1992). Ethics committees in Canadian hospitals: Report of the 1990 pilot study. *Healthcare Management Forum,* 5(1), 19–26.

Tschudin, V. (1994). *Deciding ethically: A practical approach to nursing challenges.* London: Baillière-Tindall.

Yeo, M. (1993). Toward an ethic of empowerment for health promotion. *Health promotion international.* 8(3): 225–235.

PART
FOUR

Accountability

Chapter 19

▼▼▼▼▼▼▼▼▼▼▼▼▼▼▼

Accountability, Standards, and Quality

DONNA LYNN SMITH, DONNA ARMANN-HUTTON, NOELA J. INIONS, AND DENNIS HUTTON

KEY OBJECTIVES

In this chapter, you will learn:

- That accountability is the defining aspect of professionalism and leadership.
- How accountability, standards, and quality relate to one another in health care.
- Different types of standards and the sources for their authority.
- Some similarities and differences among scientific, professional, organizational, legal, and community standards.
- The origins and evolution of interest in the concept of "quality" in health care.
- Definitions of common terms associated with "quality management."
- About efforts to improve the standards of nursing administration and health care in Canada.
- Current issues and dilemmas with respect to standards and accountability in the Canadian health system.

INTRODUCTION AND OVERVIEW

A professional education includes not only the knowledge specific to the discipline, but also awareness of the standards that are applicable to that discipline. Professionals are expected to use discretionary judgement in the application of their specific knowledge to particular situations, and the public holds them accountable for informed, ethical practice in which the well-being of clients is a priority.

The privileges enjoyed by professionals include varying degrees of self-governance, in return for which they accept an obligation to maintain and monitor professional standards through processes of peer review and discipline. In regulated professions, the professional association or college has the legal authority to administer various types of penalties to members of that profession who fail to meet expected standards. (See also Chapter 16.)

People who accept positions in leadership and management in health organizations accept responsibilities that go beyond those associated with their original professions or occupations. By virtue of the *authority* vested in their positions, they may become *responsible* for safeguarding the well-being of large groups of people, such as clients and staff of units, programs, or entire organizations; sometimes the health of whole communities, provinces or countries falls within their purview. They are also likely to be held accountable for the stewardship of funds and other resources provided by the community.

Leaders and managers generally enjoy higher incomes than do members of the general public and others in their profession. They may, in addition, receive various perquisites (or "perks"), such as greater discretionary use of their time, or the use of a company vehicle. In return, it is expected that they will behave with integrity, and will not abuse their positions of privilege.

Leaders and managers in the health-care field are particularly likely to attract criticism if they fail to live up to public expectations. Whether consumers are paying for health services directly, through rising insurance premiums, or through taxes that support universal access and payment for health services, they have grown intolerant of mistakes by health professionals and health-care managers. Members of the public are no longer prepared to accept discourteous or paternalistic behaviour from health professionals and organizational leaders, and they expect that deficiencies and inefficiencies in service and management will be prevented or promptly corrected.

There have been many variations on the theme of quality since formal programs of quality assurance began in health organizations more than three decades ago. Table 19.1 contains a list of definitions that reflect the current terminology and emphasis in a field that is now broadly defined as "quality management."

Parallel developments in business, industry, and science have influenced approaches to quality management in health care. As the costs of health care have risen and neo-conservative economic viewpoints have become popular, traditional approaches to the development and assurance of professional standards have sometimes been disparaged as costly "turf protection." Consultants and executives have successfully marketed a plethora of management interventions to save money by achieving teamwork and horizontal integration of organizational processes. Program management structures have resulted in the flattening of organizational hierarchies, a decrease in the number of middle-management positions, and the diffusion of authority and responsibility (see also Chapter 7). The positions of professional leaders have been eliminated in many organizations and the virtues of self-directed teams have been promoted. Many of these organizational experiments have been costly, not only in terms of lost expertise and morale in the professional workforce, but also in terms of liability for mistakes.

Table 19.1

DEFINITIONS OF KEY TERMS
FOR QUALITY MANAGEMENT
IN HEALTH CARE

Accountability	Answering for one's actions and the consequences of those actions; acting within the authority of one's position to accept responsibility for specifying standards, measuring performance against those standards, and making decisions as necessary to correct problems and improve quality,
Guidelines	Authoritative statements describing recommended courses of action for specific clinical situations, technical conditions, or patient populations.
Standard	A broad statement of agreed-upon quality for a given element of care.
Structures	Human and material resources; organizational frameworks, or systems. Sometimes referred to as "inputs."
Process	Activities that occur between client and care-providers while care is taking place.
Outcome	Any change that takes place in the client as a result of the inputs and interactions between client and provider; includes changes in health status and client satisfaction.
Criteria	Statements describing predetermined elements that clarify the intent of a standard, and the degree to which that standard has been accomplished.
Indicators	Observable and measurable dimensions that provide information on aspects of care.
Benchmark	A reference point signifying the highest mark of quality of certain goods, services, or processes used as a comparison point for quality in like organizations or situations.
Measurement	The process of determining whether a standard has been met.
Quality	Level of excellence, value or worth; conformance to standards that are either implicit or explicit.
Quality Management	An umbrella term encompassing all systematic approaches to the assessment and improvement of quality.
Quality Assessment and Improvement	A systematic process wherein there is a data-based, judgemental appraisal of a selected element of care and subsequent improvement; a term that is gradually replacing the more traditional term, "quality assurance" (QA).
Continuous Quality Improvement (CQI)	A collaborative team process, usually interdisciplinary and statistically supported, used to respond systematically to discrete opportunities for improvement.
Total Quality Management	A leadership paradigm that subscribes to quality as a driving value for an organization; the value is operationalized by top-down total employee commitment and participation in consumer-focused continuous-quality improvement of all work processes throughout and organization.

Source: Adapted from J. A. Schmele, *Quality Management in Nursing and Health Care* (Albany, NY: Delmar, 1996), pp. 589–91.

In recent years, the American health system has also seen a steady rise in litigation by injured or dissatisfied patients, and the United States government has implemented billions of dollars worth of elaborate regulatory mechanisms in response to escalating liability claims by health-care consumers who have suffered damages as a result of carelessness, malpractice and even fraud. In Canada, both federal and provincial governments have been hesitant to impose and monitor standards and, although it is not widely recognized, regulatory requirements for health services in Canada are minimal in comparison to the American system.

This chapter focuses on the nature and importance of professional accountability, and highlights some of the conditions that must be in place if health organizations are to be accountable to the communities they serve.

WHAT IS ACCOUNTABILITY AND WHY IS IT IMPORTANT?

Gardner and Russell (1989) have pointed out that individuals make choices to be responsible, reasonable, and responsive, and it is in making these choices that they accept accountability. Responsibility can be seen in the action taken;

> an individual or corporate entity who is 'responsible' is trustworthy, reliable, able to tell right from wrong, and able to think and act reasonably. We may not know at the time what is 'reasonable' so the accountability relationship has to include the concept of responsiveness. Responsiveness is the quality evident in activities to both receive and search out relevant information. It implies an awareness of, and sensitivity to factors in the environment that affect the ability to accomplish the task (pp. 3-4).

Ideally, standards are available to provide guidance to individuals as to when and why they should take action. But this is not always the case, making responsiveness a key element of accountability.

A FRAMEWORK FOR HEALTH-CARE STANDARDS

The work of Dr. Avedis Donabedian at the School of Public Health at the University of Michigan laid the foundation, and continues to provide a durable conceptual framework, for understanding the nature and various types of health-care standards. As shown in Table 19.2, information about structure, process and outcomes is needed to assess quality in health care.

Structural standards for nursing services might include requirements such as the following:

- All nurses employed in an agency must be eligible for licensure in the jurisdiction.

Table 19.2
TYPES OF INFORMATION REQUIRED FOR QUALITY ASSESSMENT

Structure

The attributes of settings in which care occurs (physical and organizational tools and resources). Includes:
- material resources (e.g., facilities, equipment, money);
- human resources (e.g., number and qualifications of personnel); and
- organizational structure (e.g., medical staff organization, peer-review methods).

Process

What is actually done in giving and receiving care (the activities that occur between client and provider). Includes:
- patient's activities in seeking care and carrying it out; and
- practitioner's activities in making a diagnosis, and recommending or implementing treatment.

Outcomes

The effects of care of the health status of patients and populations (the changes in status attributable to antecedent health care). Includes:
- improvements in a client's knowledge;
- changes in a client's behaviour; and
- degree of client satisfaction with care.

Source: Adapted from A. Donabedian, "Evaluating the Quality of Medical Care," *Milbank Quarterly, 44* (Supplement, 3, 1996), pp. 166–203.

- All non-licensed personnel providing client-care services must be supervised by a registered nurse.
- Current policy and procedures manuals will be available for reference by nurses on all units in the organization.
- The nurse-to-patient ratio in the ICU step-down unit will be one nurse for every two patients at all times.

Process standards for nursing services might include the following:

- All nursing personnel demonstrate kindness and respect for patients.
- Nurses ensure that no patient is permitted to suffer pain that can be alleviated by comfort measures or medication.
- Patients are instructed in the safe administration of their medications.

Outcome standards for nursing services might include the following:

- No more than two percent of incontinent patients develop pressure sores.

- In "client-satisfaction" questionnaires, patients indicate they feel they have been treated with kindness and respect by all levels and categories of staff who care for them.
- The follow-up care of patients discharged from hospital is not interrupted by a return to hospital because of problems in administering their medications.

As can be seen from these examples, *structural standards* (sometimes called "inputs") are the easiest to measure. *Process standards* are more challenging, and it is in the area of process that many total quality management programs or continuous quality improvement programs strive to make a difference.

Outcome standards, whether these include effects on the client's health status, such as a return to mobility, or whether they involve administrative "outputs," such as lengths of stay for particular client groups, are the most difficult standards to define and measure. There is a particular danger that because of this difficulty, outcome measurement will be superficially focused upon easily quantifiable indicators. Although it seems obvious that outcomes are the result of structure and process, and that gathering information and conducting quality-assurance activities in these two domains is therefore important, some leaders have advocated that "outcomes are the only thing that matters," and that therefore only outcomes should be measured. Measuring only outcomes makes it difficult to understand and interpret information about the outcomes, such as why some are achieved while others are not. Without information about structure and process in the delivery of health services, it is also difficult to interpret trends in relation to decisions made within the organization.

For example, as health organizations have been downsized and the numbers of middle managers reduced, in many settings the committees and individuals whose positions were dedicated to maintaining a system of nursing policies and procedures have vanished. Layoffs, bumping, and an increase in the numbers of casual or call-in nursing positions have destabilized the nursing workforce, leading to a loss of specialized expertise in many parts of individual organizations, and in the health system as a whole. It might be supposed that during such times, the roles of clinical educators and clinical nurse specialists would be recognized as being more important than before, and that the number of such positions would be increased. It might also be supposed that in such circumstances, the availability of reference materials such as clinical policy and procedures manuals would be considered crucial. Nevertheless, it is not uncommon for nurses in both large and small health-care organizations to confirm that clinical educators are fewer in number than ever before, and that nursing policy and procedures manuals, if available at all, have often not been revised since the early 1990s.

As freedom-of-information legislation is fully implemented, it will be relatively easy for members of the public to gain access to organizational policies and guidelines of all types. When mistakes are made, it has been common for lawyers to require that clinical policies and procedures be produced as exhibits in legal proceedings. By the time a particular case comes to trial, the executives who made decisions to eliminate key positions and resources may have moved on to other things, but the public, through the courts, will hold the organization, and its clinical professionals, accountable nevertheless.

TYPES OF HEALTH-CARE STANDARDS

Safety and quality cannot be assessed or improved in the absence of standards. In manufacturing and production, it is relatively easy to establish standards for the appearance, composition, functionality, and safety of a product. As the organizational theorist Charles Perrow (1979) has pointed out, complexity in organizations arises from differences in raw materials, structure, technology, and the environment. In manufacturing processes, the rules are built into machines, whereas in "people-changing" organizations such as schools, prisons, and health services, professional workers engage in "search behaviour" to define and solve complex problems.

Health care organizations have been described as the most complex of all organizational types, sharing features with other knowledge-based industries, but having "non-standard" raw materials in the form of human beings with health problems and physicians who are "in" the organizations but not "of" them. The education that professionals receive prepares them to use facts, principles, and information in particular situations to make discretionary judgements. For all of these reasons, determining standards for health services and measuring their achievement is a complex task. As mentioned earlier in this chapter, it is the quality of discretionary judgement that distinguishes professional work. Box 19.1 presents an example that highlights the need for discretionary judgement by professionals.

There are many different types of standards, including professional, ethical, organizational, community, and legal standards, and their authority is derived from a variety of different sources.

PROFESSIONAL STANDARDS

Scientific knowledge and professional expertise arising from science and other forms of formal learning, and experience in the art of the profession, are the sources of authority for professional standards. The knowledge base for professional practice is evolving exponentially, making it a challenge for members of all health professions to maintain standards of practice. In the past, standards were agreed upon by groups of experts who established a consensus as to what constituted acceptable or "best practice" in a particular area. Today, all health professions seek to base their practice upon scientific evidence. For example, the treatment for stomach ulcers has

---

Box 19.1

DISCRETIONARY JUDGEMENT BY PROFESSIONALS: A CASE EXAMPLE

A generally accepted legal standard is that "approved practice" must be met in the clinical setting. However, meeting this standard may not be sufficient to defend an allegation of negligence. An example arose in the case of *Anderson v. Chasney* (1949), 57 Man.R. 343, (1949) 4 D.L.R.. 71 (C.A.), aff'd (1950) 4 D.L.R.. 223 (S.C.C.), where approved practice was met as cherry swabs were used, and not counted, during a tonsillectomy and adenoidectomy procedure. The child subsequently suffocated and died from a cherry swab which was left in the lower part of his throat.

A lawsuit by the parents was successful. The court recognized that "approved practice" (that is, not to count cherry swabs) had been met in the circumstances, but ruled that this practice did not meet a reasonable standard of care and therefore was insufficient to exonerate the defendants The message in this case is that, where a precaution could be used that would entail little expenditure of time and money, and where a person with no professional training in the area would judge the precaution to be reasonable, the failure to take the precaution may be found to be negligent, even where other professionals also fail to take care. The lesson to be learned is that a court may, in rare circumstances, disagree with the adequacy of a professionally agreed upon "approved practice" and impose a higher standard. It is clear from this case that blind adherence to generally accepted practices, even when these practices have been professionally approved, is not a substitute for professional diligence and thoughtful judgement.

It is interesting to note that in this case only the surgeon was found negligent. The court held that the surgeon has the duty to check and remove all sponges, and the surgeon had access to string swabs as well as nurses to count the cherry swabs but did not request either of these precautions, as this was not the usual practice of this surgeon or of this hospital. It should be noted that this case was heard almosy fifty years ago, and that a court today would likely make a finding of negligence against the hospital staff and the hospital as well as the surgeon, due to changes in the standard of care for organizations and professional staff.

---

changed since scientific studies showed that they are caused by a bacterium and not, as was previously thought, by stress. However, a series of replicated, randomized clinical trials or the equivalent must be conducted with unequivocal results before an evidence-based standard can be established or changed.

ETHICAL STANDARDS

The authority for ethical standards is derived from moral principles. The ethical standards of the health professions affirm the obligation to provide competent, safe, and respectful care. However, the ethical codes of the health professions have some differences in emphasis. For example, codes of ethics for physicians have traditionally emphasizd issues of loyalty and collegiality in relationships with other members of the same discipline to a greater extent than the codes of some other health professions.

Some health-care administrators assume positions of leadership after being credentialled in a regulated health profession, whereas others acquire education and experience in fields where licensing, regulation of practice, and peer review are not obligatory. In the 1950s and 1960s, efforts to professionalize the administration of health services led to the development of graduate programs in health-services administration in the United States, Canada, and some other western countries. Professional associations of health administrators were formed with the objective of raising standards. The Canadian College of Health Service Executives (CCHSE) is one such organization and, like its American counterpart, it has established criteria for membership and continuing-education requirements, and it conducts and sponsors various educational activities. Members of the college who pass its certification examination may use the designation Certified Health Executive (CHE).

The CCHSE has also adopted standards of ethical conduct. These state that health executives are expected to serve as moral agents whose management decisions and actions must be assessed for their consequences on individuals, organizations, and communities, and that they must accept responsibility for the results of these decisions and actions. Further, the standards affirm that health executives have responsibilities to their profession, and must ensure that their decisions are not compromised by conflict of interest (CCHSE, 1993).

Membership in the CCHSE is not a prerequisite to employment in the field of health-care administration. In fact, many individuals have been successful in obtaining positions in health administration without any credentials in a health discipline, much less in health services administration. Despite the absence of supporting evidence, it is widely believed that those who are experienced in managing industrial or business organizations have also acquired the necessary expertise to manage the health system. The lessons of organizational theory would suggest otherwise, but until the complexities and unique knowledge requirements for health services administration are more widely appreciated, clinical professionals will continue to face the dilemma of interpreting the importance and centrality of professional and ethical standards to leaders who come from disciplines where these are not a central feature.

ORGANIZATIONAL STANDARDS

The source of authority for organizational standards in a legally autonomous health care organization is the organization's governing board—which is morally and legally accountable for the actions of all employees, medical staff, and volunteers—and the officials appointed or hired by the board. Organizational standards usually take the form of policies and procedures that guide the core or predictable aspects of operations, and also

address the unexpected—providing, for example, for the diversion of am-
bulances when emergency departments are overburdened. Some organizational standards are written down; others are expressed less formally
through the norms of the corporate culture.

Standards in health organizations have both administrative and clinical dimensions. *Administrative* policies and procedures range from staff
recruitment and hiring practices to board policies regarding the investment of reserve funds. Most organizations conduct their operations
through various committees, and the memberships and terms of reference
for the main decision-making committees are also a matter of administrative policy, whether written or unwritten. Even a graphic representation of
organizational structure is a manifestation of administrative policy, illustrating and describing the various positions where authority and responsibility are vested.

Clinical policies and procedures are those that are evidence-based and
provide guidelines for clinical staff on best practices in caring for and
treating the organization's patients and clients. It is at the point where
administrative and clinical policies intersect that conflicts can occur
in health-service organizations. Health professionals often feel that the administrative perspective does not adequately acknowledge the complexities and demands of clinical care. Such concerns may be supported by
professional associations, which are accountable to the public for setting
standards and monitoring practice within the discipline. For example,
many professional nursing associations have criticized decisions by
health-service organizations to employ more multi-skilled, non-licensed
workers, and to delegate tasks to them that were formerly the responsibility of licensed professionals or paraprofessionals—decisions that are often
touted as a way of improving care, but which are implemented to avoid or
control labour costs. However, although professional associations may express concern and disapproval about organizational policies, they have no
direct influence or control over the directions taken by individual organizations.

Nurses and other health professionals often experience a sense of conflict between the expectations of their employing organizations and the
standards and ethical obligations of their professions. This problem is
exacerbated because traditional positions of leadership in clinical departments such as "vice president, nursing," "director of rehabilitation medicine," "manager of social work," and so on, have largely disappeared.
Individuals in these positions often assisted in interpreting and reconciling the standards and expectations of professional practice with the demands of the organization, informing colleagues with non-clinical
backgrounds of facts, issues, risks, and benefits of various courses of action. Today, although medical staff organizations tend to be constituted
much as they always have been, other professionally oriented departmental structures have, for the most part, been dissolved.

LEGAL STANDARDS

The authority for legal standards derives from the legislation enacted by federal and provincial legislatures, and from government regulations. As explained in Chapter 3, numerous legal requirements must be met by individual clinical professionals and health-service organizations. The requirements expressed in the form of criminal and civil law and in government regulations arise, in part, from the expectations and values of the community, or from professional organizations (Feeny, Guyatt & Tugwell, 1986; Rozovsky, 1987). However the legislative process is complex and time-consuming and for this and other reasons, not all community standards are enshrined in law.

COMMUNITY STANDARDS

The sources of authority for community standards are the commonly held values and expectations of the community. As our society becomes more pluralistic, it is sometimes difficult to determine what the standards of the community are at any given time. However, the emergence of consensus with respect to some community standards can be recognized in legislation that has been developed over the last several decades to protect the rights of workers, require employers to maintain standards of occupational health and safety, protect civil and human rights, and prevent discrimination. Many community values are not legislated and remain implicit until a specific instance of extreme behaviour by an individual or organization calls forth a spontaneous human response to a tragedy, atrocity, or crime. Box 19.2 describes a situation in which community standards were expressed.

As members of the community become empowered by better education and numerous sources of information, they use their power as stakeholders skillfully to make greater demands on both businesses and public-sector organizations. They expect value for their money and increasingly demand that products offered for sale be safe and dependable. Manufacturers are now held liable by the public for promoting and selling products that result in egregious consequences. In recent years, for example, tobacco companies have been held liable for health problems and costs incurred by people who became addicted to smoking, and manufacturers in various other industries have offered out-of-court settlements to individuals who might otherwise bring legal action.

Public organizations and governments are not immune to the effects of evolving community standards. For example, the forced sterilization of people with mental and physical handicaps, once legal, is now abhorred. Growing expectations for accountability by public officials can be seen in widespread support for such initiatives as the prosecution of war criminals, and investigations into the contamination of the blood supply in Canada. Public officials are increasingly held accountable for knowing what is available to be known, and acting responsibly with the best information at hand to make decisions that protect public safety.

Box 19.2
WHAT, THEN, MUST I DO?
BY CHRIS LEVAN

We live in such an entertainment culture that it is sometimes startling when real life walks up and knocks on our forehead. So comfortable with being an audience, no one expects to be dragged onto the main stage as a live actor. Last month, a rare moment arrived when the curtain went up on a drama of sharp edges. It evolved before our eyes on a steamy August flight from the East. The plane was packed. On cue, the aircraft's air conditioning sputtered and quit. Humidity rose, patience fell as the captain chirped that we'd just have to get up to cruising altitude for things to cool down.

The plane was taxiing to the runway —slowly. A few rows ahead, I could hear a young child crying. Then, during a pause in the white noise, the father's stern voice carried back, "Shut up kid!" This admonition was followed by several whacks from what must have been a rolled-up newspaper. Predictably, this brought more crying and whining from the child. The mother, who was holding an infant, tried to calm dad down, but he was not to be put off his tantrum. His biting language cut into the crying child and spilled over onto the baby. The cabin became deathly still. The abuse was obvious, and it was equally clear that this fellow was oblivious to the damage he was inflicting on his family.

"What, then, must I do?" That's what we were all thinking as we buried our doubts in the flight magazine. It's the keystone ethical question. All our faithful action depends on how we answer it.

My initial reaction was to hide behind Hollywood optimism. Maybe the troublesome man will just go away or offer a public apology. Could he be calmed by the in-flight movie? Where are the Promise Keepers when you need them?

Eventually the abusive father took himself to the washroom. Immediately, a woman who was sitting in front of the family turned to the young mother and explained how her husband was being very cruel. "You don't have to take this treatment. Don't let him speak like that to your children." When the man returned to his seat, the woman confronted him about his behaviour, telling him to get help and stop exacting the price of his anger from his children. The man smiled through his teeth and sulked in his seat.

I thought it was a noble attempt to name the injustice, and my heart applauded this woman's courage—a prophetess in our midst. Having been alerted by the other passengers, the purser also came back and repeated a similar message.

Alas, these interventions didn't seem to alter the fellow's temper. When it flared again, at the small child, another passenger in front of the couple turned and quietly said, "Look, it's a hard flight for all of us. How about I take the youngster for a walk down the aisle?" No rebuke, no angry muttering, just an offer to help relieve the strain.

A saint was on that plane. This older gentleman (the best and noble label to give him) kept the child happy and laughing for three hours as he walked in the aisle with him, taking a pass or two through the first-class cabin and visits to the flight deck. After the plane had landed the language began again. The gentleman quietly spoke to the father. "I guess we've all had a long night, haven't we? The little guy is doing his best." This seemed to cool down the hot flares in the father's eyes.

Thank you—to the saint and the prophet. You've taught me again that it's not enough to have ethical thoughts— eventually they have to get out into the light of day, casting out the shadows that would otherwise overtake us.

Reprinted with permission of the author. Dr. Chris Levan is an ordained minister and the principal of St. Stephen's College in Edmonton. He writes a regular column for *The Edmonton Journal*, where this piece first appeared on September 20, 1997.

Table 19.3

STANDARDS FOR NURSING ADMINISTRATION

Standard 1	Nursing administration plans for, and implements, effective and efficient delivery of nursing services.
Standard 2	Nursing administration participates in setting and carrying out of organizational goals, priorities, and strategies.
Standard 3	Nursing administration provides for allocation, optimum use of, and evaluation of resources, such that the standards of nursing practice can be met.
Standard 4	Nursing administration maintains information systems appropriate for planning, budgeting, implementing, and monitoring the quality of nursing services.
Standard 5	Nursing administration promotes the advancement of nursing knowledge and the utilization of nursing findings.
Standard 6	Nursing administration provides leadership that is visible and proactive.
Standard 7	Nursing administration evaluates the effectiveness and efficiency of nursing services.

Source: Canadian Nurses Association, *The Role of the Nurse Administrator and Standards for Nursing Administration* (Ottawa, ON: CNA, 1988), p. 10.

STANDARDS FOR NURSING ADMINISTRATION AND HEALTH SERVICES IN CANADA

Nursing as a profession has a proud history of attending to issues of quality. In 1986, a joint statement on nursing administration prepared by the Canadian Nurses Association, the Canadian Public Health Association, the Canadian College of Health Service Executives, the Canadian Hospital Association and the Canadian Association of University Schools of Nursing supported a position paper on the role of the nurse administrator, and provided impetus to the development and publication of a document entitled *The Role of the Nurse Administrator and Standards for Nursing Administration* (Canadian Nurses Association, 1988). These standards were intended to address nursing administration in all settings, and began with the premise that nursing administration is concerned with knowledge of systems, organizations, and groups as it relates to the environment, health, and nursing. The various levels of nursing administration are depicted conceptually on a continuum that distinguishes between the professional and corporate dimensions of nursing management. In the professional dimension, the nurse administrator demonstrates knowledge and expertise with respect to professional nursing, exerts leadership in relation to the discipline, and acts as an advisor on nursing matters. In the corporate dimension, she or he participates in the organization's administrative team for the purpose of determining policies, priorities, allocation of resources, and general management issues. Highlights from the seven standards in this document are summarized in Table 19.3.

MEASURING THE QUALITY OF HEALTH SERVICES IN CANADA

The objective of providing quality health care to patients and clients is one that is cited in the mission statement of every modern health-delivery system and organization. But how much quality is enough, and how much can the organization and society afford? In this age of restructuring, regionalization, and cost reduction, how does one know that the objective of quality care is being met?

The Canadian Council of Health Services Accreditation (CCHSA) administers a voluntary accreditation program that is organized and administered by health-care professionals independently of government agencies. Members of the CCHSA corporate board include representatives from the Canadian Hospital Association, Canadian Medical Association, Canadian Nurses Association, Canadian Long Term Care Association, the Royal College of Physicians and Surgeons of Canada, and the Canadian College of Health Service Executives. The accreditation program provides an effective means whereby health-care organizations can assess their level of performance against a set of nationally applied standards. Regular sur-vey visits provide an opportunity for external peer review and validation. The focus of the accreditation program is to identify ways in which the participating health organizations can continuously improve.

The mission of CCHSA is to promote excellence in the provision of quality health care and the efficient use of the resources of health-care organizations. The CCHSA has been responsible for accrediting hospitals and developing standards for health services in Canada since 1958, but over the past ten years the process for the accreditation survey has changed. Prior to 1988, the survey was directed primarily at hospitals and organized into departmental reviews (e.g., medicine, nursing, laboratory medicine, and environmental services). More recently, the focus has been patient-centred and the current survey documents are organized to review patient-care teams, as well as a number of support areas including information management, human resources and development, environmental management, and leadership and partnerships. Standards have also been developed to address specific types of health-care facilities; namely, acute care, long-term care, small community hospitals, cancer-treatment facilities, and community programs.

Preparation for an accreditation survey entails the completion of a set of documents that shows how the organization meets the accreditation standards. Surveyors assigned by the council review the completed survey documents, visit clinical areas, and talk with staff at all levels of the organization. At the end of the survey visit, they provide "debriefing" to the administrative staff regarding some of their impressions. As soon as possible following the visit, a written report is provided to the organization. Areas of excellence are recognized and recommendations are made as to how quality can be improved.

The CCHSA continually strives to update and modify its standards so that they accurately reflect current or best practice. At all stages of the review and development process, the CCHSA involves individuals from organizations and facilities across the country who are representative of, and experts in, a particular type of health service.

Since its standards were revised in 1995, the CCHSA has continued to encourage feedback about their applicability and the usefulness of the survey process as a whole, in a concerted effort to develop standards by which health-care services can evaluate their programs and continuously improve the quality of care to patients and clients.

EMERGING INFLUENCES ON HEALTH STANDARDS, MEASUREMENT, AND ACCOUNTABILITY

For many years, health organizations have looked to national bodies such as the CCHSA for guidance and a process for measuring their compliance with standards of care. Today, two other types of systems are influencing developments in the measurement of quality and accountability in the health-care field. These are the ISO9000 system of standards, and the Effectiveness Framework and Measurement approach developed by the Canadian Comprehensive Auditing Foundation.

INTERNATIONAL STANDARDS ISO9000

The ISO9000, originally used in industry, is being introduced in the health-care environment to serve as a quality-system framework in support of quality management. To be competitive and to maintain good economic performance, organizations need to employ increasingly effective and efficient systems. Such systems should result in continual improvements in quality, and increased satisfaction of the organization's customers and other stakeholders, including employees, owners, suppliers, and society.

Customer requirements are often described as part of the "specifications" of a product. However, if there are any deficiencies in the organizational systems that supply and support the product, specifications may not in themselves guarantee that a customer's requirements will be met. This concern has led to the development of quality-system standards and guidelines that complement relevant product requirements included in the technical specifications. The International Standards in the ISO9000 family are intended to provide a generic core of quality-system standards applicable to a broad range of industry and economic sectors.

International Standards are not intended to enforce uniformity in quality systems. The International Standards in the ISO9000 family describe what elements should be encompassed in a quality system, but not how these elements must be implemented. Needs vary from one organization to another, and the design and implementation of a quality system must be guided by the objectives, products, processes, and practices of each individual organization.

The ISO9000 Standards have been adopted by more than 200,000 companies and institutions in more than 114 countries throughout the world. Thirty-five hundred of these companies are located in Canada, 15,000 in the United States, and 300 in Mexico.

There are two primary reasons for implementing a quality-assurance system. The first is the need to gain certification in order to give a product a competitive edge, and in this regard it is worth noting that ISO is quickly becoming a necessity for companies doing business in Europe. The second reason is to gain the efficiencies that a quality-assurance system offers. ISO9004–1991—Part 2 is meant to be utilized by companies in the service sector that are not intending to become ISO certified, but are interested in planning and implementing a quality system. Although ISO9004–1991—Part 2 is not designed for the purposes of official registration, it offers the benefits of quality practices if it is implemented effectively. The key aspects of a quality system as listed in ISO9004–1991—Part 2 are summarized in Table 19.4.

The standards illustrated in this table closely match what is known as Total Quality Management, and are also comparable to the standards used by the CCHSA. It should be noted that a greater emphasis on customer-service over manufacturing-process standards is expected for the remainder of the series when the next ISO9000 revision is issued, in the year 2000.

A COMPARISON OF ISO9000 AND CCHSA STANDARDS

The ISO9000 and CCHSA systems of standards have certain similarities. The twenty elements of ISO9000 can be grouped into four broad categories: 1. management/leadership involvement; 2. process and system improvement; 3. process management and control; and 4. quality system support. The categories of standards in CCHSA include: 1. governance and leadership; 2. support systems; 3. patient/client-care processes; and 4. total quality improvement.

The two systems also have basic differences. ISO9000 requires documentation of specific elements, which serve as the framework of a quality system. This ensures consistency of processes and their outcomes, but does

Table 19.4

ELEMENTS OF ISO9004-1991—PART 2

1. **Management Responsibility**
   - **General**
   - **Quality Policy**
   - **Quality Objectives**
   - **Quality Responsibility and Authority**
   - **Management Review**

2. **Personnel and Material Resources**
   - **General**
   - **Personnel**
   - **Motivation**
   - **Training and Development**
   - **Communication**
   - **Material Resources**

3. **Quality System Structure**
   - **General**
   - **Service Quality Loop**

4. **Quality Documentation and Records**
   - **Documentation System**
   - **Documentation Control**

5. **Internal Quality Audits**

not necessarily guarantee the most desirable quality of the outcome. CCHSA standards, on the other hand, describe the process required to achieve desired patient outcomes, but do not ensure consistent adherence to processes across the system, as the accreditation process is more consultative than prescriptive.

In the ISO9000 system, standards related to consistency of processes are of extreme importance. Examples of the rigid format that is expected of an ISO9000-certified entity include requirements for regular internal audits, for formalized corrective- and preventive-action processes, and for regular management review of the quality system. Such requirements are intended to ensure continuous improvement, and non-compliance results in non-certification. Within CCHSA, a health facility may be granted 1. full accreditation; 2. accreditation with report or revisit; or 3. non-accreditation. In the CCHSA standard, the process of continuous improvement is suggested, but non-compliance does not necessarily result in non-accreditation.

Widespread implementation of ISO9000 standards in industry, along with government support for the standardization process, has generated interest in the system within the health-care field, and there has been much discussion in recent years about the relative merits of the CCHSA system versus the ISO9000 system for accrediting Canadian hospitals. While one standard is not necessarily better than the other, consistency in methodology among facilities may result in important efficiencies.

The challenge for the future may be to integrate the requirements of both the CCHSA and the ISO9000 standards systems for use in health-care settings. Work will be required to "translate" ISO9000 standards into the "business" of hospitals, but as the ISO9000 is meant to be applicable to any business or process, this goal should be achievable.

Box 19.3 describes the first ISO9000 registration in a Canadian hospital.

CCAF STANDARDS APPLIED TO A HEALTH ORGANIZATION

Many systems and methods are to be found in the area of total quality management and continuous quality improvement, but one that has great promise as a means of evaluating effectiveness of health care programs and services, and promoting accountability, is proposed by the Canadian Comprehensive Audit Foundation (CCAF).This system is based on a framework of twelve *attributes of effectiveness*: management direction, appropriateness, achievement of intended results, secondary impacts, costs, productivity, responsiveness, financial results, working environment, protection of assets, monitoring, and reporting. The framework is a tool that can be used by senior management to analyze and report to the governing authority through management representations on the performance of the organization "and about which the governing body can exact accountability from management in the exercise of its [overall] responsibilities" (CCAF, 1992, p. 11).

The Effectiveness Reporting Framework was first applied in a health organization in a pilot project at the Queen Elizabeth Hospital in Toronto. A booklet and videotape available from the CCAF about this project have since been used by other health organizations to assist them in implementing the framework. The following statement from this resource booklet makes an appropriate conclusion to this chapter:

> The tendency of Boards and their management has been to focus on financial and operational data, because this is the type of information most readily available and easily interpreted.... Nonetheless, there is an increasing public awareness that the Board has to be more closely involved in monitoring quality of care issues and the results achieved through the hospital's programs and services. We can see these concerns emerging everywhere—in government policy, in regulation and accreditation, and in the discussions and literature of the health-care professions. Yet, in these areas, information is much more limited. Steps must be taken to improve this situation (CCAF, 1992, p. 6).

SUMMARY

- Accountability for decisions and actions is the defining characteristic of professionalism, and of professional leadership and management.

Box 19.3
APPLICATION OF ISO9000
IN A CANADIAN HOSPITAL

In 1998, the Cranial, Osseointegration and Maxillofacial Prosthetic Rehabilitation Unit (COMPRU) at the Misericordia Hospital in Edmonton was awarded the first ISO9000 registration of a publicly funded health care program in Canada. Preparation for the ISO9000 assessment was carried out under the umbrella of the overall total quality improvement program within the corporate organization of the Caritas Health Group of which the Misericordia Hospital is a member.

According to Gail Hufty, the Business Leader responsible for the COMPRU program, extensive staff education was required, to prepare for the rigour of the standards requirements and to achieve the "buy in" necessary for the team to commit to the process and to be successful. She believes that the certification process made the unit more efficient and confident of the quality of its program.

Under the new system, practice is consistent, and when practice does not conform to the established standard operating procedures, the reasons are documented to provide a basis for continuous improvement. Records are current, and each member of the team is familiar with the responsibilities of other team members. These requirements facilitate continuity of service, enhance the satisfaction of patient and care providers, and support achievement of the clinical outcomes of the program.

The reference materials available to staff and for examination by ISO auditors include standards and expectations relating to the unit's operations. One section, for example, outlines the roles, responsibilities and training requirements for all personnel in the program (structure), while another describes how staff will behave in relation to patients and to each other (process).

The process standards empower individuals at all levels and in all roles in the COMPRU program to accept personal and professional accountability for acting when they believe something has gone wrong, or may be about to go wrong. If the actions of the person who identified the problem are not able to prevent or correct it, that person is expected to take it to a higher authority. These *process standards* reinforced by the *structural standards* that describe accountability and responsibility, support the identification and correction of problems in care that could lead to unsuccessful *outcomes* for patients. In fact, the standards for the program specify the desired patient outcomes and are "service oriented" towards patient satisfaction.

Although quality, rather than risk management, is emphasized in the ISO9000 standards system, the example of the COMPRU program illustrates how risks can be prevented through compliance to structure, process and outcome standards. When supported by the corporate culture, the involvement of individuals at all levels of the program, and appropriate training, standards that are in compliance with ISO9000 can help to increase patient and caregivers' satisfaction, and improve treatment outcomes.

- Accepting accountability entails making choices about responsibility, reasonableness, and responsiveness.
- Public expectations require health professionals to know the standards of their disciplines, and to practice according to those standards.
- Accounting for the quality of health-care programs and services is typically based on predetermined standards that are derived from various sources of authority.

- Many types of standards exist, including professional, ethical, organizational, legal, and community standards.
- Professional associations and organizations typically establish standards both as guidelines for practitioners and for accreditation purposes.
- A traditional framework for establishing criteria for the measurement of quality in health care consists of the identification of structure, process, and outcome standards. Such standards may pertain to a particular health discipline or to an entire program or organization.
- Health-service organizations in Canada may seek voluntary accreditation from the Canadian Council for Health Services Accreditation. Standards are developed and maintained by a governing board of health-care professional associations; health agencies are surveyed by competent health-care practitioners, and an accreditation report is produced. There are four levels of accreditation rating.
- The application of ISO9000 standards to the health field is in its infancy. These standards provide a quality-system framework for promoting continuous improvements in efficiency, effectiveness, and customer satisfaction. An advantage to this type of system is the requirement that errors or problems be immediately corrected, thus ensuring accountability and responsibility.
- Increasing emphasis is being given to measurement of health-care outcomes. The CCAF is an example of a tool for senior management in determining the effectiveness of organizational performance. Although not widely implemented in the health-care field, the system has potential for monitoring quality-of-care issues and achievement of results in programs and services.

FURTHER READINGS AND RESOURCES

Schmele, J.A. (1996). *Quality management in nursing and health care.* Albany, NY: Delmar. This book was written in response to the need for an "upper-level textbook for Quality Management courses in nursing and other health care disciplines" (p. xix). It contains strong historical and theoretical information as well as extensive references not found in the many practice- or business-oriented books on the subject. Incorporating international and interdisciplinary perspectives, the distinguished contributors to this edited book discuss key topics such as the role of consumers in quality management, accountability, the organizational context for quality, utilization management, infection control, and risk management. Although each chapter is designed to stand alone, thereby increasing the value of the book as a reference, common themes, values and trends are highlighted.

Sibbald, B. (1997). A right to be heard. *Canadian Nurse, 93*(10), 23–30. This is an account of the testimony given by a group of operating room nurses at the Winnipeg Health Sciences Centre Children's Hospital, at the inquest into the deaths of babies undergoing open-heart surgery under their care. The mortality rate for these babies was reported to be more than twice as high as the mortality rate for such babies at the Sick Children's Hospital in Toronto. Among the many issues that the nurses cited at the inquest were lack of surgical leadership and skill, lack of accountability, lack of communication, a confused chain of command, and most importantly, no way of assessing the open-heart surgical program (p. 28). This case illustrates how important it is for all registered and student nurses to understand the concepts discussed in this chapter, especially the concept of professional responsibility. Readers of Sibbald's article should consider the issues and underlying problems in the case, what other actions the nurses could have taken to make their voices heard, what organizational supports need to be in place to assist nurses and other health professionals to fulfil their professional responsibilities in relation to such cases, and what administrative actions might have prevented the infant deaths. The inquest concluded in October, 1998 and the report and recommendations arising from it will be instructive to all heath professionals and adminstrators.

REFERENCES

Anderson v. Chasney (1949), 57 Man.R. 343, (1949) 4 D.L.R.. 71 (C.A.), aff'd (1950) 4 D.L.R. 223 (S.C.C.)

Canadian Comprehensive Auditing Foundation (1992). *Reporting on effectiveness: The experience of the Queen Elizabeth Hospital.* Ottawa, ON: CCAF.

Canadian College of Health Service Executives (1993). *Standards of ethical conduct for health service executives.* Ottawa, ON: CCHSE. Mimeograph.

Canadian Nurses Association. (1988). *The role of nurse administrator and standards for nursing administration.* Ottawa, ON: CNA.

Donabedian, A. (1966). Evaluating the quality of medical care. *Milbank Quarterly,* 44 (Supplement, 3), 166–203.

Feeny, D., Guyatt, G. & Tugwell, P. (1986). *Health care technology: Effectiveness, efficiency and public policy.* Montreal, QC: Institute for Research on Public Policy.

Gardner, L., & Russell, A. (1989). *The concept of accountability: A discussion paper.* Edmonton, AB: Policy Development Division, Alberta Health. Mimeograph.

Levan, C. (1997). What, then, must I do? *Edmonton Journal,* September 20.

Perrow, C. (1979). *Complex organizations: A critical essay* (2nd ed.). Glenview, IL: Scott, Foresman and Company.

Rozovsky, L.E., & Rozovsky, F.A. (1987). How CCHA guidelines have evolved into law. *Health Care,* 29(8), 62.

Chapter 20

▼▼▼▼▼▼▼▼▼▼▼▼▼▼

Recruiting, Selecting, and Developing Staff

ARDENE ROBINSON VOLLMAN

KEY OBJECTIVES

In this chapter, you will learn that:

- Recruiting, selecting, and developing staff is one of the most vital duties of a nurse manager.
- Performance management of personnel can be examined through a human resources planning process, which involves the nurse manager in job analysis, including analysis of both job requirements and job performance.
- Job requirements are analyzed through job descriptions, performance standards, personnel policies, and market analysis, and form the basis for recruitment, selection, hiring, and orientation of staff.
- Job performance is measured through data collected about employee behaviour and achievements through supervisor, self, and peer appraisal.
- Performance development is enhanced by coaching, training, and staff development.
- Appraisal information and feedback are provided to employees as part of a developing work plan for performance maintenance and enhancement against which the next work cycle will be analyzed.

INTRODUCTION

Health is a labour-intensive industry; 75 to 80 percent of total Canadian health-care expenditures are allocated to human resources (Martin, 1990). Competition for funding in today's environment is intense, and health-care organizations are faced with the challenge of getting the highest performance from every employee so they may provide quality service and effect positive patient outcomes. Performance management is the process that supports this challenge; it is but one part of overall organizational management, a complex system that includes management of personnel, finance, material, and program components.

Recruitment and retention of qualified professional nursing staff is one of the key issues facing nurse managers today. To maintain quality care, nurse managers must focus efforts to meet this challenge. This task cannot be undertaken by nurse managers alone; it requires the efforts and talents of the entire organization. The nurse manager's participation is integral to its success, however. To be successful, managers must know where needs exist, where the vacancies are, how many vacancies need to be filled at the time, the best staff mix, and the budget implications of any choices being considered. Crucial to this analysis is the internal environmental scan which ensures that service-delivery component (nursing care) is consistent with the mission, vision, and goals of the agency.

A CONCEPTUAL FRAMEWORK FOR PERFORMANCE MANAGEMENT

Organizations today publish documents that outline their corporate vision, mission, values, goals, and objectives. These form the basis for organizational structures, which appear in the form of charts and statements of departmental roles, functions, and responsibilities.

Human resource management aims at improving the productive contribution of organizations while simultaneously attempting to attain other societal or personal objectives. Performance management provides an organization with an effective workforce, and, to achieve this purpose, involves analysis of how employers obtain, develop, utilize, evaluate, maintain, and retain the right numbers and types of workers (Werther, Davis, Schwind, & Das, 1990; p. 9). Within any organization, the four resources (personnel, finances, materials, and services or programs) are managed and evaluated through standardized procedures appropriate to each resource and to each organization. This system is illustrated in Figure 20.1. The personnel, or human resource management system, shown on the right side of the model, will be used as a framework for further discussion.

PERFORMANCE MANAGEMENT SYSTEM

Performance management is widely—and correctly—regarded as crucial to the successful achievement of an agency's strategic goals. Performance management means deploying a comprehensive, strategy-linked framework for measuring performance across the entire enterprise, and then using the results to make informed, evidence-based decisions about important issues and to identify and address areas where structural or process changes are needed (Kruzner & Trollinger, 1996).

The ultimate goal of performance management is to develop, sustain, and amplify service quality over the long term to deliver tangible benefits to the mission (patient outcomes). Kruzner and Trollinger (1996) identify

Figure 20.1

PERFORMANCE MANAGEMENT SYSTEM

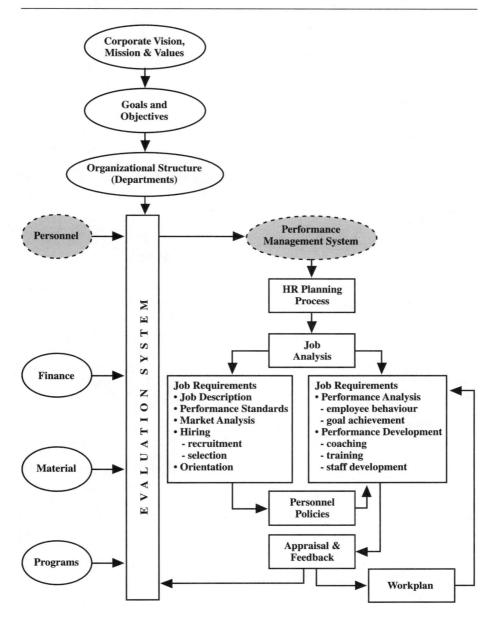

six key elements to successful performance management: strong executive support; linkages between performance measures and strategic goals; measures that cross traditional work boundaries; reward schemes to reinforce co-operation; performance measures tailored to special roles of each unit/ program; and focus of information on the user, not on technology. These elements are key to the organization's staff recruitment, selection, appraisal, and development functions.

Before any staffing action can be initiated, a nurse manager must be certain that the job analysis is current and relevant, and takes into account future needs. This total process is called the "human resource (HR) planning process," and it is not an easy operation to carry out in this rapidly changing health-care environment. Human resource planning generally begins with a thorough job analysis.

Job analysis is the process of collecting information about the work performed and the characteristics of the staff member (nurse) required to perform the role. Particularly where health settings are in transition, the nurse manager ignores this step at his or her peril. Job analysis has two components: *job requirements* and *job performance,* and both are mitigated by the personnel policies in place. As it is important for nurse managers to be familiar with these functions, they are examined in detail in the next sections of this chapter.

ANALYZING JOB REQUIREMENTS

Analysis of job requirements has several stages (see Figure 20.1). The first three aspects of this task—the development of job descriptions and performance standards, and market analysis—are usually co-operative efforts at the managerial levels and not the prerogative of a single nurse manager. For example, some facets of job descriptions for staff nurses may be part of the whole contract negotiation between unions and management. However, each nurse manager needs to be familiar with these three aspects because some job requirements are specific to departments or units.

JOB DESCRIPTION, PERFORMANCE STANDARDS, AND MARKET ANALYSIS

An obvious beginning in the analysis of job requirements is to consider education and prior experience needed for the job; these lead to a clear, detailed *job description.* It is important to consider whether the proposed description is realistic and reasonable, and whether it takes into account the direction of the organization, of current health-care issues, and of the health professions.

The human resource department can help the manager determine if the job descriptions and the unit's requirements "fit" with *performance standards* supplied by professional organizations and other similar institutions; often these have legal implications. Managers must remember also that every newly hired staff member has the potential to affect patient outcomes as well as the success of the work team and the organization. Table 20.1 shows five steps a nurse manager should consider as he or she prepares for

---

Table 20.1
PREPARATION FOR PERFORMANCE MANAGEMENT SYSTEM REVIEW

---

1. Set the organizational context.

- Review organizational and departmental documents, economic and job forecasts, and trends in service delivery.
- Survey the literature regularly.
- Maintain an active professional network to use in benchmarking and planning activities. (Vaziri, 1992)

2. Analyze the job.

- Describe what the work seeks to accomplish.
- Describe the necessary employee activities or behaviour required by the job.
- List the equipment used to perform the job.
- Determine factors in the work environment deemed essential for acceptable job performance. (Dolan & Schuler, 1987)

3. Determine job requirements.

- Collate and review job descriptions in light of the job analysis, provincial standards of practice, and special professional interest groups' recommended guidelines.
- Articulate the human requirements necessary to perform the functions of the job.
- Assess the efficacy of the systems internal to the organization that disseminate information and communicate expected standards.

4. Examine environmental influences.

- Review policies, regulations, procedures, and standards of care.
- Ensure that they are current, relevant, realistic and readily available to staff.
- Inspect facilities, resources, and equipment to ensure they are maintained and available for staff to fulfil their roles effectively.
- Assess whether staff have opportunities to learn.
- Review staff development and training processes.

5. Consider legal implications.

- Review and understand the employment contracts, labour codes, and other relevant regulations.
- Ensure that the components of the performance management system are written, job-related, objective, easily understood, and up-to-date, with provision for staff input at all stages. (Martin & Bartol, 1991)

a review of the performance management system before staff changes are made. If these steps are done well at this stage, they also will provide a framework for developing evaluation criteria that will be needed in later stages of performance management (e.g., appraisal, evaluation, feedback).

At each phase of this preliminary preparation process, a nurse manager will be challenged to articulate his or her own philosophies and compare these with the organization's performance management practices and values. If discrepancies come to light, the manager will need either to resolve them by acting within the organizational structure to effect change (a lengthy process) or, after discussion with senior management colleagues and staff, to work within the present system while acknowledging its shortcomings and continuing to advocate for administrative changes. Reviewing and analyzing the performance management system gives a nurse manager an understanding of the organization's goals, values, structure, and personnel policies relevant to the process. This will assist in the recruitment, selection, performance analysis, and performance development functions of the management role.

Once employment needs have been established and the environment assessed, *market analysis* is the next step. Supply can be determined by the number of applicants available. Supply includes new graduates from local basic or degree nursing programs or from advanced certificate or postgraduate nursing preparation, nurses who are moving into the area, nurses who may be unemployed or under-employed, former staff who have been laid off, and former staff who dropped out of full-time work for family or personal reasons and now wish to return. Relocation costs to bring in nurses from other areas can be high, so recruitment from other locales is frequently not conducted until the local market has been tapped or exhausted.

Knowing what and who you need, matching person-position disparities, determining short- and long-term requirements, and knowing where nurses can be found are the foundations of human resource planning. The next step in analyzing job requirements involves finding the right people for the right positions.

Once these steps have been taken, the manager can proceed with *hiring* (recruitment, search, selection) and *orientation*. As these two stages have a major impact for a nurse manager, each is examined in more detail.

HIRING

The process of hiring staff includes both recruiting applicants and selecting the one(s) who best fit your needs. The success or failure of a manager is often measured by the results achieved in these two phases of the whole performance management process.

Recruitment

Recruitment is a marketing process whereby qualified and interested people are attracted to an agency for employment in a manner that facilitates the work of the organization. It represents a significant part of the whole human resource planning process; selection of qualified personnel can only be as good as the recruitment process allows.

Recruitment is not an easy process. Nursing work can be highly specialized. Turnover is expensive. Under- or over-utilization of staff impacts morale, job satisfaction, and the future recruiting efforts of the organization. Errors in judgement can have a negative impact on the work, goals, and survival of the organization.

Because recruitment can be so expensive, efforts to retain staff should be considered (Norton & Crissman, 1992). Analyzing reasons for turnover (e.g., through exit interviews and employment data systems) is an important strategy. Has everything been done to retain those excellent nurses already in the agency? Retraining or adapting existing staff through remediation, inservice, or education is an avenue that can be explored within the context of staff development. Job restructuring or modification is another means.

As part of a long-term recruitment program, applicant sources outside the organization must be developed. Besides advertising to attract those nurses who are currently not in the work force or who are employed elsewhere, universities and college nursing programs should be regarded as important sources of new nurses. The clinical placement of students on a manager's unit provides opportunities to observe them and assess their potential as future employees. Other external sources include professional conferences, where word of mouth and direct recruitment can be effective strategies. And finally, current employees may be encouraged to use their professional contacts to recruit new staff members.

Recruitment efforts can be evaluated through two basic questions: Does the recruitment program attract good applicants? Do those nurses selected become good employees? When you interview, ask applicants how they heard about your agency. If you keep this information on file and review it regularly, you will gain valuable information about which strategies were effective, and how those nurses fared in terms of job performance and satisfaction.

Selection

Once a pool of applicants is generated, the selection process begins. Selection is defined as the process by which an identified candidate is chosen for a particular position. It is a focal point of the human resource planning process, and represents one of the most visible outcomes. Selection processes are intended to investigate applicants' values to see if these are congruent with the professional practice environment. As well, they are means of exploring the clinical expertise of applicants.

Pre-screening, a first stage of the selection process, is accomplished through review of résumés, application forms, and biographical data. Occasionally, a pre-screening interview is conducted in anticipation of a more formal interview and reference checking.

Although many applicants send or bring résumés at the time they apply for a position, using an application form provides three main advantages: it can be used to determine whether a candidate meets the job specifications by focusing on pertinent information (e.g., job history with dates) that may be missed in a résumé; it can be analyzed quickly and in detail and compared with those of other applicants to rank candidates for the next phase of the selection process; and it can be used in preparation for the selection interview (Norton & Crissman, 1992). Applicants are often asked to sign a statement attesting to the veracity of their claims, allowing the manager to verify the information on the understanding that, if hired, they may be dismissed should any information they have provided be proven false.

Large amounts of complex information may be generated during this stage, and electronic checklists, spreadsheets, and databases (in increasing order of technological complexity) can be useful for collecting and analyzing such information (Bowles, 1995).

The interview is the most common process for staff selection and is considered by many to be the only method by which the personal characteristics and true nature of the candidate can be accurately identified. An interview takes place after pre-screening has been completed. The usefulness of the interview process depends on good preparation and sound implementation.

Many selection interviews are conducted by teams—both to spread the responsibility for decisions, and also to allow team members to whom a candidate will later be accountable to have some say in the process. Norton and Crissman (1992) advise that the lead interviewer should plan the process. In the case of a staff nurse position, this lead interviewer is most often the head nurse or unit manager. When hiring staff from disciplines other than nursing, the wise nurse manager ensures the selection committee represents a cross-section of relevant disciplines.

Norton and Crissman (1992) advise that the applicant's job history be reviewed during the interview. Questions that address specifics in the job description and performance standards should be prepared and assigned to members of the team. Many questions can be standardized if several applicants are being interviewed for the same (or a similar) position.

The lead interviewer has several responsibilities: training members of the interview team; developing standardized interview questions and/or practice scenarios; screening applicants by telephone or in person; determining who should ask what questions and when; comparing internal and external applicants; checking references; and following up with all applicants, successful or not. As well, human resource departments often have guidelines related to interviews, and these should be honoured.

According to Norton and Crissman (1992), an effective interviewer should create an open communication atmosphere, deliver standardized questions consistently, avoid questions or conversation not related to the applicant's ability to do the job (e.g., marital status, religion), maintain control over the interview, be a good listener and take good notes, keep

Box 20.1

COMMON QUESTIONS FOR
CHECKING REFERENCES

1. Can you give me an example of how [the candidate] approached new assignments?
2. What adjectives would you use to describe the interactions of [the candidate] with (1) colleagues, (2) clients, (3) others [as relevant]?
3. How often was [the candidate] absent from work?
4. How frequently was sick time taken? Were there any noticeable patterns in absences?
5. What types of training and development were undertaken while [the candidate] was employed by you? Was this at [the candidate's] initiative, or at the suggestion of the supervisor? Who bore the costs?
6. What are the reasons why [the applicant] left your employ? Would you rehire this person?
7. Is there anything you would like to add to what you've already told me?

conversations flowing without leading the candidate, appropriately interpret non-verbal cues, and ask good follow-up questions to evaluate the use of higher level cognitive skills (p. 274).

Unstructured interviews lack consistent frameworks and are difficult to analyze, particularly when there are several applicants, as there are often no predetermined response criteria or recording systems. For this reason, structured or focused interviews are more popular. Individual interviewers may still be biased, but bias can be minimized by using an interview panel, by using standardized questions, and by scoring the applicant against predetermined criteria that are consistent with the job description (Bowles, 1995).

Be wary of first impressions! Ootim (1995) suggests three factors make impressions on interviewers: appearance (55% of the impression made), voice (38%), and actual words (7%). These impressions are created in the first four minutes of the interview and, at times, may contaminate the process, preventing fair review of an applicant.

Always debrief the team immediately following each interview, and meet to rank all applicants following completion of all interviews. Do not rush to make the decision until you have reviewed and investigated thoroughly the references provided by all applicants.

Checking references, which is increasingly done by phone, takes skill and intuition on the part of the manager. Since the applicant provides the names of references, it can be assumed that these people generally will be favourable to the applicant. The nurse manager can, however, couch questions in such a way as to delve below the surface of clichés and standard responses. A checklist of standard questions is a valuable tool (see Box 20.1). However, it is critical to be aware of cues, so that probes can be used to solicit more information or specific examples of practice. Often, asking for examples in your request for specific descriptions of behaviours can elicit important information about an applicant's characteristic responses in usual work-related situations.

It is generally not acceptable practice to contact references other than those provided. If an applicant requests that his or her current employer not be contacted, this request should be respected. Those who provide references are also becoming aware of the legal consequences of dishonesty (e.g., giving an excellent reference to rid themselves of a problem employee can lead to a lawsuit for negligence). As a result, human resource departments rarely disclose more than dates of employment, so personal references become a most valuable source of information for the manager.

Once a decision has been made, the nurse manager will collaborate with the human resource department to make an offer of employment and do the necessary administrative work to support the appointment process. Once the job offer has been successful, the nurse manager should advise unsuccessful candidates of the decision. Those not offered a job may want feedback from the interviewer about their performance during the process, so the nurse manager should be prepared to offer some examples of what they did well and what they might strengthen before their next opportunity. The nurse manager should also find out if unsuccessful candidates would like their applications kept on file for future openings.

ORIENTATION

A complete introduction to the organization and the work unit are essential to ensure that a new employee will be both productive and satisfied. Orientation is more than simply a checklist of meetings, seminars, work-relevant activities, and so forth; it sets the stage for future job success and is, therefore, a critical component of the total job requirement process. A good orientation will reduce the possibility of errors, save time, and present clear and realistic job expectations. The new employee will begin to understand the technical, social, and cultural aspects of the agency and the unit.

The organization, usually through its human resources or personnel department, is responsible for a generic orientation that presents the agency, its mission, vision, goals, and objectives. The structure and the people who form the upper administration are introduced. Physical facilities, regulations, policies, and so on are presented, and often employees are given a handbook to keep. Benefits, pay issues, vacations, and probationary periods are discussed.

Once the new employee is introduced to his or her supervisor and co-workers, the on-job orientation begins. The nurse manager must be intimately involved in seeing that it goes well. Relevant job experiences, tasks, and activities should be explained, and training, if required, should be offered. As well, the social side of unit life should be introduced in the interests of team development. A "buddy system" is frequently used to complement the supervisor's role in orientation. An experienced manager knows, however, that delegating the entire orientation to a co-worker may interfere with development of positive relationships with a new staff member.

As with all aspects of management, an evaluation process should be in place to ensure the new employee has all the information needed to do the job well. Sometimes information given at formal meetings in the early phases is not recalled; it may have seemed unimportant or irrelevant at the time. An orientation team should survey new staff to make certain that the process went smoothly, information was complete and relevant, and that the new employee feels satisfied.

During the probationary period, the manager must also monitor the process by taking time to answer questions, provide feedback, and offer relevant information or support. This should not simply involve rushing past a new employee and asking, "Is everything okay?"; instead, time should be set aside to build rapport and let questions and suggestions emerge. This investment will pay off later in a staff member who feels welcome and nurtured.

JOB PERFORMANCE

In addition to analysis of job requirements and attraction of new staff, the nurse manager is constantly involved in the ongoing analysis of job performance. (See Figure 20.1, noting the box to the right.) Analysis of job performance is required for all employees as well as for new staff, although appraisal and feedback (evaluation) for new workers usually take place more frequently during the orientation and probationary phases of employment.

PERFORMANCE ANALYSIS

The process of monitoring job performance begins with performance analysis (Werther et al., 1990). It is a process of gathering, analyzing, evaluating, and communicating information about how an employee's behaviours and subsequent outcomes of those behaviours contribute to the achievement of corporate goals and compare to managerial expectations or established standards of practice.

Performance analysis can be formal or informal. Examples of formal analysis are the end-of-probation or appraisal interview for new employees, and annual performance evaluations for long-term employees. Informal performance analysis may take the form of words of praise to commend a staff member for a task well done, or a reprimand to someone for failing to follow a policy or procedure. However, all informal feedback should be documented for your records and to help recollection when preparing formal appraisals.

Nurse managers play a key role in ensuring optimal employee performance and, thereby, effective client care. The Canadian Nurses Association (1988) states that nurse managers should provide for "the allocation, optimum use of, and evaluation of resources such that the standards of nursing practice can be met" (p. 12). Nurse managers must understand clearly the need, purposes, and developmental function of performance analysis and its relationship to other human resource functions (e.g., compensation, benefits).

The purpose for which performance analysis is used has significant implications for nurse managers (see Table 20.2). The evaluative and monitoring functions of performance appraisal are retrospective in nature. The nurse manager judges and assesses the value of the staff member's performance in light of previous behaviours and outcomes. Consequently, the role of the staff member in this process is passive or defensive. On the other hand, the developmental function of performance appraisal is prospective. The appraisal is no longer the sole territory of the manager; staff play an integral role to make the exercise interactive and meaningful.

Many nurse managers—both new and experienced—are intimidated by job performance analysis. It takes time, it generates discomfort when one sits in judgement of another, it raises barriers against rapport, and it requires skills for which many managers feel ill-prepared.

PERFORMANCE DEVELOPMENT

Mastery of the performance development aspect should excite nurse managers if they aspire to excellence both for themselves and for their staff. Performance development is the process of enhancing employee productivity and work quality through motivation and education in response to the strategic needs of the whole organization. A developmental approach to performance improvement will foster acceptance of change and a willingness or confidence to explore new practice options; this is essential today because of the prevailing climate of fiscal constraint. In addition, with changing work structures, managers may have an extraordinary number of individuals to supervise and appraise, making the required attention to detail an impossible task.

Blitzer, Petersen, and Rogers (1993) identified several benefits of a development-oriented improvement system that help to improve individual and corporate performance. Such a system:

- Makes people feel uniquely valuable by creating an environment where staff members feel comfortable expressing their emotions or opinions and by rewarding ideas, efforts, and achievements.
- Makes people feel competent by helping to monitor their progress towards achieving established goals and helping them to develop through mistakes.
- Helps people feel secure by openly communicating what is happening in the organization.
- Empowers people when a nurse manager demonstrates awareness of and interest in their personal development goals and finds opportunities for them to expand their horizons.
- Connects people to the team when the nurse manager enhances feelings of acceptance, appreciation, and respect among staff.

Table 20.2

PURPOSES OF PERFORMANCE ANALYSIS

---

1. **Evaluate individuals, teams, and programs**	**Document, communicate, and use information about employee performance to support administrative decisions.**
2. **Develop and train staff**	**Identify areas for employee growth and recommend ways of improving performance or enhancing the potential for performance.**
3. **Monitor work quality**	**Collect and analyze data in order to validate that selection procedures and training and development programs are maintaining acceptable standards of performance.**

Performance development (See Figure 20.1) is the ongoing relationship between individual staff members and their employing institutions. Short-term development, often referred to as training, is usually dominated by the building of knowledge, skill, and expertise, while longer-term development responds to an individual's goals and aspirations as well as to the institution's anticipated strategic requirements.

An example of training would be a hospital that introduces a new technology on the antenatal unit and provides inservice education and on-job coaching for staff who are affected by the change. New employees are provided with training as part of orientation. Regular employees may need to show proof of ongoing training, such as recertification. As well, there may be staff-development initiatives; for example, when a hospital introduced a new policy to give preference to advance practice nurses for promotions to head nurse, it was necessary to examine support packages for nurses wishing to continue their education at the Master's level.

Training and development can take the form of formal and informal learning through lectures, courses, books, audio-visual methods, electronic means (e.g., access for staff to the world-wide web or to interactive CD-ROM technology), and distance or correspondence courses. Experiential development through on-job coaching and job rotation can be informal or formal, depending on the mentorship available and the institutionalization of such programs. In any event, job assignments that allow and encourage performance of new skills and competencies is an integral component of the development process. A transfer of learning from theoretical to practical can be fostered through appropriate recognition, monitoring, evaluation, and reward of positive performance. Evaluation of training and development must be a continuous process, not a one-time terminal event, if effectiveness of learning is to be facilitated.

Nurse managers who are purchasing or planning a development or training program must evaluate the program carefully to determine whether the contents suit the employee profile and the needs of the agency. Among the components to be considered are: goals and objectives; breadth of coverage of content; depth of information; training methods used; sequencing of activities; evaluation procedures; monitoring and feedback systems; resources required; cost; and temporal considerations.

APPRAISAL AND FEEDBACK

Appraisal and feedback form a vital part of the total performance management system—and they are frequently problematic for nurse managers. Review of the job analysis steps and strategies can help managers address these points, which are often affected by the complex nature of nursing work. Ambiguous definitions and descriptions for job requirements and job performance threaten the reliability and validity of measurement (Brown, 1988; Carroll & Schneier, 1982; Stone & Meltz, 1988). Clear objectives lead to satisfactory implementation, ease of subsequent measurement, and straightforward performance review and analysis. Ambiguous goals and tasks result in conflict and disagreement.

In many cases, conclusions about performance are affected by such factors as time lag between a nursing intervention and client outcome, involvement of multiple personnel, and social characteristics of the environment. For example, a single task may entail many activities and have several outcomes. Therefore, the need for appropriate data collection, documentation, and communication is central to the effectiveness of any system. Performance analysis strategies, however difficult to construct, can be devised to meet the needs of the organization to evaluate performance, identify performance gaps, reward exemplary staff, and plan development strategies for individuals and the organization.

In general, managers need to assess two aspects of performance: employee behaviour and achievement of goals (Goodale, 1992). The nurse manager should determine not merely what took place, but what problems ensued and what actions a staff member took to try to overcome them (Burdett, 1988). Goals, objectives, and performance can then be placed in context.

Employees may be measured or compared against themselves, other employees, or some absolute standard (Dolan & Schuler, 1987). When a manager states "X is an excellent employee" it means X is being compared with others; "X has improved herself" means the nurse has done better on some criterion than at the last performance appraisal; "X meets the job requirements" means that, compared to the standard set for that task or role, X meets the criteria. These statements contain different underlying conceptual or philosophical frameworks and require different methods of measurement.

In most organizations, a combination of methods are used. In health service settings, using a multi-faceted approach will make it easier for a nurse manager to provide staff with a reliable and valid performance analysis that addresses most dimensions of the complex and dynamic nature of nursing work.

Gathering information for appraisal and feedback is an ongoing process. A file system of some sort should be put in place that will allow the manager to record critical incidents and other anecdotal notes (e.g., instances where positive or critical feedback was given) that illustrate staff behaviours relating to the tasks and activities inherent to the job. This may be an informal system for the satisfactory staff member, or more formal if specific documentation is required for disciplinary purposes (see also Chapter 26). Nevertheless, both types of file systems can provide an effective paper trail in the event that a performance-related issue is challenged by a staff member (Scholtes, 1993).

Information should be collected from as many sources as possible. In many health institutions, systems track quantitative data on individuals (e.g., attendance), work units, and the department. Getting input from multiple sources provides a larger data base for decision-making and enhances the reliability of job performance data, by making it possible to capture the essence of nursing work. Client satisfaction and unsolicited "beefs and bouquets" from professional colleagues within and external to the workgroup are helpful data sources. Self-appraisal and peer review are two approaches that might be considered.

SELF-APPRAISAL

As organizations become flatter, managers need to encourage self-appraisal, personal and team goal setting, and team accountability. Self-appraisal is becoming a common component of performance analysis and part of the trend towards participative management. It enhances staff involvement in and commitment to performance improvement.

Self-appraisal can be beneficial if the performance-appraisal process in the organization focuses on professional development and personal growth. Managers can ensure the success of a self-appraisal process by:

- Maximizing the amount of performance standard and feedback information given to staff.
- Fostering an environment that affirms critical feedback as useful to the improvement process.
- Balancing professional development and personal growth needs of employees with the organization's mission and corporate goals.
- Mentoring, coaching, and role modelling in order to instil realism into staff opinions of their skills, capabilities, and contributions.
- Making self-appraisal a daily process.

PEER REVIEW

Peer review is the process of having work performance analyzed and evaluated by co-workers or colleagues of equal rank against established criteria or competencies. It is based on the principles of professional autonomy, accountability, and collegiality. While there are both advantages to and concerns about the peer-review process, peer review in nursing can be an excellent method of quality control and consumer protection (Gerstner, McAllister, Wagner, & Kraus, 1988).

The degree to which staff members are comfortable with the peer-review process depends upon the history of the work unit, the extent to which it has developed as a team, and the level of trust staff members have in each other and in their supervisor. Effective interpersonal communication is the foundation of a constructive appraisal process; reciprocal responsibilities of team members and supervisors are key factors in achieving the ultimate goals of performance review. Although the potential advantages of peer and self ratings are well-documented in the literature, they remain largely under-utilized as tools for responding to the performance pressures of the 1990s (Bader & Bloom, 1992; Buhalo, 1991).

DOCUMENTING PERFORMANCE

The role of documentation in assessment is critical: the benefits to the organization of well-documented performance analyses are great, the risks of poor documentation are high. The trend for employers to use performance analysis data when making significant human resource decisions creates the potential for conflict and misunderstanding between employer and staff, and is a factor in the trend towards increasing litigation (Martin & Bartol, 1991). In general, employers are better able to mount convincing arguments for the legitimacy of their actions when they have performance analysis documentation on file. Since employers can also be legally challenged on the basis of what nurse managers write in staff members' performance appraisals, potential problems can be minimized if statements are based on performance criteria that are concise, objective, and easily understood by all parties involved (Saxe, 1988), and are openly addressed by both parties.

The nurse manager's written comments must reflect a thorough, clear, and precise analysis of the staff member's performance strengths and weaknesses. Generalizations tend to take weaknesses out of context and over-emphasize them; ambiguous wording can lead to an inaccurate and incomplete summary of performance. When a behaviour occurs once, it is an incident; twice is a coincidence; three times is a pattern (Smith, 1993). The activity, task, or responsibility under discussion should be part of an observed pattern, not an isolated incident or a one-time uncharacteristic behaviour (Ilgen & Feldman, 1990).

Cyr (1993) outlines a seven-step process to guide a nurse manager in preparing written comments:

1. Select and focus on a job activity, an individual, or an observable responsibility or task.

2. Indicate the degree to which this activity, responsibility, or task is performed.

3. Describe when or where the observed performance happens, with whom it happens, under what circumstances, and during what type of activity.

4. Suggest an influential factor that positively or negatively affects the activity, responsibility, or task in question. These factors may stem from the individual staff member, the organization, or the external environment. Be careful not to make inaccurate inferences or draw false conclusions.

5. Point out trends in the improvement, decline, or maintenance of job performance levels.

6. Give an example—a "representative instance" of a situation—that involves the activity, task, or responsibility under discussion and that is drawn from an observed trend in job performance.

7. Show consequences—short- and long-term outcomes—so that the nurse sees the work in terms of its effect on others and how it contributes to overall organizational success.

COMMUNICATING JOB PERFORMANCE

The formal appraisal interview is the principal component of the performance appraisal process—and one of a nurse manager's most challenging experiences (McAlister, 1993). Nurse managers must prepare carefully for this interview. If it is not conducted properly, staff members will not know any more about where they stand after the session than they did before, and opportunities to promote or enhance professional development and personal growth will be missed.

The appraisal interview is the culmination of informal meetings with an individual, as well as informal and formal positive and critical feedback given since the previous performance interview. There should be no surprises in this session! By the time the formal appraisal interview is held, both the nurse manager and the staff member should have a good idea of how things have gone, or are going, in relation to their personal and unit objectives.

Taking time to do a complete analysis of the employee in relation to the job enables a nurse manager to assess better the training and development needs of the employee and of the work unit itself. Training and development should focus not only on the employee's weaknesses, they should focus also on the employee's strengths and interests, and on corporate goals and objectives.

The outcome of this performance analysis leads to the development of a personalized work plan for the coming months (see Figure 20.1). The work plan provides a road map for employee and team activities in performance maintenance and enhancement, and becomes the basis for future performance reviews.

CONCLUSION

In the health sector, where staffing costs can reach 70 to 80 percent of an agency's total budget, it is vital that personnel perform optimally. It is, therefore, critical for nurse managers to allocate dollars, time, and energy where they can have the most impact on organizational effectiveness and efficiency. A performance management system that reflects the organization's mission, vision, values, goals, and objectives as well as recognizing shifting paradigms in management and organizational processes and structures is key to ensuring optimum health outcomes for clients.

SUMMARY

- Performance management starts with a human resources planning process and careful job analysis.
- Job analysis has two parallel aspects: job requirements and job performance.
- Job requirements involve development of job descriptions and performance standards, followed by a careful market analysis. Hiring is the next stage, and involves recruitment and selection. Orientation follows.
- Once people are in place, analysis of job performance of individuals, work teams, and programs is instituted and, ideally, conducted on a regular basis. Job performance review includes performance analysis, documentation, communication, training, and development.

FURTHER READINGS AND RESOURCES

Brooks, S. B., Olsen, P., Reiger-Kligys, S., & Mooney, L. (1995). Peer review: An approach to performance evaluation in a professional practice model. *Critical Care Nursing Quarterly, 18*(3); 36–47. Role expectations of staff nurses are changing and nurses must become empowered and actively involved in facilitating change, rather than having change foisted on them. This article provides graphic representation of a practice model as well as suggested forms for use of performance evaluation.

Dunn, M. G., Norby, R., Cournoyer, P., Hudec, S., O'Donnell, J., & Snider, M. D. (1995). Expert panel method for nurse staffing and management. *Journal of Nursing Administration, 25*(10); 61–7. The method described in this article represents a bold new approach for the identification of nurse staffing requirements and the management of resources.

REFERENCES

Bader, G. E., & Bloom, A. E. (1992). How to do peer review. *Training & Development, 46*(6), 61–2, 64–6.

Blitzer, R. J., Petersen, C., & Rogers, L. (1993). How to build self-esteem. *Training & Development, 47*(2), 58–60.

Brown, R. D. (1988). *Performance appraisal as a tool for staff development.* San Francisco: Jossey-Bass.

Bowles, N. (1995). Methods of nurse selection: A review. *Nursing Standard, 9*(15), 25–9.

Buhalo, I. H. (1991). You sign my report card I'll sign yours. *Personnel, 68,* 23.

Burdett, J. (1988). Results driven performance appraisal. *The Human Resource, 5*(1), 19–21.

Canadian Nurses Association. (1988). *The role of the nurse administrator and standards for nursing administration.* Ottawa: Canadian Nurses Association.

Carroll, S. J., & Schneier, C. E. (1982). *Performance appraisal and review systems.* Glenview, IL: Scott, Foresman.

Cyr, R. (1993). Seven steps to better performance appraisals. *Training & Development, 47*(1), 18–9.

Dolan, S. L., & Schuler, R. S. (1987). *Personnel and human resource management in Canada.* St. Paul, MN: West.

Gerstner, M., McAllister, L., Wagner, P. L., & Kraus, C. (1988). Peer review. In S. E. Pinkerton & P. Schroeder (Eds.), *Commitment to excellence: Developing a professional nursing staff* (pp. 199–209). Rockville, MD: Aspen.

Goodale, J. G. (1992). Improving performance appraisal. *Business Quarterly, 57*(2), 65–70.

Ilgen, D. R., & Feldman, J. M. (1990). Performance appraisal: A process focus. In L. L. Cummings & B. M. Staw (Eds.). *Evaluation and employment in organizations* (pp. 1–57). Greenwich, CT: JAI Press.

Kruzner, D., & Trollinger, R. (1996, Nov. 11). Performance management vital in implementing new strategies. *Oil and Gas Journal,* pp. 66–72.

Martin, D.C., & Bartol, K.M. (1991). The legal ramifications of performance appraisal: An update. *Employee Relations Law Journal, 17*(2), 257–286.

Martin, J.-C. (1990). Executive in Residence, Faculty of Administration, University of Ottawa, personal communication, Oct. 10, 1990.

McAlister, J. (1993, April). Appraisal interviews do's and don'ts. *Supervisory Management,* p. 12.

Norton, S. D., & Crissman, S. (1992). Staffing, recruiting, and selecting. In P. J. Decker & E. J. Sullivan (Eds.), *Nursing administration: A micro/macro approach for effective nurse executives* (pp. 257–280). East Norwalk, CT: Appleton & Lange.

Ootim, B. (1995). So you think that you can interview? *Nursing Management, 2*(6), 20–1.

Saxe, S. D. (1988). Do performance appraisals violate the Human Rights Code? *The Human Resource, 5*(2), 18–9.

Scholtes, P. R. (1993, Summer). Total quality or performance appraisal: Choose one. *National Productivity Review,* pp. 349–363.

Smith, M. L. (1993, February). Give feedback, not criticism. *Supervisory Management,* p. 4.

Stone, T. H., & Meltz, N. M. (1988). *Human resource management in Canada* (2nd ed) (pp. 331–379). Toronto: Holt, Rinehart and Winston.

Vaziri, H. K. (1992, October). Using competitive benchmarking to set goals. *Quality Progress,* pp. 81–85.

Werther, W., Davis, K., Schwind, H., & Das, H. (1990). *Canadian human resource management.* (3rd ed). Toronto: McGraw-Hill Ryerson.

CASE STUDY

In response to your hospital's strategic planning priorities, a call for proposals went out to all managers for programs that address the goals of the institution. You responded by preparing a successful proposal for a new program component—specifically, the hiring of a community-outreach and education nurse to facilitate service delivery by the general medical unit.

You have received funding to move forward. Your literature search and consultations with experts in the field have given you confidence that you have set accurate job specifications and clear performance indicators consistent with the philosophy of the nursing division.

Your next task is to recruit a nurse into this position. You have extra funds for the first year of the program as part of administration's commitment to success.

1. Describe the methods and personnel you would use to locate appropriately trained applicants and select the right candidate.
2. Detail how you would plan for this candidate's orientation to the organization, the work team on the general medical unit you manage, and this new role.
3. What monitoring and evaluation strategies might you consider putting in place to assess employee behaviour and performance?
4. Who might need training or development to support this new initiative?

Chapter 21

▼▼▼▼▼▼▼▼▼▼▼▼▼▼▼▼

Human Resource Allocation: Staffing and Scheduling

GERMAINE M. DECHANT

KEY OBJECTIVES

In this chapter, you will learn:

- To define common terms used in staffing.
- A step-by-step approach to staffing that identifies the key variables to consider and the information needed.
- To develop a basic staffing plan.
- To describe the role of the first-level manager in scheduling.
- Approaches and variables to consider in the process of scheduling.
- To present a basic schedule.
- Creative approaches to scheduling.
- Some of the legal and ethical issues inherent in staffing and scheduling.

> *"The basic role of the leader is to build a complementary team where each strength is made productive, and each weakness made irrelevant." (Steven Covey, Principle-Centered Leadership, 1992, p.246).*

INTRODUCTION

Mastery of resource allocation and financial management is clearly among the conditions of survival for first-level managers in the new environment of health-care reform, with its flattened organizations and its philosophy of decentralized decisions made at the point of service delivery, where the impact is felt. This theme is recurrent in the health-care literature, where one finds general agreement that an integral and key component of the first-level manager's role is the allocation and management of resources of all kinds, including equipment, supplies and services, and human resources. The manager sets the standards and direction for practice and is directly responsible and accountable for all aspects of the management of the staff delivering the care. This represents a significant change in the role of the first-level manager, and requires the development of a skill set once associated exclusively with the mandates of directors of nursing services and other senior administrative personnel. This new direction presents challenges at once intimidating and exciting, and enriches the role of the first-level manager.

Because human resources represent the largest portion of the total operating budget in any health-care unit, managerial success in the area of fiscal management begins with an understanding that expertise in staffing and scheduling is fundamental to effectiveness in human resource allocation, and that variables in one of these areas cannot be successfully manipulated without due consideration to the impact on the other variables. This chapter promotes an understanding of the complexity of staffing and scheduling, and provides an opportunity for the reader to develop basic skills in this area in order to begin to build a comprehensive approach to human resource allocation. It presents an approach to staffing and scheduling that is, if not scientific, at least systematic.

STAFFING AND ITS CRITICAL VARIABLES

"Staffing" is the process used to determine the acceptable number and skill mix of personnel needed to meet the treatment and care requirements of patients in a program or unit in any setting, whether it is a community agency, an ambulatory-care clinic, an emergency department, or a continuing-care unit. Matching appropriately-skilled staff with patient needs for quality care, and doing so within the parameters of available resources, is an ongoing challenge for the manager. In developing the staffing plan, it is imperative that the manager consider the following key variables and understand their interdependence:

1. Philosophical framework for practice
2. Characteristics of the patient population
3. Environmental factors
4. Personnel characteristics

PHILOSOPHICAL FRAMEWORK FOR PRACTICE

A unit or program's vision, mission, values, philosophy, goals, and objectives directly affect the staffing plan. These need to be precise statements so that service implications are clear in terms of what the patient can expect, and also to guide quality standards, policies, procedures, and strategies for service delivery. A statement of vision, for instance, may necessitate activity changes, while a mission that includes patient and family education and a focus on health promotion will have workload implications for unit personnel. This will also be the case for a management philosophy that promotes continuous service improvement; staff development; decentralized decision-making; or staff participation in such activities as clinical research, program planning and evaluation, community liaison, and service-access co-ordination.

The choice of a model for the delivery of care will also be guided by the philosophical framework of the unit, and the model will in turn have a tremendous impact on the approach to service delivery and decisions regarding staff mix. For example, the choice of patient-focused care over primary nursing, team nursing, or functional nursing as a model will influence the type and number of professionals selected to staff the unit (see also Chapter 8). Services organized around a medical model with medical dominance, or on an interdisciplinary team model in which the physician serves as a team member and consultant, will determine to a great extent the unit's direction in staff team configuration and recruitment plans.

Of importance, as well, are the unique blend of history and traditions that may be enmeshed—often at a subconscious level—with the unit's approaches to service delivery. Knowledge of the unit's culture is very useful, and in some cases a change in paradigm may be needed to simplify practice and lead to adjustments in staffing mix.

The unit's status as a teaching unit is also an important factor for staffing. The types and levels of students and the extent of staff involvement with student teaching and supervision must be considered.

CHARACTERISTICS OF THE PATIENT POPULATION

The type of patient admitted to a unit is a factor of obvious importance in the development of a staffing plan. Collection and analysis of data about this patient population is an essential first step in the process of staffing. The following elements need to be identified—either as projections on the basis of the literature available on this clinical population and on the experience of other similar units, or as actual data based on the previous years' experience:

- Number of patients and demand for service (unit average occupancy)
- Patterns and trends in census
- Admission and discharge rates or number and length of visits to the clinic
- Average length of stay (ALOS)
- The conditions or illnesses experienced by patients e.g. medical, surgical, psychiatric, oncology
- Level or complexity of treatment needs, as well as direct and indirect care requirements (patient classification)
- Patient demographics: age; education level; socio-economic factors influencing health-care needs; physical, psychological, spiritual, cultural, and recreational needs (see Chapter 2 for a discussion of the importance of demographic and epidemiologic information)

- Patient expectations for services (patient satisfaction results)
- Needs of patients' families and/or significant others

ENVIRONMENTAL FACTORS

It is well known that management decision-making is influenced by the environmental factors that impinge on a unit or program. That knowledge needs to be applied to the development of a unit's staffing plan. Consider the following factors:

- The number of patient beds or clinic spaces.
- The number of hours the unit or clinic is open.
- The design of the unit. For example, a medical unit made up exclusively of private rooms may be preferable from the patient's perspective; however, such a physical layout has definite implications for workload and staff assignment patterns.
- The unit's fit in the total organization. For example, is the unit a stand-alone, isolated clinic, or one of several units within a large organization where human resources are supported and shared across units? This would be a significant staffing factor in a situation in which, for example, the patient census indicates that adequate care could be provided by one caregiver, but issues of staff and patient safety indicate that the unit cannot be staffed by one person alone. In this situation, two units in close proximity may be able to provide safe coverage for each other.
- The unit's fit within the community. Is the unit functioning within an integrated network of agencies upon which one can call others for support?
- Availability of equipment and supplies.
- Technological advances.
- New drugs or treatment approaches.
- Number of staff physicians and residents on the unit, their expectations, and their approaches to practice.
- Legal considerations, such as contractual agreements.
- Service boundaries. For exactly what services is the unit responsible? Do its responsibilities include traditional laboratory functions, such as blood collection? Is it responsible for covering dietary and pharmacy services on evening or night shifts?

PERSONNEL CHARACTERISTICS

Among the factors affecting staffing are the characteristics of the pool of professionals available to the unit as caregivers. A unit's ability to meet service-delivery requirements rests to a great extent on the individual competence of the caregivers—competence that results from education, experience, motivation, health, attitude, and perhaps a variety of other personal factors. In practice, individual differences in competence among caregivers in the same classification are extremely important and cannot be ignored. A comprehensive personnel inventory should include the following factors:

- the skill mixes available;
- the role functions and professional mandate of each group;
- the competitive markets for staff in the larger community, and the unit's potential for success in recruitment;
- education;
- classification;
- experience;
- length of service;
- individual aspirations, goals and objectives;
- level of expertise;
- age;
- gender;
- social and ethnic background;
- use of staff versus line positions, for example, clinical specialist or senior therapists; and
- access to staff resources from other departments, such as physiotherapy and respiratory therapy.

Critical variables to consider in the staffing process are summarized in Box 21.1.

THE STAFFING PLAN

Having analyzed the critical staff variables, the first-level manager now has the information needed to develop a staffing plan. The staffing plan includes the basic number of staff in each discipline required to adequately staff the unit on each shift. The staff may be all nurses, nurses working with licensed practical nurses (LPNs), or a combination of several types of professionals working together as a multidisciplinary team.

Where a workload-measurement system is in place, the manager must consider its results seriously as a guide in the process of developing a staffing plan. Workload-measurement systems first emerged in the 1960s as patient-classification systems were developed, and they were used primarily to identify the nursing-care needs of patients and the nursing resources necessary to meet those needs. Workload-measurement systems typically identify the following: direct nursing care requirements of patients (often referred to as levels of patient acuity); indirect nursing care (i.e., care activities carried out on behalf of patients, but not in their presence, such as charting) and activities that are unit-related but not necessarily patient-contact related (such as the narcotic count). Patients are assigned to categories of care, and staffing is then determined according to specific decision rules.

There is a large body of literature available on the topic of workload-measurement systems to which the reader is referred (see, for example, Giovannetti, 1994). The brief mention included here is intended to underscore the fact that although a first-level manager cannot rely exclusively on

Box 21.1
STAFFING VARIABLES CHECKLIST

Philosophical Framework for Practice

Vision
Mission
Values
Goals
Objectives
Quality Standards
Policies and Procedures
Patient-care Model
Culture
Staff Participation In:
    Teaching
    Continuous Service
Improvement:
    Decision-Making
    Clinical Research
    Program Planning
    Program Evaluation
    Community Liaison
    Service-access Co-ordination

Characteristics of the Patient Population

Number of Patients
Average Occupancy
Patterns and Trends in Census
Admission Rates
Average Length of Stay
Patient Conditions/Illnesses
Patient Classification
    Requirements
Patient Demographics:
    Age
    Education
    Socio-economic Factors
    Physical Needs
    Psychological Needs
    Spiritual Needs
    Recreational Needs
    Cultural Needs
Patient Expectations for Service
Family Support Needs

Environmental Factors

Number of Beds/Clinic Spaces
Number of Hours
Unit Design
Unit's Fit in Organization
Unit's Fit in Community Network
Equipment and Supplies
Technology
Service Boundaries
Union Contracts

Personnel Characteristics

Skill Mix
Roles and Professional Mandate
Availability
Education
Classification
Experience
Individual aspirations, goals and objectives
Length of Service
Expertise
Age
Gender
Social and Ethnic Background
Staff vs Line Positions
Support Resources

the organization's workload-measurement system to generate a staffing plan, the workload indicators reflective of nursing care requirements and indirect staff activities provide very useful information. Managers are well advised to familiarize themselves with their organization's specific workload-measurement system in order to determine the extent of its usefulness in reliably predicting workload and therefore staffing requirements.

Table 21.1 presents a staffing plan for a residential treatment centre for adolescents who suffer from mental illness. This tertiary-care centre is one of the community-based programs offered through Child and Adolescent Services Association (CASA).

Table 21.1

BASIC STAFFING PLAN FOR A TEN-BED RESIDENTIAL TREATMENT CENTRE FOR ADOLESCENTS

Staff Classification	SHIFT		
	Day	Evening	Night
RPN/RN	4	1	0
Child-care Counsellors	1	3	2
Senior Therapist	1	0	0
Secretary	1	0	0
Total Staff	7	4	2

You will notice that this staffing plan shows very clearly the number and classification of staff needed for a required staffing complement for all three shifts. What this plan does not show, however, is the number of individual employees you need to hire in order to have in attendance four nurses on days and one on evenings, or one child-care counsellor on days, three on evenings, and two on nights. The key question is this: "How many individuals would need to be hired if you wanted to have in attendance one individual 24 hours per day, 365 days per year?"

To answer this question, the first-level manager must understand the difference between paid hours and effective hours of work.

- *Paid hours* reflect the number of hours for which the employee is remunerated, and incorporates worked hours, benefits hours, and activities for which the employee is paid while away from the work place.
- *Effective hours* is another term for "worked hours." That is, effective hours represent the number of hours during which the employee is providing either direct care to patients or is engaged in indirect activities. Direct care is generally defined as time spent with the patient (e.g. in group therapy), and indirect time is the time spent preparing for or following up on a direct activity (e.g. post-group debriefing). Which activities are considered "direct" and which are considered "indirect" differs by facility, so it is important for the manager to be familiar with the local policy or practice. Effective hours are determined by subtracting the benefit hours from the paid hours.
- *Benefit hours* include sick days, vacation days, statutory holidays, education days, and leaves without pay, such as bereavement leave. Benefit hours are determined by the agency's personnel policies and the terms of the applicable collective agreement. In an agency where there are no collective agreements, personnel policies guide decision-making. Historical patterns of use, for example with sick time, must also be taken into consideration.

Table 21.2

DETERMINING BENEFIT HOURS

Benefit Hours	Days Per Year	Hours Per Day	Total Hours Per Year
Vacation	15	7.75	116.25
Statutory Holidays	11	7.75	85.25
Paid Education Days	2	7.75	15.50
Average Paid Sick Days	4	7.75	31.00
Totals	32	7.75	248.00

The benefit hours calculated in Table 21.2 are those applicable to the ten-bed residential treatment centre presented in Table 21.1. Now that we know the benefit hours, we can calculate effective hours.

Calculating Effective Hours

Effective hours can be calculated in two different ways, using either benefit days or benefit hours.

Using Benefit Days

Total days per year	365
Less total benefit days per year	32
	333
Less total number of days off per year (2 3 52 weeks)	104
days:	229
hrs/day:	× 7.75
Worked or Effective Hours	1774.75

Using Benefit Hours

Total hours per year (365 × 7.75)	2,828.75
Less total benefit hours per year	248.00
	2,580.75
Less total number of hours off per year (104 3 7.75)	806.00
Worked or Effective Hours	1,774.75

Calculating Paid Hours

Paid hours include worked hours plus benefit hours.
In the residential treatment centre example:

Worked Hours	1,774.75
Plus benefit hours	248.00
Paid hours	2,022.75

An employee in this residential treatment centre is therefore paid for 2,022.75 hours while actually working 1,774.75 hours. For a clinical unit open 24 hours a day, every day of the year, 8,760 hours (365 × 24 hours) per year require coverage. If one employee provides 1,774.75 hours per year, a simple process of division shows that 4.94 (8,760/1,774.75) staff members are needed for one staff member to be available 24 hours a day, 365 days of the year.

The residential treatment centre, however, is closed on weekends. Once again, a simple process of division shows that for this centre, 3.53 (261 days × 24 hrs = 6,264 hours/1,774.75) staff members are needed for one staff member to be available 24 hours a day, 261 days of the year.

It is essential at this stage to calculate staffing requirements for each classification applying the reality of each particular unit. Let us go back once again to the ten-bed residential treatment centre example, in which four nurses are needed on days, and one on evenings.

In an environment where a combination of full-time and part-time employment is common, the terminology used to describe staff totals can be confusing. To minimize confusion, staff positions are usually expressed as full-time equivalents (FTEs). A full-time equivalent represents the **paid** hours of work. In the example used above, one FTE = 2,022.75 paid hours. For this same example, then, the following calculation is applied to determine the number of FTEs required:

Minimum Staff Requirement	5.00 FTE
Relief Staff (1,240 ÷ 2,022.75)	0.61 FTE
Total RPN/RN FTE Requirement	5.61 FTE

It is important to note that these 5.61 FTEs could be comprised of any combination of full- and part-time staff. The mix of full- and part-time positions should be decided on the basis of what configuration best meets the operational needs of the unit. Table 21.3 illustrates how the RN/RPN staffing requirements for the residential treatment centre are calculated.

It is important to note as an aside that the manager who completes this calculation process for all classifications in a specific unit has also completed the fundamental work required for budget preparation e.g. 5.61 FTEs × Average Hourly Rate = Budget required. Simple? Yes!

STAFF SCHEDULING

Staff scheduling is the process of distributing budgeted days of work and days off for personnel, in the pattern identified in the basic staffing plan, so that requisite patient-care needs are met on all shifts. Scheduling is time-consuming, and can be fraught with frustration; however, it is also a very important process which deserves attention and effort so that effective and efficient practices are developed. The objectives of a staff schedule are as follows:

1. To meet patient care requirements;
2. To operate within the parameters of the allocated budget;
3. To maintain fairness and flexibility; and
4. To consider the personal needs of individual staff members.

Table 21.3

STAFFING REQUIREMENT BY CLASSIFICATION, TEN-BED RESIDENTIAL TREATMENT CENTRE

Staff Classification	Shifts	M	T	W	T	F	S	S	Total
Registered Psychiatric Nurse or	Days	4	4	4	4	4	0	0	20
Registered Nurse	Evenings	1	1	1	1	0	0	1	5
	Nights	0	0	0	0	0	0	0	0

	Total	25
Each Nurse has 2 days off, therefore, ÷		5
Minimum Staff Requirement		5 RPN/RN
Convert to Effective Hours	×	1,774.75
Total Effective Hours		8,873.75
Paid Hours (5 × 2,022.75)		10,113.75
Relief Hours (10,113.75 − 8,873.75)		1,240.00

Many factors influence staff scheduling and how it is approached. A unit's staff schedules must, for example, accommodate the requirements of local collective agreements, reflect personnel policies and procedures, and at the same time be responsive to greater and lesser workload demands on the unit itself. Scheduling is, without question, a complex and challenging process for the first-level manager.

Box 21.2 provides a comprehensive list of factors that should be considered in staff scheduling. Many are driven by the requirements of the collective agreement. Where there is no collective agreement, local personnel policies and labour laws can provide guidance.

For every shift of every day, first-level managers must juggle many complex factors to project workload requirements, and determine an appropriate assignment of staff to ensure that adequate services are delivered. The successful achievement of this goal is an admirable accomplishment, especially when one considers the number of unexpected events that can occur in any clinical environment. Any method, technique, or approach that can be applied to simplify this process, while keeping it integrated with other critical factors such as quality of care, good staff morale, and efficiency, will be of assistance to the manager.

APPROACHES TO STAFF SCHEDULING

The three major approaches to staff scheduling are the traditional approach, cyclical scheduling, and self-scheduling. All three approaches may be assisted or supported by the range of scheduling enhancements that are now offered by computers.

Box 21.2

FACTORS FOR CONSIDERATION IN STAFF-SCHEDULING DECISIONS

Staff Factors

Availability
Mix needed
- Discipline mix, e.g. RN/LPN ratio
- Male/female ratio
- Full time/part time
Expertise needed
Supervisory needs
Continuity of care requirements

Scheduling Model

Eight hours or extended shifts
Hours worked per schedule
Weekends worked per schedule
Maximum number of days worked before days off
Length of cycle rotation
Posting time requirements

Staff Special Requests

Procedure for shift trades; leaves of absence; vacation and paid holidays:
- Requests
- Response to requests
- Approval guidelines
- Time frame

Casual or Float Pool

Guidelines re:
- Structure of pool: central or unit-based
- Availability requirements
- Assignment method
- Orientation requirements
- Supervision and performance review
- Compensation

Unusual Staff Occurrences

Procedure for:
- Tardiness
- Absenteeism without notice
- Absenteeism program in the organization

Irregular Hours of Work

On-call and overtime guidelines for:
- Availability
- Authorization
Guidelines for being:
- Called after shift begins
- Returning staff home after they have reported to work
- Split shifts
- Call back

Temporary Reassignment

Guidelines for:
- Equity in deciding who will float
- Assignment method
- Orientation
- Supervision and performance review
- Feedback and recognition

TRADITIONAL APPROACH

The traditional approach to staff scheduling is one in which the manager develops a new schedule from scratch each month, taking all appropriate factors into consideration. The major advantage of this approach is its flexibility, since it allows for the impacts of changes to be addressed. The traditional approach has major disadvantages, however, including the fact that it is extremely time-consuming for the manager, and therefore costly. Most, although not all, managers have opted for more effective and efficient approaches.

CYCLICAL SCHEDULING

In cyclical scheduling, a schedule which provides desired coverage is developed for the unit for a number of weeks. (Six weeks is a typical time frame.) The schedule then repeats itself in cycles. A cyclical schedule must be designed to meet collective-agreement requirements and to accommodate rotating, permanent or mixed shifts, as well as fixed days off, such as four or five day weekends. Its design will also vary depending on whether the unit uses regular or extended hours of work, or a combination of the two.

Advantages of cyclical scheduling include its stability, in that once it is set up, it undergoes only minor changes; its lower cost, since the manager is not starting over again each month; and the enhanced staff satisfaction that results when staff know what their schedule will be for many months in advance, and can make personal plans.

Figure 21.1 presents an example of a simple cyclical schedule. This schedule is the actual one used in the residential treatment centre for adolescents discussed earlier in this chapter.

The major disadvantage of cyclical schedules is that they are inflexible. Days on and off are fixed, and the changing workload requirements which characterize most patient-care environments are not easily accommodated. The effect of this inflexibility can be minimized through a system that allows for staff shift exchanges, and for staffing adjustments on a shift-by-shift basis as workload requirements dictate. The manager has the responsibility to establish the protocol that allows this to happen.

SELF-SCHEDULING

Self-scheduling is a process in which staff on a unit collectively develop and implement the work schedule. This approach was developed in the hospital environment, in response to the recognition that work schedules were typically a major source of discontent among nurses. The approach is designed to provide staff with control over decisions which have an obviously significant impact on their professional and personal lives. The goals of self-scheduling are:

1. To increase staff autonomy through control over the work schedule;
2. To promote staff retention by providing increased flexibility and creativity in scheduling;
3. To decrease absenteeism through the introduction of a self-coverage plan for illness; and
4. To support team development through a heightened sense of accountability to one another, as negotiations take place among staff members.

For self-scheduling to succeed, unit staff must either provide the impetus for, or display a high level of commitment to, this approach. The manager and the unit staff need time to learn the model before deciding to move ahead with implementation. Keys to successful implementation include:

- strong support for the concept by the manager;
- staff participation in every aspect of the changeover; and
- union support for the concept.

F i g u r e   2 1 . 1

**E X A M P L E   O F   A
C Y C L I C A L   S C H E D U L E**

		S	M	T	W	T	F	S	S	M	T	W	T	F	S
Senior Therapist		X	P	S	P-	P	S	X	X	P	P	P-	P	S	X
Primary Therapist		X	D	D	D	D	D	X	X	D	D	D	D	D	X
Primary Therapist		X	D	D	D	D	D	X	X	D	D	D	D	D	X
Primary Therapist		X	S	S	S	S	S	X	X	S	S	S	S	S	X
Charge Nurse		B	E	E	K	I	X	X	B	E	E	K	I	X	X
Associate Therapist		B	E	I	K	E	X	X	B	E	I	K	E	X	X
Associate Therapist		B	E	I	K	E	X	X	B	E	I	K	E	X	X
Recreation		B	E	E	K	I	X	X	B	E	E	K	I	X	X
Permanent Nights		X	N	N	N	N	N	X	X	N	N	N	N	N	X
Permanent Nights		X	N	N	N	N	N	X	X	N	N	N	N	N	X
Cook		X	C	C	C	C	W	X	X	C	C	C	C	W	X
Secretary		X	S	S	S	Y	S	X	X	S	S	S	Y	S	X

Source: **Ten-bed Residential Treatment Centre for Adolescents (CASA)**
**Every person repeats the same two-week schedule continuously. This two
week schedule averages 38.75 hours per week per person. The longest work
span is five days. Long weekends off and special leaves, as well as vacation
and other absences are covered by individuals in a unit-based casual pool.**

Key: RN = Registered   CCC = Child Care   B = 1900 to   C = 0845 to
           D = 0700 to 1515   E = 1400 to 2315   I = 1430 to   K = 1430 to
           N = 2300 to 0700   P = 0845 to 1515   S = 0815 to   T = 1800 to
           W = 0845 to 1600   Y = 0900 to 1715   P-T = Split   X = Days Off

A fair pilot should be at least six months long. The first three months are extremely demanding because of the magnitude of the change, and the fact that much teaching and coaching is required. Development of a plan reflecting the entire implementation process provides staff with a better understanding of what to expect, and allows the manager to plan, monitor, and evaluate the change process very carefully (Dechant, 1989).

The impact of this approach on the first-level manager is considerable. The manager in this scenario becomes a facilitator of the process—a coach rather than a supervisor, empowering staff to make effective choices as members of a self-directed team. This approach is consistent with modern principles of leadership and with a philosophy of decentralized decision-making and shared governance.

Despite its potential benefits, self-scheduling is rarely used. Possible reasons include the reality that first-level managers are in many cases overwhelmed with work, and this is a very time-consuming approach to introduce. Staff, as well, may be unwilling to add to their already onerous workloads, and may see scheduling as the manager's responsibility. Responsibility to work out the inevitable conflicts rests with staff who may feel considerable stress related to the assertiveness required to ensure that they get a fair schedule.

Self-scheduling appears to be a very creative way to increase staff dignity and job satisfaction. It reflects a change in how we think (not just in how we do things) about staff, and about the role of the manager. Self-scheduling may be termed a "power strategy": it empowers staff by allocating to them the responsibility, the authority, and the accountability to gain and retain control over an aspect of their work that is vitally important to their lives. This approach is well worth the manager's consideration.

COMPUTERS

The capability of computers to assist in staff scheduling is well worth investigation by the manager. Sophisticated systems are now available that sift through large databases, take a variety of individual and system constraints into account, reject data which do not fit constraints, and print out an optimal detailed schedule. Today's manager may find such a system to be an invaluable support, and the time required to complete a cost-benefit analysis may be time that is well spent.

STAFFING ADJUSTMENTS

Patient-care needs vary from shift to shift, and unfortunately such variations often cannot be anticipated or accurately forecast. This generates a need for staffing adjustments. Staffing adjustments should not be confused with regular staff scheduling. While the goal of staff scheduling is to plan for staff allocation throughout the year on the basis of predictable factors, staffing adjustments are driven by unexpected conditions that result either in over- or under-staffing. These conditions result in an adjustment process that occurs on each shift by means of various approaches, of which perhaps the best known is the float pool.

Float pools consist of casual or relief staff who are employed by an organization to work on an as-needed basis. Expectations of these float staff members vary from one organization to another. The parameters in most cases are defined by the collective agreement. The structure of float pools also varies. In some organizations, float personnel are unit-based and managed by the first-level manager. In others, float personnel are based in a centralized pool that is managed by a staffing co-ordinator. A unit-based, casual-relief-staff structure is generally thought to have the advantages of including a small number of flexible staff under the direct supervision of a manager, and developing in this staff a high level of commitment to the unit. Expectations of relief staff members in this situation are generally the same as those of the full-time staff in terms of performance standards and ongoing professional development. In many organizations, unit-based relief staff also work through the centralized float pool when their commitment to their unit of origin is fulfilled and they desire extra work.

Cross-utilization is an enhancement of the historical approach of floating. "Floating" refers to a process where shift by shift, in response to patient need, nurses permanently assigned to a unit are reassigned to another unit or department with which they may not be familiar. "Cross-utilization" partners groups or units with similar patient populations requiring similar nursing skills (American Organization of Nurse Executives, 1993). As the individual units in the group experience variations in census and acuity, skilled staff move from one unit to the other. This process benefits patients and staff because patients receive care from personnel with the appropriate skill mix, and nursing staff become familiar with colleagues in the group and feel more inclined to include these "floating" nurses in unit and social activities. In cross-utilization, the nurse manager must ensure that there are appropriate supports through policies and standards of care, and that there is a clear structure for accountability and decision-making.

The management of overstaffing is a challenge. It is imperative that staff-reduction strategies be developed in advance of need. Managers must understand the process, and the financial and other implications of, for example, sending a staff member home after the start of a shift. It is also important for these strategies to be consistent with collective-agreement requirements, and to be supported by the organization.

JOB SHARING

Job sharing is a term used to refer to a situation in which two or more part-time staff members fill one full-time equivalent position. These individuals provide coverage on the shifts required for a full-time position and cover for each other's vacations and other absences. Today's managers generally stay away from traditional job-sharing contracts, and address the need for scheduling flexibility by developing a balance of full- and part-time positions in their complement of FTEs. The manager must be aware of the increased benefit costs associated with part-time positions.

PATIENT-FOCUSED CARE

"Patient-focused care," also known as "patient-centred care," is a hospital care-delivery philosophy that has important implications for staffing and scheduling. Patient-focused care is based on the belief that the traditional health-care system has become so specialized that it is difficult for patients to receive timely, personalized care when, for example, they may need to see fifteen or more staff during the admitting process alone. (See Chapter 8.)

A patient-focused hospital reduces the number of people and places a patient encounters during a hospital stay. It does this through cross-training, a system that also increases staff productivity by reducing "down" time. Cross-training requires a staff member with one skill set to learn and assume responsibility for an additional set of skills.

Patient-focused care models also frequently require the redesign of units. Each patient-care unit might, for example, be equipped with an admitting area, diagnostic laboratory, satellite pharmacy, and rehabilitation room. The Lakeland Regional Medical Center, where the Booz-Allen model of hospital decompartmentalization was first elaborated, had bedside care provided by teams of multi-skilled practitioners made up of a care pair of registered nurse and technician; this pair was backed by a unit-based pharmacist, unit clerk, and unit-support aide (Weber, 1991).

The movement to patient-focused care holds appeal because its design focuses on decreasing the number of personnel, the amount of waiting time, and the amount of travel time patients experience in the daily process of care. Most organizations in the Canadian health-care systems would require redesign of their current patient care units to accommodate the increased number of functions in one geographic area that are required by this model. The impact of cross-training on professional standards of practice also needs to be examined. If implementation of this new trend is more than a fad, first-level managers will need to become very knowledgeable regarding its implications on human resource allocation.

ETHICAL AND LEGAL ISSUES IN STAFFING AND SCHEDULING

The primary legal and ethical obligation of the first-level manager in relation to staffing and scheduling is to provide safe patient care within professionally defined standards of practice and organizational policies and procedures. This underscores the need for the manager to have an excellent understanding of all the variables highlighted in this chapter, as well as the ability to integrate these variables in an effective staffing plan and in scheduling practices. It is important to remember that in scheduling, the first-level manager is legally bound to integrate the requirements of the collective agreement, and is not free to negotiate with individual staff members any special arrangements that would be in breach of the collective agreement.

In addition to the patient-care imperative, first-level managers must recognize their obligation to examine, analyze and shape the environment within which staff practices, and to continually strive for improvement. Staff input and feedback in the process of staffing and scheduling is consistent with an approach that fosters individual autonomy and promotes opportunities for professional contribution. Continuing learning and growth are hallmarks of the professional.

The first-level manager also has an ethical imperative to optimize outcomes in patient care and staff satisfaction while balancing these with judicious use of the limited resources in the unit or program budget. Finally, the manager has an ethical responsibility to advocate as appropriate for the resources required to deliver the unit's mission. Both of these final points have implications for staffing and scheduling.

CONCLUSION

The allocation of human resources is an exacting and integral component of the role of the first-level manager. To discharge this role effectively and efficiently, the manager must be able to integrate and manipulate many interrelated variables. This is accomplished through a complex process which presents many challenges. Managers who rise to these challenges are those who know intimately the unit or program for which they are accountable, and recognize that they have the power to influence and shape this environment through their approach to staffing and scheduling.

The manager with expertise in human resource allocation has an opportunity to create effective teams and to implement flexible strategies designed to cope with rapidly changing and unpredictable environments that undergo wide variations in workload demands. The manager's success in this area has a direct impact on the quality of care patients receive. Successful staffing and scheduling also fosters a healthy environment for care givers. These are goals of indisputable importance, and the manager who excels in this complex process deserves admiration and respect.

SUMMARY

- Staffing is the process used to determine the acceptable number and skill mix of personnel needed to meet the treatment and care requirements of patients in a program or unit in any health-care setting.
- Key variables that directly affect a unit or program's staffing plan include the philosophical framework for practice; the characteristics of the patient population; environmental factors; and personnel characteristics.
- To develop a basic staffing plan, the first-level manager must be able to calculate paid hours, effective or worked hours, and benefit hours.
- Staff scheduling is the process of distributing budgeted personnel days of work and days off in the pattern identified in the basic staffing plan, in order to meet the requisite patient-care needs on all shifts.
- Many complex factors influence staff-scheduling decisions and choice of approaches. The staff schedule, however, must have as its objectives to meet patient-care requirements; operate within the parameters of the allocated budget; and maintain fairness, flexibility, and consideration of individual personnel quality-of-life needs.
- Key factors to consider in staff-scheduling decisions include: staff factors; the scheduling model in use; staff special requests; casual or float pool availability; structure and guidelines; unusual staff occurrences; irregular hours of work; and guidelines for temporary reassignments.

- The most commonly used approach to staff scheduling is the cyclical schedule, which provides the desired coverage over a number of weeks and then repeats itself in cycles.
- The primary legal and ethical obligation of the first-level manager, in relation to staffing and scheduling, is to provide safe patient care within professionally defined clinical standards; standards of practice and organizational policies and procedures. This underscores the need for the manager to have an excellent understanding of all the variables highlighted in this chapter and the ability to integrate these variables in an effective staffing plan and scheduling practices.

FURTHER READINGS & RESOURCES

Arnold, B., & Mills, E. (1983). Care-12: Implementation of flexible scheduling. *Journal of Nursing Administration, 13*(7/8), 9–14.

Beaman, A. (1986). What do first-line managers do? *Journal of Nursing Administration, 15*(5), 6–9.

Beauchamp, T., & Childress, J. (1989) *Principles of Biomedical Ethics*. New York: Oxford University Press.

Bechtel, G. & Printz, V. (1994). Evaluating quality of care using modular nursing on a multispecialty unit. *Clinical Nurse Specialist, 8*(2) 81–84.

Behner, K. G., Fogg, L. F., Fournier, L. C., Frankenbach, J. T., & Robertson, S. B. (1990). Nursing resource management: Analysing the relationship between costs and quality in staffing decisions. *Health Care Management Review, 15*(4), 63–71.

Bioethics Centre Interdisciplinary Committee (1994). *A Handbook of Health Care Ethics and Institutional Ethics for Staff in Health Care Institutions*. Edmonton, AB: University of Alberta Hospitals.

Braddy, P. (1987). Scheduling alternatives for administrators. *Nurse Forum, 23*(2), 70–77.

Budd, M. & Propotnik, T. (1989). A computerized system for staffing, billing, and productivity measurement. *Journal of Nursing Administration, 19*(7), 17–23.

Cockerill, R. W., & O'Brien-Pallas, L. L. (1990). Satisfaction with nursing workload systems: Report of a survey of Canadian hospitals. Part A. *Canadian Journal of Nursing Administration, 3*(2), 17–22.

De Groot, H. A. (1989a). Patient classification system evaluation. Part 1: Essential system elements. *Journal of Nursing Administration, 19*(6), 30–35.

De Groot, H. A. (1989b). Patient classification system evaluation. Part 2: System selection and implementation. *Journal of Nursing Administration, 19*(7), 24–30.

Douglas D., & Mayewski, J. (1996). Census variation staffing. *Nursing Management, 27*(2) 32–36.

Elliott, T. L. (1989). Cost analysis of alternative scheduling. *Nursing Management, 20*(4), 42–43.

Giovannetti, P., & Johnson, J.M. (1990). A new generation patient classification system. *Journal of Nursing Administration, 20*(5), 33–40.

Hays, P. (1989). a change of pace: Alternative work schedule options. *Clinical Management in Physical Therapy, 9*(2), 26–29.

Hung, R. (1991). A cyclical schedule of 10 hour, 4 day workweeks. *Nursing Management, 22*(9), 30–33.

Imig, S. I., Powell, J. A., & Thorman, K. (1984). Primary nursing and flexi-staffing: Do they mix? *Nursing Management, 15*(8), 39–42.

Kutash, M. B., & Nelson, D. (1993). Optimizing the use of nursing pool resources. *Journal of Nursing Administration, 23*(1) 65–68.

Lant, T. W., & Gregory, D. (1984). The impact of the 12-hour shift: An analysis. *Nursing Management, 34*, A-B, D-F, H.

McGuire, J. B., & Liro, J. R. (1986). Flexible work schedules, work attitudes, and perceptions of productivity. *Public Personnel Management, 15*(1), 65–73).

O'Brien-Pallas, L. L., & Cockerill, R. W. (1990). Satisfaction with nursing workload systems: Report of a survey of Canadian hospitals. Part B. *Canadian Journal of Nursing Administration, 3*(2), 23–26.

O'Brien-Pallas, L. L., Cockerill, R., & Leatt, P. (1992). Different systems, different costs? *Journal of Nursing Administration, 22*(12), 17–22.

Ringl, K. K., & Dotson, L. D. (1989). Self-scheduling for professional nurses. *Nursing Management, 20*(2), 42–44.

Ritz, D., & Dugan, M. (1990). 12-hour shifts—a scheduling alternative for ORs. *AORN Journal, 51*(3), 810–815.

Velianoff, G. D. (1191). Establishing a 10-hour schedule. *Nursing Management, 22*(9), 36–38.

REFERENCES

American Organization of Nurse Executives (1993). Cross-utilization of nursing staff. *Nursing Management, 13*(7), 38–39.

Dechant, G. (1989). Self-scheduling for nursing staff. *AARN Newsletter, 46*(5), 4,6,8.

Giovannetti, P. (1994). Measurement of nursing workload. In J. M. Hibberd & M. E. Kyle (Eds.). *Nursing management in Canada* (pp. 331–349). Toronto: W. B. Saunders.

Weber, D. O. (1991). Six models of patient-focused care. *Health Care Forum Journal, 34*(4), 23–31.

CASE STUDY

A regional health authority has just released its business plan for the next three years. One of its goals is to establish a sub-acute-care unit in its long-term-care facility. The principal objective of the sub-acute-care unit is to permit movement of patients who are not yet ready for home-care services out of the acute-care hospitals, thus freeing up beds for more acute and intensive care services.

John Stanych, BScN is currently the manager of three 30-bed units that offer a variety of programs for long-term-care clients. One of these units is to be designated as sub-acute care, and it will therefore have a liaison role with the local acute-care hospitals. Mr. Stanych recognizes that he must review his staffing plan and work schedule to accommodate the needs of a different client population. Using the examples provided in this chapter, consider the following questions:

1. What difference will a change in client population make to the staffing of this unit?
2. Identify environmental and personnel factors that John Stanych must take into consideration in a revised staffing plan.
3 Establish the number of paid hours, effective hours, and benefit hours that will apply to full-time equivalent staff positions (FTEs) on this unit.
4. What type of staffing mix will Mr. Stanych try to secure from senior management?
5. Estimate the number of staff needed to provide services 24 hours per week, seven days per week, and draft a staff schedule.
6. Identify the factors to take into account in designing a staff schedule for this unit.

Chapter 22

▼▼▼▼▼▼▼▼▼▼▼▼▼▼▼

Business Planning and Budget Preparation

LINDA M. DOODY & MOIRA HENNESSEY

KEY OBJECTIVES

In this chapter, you will learn:

- How budgeting is part of the business-plan approach to health-services management.
- Key budgeting concepts, including how capital and operating budgets work.
- How to develop and manage an operating budget for a thirty-bed nursing unit.
- The importance of financial controls and reporting at the middle-management level in a health organization.
- Cost-containment initiatives and resource management.

INTRODUCTION

The health-care industry consumes ten percent of Canada's gross national product. To preserve this social program within available financial resources, restructuring of the health-care system has been necessary. This restructuring has placed increased emphasis on regionalization and the devolution of service authority to the local level.

Provincial governments are establishing broad directions and guiding principles for the comprehensive and effective delivery of health programs and services, consistent with the tenets of the *Canada Health Act*. Guiding principles for the provision of reasonable access to primary, secondary, and tertiary services for all residents have been developed. Implementation of these principles vary from province to province, depending on size and geography.

In some provinces, regional health authorities (RHAs) or regional boards have been formed to administer programs and services to residents within defined geographic areas. These organizations are adopting a business approach to managing health services, based on the development of a business plan which is a blueprint for the future delivery of programs and services.

In this chapter, budget preparation is discussed as an integral element of overall business planning for health organizations and regions. The responsibilities of the nurse manager are discussed with respect to matching the health needs of the clients served with available financial resources. A case example and analysis is presented to assist the nurse manager in applying the basic concepts of budgeting for capital and operating expenditures. Variance reporting and cost-containment initiatives are outlined in relation to the nurse manager's responsibility for providing high quality health services within the fiscal realities.

THE BUSINESS PLAN

In one Canadian province, a business plan has been defined as a set of statements about the mission, goals, and strategies of an organization that are accomplished within a set period of time (Oberg & Wagner, 1994). The plan must be based on the strategic directions established by the province and must provide a seamless continuum of health services. Ideally, a health business plan will have input from consumers and key stakeholders. It must ensure that core health services are available, accessible, and affordable, and must meet the financial targets established for the region by the department of health. A business plan may include the following elements:

- health-care needs assessment;
- vision, mission, and values;
- guiding principles;
- goals, objectives, priorities, and strategies for service delivery; and
- human, structural, and financial resources.

HEALTH-CARE NEEDS ASSESSMENT

The *health-care needs assessment* includes an inventory of current health programs and services offered in the region; a demographic and health-status profile of the catchment population; consumer expectations regarding health services; and gaps in programs and service delivery (Refer to Chapter 2 on demographic and epidemiologic information). This information can be obtained from reports such as Statistics Canada census data and Canadian Institute for Health Information data, proposals for new health services submitted by special-interest groups, customer-satisfaction surveys, and by means of focus groups and community meetings.

As part of the senior management team, the senior nursing executive is actively involved in conducting the health-care needs assessment by collecting and analyzing data, and by participating in focus groups and community meetings. Managers in charge of nursing at the unit level provide data to the senior nursing executive, and are involved in discussing the program or services they manage from utilization, consumer-demand, human, and financial perspectives.

For example, the nurse manager of an eight-station dialysis unit notes that patients are not being dialysed properly, in that some patients who need three treatments weekly are receiving only two treatments because the patient workload has increased beyond the available capacity. A waiting list for this service also exists and residents who require dialysis treatments are relocating to other areas that provide renal dialysis services. A review of five years' historical workload indicates that the number of patients receiving the treatment has doubled. The nurse manager's responsibility in contributing to the health business plan might be to lead or work with a team of colleagues to develop a proposal to expand the renal dialysis service to meet the health needs of the population in the region.

VISION, MISSION, AND VALUES

The *vision statement* considers the health-care needs assessment and states health ideals for the organization. It reflects the values of the organization and provides a common direction for the provision of health services. A vision statement might include a goal such as the following: "to assist communities and individuals achieve the highest level of health possible."

The *mission statement* describes how the organization will fulfil its vision. It is the driving force for all actions within the organization. It should be brief, succinct, and clear. The following is an example of a mission statement: "Working in partnership with other health-service providers, communities, individuals, families, groups, and organizations, the regional health authority is responsible for the delivery of institutional acute- and long-term-care services."

To assist them in achieving their mission and interpreting the vision for their organization, the board may affirm a set of *values*. These values assist the organization in decision-making and other relevant activities. Some common values are: respect for persons, a caring community, justice and fairness, collaboration, and the pursuit of excellence. One of the value statements of the Health Care Corporation of St. John's (1996), for example, focuses on respect for persons:

> "The Corporation respects the needs and rights of clients/patients and their families, staff members including physicians, volunteers and others. We believe in keeping client information confidential and in providing the client with information to make informed choices. We value the needs of the whole person and we place the clients and their families at the centre of our service."

The vision, mission, and value statements provide broad policy directions and a framework for choosing, developing, and evaluating programs and services. The nurse manager must be cognizant of these ideals and reflect them in the delivery of services at the unit level.

GUIDING PRINCIPLES

Guiding principles are derived from the vision and mission statements. Examples of some guiding principles for an RHA are the following:

- To ensure that the RHA, in collaboration with other health providers, delivers comprehensive health-care services for individuals and groups of clients as part of a health continuum.
- To be accountable to the community and government for the delivery of effective programs and services within available financial resources.

GOALS, OBJECTIVES, AND STRATEGIES FOR SERVICE DELIVERY

The organization must establish *goals* consistent with its mission and vision. Examples of goals might be:

- To provide a continuum of affordable, accessible, and appropriate quality care;
- To enable the consumer to lead a healthy and independent life.

Objectives are the key to achieving goals, and *strategies* are the means by which the objectives are accomplished. In terms of the first goal, i.e. providing a continuum of quality care, a specific objective might be the development of lower cost ambulatory-care programs. A strategy that the board might use to achieve this objective would be to close inpatient beds and enhance outpatient and community support services within the current approved budget. Extending this example to the nursing-unit level, a strategy that the nurse manager could use would be piloting a pre-admission clinic to reduce lengths of stay and improve accessibility to fewer inpatient beds.

Another example that shows the relationship between goals and objectives concerns a comprehensive mental-health program which has inpatient and day-care activities. The patient census for the day-care program is low, and staffing costs are high. Because the organization has a mandate to provide a comprehensive mental-health program, the nurse manager cannot unilaterally make a decision to discontinue the day-care program. However, she or he can review the utilization data and the mental-health needs of the catchment population to make recommendations to the senior nursing executive regarding proposed changes for the day-care service. These might include discontinuing the program, extending services to residents of another region, or changing the types of activities offered in the day-care program to better address actual needs.

In terms of the second goal, enabling the consumer to adopt a healthier lifestyle, a board objective might be to offer educational services to the consumer regarding healthy living habits to cope with factors affecting their health, such as obesity, stress, or diabetes. In this example, a strategy for the nurse manager would be to facilitate the development of a teaching program, pamphlets, and other educational material on these subjects.

HUMAN, STRUCTURAL, AND FINANCIAL RESOURCES

In this element of the business plan, the vision, mission, objectives, and strategies are translated into concrete, tangible terms, such as staffing, facilities, and finances.

Human Resources

The organization must develop a workforce plan that includes the number and type of staff required to carry out its service-delivery plan. In health organizations, salaries and related costs represent about 80 percent of the total operating budget. The human resources plan identifies management personnel and staff who provide direct care and support services. It may also forecast needs for certain types of personnel and incorporate strategies for recruiting and training them. (See Chapters 20 and 21.)

Structural Resources

Structural resources include equipment and physical facilities. In developing the business plan, the organization must identify the need for new equipment, and areas where new facilities are needed, or where existing facilities require upgrading or renovation. In times of financial scarcity, facility renovations and redevelopment are normally limited to those projects that address safety issues or improve service delivery.

Financial Resources

The budget is a financial plan that allocates available resources to specific goals, areas, and activities. Expenditures are then monitored against financial targets. The budget is often a basis for evaluation of organizational effectiveness as it is an indicator of how well resources are utilized.

Most health organizations prefer to use a participatory approach to the budgeting process. Although the co-ordination and assembly of a range of input takes considerable time and effort, this approach is well worth the effort. McConnell (1993) cites the following advantages associated with a participatory budgeting process:

- the end result is a more realistic and workable budget because front, line supervisors are familiar with the day-to-day operations and the financial resources needed to manage programs and services;
- there is increased commitment and ownership to managing the budget due to active involvement in its preparation;
- interdepartmental and intradepartmental relationships improve because front-line supervisors obtain a better understanding of the total picture and the various responsibilities of the individual players; and
- a team spirit is created where all managers are working together for a common goal.

Budgets are usually prepared for the fiscal year which begins April 1 and ends March 31. They are based on a combination of past activity, current trends, and whatever knowledge is available regarding future situations. The budget is the best estimate of the financial resources needed to carry out the projected work activity for the fiscal year. It must be realistic and reflective of the economic and political environment.

The board of the organization is ultimately responsible for the budget. It does not prepare the budget but must understand, support, and approve financial proposals developed by the executive team.

DEVELOPING AND MANAGING A BUDGET

A cost centre is the smallest organizational unit for which a budget is prepared (McConnell, 1993). Budgets for individual cost centres are prepared by unit supervisors and assembled by middle- or senior-level managers for their total area of responsibility. The budgets for nursing and laboratory may be organized functionally, for example, while mental-health and cancer care may be treated with a program approach. The budgets for functional centres and programs are then compiled and summarized into a budget for all institutions, programs, and services in the region.

There are two basic types of budgets—capital budgets and operating budgets. The capital budget relates to fixed assets such as equipment, furnishings, land, and buildings. The operating budget includes all revenue and expenses related to the day-to-day operations of the programs and services offered by the organization.

CAPITAL BUDGETS

In health organizations, there are two components to capital budgeting: capital equipment and capital projects. *Capital equipment* includes large items such as CT scanners, ventilators, dialysis stations, or electric beds. Items that usually cost more than $1,000 or have an expected life span that is longer than three to five years are included in the capital-equipment budget. Smaller items such as intravenous poles and medical trays that normally cost less than $1,000 are included as part of supplies in the operating budget.

Capital equipment can be either purchased or leased. If the equipment is purchased, the cost is included in the capital-equipment budget. If the equipment is leased, as IV pumps may be, for example, the annual lease payments are included in the operating budget.

Sometimes, organizations will enter into cost-sharing arrangements with the provincial government for equipment which requires a large investment of money. These cost-sharing arrangements may extend over three to five years. For example, the organization may cost-share the replacement of standard beds with electric beds over a three-year period in a long-term-care facility.

Managers of programs or patient-care units are usually involved in preparing capital-equipment budgets. Requests for capital equipment frequently exceed available financial resources. The nurse manager may receive individual requests for equipment from the medical staff and allied health professionals working on the unit. Some requests to replace or purchase new equipment are essential to the safe operation of the program or service, whereas other requests may be less oriented to safety than to an interest in having the most recent technology.

Development of a capital-equipment budget should include short- and long-range plans for equipment. The process requires the preparation of a capital-equipment inventory. This inventory will include the age, condition and life expectancy of each piece of equipment. A three-year capital-equipment plan should be developed which outlines equipment purchases in order of priority. This plan should include costs of inflation and a contingency factor for unexpected replacement of equipment. In most health organizations, this process is co-ordinated through one division of the organization, such as materiels management (also known as purchasing) or biomedical engineering. Increasingly, nurse managers participate in formal product evaluation or technology assessment committees.

Capital projects include renovations to existing buildings or the construction of new buildings. Some examples are renovations to an existing nursing unit to include rehabilitative space, upgrading of electrical equipment to requirements defined by the Canadian Standards Association (CSA), or replacement of windows or a roof. Program or nurse managers are not usually involved in preparing cost estimates for capital projects, but as members of planning or "user" groups, they contribute to an identification of needs and operational requirements.

OPERATING BUDGETS

The operating budget consists of revenue and expenses. *Revenue* includes funding that is provided by the provincial government; third-party payers such as Veterans Affairs Canada or the RCMP, monies from private-room accommodations, and money from other sources. Expenses include compensation in the form of salaries and employee benefits, and supplies, including medical and surgical items, drugs, oxygen, and food.

Many organizations now develop operating budgets and report financial, statistical, and clinical data according to Management Information Systems (MIS) guidelines. These guidelines were developed through the co-operative effort of provincial and national governments and health-care associations. The MIS guidelines reflect management-information principles and provide a conceptual framework for the collection, integration, and reporting of financial, statistical, and clinical data. MIS guidelines specify what data to collect, how to group and process the data, and how to use the data to support management functions of decision, making, planning, budgeting, controlling, and evaluating (Candian Institute of Health Information, 1994).

According to the MIS guidelines, data can be reported at departmental and/or global levels. The departmental approach includes the resources used to provide a specific service within a specific functional centre— for example, surgery as a part of nursing inpatient services. The global approach identifies the resources used to provide a specific service to a specific patient or group of patients. Global costs would include staffing and supplies for *all* aspects of patient care, including not only nursing, for example, but also dietetics, social work, and housekeeping. In a global reporting system, the total cost of a surgical procedure such as a coronary artery bypass graft can be determined.

Key components of departmental reporting, the system used most often in Canadian health facilities, are financial data, statistical data, indicators, and variances. *Financial data* consists of all revenue and expenses associated with a service or program. On a nursing unit, the revenue generated is usually income associated with private and semi-private accommodations. Expenses on a nursing unit include direct operating costs such as salaries, employee benefits and supplies, and indirect operating costs such as housekeeping and laundry services.

Statistics always accompany an operational budget. In preparing the operational budget, the manager must compile and summarize data from the previous twelve months and make projections for the next financial year. Some common statistics include patient activity, workloads, and staffing. Patient activity on a nursing unit may include average occupancy, total patient days, number of admissions, and discharges and transfers, as well as a summary of workload measurement.

Workload measurement and patient-classification systems are tools that assist the manager in providing an appropriate level of staffing to meet the expected demand for nursing care (see also Chapter 21). Prior to the development of patient-classification systems, staffing levels were determined by global standards; for example, 2.5 hours of direct nursing care were estimated to be required per patient per day, or one RN was estimated to be needed in order to care for three patients. These global standards did not reflect variations in care requirements among patients. Patient-classification systems were designed to provide a more accurate estimate of nursing workloads by using critical indicators of care, such as bathing, ambulation, and feeding. Workload-measurement systems, if well-designed and maintained, may provide a reliable and valid assessment of patient-care needs which can then be used to help the nurse manager allocate staff to patients efficiently. Data generated by a workload-measurement system should be part of the permanent clinical record, and should be summarized and reviewed from time to time to assess changing trends in patient-care requirements.

MIS guidelines require the use of *indicators* so that managers may evaluate and control current operations, and plan for the future. Indicators are calculated using financial and statistical data which produce various ratios and percentages. For example, an outpatient visit may be considered a unit of service for which the direct cost can be calculated. If the direct cost per unit of service is known (e.g., a clinic visit), it can be monitored over time and compared with other similar units of service. Such indicators assist managers in controlling expenditures.

Another example of an indicator is the productivity of nursing staff. Productivity is calculated by dividing the required hours of care (as esti-

---

Box 2 2 . 1

UNIT CHARACTERISTICS

Bed allocation:

2 private, 10 semi-private, and 2 wards consisting of 4 beds each

Most common
surgical diagnoses:

gynecological procedures such as hysterectomies and ovarian cysts; mastectomies; abdominal peritoneal resections; cholecystectomies

Most common
medical diagnoses:

cardiac and pulmonary disorders, including chronic obstructive lung disease, myocardial infarction, angina, pneumonia, peripheral vascular disease, and diabetes

Other characteristics:

Two patients on the unit are medically discharged and awaiting placement in a nursing home: one has been on the unit for two years, and the other has been on the unit for eighteen months.

In the year prior to the budget year, there were 10,400 patient days.

The average patient requires 4.0 hours of nursing care per 24 hours.

---

mated by the workload-measurement system) by the actual hours of care provided (i.e., payroll data), and multiplying the quotient by 100. A productivity rate of 100 percent indicates that the actual hours of care match the required hours of care. A rate greater than 100 percent indicates that actual hours provided were less than required, while a rate less than 100 percent indicates that more hours of care were provided than were necessary. Most facilities set acceptable productivity ranges at 85 to 115 percent.

The final key component of the MIS departmental reporting system is variances. A *variance* refers to the difference between the budgeted cost and the actual cost of an item—for example, the cost of paying overtime to nurses. Variances can be positive or negative, and these will be discussed later in the chapter.

DEVELOPING THE BUDGET

To assist the reader in understanding and applying key concepts in developing an operating budget, a case example of a 30-bed medical/surgical unit in a regional hospital is presented as an example in Box 22.1. To develop the operating budget for this nursing unit, the nurse manager must determine the human resource/staffing costs, supply costs, and revenue.

HUMAN RESOURCE COSTS

The bed allocation, patient days, and average hours of nursing care are used to determine the human resource/staffing costs of caring for patients on this nursing unit (see Box 22.2).

Human resources or staffing consists of management and operational support, and unit producing personnel (UPP). Management and operational support personnel are those whose primary function is the management and

Box 22.2

**HUMAN RESOURCES/
STAFFING CHARACTERISTICS**

- Management and operational support personnel consists of one nurse manager and one unit clerk.
- The unit producing personnel includes registered nurses and registered nursing assistants.
- The average annual salary for the nurse manager is $48,000.
- The average hourly rate for remaining staff is:

Registered Nurse	$20.51
Registered Nursing Assistant	$12.82
Unit Clerk	$10.26

- The skill mix for the unit producing personnel is 70% RNs and 30% RNAs.
- Benefit salaries are 20% of regular salaries.
- The benefit contribution expense is 19.5% of regular salaries plus benefit salaries.

clerical support of the nursing unit. In this case, management and operational support personnel include the nurse manager and the unit clerk. Also in this case, the UPP are RNs and RNAs whose primary function is to carry out activities directly related to the care of the patient.

In preparing the budget, management/operational support, and unit producing personnel are expressed as full-time equivalent (FTE) positions. An FTE measures the total number of personnel in terms of a specified work week, e.g., 40 hours. The work week may vary from province to province as it is usually negotiated during the collective-bargaining process. In Newfoundland, for example, one FTE position is equivalent to 37.5 hours per week or 7.5 hours daily, for a total of 1950 earned hours per year. These earned hours include worked hours (the hours a nurse actually works) plus benefit hours, such as sick leave and vacation leave. An FTE may be a full-time staff member who earns 1950 hours per year, or it may be two or three staff members who together earn 1950 hours per year. FTEs may be determined in terms of hours or shifts. For example, a person who works half time or 975 hours per year is 0.5 FTE, a person who works 800 hours per year is 0.4 FTE, and a person working one shift per week or 7.5 hours per week is 0.2 FTE. The total number of FTEs is not usually the same as the total number of staff. For example, a nursing budget may have 16.4 FTEs but may consist of 21 staff.

Regular Salaries: Unit Producing Personnel

To calculate the unit producing personnel for this 30-bed unit, the nurse manager must first determine the occupancy rate. The occupancy rate is the ratio of occupied beds to the total number of beds on the unit. This 30-bed unit has the potential for 10,950 patient days (i.e. 30 beds × 365 days) per year. In this case, however, there were 10,400 patient days in 1996/97. To calculate the occupancy rate, the following formula is used:

$$\text{Occupancy Rate} = \frac{\text{Actual Patient Days}}{\text{No. of beds} \times 365 \text{ days/year}} = \frac{10,400}{30 \times 365} = 95\%$$

A 95 percent occupancy rate for this unit means that there are an average of 28.5 beds occupied each day.

To determine the total number of unit producing FTEs required for this 30-bed nursing unit, the occupancy rate or number of beds occupied is used in conjunction with the average hours of care per patient per 24-hour period. The formula is as follows:

$$\text{No. of FTEs} = \frac{\text{No. of beds occupied} \times \text{hours of care per patient per 24 hrs.} \times 365 \text{ days}}{\text{Earned hours per FTE}}$$

$$= \frac{28.5 \times 4.0 \text{ hours} \times 365}{1950 \text{ hours}}$$

$$= 21.3$$

Based on a skill mix of 70 percent registered nurses (RN) and 30 percent registered nursing assistants (RNA), the 21.3 FTEs would consist of 14.9 RN and 6.4 RNA. Regular salaries for nursing personnel are based on a salary scale negotiated through collective agreements. Based on an average hourly rate of $20.51 for a registered nurse and $12.82 for a registered nursing assistant, regular salaries are calculated as follows:

14.9 RNs @	$20.51/hour × 1950 hours/year	=	$595,918
6.4 RNAs @	$12.82/hour × 1950 hours/year	=	$159,994
			$755,912

Note: All catculation are rounded up to nearest dollar.

Benefits: Unit Producing Personnel

According to the MIS guidelines, direct benefits are referred to as benefit salaries and include relief for vacation, sick leave, and statutory holidays, as well as overtime, in-charge pay, shift differential, and educational allowance. These benefits are generally negotiated through the collective-bargaining process and vary from province to province. In recent years, fiscal realities have led to minimum staffing levels on many nursing units. This reduced staffing has resulted in one-to-one replacement of nursing staff, which results in higher benefit-salary costs. Benefit-salary costs may be calculated individually, or estimated as a percentage of regular salaries. Benefit salaries are estimated at 20 percent of regular salaries. In this case example, regular salaries are $755,912; therefore, benefit salaries are $151,182 ($755,912.00 × 0.20). Regular salaries and benefit salaries must be added together before calculating the benefit-contribution expense.

Indirect benefits are referred to as the benefit contribution expense and they represent the facility's contribution to benefits such as Canada Pension Plan (CPP), Employment Insurance (EI), provincial pension, and health insurance. Benefits such as CPP and EI are constant among the provinces; other benefits may vary slightly. Benefit contribution expense is calculated as a percentage of regular salaries plus benefit salaries. In this case example, the benefit contribution expense is estimated at 19.5 percent of these costs or $176,883 [($755,912 + $151,182) × .195].

Regular Salaries and Benefits: Management and Operational Support Personnel

To calculate the management and operational support personnel costs for this 30-bed unit, the nurse manager's salary and the unit clerk's salary are added together. Based on an average salary of $48,000 for the nurse manager and an average hourly wage of $10.26 for the unit clerk, regular salaries for these personnel are calculated as follows:

Nurse Manager	=	$48,000
Unit Clerk @ $10.26/hour × 1950 hours	=	$20,007
		$68,007

Because these staff members are not replaced when absent for vacation or sickness, there are no benefit salaries associated with the positions. Employee benefit contributions amount to 19.5 percent of regular salaries or $13,261 ($68,007 × .195).

Other Compensation Considerations

When calculating regular salaries for all personnel working on the unit, the nurse manager must be aware of future changes such as step progressions (i.e., increments on the salary scale), and wage increases. Step progressions will vary from employee to employee on an annual basis; wage increases may vary by job classification. Occasionally, an employee will leave or retire who is entitled to accumulated annual leave and/or severance pay. Severance pay is a termination bonus based on years of service and is a benefit accrued in some provinces. The funding allocated for these benefits is a one-time cost that should be included in budget projections in the year the costs will be incurred.

The total compensation expense for management and operational support as well as unit producing personnel for this 30-bed nursing unit is calculated in Table 22.1.

SUPPLIES

According to the MIS guidelines, supplies are divided into various categories such as medical and surgical supplies, drugs, medical gases, printing and office supplies, laundry, and linen. Supplies usually represent about 20 percent of the total operating budget.

In many cases, nurse managers are responsible only for determining the budget allocation for supplies that are used directly for patient care, such as medical/surgical supplies, drugs, and medical gases. Medical/surgical supplies include items such as dressings, catheters, needles, syringes, and gloves. Drugs are subdivided into categories such as IV solutions, anti-neoplastics,

Table 22.1

CALCULATING COMPENSATION

Management and Operational Support Personnel		
Regular Salaries	$68,007	
Benefit Salaries	0	
Employee Benefit Contributions	13,261	81,268

Unit Producing Personnel		
Regular Salaries	755,912	
Benefit Salaries	151,182	
Employee Benefit Contributions	176,883	1,083,977

Total Compensation Expense		**$1,165,245**

total parenteral nutrition, and antibiotics. Medical gases include anaesthetic gases and oxygen. Other supply costs include laundry and linen, which may be determined by other departmental managers.

In determining the current year's budget for supplies, the nurse manager should review actual costs for the previous year, and adjust these amounts for inflation and workload changes such as bed closures, a new physician, or increased patient acuity. Such changes may be interdependent. For example, a new physician can effect a change in the patient profile by performing more complicated surgeries or admitting patients who require higher levels of care, thereby increasing patient acuity. The change in patient acuity will result in increased usage of more costly medical/surgical supplies and drugs.

To calculate the supply costs in this case example, the nurse manager must make an adjustment for inflation, as all other factors remained constant including number of beds, occupancy rate, and other factors. Inflation is based on the Consumer Price Index and is provided on an annual basis by Statistics Canada. If the inflation rate for the budget year is estimated at three percent, and the actual cost for the previous year was $262,000, the projected costs for the budget year's supplies would be $270,000 ($262,000 × 1.03). The allocation of these supply costs is shown in Table 22.2.

REVENUE

Revenue for this 30-bed nursing unit is limited to income from patients in the private and semi-private rooms. The daily rates that patients are charged for these rooms are usually established by the province. In this example, revenue is generated from the two private and ten semi-private rooms; the room rates are $75 for a private room and $60 for a semi-private room. Based on the 95 percent occupancy rate on this nursing unit, the revenue is calculated as follows:

Table 22.2

CALCULATING SUPPLY COSTS

Supply Item	Previous Year	Budget Year
Medical Surgical Supplies	$104,000	$107,200
Drugs	$136,000	$140,100
Medical Gases	$ 22,000	$ 22,700
Total	$262,000	$270,000

Private: 2 rooms @ $75 per day $\times$ 365 days $\times$ .95 = $ 52,013
Semi-private: 10 rooms $\times$ 2 people @ $60 per day $\times$
               365 days $\times$ .95   = $416,100
                                                                $468,113

The invoices for recovering this revenue are usually generated by the accounting office and given to patients upon discharge. As revenue calculations are completed by staff in the finance department, the nurse manager is not usually involved in the revenue recovery process.

A summary of the whole operating budget appears in Table 22.3.

FINANCIAL CONTROL AND REPORTING

While reviewing the monthly budget reports, managers should seek clarification from accounting staff regarding areas of concern, or instances where details seem to be unclear. Developing a good working relationship with accounting staff will assist the nurse manager in becoming more knowledgeable about variance reporting, and will enable the manager to alter expenditure patterns to address unfavourable trends which may be developing.

Variances are the differences between budgeted or expected performance and actual performance. Under a participative budgeting process, managers are provided with a monthly report that shows a comparison of budget projections and operating results for the month, and a variance column displaying the differences between actual and budget projections. A negative variance occurs if actual costs are greater than budgeted costs; a positive variance occurs if actual costs are less than budgeted costs. Negative variances are sometimes indicated in parentheses. Both negative and positive variances are demonstrated in the example of a budget report for the month of August in Table 22.4.

Budget reports also provide a year-to-date summary of actual and budget expenditures, and sometimes include information about workload and patient activity. Managers should examine these monthly reports and

Table 22.3

OPERATING BUDGET FOR A 30-BED
MEDICAL/SURGICAL UNIT

Nursing Unit
One-Year Operating Budget

COMPENSATION		
Management and Operational Support Personnel		
Regular Salaries	$ 68,007	
Benefit Salaries	0	
Employee Benefit Contributions	13,261	81,268
Unit Producing Personnel		
Regular Salaries	755,912	
Benefit Salaries	151,182	
Employee Benefit Contributions	176,883	1,083,977
Total Compensation Expense		**1,165,245**

SUPPLIES		
Medical and Surgical Supplies	107,200	
Drugs	140,100	
Medical Gases	22,700	
		Total Supplies
270,000		
Total Expenses		**1,435,245**
Less Revenue		
Accommodations		
Private	(52,013)	
Semi-Private	(416,000)	(468,113)

Total Operating Budget		**$967,132**

should be able to justify variances outside the expected range. Ongoing negative variances may indicate trends which require the intervention of managers and front-line supervisors. For instance, if the volume of work is increasing and the worked hours remain constant, the manager may need to make a temporary increase in the number of staff for peak periods. Note that in Table 22.4, there is a negative variance for unit producing personnel for both the month of August and the year-to-date. If the variance continues much longer, a permanent staffing adjustment may need to be made.

Managers are usually expected to answer to their immediate supervisors for budget variances. According to McConnell (1993), "answering to variances under budget is almost as important as answering to variances over budget" (p. 327). Being under budget may be due to a seasonal variation in expenses, and does not necessarily mean a cost savings. For example, the

Table 22.4
BUDGET REPORT FOR THE MONTH OF AUGUST

| | AUGUST | | | YEAR-TO-DATE | | |
	Budget	Actual	Variance	Budget	Actual	Variance
Item						
Compensation:						
Management/support	6,772	6,772	—	33,860	33,860	—
Unit producing staff	90,331	93,000	(2,669)	451,655	476,200	(24,545)
Supplies:						
Med/Surg	8,933	9,000	(67)	44,665	42,600	2,065
Drugs	11,675	10,700	975	56,375	60,725	(4,350)
Medical gases	1,841	1,500	341	9,455	8,050	1,405
Total	**119,552**	**120,972**	**(1,420)**	**596,010**	**621,435**	**(25,425)**

Patient Care Unit: 30-bed medical/surgical

vacation relief budget for nursing staff may be distributed equally over a twelve-month period, but there may not be any actual expenses incurred for vacation relief during the winter months.

RESOURCE MANAGEMENT

According to Buchan (1992), "cost containment is the key concept that nurses must grasp in this time of shrinking budgets and growing demands for health care. As health-care budgets come under increased scrutiny, nurses must prove their cost effectiveness" (p.117). If nurses ignore this issue, important decisions on resource allocation will be made by administrators who have a strong knowledge of costing but a weak appreciation of the impact of cost containment strategies on the quality of nursing care.

Nurse managers need to be aware of the costs of staffing, supplies, and equipment used to provide health services. The most costly input in the provision of nursing care is staffing, which represents approximately 70 percent of the operating budget. As noted earlier, workload-measurement systems can be used to control staffing costs by assigning staff according to the actual demand for nursing care. However, patient-care requirements often fluctuate, and the nursing manager must monitor these changes in patient acuity and adjust the staffing levels accordingly. This may be done, for example, by calling in casual staff to meet increased demands, or by floating excess staff to understaffed units (refer also to Chapter 21 on staffing). If staff are transferred to another nursing unit, the unit manager must ensure that costs are allocated to the unit where the staff actually performs the work.

It is important that the mix of nursing skills matches patient-care requirements. Nursing workload-measurement systems do not solve the question of what category of nursing staff to assign to patients—that decision requires nursing judgement. In general, work should be assigned to the least costly personnel capable of doing the work. Professional staff should be assigned to work requiring their expertise. For example, the registration function in an outpatient clinic should be assigned to clerks, rather than to registered nursing assistants, while patient assessment is the function of RNs. The skill mix of nursing staff differs from unit to unit. Some specialized areas like obstetrics, emergency, and critical care are generally staffed by RNs only, whereas general medical surgical units may have a mix of RNs and RNAs. Nurse managers must be constantly monitoring the profiles of patients on the unit and adjusting the staffing complement and skill mix to match patient need.

Managers can also control input costs through the judicious use of supplies and equipment, by selecting products that have the desired qualities at the lowest price, for example. Most facilities have a product-evaluation committee that considers new products from quality and cost perspectives. The committee's findings regarding various products will assist the manager in choosing quality supplies and equipment at a reasonable price. Supply costs can also be controlled by closely monitoring the amount used. Managers should encourage practices that control waste and prevent pilferage; for example, equipment that is reusable should not be treated as if it were disposable.

McKay, cited by Edwardson (1988) suggests that increasing the cost sensitivity among nursing personnel is another means of controlling supply costs. McVay further states that "one nurse manager was able to produce large savings by simply placing price tags on chargeable supplies. Nurses in the study hospital discovered that they could substitute less costly items with no untoward effects and avoid using some items altogether" (p. 84).

Nurse managers must also look at utilization indicators as a way to monitor costs while providing quality care. A review of indicators such as occupancy and average length of stay over a specified time period will reveal trends that can assist the nurse manager in making decisions regarding appropriate bed utilization. The use of care maps, for instance, allows managers to monitor the average length of stay for selected diagnostic groups of patients.

To manage resources effectively, nurse managers must also examine the process used in providing care. A nurse manager should ask, for example, whether some of the routine tests and procedures for patients could be done more efficiently. Many hospitals have introduced pre-admission clinics and same-day admission programs whereby elective patients receive their diagnostic tests as outpatients one or two days before admission. Pre-admission clinics reduce the average length of stay for patients and improve their quality of life by reducing their time spent away from home. It is worth noting, however, that while pre-admission programs increase the number of patients who can be admitted, the patients who are admitted to hospital are on average more acutely ill while in hospital, and will therefore likely increase the overall cost of care provided by the facility.

The nurse manager must work closely with other health-care providers, including medical staff and allied health professionals, to assess the utilization of services. Working as a team, these individuals can determine whether services and programs should be introduced, continued, or discontinued. Efforts should be made to ensure that more effective use of resources is accompanied by an improvement in the quality of care provided.

SUMMARY

- Fiscal restraint has resulted in the restructuring of health-care organizations throughout Canada, and health agencies are adopting business strategies to deliver services to patients and clients.
- A business plan is a set of statements about the mission, goals, and strategies of an organization to be accomplished within a set period of time.
- Budgeting and financial management are integral components of a business plan.
- Nursing services generally consume 70 to 80 percent of the total operating budgets of hospitals.
- Managers are responsible for two types of budgets, capital budgets and operating budgets.
- Management Information Systems (MIS) guidelines are used across Canada to standardize financial reporting and statistics related to health-care costs.
- Budgets are used to control costs through regular monitoring of variances, such as the difference between expected performance and actual performance.
- Cost containment is the responsibility of managers and staff, and can be achieved by re-examining all aspects of patient-care delivery to ensure efficient use of human and material resources.

FURTHER READINGS AND RESOURCES

Brazil, K., & Anderson, M. (1996). Assessing health service needs: Tools for health planning. *Health Care Management Forum, 9*(1), 22–27.

Edwardson, S. R. (1998) Productivity. In E. J. Sullivan & P. J. Decker (Eds.). *Effective management in nursing* (pp. 71–92). Menlo Park, CA: Addison-Wesley.

Harber, B., & Miller, S. (1994). Program management and health care informatics: Defining relationships. *Healthcare Management, 7*(4), 28–35.

Health Care Corporation of St. John's (1996). Mission statment. St. John's, Newfoundland: Author. (Mimeograph)

Hodges, L. C., & Poteet, G. W. (1991). Financial responsibility and budget decision making. *Journal of Nursing Administration,* 21 (10), 30–33.

Keddy, W., & Wolnik, S., (1989). Monitoring and evaluating organizational effectiveness In Canadian Hospital Association (Ed.). *Introduction to nursing management: A Canadian perspective* (pp. 125–145). Ottawa: Canadian Hospital Association.

Krissman, R. A. (1992). Meaningful information for decision making. In A. E. Barnett & G. G. Mayer (Eds.), *Ambulatory care management and practice.* (pp. 185–194). Gaithersburg, MD: Aspen.

Levine-Ariff, J., Hartmann, M., & Wojcicki, T. (1988). Budgeting and resource allocation. In E. J. Sullivan & P. J. Decker (Eds.) (pp. 443–462). Menlo Park, CA: Addison-Wesley.

McFaul, W. J., & Lyons D. M., (1996). Strategic resource management. *Journal of Healthcare Resource Management, 15*(10), 9–13.

Monaghan, B. J., Alton, L., & Allen, A. D. (1992). Transition to program management. *Leadership in Health Services, 1*(5), 33–37.

Newfoundland Provincial MIS Nursing/Ambulatory Care Steering Committee, (1995). *Nursing inpatient service: Statistics and indicators.* Available from Newfoundland and Labrador Centre for Health Information, St. John's, Newfoundland.

Olsen, J. (1995). What is resource management. *Journal of Healthcare Resource Management, 13*(1), 11–13.

White, J., & Yates, R. (1994). The effect of program management on nursing services. *Canadian Nursing Management,* No. 75, 5–8.

REFERENCES

Buchan, J. (1992). Cost effective caring. *International Nursing Review, 39*(4), 117–120.

Canadian Institute of Health Information (1994). Nursing inpatient services. In *Guidelines for Management Information Systems in Canadian Health Care Facilities.* Ottawa: Canadian Institute of Health Information.

Edwardson, S. R. (1988). Productivity. In E.J. Sullivan &P.J. Decker (Eds.) *Effective Management in Nursing (2nd ed.)* (pp. 71-92). Memlo Park, CA: Addison-Wesley.

McConnell, C. R. (1993). *The Effective Health Care Supervisor.* Gaithersburg, MD: Aspen.

Oberg, L., & Wagner, N. (1994). *Getting started II: Health business plan guidebook.* Edmonton, AB: Alberta Health.

CASE STUDY

Kim Kwan and Jodie Simcoe graduated from the same BScN program ten years ago, and they meet each other unexpectedly at a job fair. They were good friends at university and have kept in touch sporadically over the years. Both are victims of regionalization and downsizing. Their jobs disappeared in mergers of health agencies, and they were terminated from their positions and given severance packages. Both are now in the process of reassessing their prospects and career options. They decide to have coffee together and this leads to a lively brainstorming session, resulting in a decision to develop a plan to go into independent nursing practice together.

Together they identify a wide range of skills and expertise they could contribute to a joint nursing-service practice. Kim Kwan has experience in public-health nursing, specializing in health promotion and maternal and child services, and she has five years as case manager in a home-care service. Jodie Simcoe has several years of mental-health nursing and supervisory experience, and for the last three years she was a unit-based educator on a 25-bed active rehabilitation unit for traumatic brain-injured clients and post-stroke clients. She considers herself to have had valuable experience in inter-professional co-operation and teamwork. Both registered nurses have personal friends in the legal and accounting professions, and feel they can obtain enough informal advice to help them draw up a business plan for the first year of operating their independent nursing practice.

Creative exercise. Applying the concepts discussed in this chapter, draft a business plan for the proposed Kwan/Simcoe enterprise, including vision and mission statements, goals and strategies for the first year of operation. Develop both capital and operating budgets, identifying sources of revenue, direct and indirect costs. What additional budget items would be needed by nurses in independent practice not mentioned in this chapter?

PART FIVE

Tool Kit for Managers

Chapter 23

▼▼▼▼▼▼▼▼▼▼▼▼▼▼▼▼

Managing Change

Judith Skelton-Green

KEY OBJECTIVES

In this chapter, you will learn:

- Changes affecting the health-care system, and their effects.
- Basic types of change, and different models of change management.
- The difference between change and transition, and their interdependence.
- The processes which a nurse manager may use in responding to, and championing, change.
- Strategies and tools that may be used to implement change.

INTRODUCTION

Change is affecting people at all levels of the health-care system. The purpose of this chapter is to provide an overview of those changes; to explore the common issues and challenges change presents to nurse managers; and to suggest tools and strategies for the effective management of change.

CHANGES AFFECTING THE HEALTH-CARE SYSTEM

Like all businesses in North America, the Canadian health-care system is experiencing a period of significant and widespread change. The catalysts have been many and varied; this section outlines some of the most significant.

CHANGES IN FUNDING METHODS

Over the past several years, the federal government has dramatically reduced the amount of money it transfers to the provinces for health care. Provincial governments, struggling with their own debt and deficit problems, have decreased health-care funding in most, if not all, sectors. In some provinces, the government is devolving funding responsibility to municipalities by creating funding "envelopes" that are held and managed by boards located in smaller geographic regions.

CHANGES IN SERVICE DELIVERY

Restructuring of the Canadian health-care system has been initiated at a variety of levels to achieve a number of basic objectives, most of which can be summarized as either *increasing the efficiency* or *increasing the effectiveness of health care*. Some of the key strategies of system restructuring are:

- Co-ordinating and integrating all aspects of the care-delivery system, from the activities of physicians to the responsibilities of institutions, community-care agencies, and mental-health agencies. These changes are intended to ensure appropriate patient care is delivered in a timely manner, while reducing unnecessary or redundant use of the system.
- Providing the governance and funding structures necessary to support a shift in focus from the reactive treatment of illness to the proactive promotion of health, and to assist in the transition from inpatient care to community care.
- Establishing clear health policy and funding frameworks that support the goals of the provincial and federal health-care systems.
- Decentralizing health care to ensure that health planning and delivery are more closely associated with a population's specific needs, while increasing the accountability of the region.
- Increasing the accountability of caregivers by introducing modified funding structures that are designed to provide financial incentives for improved health outcomes, preventive care, and appropriate system utilization.
- Increasing the accountability of patients or taxpayers by providing access to health information and by demanding "contracts for care" with the primary-care provider of choice.
- Providing caregivers consistent and co-ordinated access to patient information through electronic health records.
- Establishing partnerships and alliances to capitalize on the unique capabilities of the private sector and to increase the competitive pressures of health-care delivery (Canadian College of Health Service Executives, 1997).

NEW EMPHASIS ON HEALTH PROMOTION AND WELLNESS

The benefits of health promotion and wellness are becoming driving forces for system restructuring. A plethora of literature outlines the benefits, both tangible and intangible, of health promotion and illness prevention. Appropriate patient screening, education, and monitoring are all key components to avoiding unnecessary illness, hospitalization, or disability. Additionally, improved access to health information and health education permits improved management and early identification of individuals in the community who may be at risk.

NEW FOCUS ON HOME CARE AND EARLY DISCHARGE

Technological advances in communication and monitoring equipment now permit effective home-management of patients previously requiring hospitalization. More and more, the provincial health systems are searching for ways to shift the focus of care from inpatient care to outpatient management, and from illness to wellness-based modalities.

EXPANDING ROLES FOR INFORMATION TECHNOLOGY AND TELECOMMUNICATIONS

Virtually all of the studies of health reform in Canada have emphasized the crucial link between health-care reform and the effective use of information technology. Indeed, many believe that the needed reforms can *only* be achieved through the effective application of new information and telecommunications technologies. As a result, many provinces are currently working towards the development of core health-information network infrastructures, around which a wide variety of services and patient-based applications can be developed and delivered.

Beyond provincial expansion opportunities, it is recognized that there is a significant need for a nation-wide information network that would not only incorporate provincial networks, but would also transcend traditional organizational, program, and geographic boundaries to integrate the health-related information services offered by a wide range of providers, thereby meeting the needs of a wide range of users, including health providers, researchers, policy makers, and the general public.

PREPARING TO MANAGE CHANGE

The five factors listed above, along with other changes in the health-care system and the world at large, place unprecedented pressure on health-service organizations, and have particular impact on the ways in which these organizations are led and managed. Vaill (1989) uses the image of "permanent white water" to describe the environment of chaotic change in which most organizations currently find themselves. This image is intended to capture the speed, unpredictability, novelty, complexity and excitement of the world in which business exists today. Those involved in the health-care system often feel they are caught in white-water situations, and as if they are paddling upstream. Today and for the future, nurse managers require an ability to deal with change positively. They are challenged to embrace change in a way that will allow them to position themselves and their organizations effectively for the future.

Nurse managers who wish to promote and facilitate change need a variety of tools, including knowledge about change and change management;

the ability to differentiate between change and transition, and to provide leadership for both; a positive attitude towards change; and a set of strategies and techniques which they can apply to the specific changes they encounter.

TYPES OF CHANGE

Change takes three forms: it may be developmental, spontaneous, or carefully planned.

DEVELOPMENTAL CHANGE

The manager can prepare for the potential *results* of developmental or spontaneous change, but cannot actually plan for these changes in a systematically controlled manner the way he or she can with planned change.

Developmental change occurs as an organism or organization grows and becomes more complex. Like human embryos, organizations grow and develop on the basis of their needs, often in highly predictable ways. Imagine, for example, that a small clinic opens in a rural community, and that it is staffed for eight hours a day by one full-time registered nurse and a full-time receptionist/secretary. A physician is available two days a week. Staff communication is simple, usually one to one, and problems are generally discussed over lunch and solved in a collaborative manner. Staff members are enthusiastic about the potential role for the clinic in community health promotion, and their efforts in this regard prove highly successful. Over time, several members are added to the staff to provide support for a variety of new services. Staff communication patterns become more complex and often break down; "turf-protection" begins; the receptionist feels overworked and angry at being "everybody's servant"; and clients are heard to remark that "the place is less user-friendly." These unwanted changes are the result of the evolution of a larger and therefore more complex organization. Change was necessary to meet predefined objectives, and could not be avoided. Nonetheless, the manager could, and should, have anticipated some of the changes and planned to minimize their negative outcomes.

SPONTANEOUS CHANGE

Spontaneous change is often called a "reaction," and may be compared to the invasion of a human organism by a cold virus. Such an invasion may cause major disruption to the health of one person but prove only a minor inconvenience to another, depending on the overall condition, both physical and psychological, of the host.

Unexpected invasions of health-care organizations take various forms. These may be events with short-term repercussions, such as an air crash near a small regional hospital, a wildcat strike that virtually closes acute-care beds in a region, or an unusually heavy snow storm in a widespread rural community served by the Victorian Order of Nurses. Long-term events can also create reactive change: a recent one is the dramatic impact of HIV on the policies and practices of health-care agencies; another is the prolonged effect of fiscal restraint on the health system.

An organization can neither fully anticipate nor avoid spontaneous change, and therefore has little or no time to plan its response. Managers can reduce reactive impact through general planning, using such mechanisms as disaster plans and assorted communication strategies. Successful responses to spontaneous change require flexibility, cohesiveness, and a level of trust within the organization

PLANNED CHANGE

In planned change, a desired future result is achieved by deliberately determining deficiencies within the current state, deciding on one or more possible improvements, and enacting a plan to achieve them. Individuals use "planned change" when they read to gain new knowledge, or take courses to develop their management skills, or decide to improve their health through exercise and better eating habits.

Organizations are constantly involved in planned change. Changes may be department-specific, such as when, for example, a unit in a long-term-care facility moves to a "no-restraint" policy; organization-wide, such as the decision to expand the services of a visiting-nurse association; or cross-institutional, such as the decision by a number of health-care organizations to merge their operations to form an integrated delivery system. Success in bringing about planned change is a major part of any nurse manager's role.

MODELS OF CHANGE MANAGEMENT

Four contemporary models of change management are particularly useful to nurse managers today. They are generally referred to by the names of the authors who first described and tested them.

LEWIN

Classical change theory has its origins in the work of Kurt Lewin (1951) who described change in terms of "field" and "force." In applying Lewin's theory of change to an organization, the organization is considered an open system. In the *unfreezing phase* the desired change or problem is identified or realized by organizational members. A "force-field analysis" is conducted to gather preliminary data regarding the problem or desired change, and to gain information about the driving and restraining forces. Figure 23.1 shows a sample force-field analysis for use by a nurse manager who is considering a change to a primary nursing-care delivery system, as a result of staff and patient dissatisfaction with the existing team-nursing system.

Figure 23.1

FORCE-FIELD ANALYSIS OF CHANGE IN NURSING-CARE DELIVERY SYSTEM

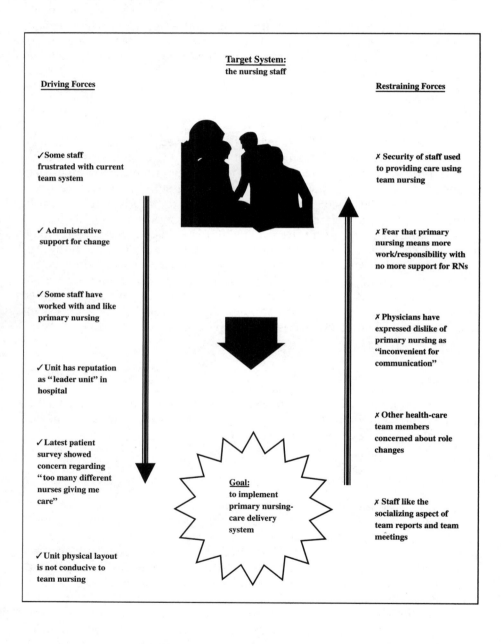

Target System:
the nursing staff

Driving Forces

Restraining Forces

✓Some staff frustrated with current team system

✓ Administrative support for change

✓ Some staff have worked with and like primary nursing

✓ Unit has reputation as "leader unit" in hospital

✓ Latest patient survey showed concern regarding "too many different nurses giving me care"

✓ Unit physical layout is not conducive to team nursing

Goal:
to implement primary nursing-care delivery system

✗ Security of staff used to providing care using team nursing

✗ Fear that primary nursing means more work/responsibility with no more support for RNs

✗ Physicians have expressed dislike of primary nursing as "inconvenient for communication"

✗ Other health-care team members concerned about role changes

✗ Staff like the socializing aspect of team reports and team meetings

Following the force-field analysis, the change agent shares initial data with the target group so a joint diagnosis of the change issue can be made. A joint action plan is developed and directed towards achieving the desired change. The focus of the action plan is to increase the forces facilitating change, and/or to decrease those inhibiting it.

In the *moving phase* actions identified within the action plan are carried out. Change begins as the system moves from its present state to its envisioned future state.

The goal of the *refreezing phase* is to integrate and stabilize the change and withdraw the change agent from the system. Data is gathered to provide the organization with the necessary information to evaluate the outcomes of the process. If the change is to remain in place, the driving and restraining forces must be re-evaluated. Analysis of the data may lead to a rediagnosis and renewed change activity.

ROGERS AND SHOEMAKER

Rogers and Shoemaker (1971) also describe a three-phase model of change. It focuses on the goal of change and the communication of that goal to all concerned. The three phases consist of: *invention of the change, diffusion or communication* of information regarding the change, and *consequence* which is either an adoption or rejection of the change. Within this model, Rogers and Shoemaker describe individual behaviours that characterize how people respond to change:

- *Innovators* actively seek and look forward to change.
- *Early adopters* help make change possible.
- *The early majority* provides a support system for the change.
- *The late majority* provides peer pressure to support the change.
- *Laggards* strive to keep doing things the way they have been done before.
- *Rejectors* work actively against the change.

The Roger and Shoemaker model is based on the assumption that people are rational and will adopt change if it is logically justified and they can see some possible gain in making the change. The focus of the approach is in providing the knowledge necessary for making a rational choice.

KANTER

In *The Change Masters* (1983), Rosabeth Moss Kanter describes a model of change that is designed to guide executives in promoting innovation and entrepreneurship within their organizations. Kanter argues that innovation and change can be fostered, promoted, and initiated at all levels within the organization. Innovation is found to flourish in organizations that possess a culture of pride that encourages teamwork, consensus building, and communication, and fosters a sense of personal value. In contrast, organizations that inhibit innovation tend to advocate a top-down approach characterized by multiple, formal structures. Kanter concludes that change initiated in this way reinforces a culture of inferiority that breeds in organizational members a sense of complacency, anxiety, and distrust.

Kanter describes three sequential "waves of activity" that characterize innovation leading to change: problem definition, coalition building, and mobilization. During the *problem definition* wave, information is gathered to shape a feasible, focused project for action. Through communication and collaboration within the organization, *coalition building* occurs to garner support and resources for the project. During the *mobilization* wave, the resources are invested to bring the innovation from idea to reality.

Inherent in Kanter's conceptualization of innovation is the concept of *empowerment*. She argues that leaders who wish to effect innovation should do so using a collaborative and participative approach that involves persuading rather than ordering, as well as team building, seeking input, demonstrating a sensitivity to the interests and priorities of others, and sharing rewards and recognition.

F E R G U S O N

Ferguson (1980) offers hope for those who feel that the "forces" stimulating and shaping change are overwhelming and uncontrollable. He suggests that people and organizations "change" in four ways when they receive new and conflicting information:

- *Change by Exception*: keeping old, time-honoured belief systems intact, but allowing for a handful of anomalies.
- *Incremental Change*: changing so slowly that affected individuals are often not even aware that change has occurred.
- *Pendulum Change*: abandoning one closed and certain system of beliefs in favour of another.
- *Paradigm* or *Transformational Change*: engaging in a conscious process which results in new insight or perspective.

In the transformational change mode, participants recognize that their previous understanding was only part of the picture—and further, that what they now comprehend is only part of what they will learn at some later point. Through transformational change, managers realize that there are new and better ways of "being" in the world. And through transformational change, we discover other individuals, other sources of power, other applications of our learning for the greater good of the system—and, indeed, of society.

Undoubtedly, the most significant impact of Ferguson's writing is the notion that by changing their thinking and attitudes, *individual* human beings have the power to provoke profound changes in their lives and in the world. For the nursing manager feeling very alone in a large and seemingly oppressive system, Ferguson's work offers inspiration to attempt change alone, "on the home front," with the hope and expectation that one's actions (however small) can, indeed, "make a difference."

CHANGE VERSUS TRANSITION

In reviewing the literature on change, several authors emphasize the importance of attending to the human side of change in organizations. The most comprehensive work in this area is that of William Bridges, a leading expert on organizational transition.

Bridges (1991) differentiates between organizational change and transition. Change, he says, can be planned and managed using a "more or less" rational model. Transition, in contrast, is a three-part psychosocial process that extends over a long period of time and cannot be managed in the same rational manner that works for change.

Bridges describes three phases in the transition experience. The first is the *ending phase,* which involves letting go of the old situation and the old identity that went with it. The second is the *neutral zone,* which exists between the old reality and a new reality that is yet very unclear. The third is the *new beginning,* a time of vision. Timing of these phases depends upon the nature of the change, and how significantly it affects a person's life.

The *ending phase* consists of three aspects: disengagement, disidentification, and disenchantment.

1. *Disengagement* can be viewed as a separation of the individual from the subjective world he or she took for granted. Bridges asserts that people whose identity is tied to relationships and feelings of belonging, or to status and role, have a particularly difficult time with disengagement. Since people in disengagement are experiencing a loss, expected behaviours may include denial, anger, bargaining, and despair.
2. *Disidentification* involves letting go of the old identity which may be a painful or even terrifying experience. Bridges suggests that people can be assisted in achieving disidentification by being given the opportunity to redefine themselves and their future.
3. *Disenchantment* is a feeling that things do not make sense anymore. A person may suspect that their job has been a "sham" or that they have been deceived all along. Bridges indicates that the only way to deal with disenchantment is to allow the pain to be expressed internally, within the organization. Open communication on the part of managers is essential at this phase.

According to Bridges, it is not clear where the ending phase of transition ends and the second phase, the *neutral zone* begins. As its name suggests, the neutral zone is an in-between time where the old way of being is no longer an option, and yet a person is not totally clear about where he or she is headed. Bridges characterizes the neutral zone as having three conditions: disorientation, disintegration, and discovery.

1. *Disorientation* occurs because the neutral zone is an interim period between one orientation that is no longer valid, and another that does not yet exist.

2. *Disintegration* is characterized by a feeling that everything is falling apart. These feelings can be so powerful that there is a real risk that a person may leave the organization. However, Bridges indicates that if they can recognize this as a symptom of transition that will pass, most people will be able to move beyond it.

3. A new *discovery* of oneself is a positive outcome of the neutral zone.

Just as an organizational transition begins with an ending, it ends with a new beginning. In the *new beginnings* phase, one completes the emotional adjustment to the change. There is a clear sense of where one is going and a new energy and motivation to get there. New beginnings are the natural outcome of the whole transition process.

In the example shown in Figure 23.1, the process of moving from team- to primary-care nursing means that the manager will be asking the staff to give up familiar routines, disrupt comfortable work habits, and develop new modes of communication—in effect to disengage themselves from the familiar past for the uncertain future. All of the characteristics of transition should be anticipated by the manager in this case, who should be prepared for the emotional reactions, and should know how to support the staff during this change.

PROMOTING CHANGE THROUGH POSITIVE ATTITUDES

Humans frequently resist change when it is imposed by others, feeling that it will be disruptive and time-consuming, and that it will result in conflict and perhaps lead to a new state which is less desirable than the present one. Such attitudes can seriously handicap an organization's efforts to move forward.

Morgan (1988) summarizes the fundamental shifts in attitude that managers must make if they are to embrace—rather than to resist—change:

- They must adopt a much more proactive, positive, and optimistic view of the future, by anticipating emerging problems, reframing them as opportunities, and planning ahead for them.
- They must learn to see their organizations "from the outside in," by identifying strengths and weaknesses from the perspective of their external customers, and developing competencies to address the deficits.
- They must constantly stimulate new initiatives, and explore new directions, by promoting, celebrating, and rewarding creativity, learning, and innovation of individuals and groups within the organization.
- They must identify and forge new partnerships with diverse stakeholders (both internal and external), in order to mobilize meaningful action on shared problems.
- They must develop and demonstrate a much greater sense of social responsibility than they have in the past.

PROCESSES FOR MANAGING CHANGE

Of equal importance with attitudes are the *processes* which managers and their organizations utilize in addressing change. Ernst & Young, a large Canadian health-care consulting firm, describes a four-phase process for successful business change:

- *Align:* Alignment involves creating the context, and the case for change. It includes obtaining executive sponsorship for the change, and developing the front-line leadership capabilities to carry it out. And it requires that one assess and attend to the risks of the change, and to the stakeholders' readiness to participate.
- *Mobilize:* In mobilizing, the manager will create a road map for both the change and the transition. This will involve developing change skills and competencies (in both self and others), identifying short-term opportunities which can produce quick and positive results, and deploying the necessary resources (such as people, time, space, and money) needed to assure that the change can be effectively carried out.
- *Implement:* In the implementation phase, the manager will actually steer the team through the planned phases of the change: ensuring short-term wins; supporting transition and managing resistance; and applying knowledge to correct the course when necessary, to avoid the potholes along the way.
- *Leverage:* Leverage is the final phase of change, the phase during which the manager ensures the stability and ongoing vitality of the change. Processes involved in leverage include promotion and transfer of knowledge and skills to those who will maintain the changed state; celebrating successes; and sustaining the momentum through continuous improvement (Ernst & Young, 1997).

John Kotter (1996), a professor of leadership at the Harvard Business School, describes an eight-stage process for creating major change. His analysis of why efforts to change and transform organizations often fail led to development of the change process illustrated in Figure 23.2.

STRATEGIES AND TOOLS TO IMPLEMENT CHANGE

Successful nurse managers will be those who recognize that change can be more of an opportunity than a threat, and can demonstrate this knowledge to others. They create a trusting environment for risk-taking, in which nurses are ready to be active participants in change, and they make use of the range of strategies and tools to help them implement change. In essence, managers become what Tichy and Devanna (1990) refer to as transformational leaders: individuals who can assist their followers to move

Figure 23.2

THE EIGHT-STAGE PROCESS OF
CREATING MAJOR CHANGE

---

1 ESTABLISHING A SENSE OF URGENCY
- ➢ Examining the market and competitive realities
- ➢ Identifying and discussing crises, potential crises, or major opportunities

⬇

2 CREATING THE GUIDING COALITION
- ➢ Putting together a group with enough power to lead the change
- ➢ Getting the group to work together like a team

⬇

3 DEVELOPING A VISION AND STRATEGY
- ➢ Creating a vision to help direct the change effort
- ➢ Developing strategies for achieving that vision

⬇

4 COMMUNICATING THE CHANGE VISION
- ➢ Using every vehicle possible to constantly communicate the new vision and strategies
- ➢ Having the guiding coalition role model the behavior expected of employees

⬇

5 EMPOWERING BROAD-BASED ACTION
- ➢ Getting rid of obstacles
- ➢ Changing systems or structures that undermine the change vision
- ➢ Encouraging risk taking and nontraditional ideas, activities, and actions

⬇

6 GENERATING SHORT-TERM WINS
- ➢ Planning for visible improvements in performance, or "wins"
- ➢ Creating those wins
- ➢ Visibly recognizing and rewarding people who made the wins possible

⬇

7 CONSOLIDATING GAINS AND PRODUCING MORE CHANGE
- ➢ Using increased credibility to change all systems, structures, and policies that don't fit together and don't fit the transformation vision
- ➢ Hiring, promoting, and developing people who can implement the change vision
- ➢ Reinvigorating the process with new projects, themes, and change agents

⬇

8 ANCHORING NEW APPROACHES IN THE CULTURE
- ➢ Creating better performance through customer- and productivity-oriented behavior, more and better leadership, and more effective management
- ➢ Articulating the connections between new behaviors and organizational success
- ➢ Developing means to ensure leadership development and succession

---

Source: Adapted from John P. Kotter, "Why Transformation Efforts Fail," *Harvard Business Review* (March–April 1995): 61. Reprinted with permission. Copyright © 1995 by the President and Fellows of Harvard College; all rights reserved.

from vision to action. They do this by creating a blueprint which allows development of the long-term and enduring new behaviours that are necessary to sustain the change.

Kriegel and Brandt (1996) state that managers who wish to overcome resistance to change must deliberately cultivate a fundamental attitude of *change readiness* in themselves and their staff members. Change readiness, they say, is an attitude that is: open and receptive to new ideas; excited rather than anxious about change; challenged, not threatened, by transitions; and committed to change as an ongoing process. Beyond this, they emphasize that change readiness is evidenced by individuals and teams who anticipate and initiate change; challenge the status quo; create instead of react to change; and lead rather than follow (pp. 8-9). The authors suggest a number of *strategies* for managers to use in coaching themselves and their staff to be change-ready:

- *Rounding up "Sacred Cows":* Challenging traditional beliefs, assumptions, and practices, in order to ferret out and discard those that are no longer useful.
- *Developing a Change-Ready Environment:* Changing the focus of the style of management from controlling to coaching, and building a work environment that is characterized by trust and caring. A trusting environment is one built on honesty, integrity, and reliability. Caring involves treating individuals with respect and empathy, and acknowledging their efforts and contributions.
- *Turning Resistance into Readiness:* Coaching self and staff to recognize and overcome the four major forms of resistance to change: fear, powerlessness, inertia, and absence of self-interest (or inability to see "what's in it for me?").
- *Motivating People to Change:* Deliberately setting out to get people excited about change, and motivating them to get on with it, through use of urgency, inspiration, ownership, and rewards and recognition.
- *Continuously Developing Traits of Change Readiness:* These traits are resourcefulness, optimism, adventurousness, drive, adaptability, confidence, and a tolerance for ambiguity.

Oakley and Krug (1991) suggest that the most powerful tool a manager can use to promote change is the EQ, or Effective Question. Effective questions, they say, are those that empower people, release their positive energy, and get them thinking and acting proactively, rather than reactively. Table 23.1 contrasts ineffective with effective questions.

The fundamental "tools" which a nurse manager has at hand to invest in innovation (or change) are threefold: information (including data, technical knowledge, political intuition, and expertise); resources (people, materials, space, time, funds); and support (endorsement, backing, approval) (Kanter, 1983, p.159). Beyond these fundamentals, the literature today provides a plethora of very specific tools and techniques to use in change situations, including change-readiness questionnaires, exercises to stimulate creativity, and team-building initiatives, as well as many others.

Table 23.1

INEFFECTIVE VS. EFFECTIVE QUESTIONS AS A TOOL FOR CHANGE

Ineffective Questions	Effective Questions
✗ What is wrong with this situation?	✓ What is already working? (Here? Other places?)
✗ Why does this always happen to us?	✓ What makes it work?
✗ Who's to blame for this? Or, How can we avoid being blamed for this?	✓ What is the objective of this change?
✗ How is this going to hurt me/us?	✓ What are the benefits of achieving this objective?
✗ What do we have to do to fix the problem?	✓ What can we do to move closer to our objective?

Source: Based on Ed Oakley & Doug Krug, *Enlightened Leadership: Getting to the Heart of Change* (New York: Simon & Schuster, 1991), pp. 137–166. Adapted with permission.

CONCLUSION

Nurse managers are functioning in complex corporations and in white-water environments which are placing ever increasing demands for change upon them: demands from multiple constituencies, from the outside environment, from changing values (of society and of its workers) and from increasingly complex tasks. In the words of Kanter (1983), they need to become change masters:

> Change masters are—literally—the right people in the right place at the right time...
> The right people are the ones with the ideas that move beyond the organization's established practices, ideas they can form into visions...
> The right places are the integrative environments that support innovation, encourage the building of coalitions and teams to support and implement visions...
> The right times are those moments in the flow of organizational history when it is possible to reconstruct reality on the basis of accumulated innovations to shape a more productive and successful future (Kanter, p. 306).

SUMMARY

To behave proactively, rather than reactively, in a changing environment, the nurse manager must:

- Recognize that there are different types of change—developmental, spontaneous, and planned—and that different approaches are required for each.
- Become familiar with some common models and terminology of change, so that comfort with change is increased, and the best model is selected for a given situation.
- Understand the difference between change and transition (the human reaction to that change), and attend carefully to both.
- Develop, and cultivate in others, a positive attitude towards change.
- Recognize that change is a complex process, which requires a planned approach and attention to numerous risk factors, if success is to be ensured.
- Identify and use strategies and tools, not only to advance a particular change effort, but also to create an environment that is consistently friendly towards, and ready for, change.

FURTHER READINGS AND RESOURCES

Bridges, W. (1991). *Managing transitions: Making the most of change.* Reading, MA: Addison-Wesley. Bridges differentiates change (the event) from transition (our reaction to it). In so doing, he helps managers to understand how change affects staff, how staff are likely to react to change, and what can be done by managers to minimize the distress and disruptions.

Kanter, R.M. (1983). *The change masters: Innovation and entrepreneurship in the American corporation.* New York: Touchstone. Kanter's book is a classic in change management. It makes the argument that the revitalizing of American corporations depends on innovation, entrepreneurship, and the development of participative management skills which encourage the use of new ideas arising from within the organization itself. This book contains many useful examples from well-known companies.

Kriegel, R. & Brandt, D. (1996). *Sacred cows make the best burgers: Paradigm-busting strategies for developing change-ready people and organizations.* New York: Warner Books. As the title implies, this is a humorous, highly-readable book, which is packed with straight-forward, practical examples and suggestions for how to lead people through the many changes and challenges confronting today's organizations. The book contains many real-world examples of successes and failures that have involved change.

Oakley, E. & Krug, D. (1991). *Enlightened leadership: Getting to the heart of change.* New York: Simon & Schuster. Oakley and Krug argue that the key to successful change lies in showing change agents how to capitalize on the under-utilized talent and energy of existing staff. The book provides numerous practical techniques, including planning, communication, and motivation tools.

REFERENCES

Bridges, W. (1991). *Managing transitions: Making the most of change.* Reading, MA: Addison-Wesley.

Canadian College of Health Service Executives (1997). *Health Reform Update, 1996–97.* Ottawa, ON: Canadian College of Health Service Executives.

Ernst & Young (1997). *Framework for change.* Unpublished document.

Ferguson, M. (1980). *The Aquarian conspiracy: Personal and social transformation in the 1980s.* Boston: J. P. Tarcher.

Kanter, R. M. (1983). *The change masters: Innovation and entrepreneurship in the American corporation.* New York: Touchstone.

Kotter, J. (1996). *Leading change.* Boston: Harvard University Press.

Kriegel, R., & Brandt, D. (1996) *Sacred Cows Make the Best Burgers; Paradigm-busting strategies for developing change-ready people and organizations.* New York; Warner Books.

Lewin, K. (1951). *Field theory in social science.* New York: Harper & Row.

Morgan, G. (1988). *Riding the waves of change: Developing managerial competencies for a turbulent world.* San Francisco: Jossey-Bass.

Oakley, E. & Krug, D. (1991). *Enlightened leadership: Getting to the heart of change.* New York: Simon & Schuster.

Rogers, E., & Shoemaker, S. (1971). *Communication of innovations.* Glencoe, NY: Free Press.

Tichy, N. & Devanna, M. A. (1990). *The transformational leader.* New York: John Wiley & Sons.

Vaill, P. B. (1989). *Managing as a performing art: New ideas for a world of chaotic change.* San Francisco: Jossey-Bass.

Chapter 24

▼▼▼▼▼▼▼▼▼▼▼▼▼▼▼

Project Management

DONNA LYNN SMITH

KEY OBJECTIVES

In this chapter, you will learn:

- The characteristics of a project, and some of the features that distinguish projects from routine organizational operations.
- How and why projects are initiated.
- Some of the structural elements of projects and why these are important to the success of a project.
- The roles of a project sponsor, project manager, and project team.
- The importance of planning, scheduling and evaluation as they pertain to project development and management.
- Some key elements of a project work plan.
- How to recognize situations or examples in which the project management approach might be applicable.
- Some features of the culture of projects.

INTRODUCTION

Organizations in the health system are being challenged to maintain and improve upon the services they offer while responding to the pressures created by emerging scientific developments and new technologies, changes in clients' expectations, changing social values, and financial restraint. Managers at all organizational levels often feel that they should be spending more time on planning and innovation, but find it difficult to do so because of the relentless pressures of their everyday work. While some aspects of this dilemma can be dealt with by using time-management strategies, it may also be the case that some planning and change-management strategies cannot be effectively accomplished without dedicated time and resource people. Organizations must find ways to maintain and continuously improve upon their routine operations through a process of incremental change. Paradoxically, they must also find ways to make strategic and innovative responses to rapidly changing external circumstances. Projects are temporary management structures that are often established to energize and speed up the process of diffusing innovations through an organization, or of accelerating the pace of change.

Matrix structures and project management technologies were initially developed in the 1950s and 1960s in the aerospace, defence, and construction industries. They began to appear in business and public-sector organizations in the 1970s, and since that time they have contributed to what Kerzner (1984) has described as an "organizational revolution." He explains that "commonly used organizational structures proved inadequate in responding to an ever changing environment," and that the complexities faced by organizations forced them to consider and implement structures that could facilitate more timely responsibilities to external pressures (p. 307). The discussion of management theory in Chapter 5 of this book provides a conceptual rationale for considering different managerial approaches for different types of tasks, activities, and environmental contingencies.

In this chapter, the characteristics of a project are described and some reasons for use of a project management approach are presented. Considerations in structuring and setting up a project, and the roles and responsibilities of project managers and project team members are then discussed. Other roles important to the success of projects, such as those of executive champions and line managers in the organization, are also considered. The chapter concludes with a discussion of some of the benefits of using and participating in project teams, and a discussion of some characteristics of the culture of projects.

WHAT IS A PROJECT?

A project can be thought of as a form of temporary management structure. There are many different variations to the design of organizational matrices and projects. A common feature of all is that they cut across the departmental and functional lines of an organization to bring together groups or people or activities in a manner that will achieve specific goals and objectives within predetermined time frames. By designing this type of temporary structure and allocating resources to facilitate its work, organizations can overcome the tendency of line departments and functional areas to make change slowly and incrementally. Projects are often created to "fast track" one or more changes considered strategically necessary for organizational adaptation and survival.

Organizations have central or core processes, many of which involve recurring activities or patterns of activities. Although these processes take place in an environment of change, and are constantly undergoing change and development, the change process is often incremental, taking place gradually and continuously. Within the core activities of an organization there may also be unplanned or unexpected change resulting from changes in the external environment, such as those involving policies or funding practices of government agencies, or public expectations. Often, however, there is a need to accelerate the change process: to introduce or develop new technologies or programs; to reposition an organization or program so that it can become more effective; to develop new competencies within an organization, program, or unit; or to plan and operationalize new systems and structures. In these circumstances, there is a need for a concentrated effort to achieve specific and predetermined results (sometimes called "deliverables") within a defined period of time, and a specified budget. These conditions define a project, and differentiate it from the more routine activities of an organization.

HOW ARE PROJECTS INITIATED?

The need for a project can be recognized at any level of an organization, or for that matter, by groups external to the organization. For example, as client groups become more effective in making their needs known through a variety of communication and public relations activities, they may put pressure on health organizations to become more responsive to clients who might previously have been a relatively low priority.

Advocacy organizations for victims of sexual assault and domestic violence, for example, may wish to encourage police departments, hospital emergency services, and health professionals to initiate educational programs and develop customized approaches that address the needs of these clients in a more focused and competent manner. These groups could accomplish their goals through a project. As with most project activities, there would be a number of different stakeholders, each of whom would have an interest in how the project would be structured; what its objectives would be; what resources would be allocated to it; and what the work plan and timelines for completion would entail. Stakeholders may be involved in such mechanisms as steering or advisory committees, and their involvement in initiating and monitoring the project is often a crucial factor in achieving project goals and diffusing the knowledge and experience developed through the project to other parts of the organization, or to other organizations.

A project might also be proposed by a group of staff within a program or work unit. For example the nurses within an extended-care unit might propose that a self-medication program be implemented. With the support of their leader, they might form a committee and develop plans for implementing the program. Their leader might assist them in communicating the objectives and potential benefits of the program to the senior level of the organization. This leader might help to facilitate the work of the group through the staff scheduling process, or by financing some planning and learning time for the committee, or by obtaining commitments for such things as renovations, supplies, and expert consultation. If the goals and plans of the committee are supported and formalized, and human or financial resources are allocated to it with the idea of accomplishing the goals within a particular time frame, the innovative idea will have become a project.

As health organizations experience dramatic structural change in a climate of increased demand and shrinking resources, projects are often initiated at the executive level of the organization. Examples of such projects might be the initiation of a Total Quality Management Program; planning and implementing new information systems; decentralizing pharmacy or other clinical services; and work redesign, customer service, or injury-prevention programs. New buildings, systems, or programs are usually planned and implemented by means of a project management structure.

STRUCTURAL ELEMENTS OF PROJECTS

The structural elements of projects include such things as a sponsor and re-porting mechanism, a committee structure for planning and monitoring the project, a project manager, and a project team.

Other structural elements are the goals and objectives, budget, and work plan of a project. The work plan identifies the expected outcomes or deliverables of the project, the activities required to complete them, and the completion dates for all activities and deliverables. Often a monitoring or evaluation process is set up parallel to a project, sometimes being com-pleted with the assistance of experts and stakeholders who are outside of the project so that impartial audits and assessments of project management and results can be obtained. In large and costly projects that take place over a period of several years, such parallel monitoring mechanisms are often critical to a successful outcome.

SPONSORSHIP AND REPORTING STRUCTURE

A project must often be "marketed" throughout the organization, particu-larly if resources in the form of staff time, expert consultation, or special funding are needed to initiate and complete it. What begins as a good idea must go beyond the idea stage to become a formally approved organiza-tional priority and investment. Organizational endorsement is important even if the amount of money required to initiate and manage the project is minimal, because the project will consume time and intellectual capital, and will therefore be a distraction from other corporate objectives.

The term "executive champion" is sometimes used to describe the role of a person at the executive level of an organization who can communicate and interpret the goals and benefits of a project to the executive team, as-sign or obtain resources needed for a project, enlist and sustain the support of other departments of stakeholder groups, remove barriers, provide recognition, and assist in disseminating the results and adopting the new knowledge developed by and through a project. Some projects begin as the ideas of an executive champion, but others originate elsewhere in the orga-nization, perhaps arising from first-line leaders or work teams. In the latter case, for the project to succeed, someone at a more senior level of the or-ganization must be persuaded to become an advocate for the project on be-half of a unit or workgroup, as in the example of the self-medication program described above. In such instances, obtaining the interest and support of an executive champion is usually key to the success of the project. Projects that are congruent with corporate vision and overall management strategy are most likely to attract corporate support; however, some organizations purposely accommodate a few low-key and inexpensive grass-roots projects as a way of allowing innovation and creativity to flourish. The term "skunk works" is sometimes used to describe unofficial projects of this nature (Kanter, 1989, p. 211), although they have also been referred to as "havens for safe learning"(Galbraith, 1982).

To be successful, most projects require a broader base of support than can be provided by an individual project leader or even a single executive champion. Most projects either have an influence and potential impact across more than one organizational unit, or they need support from other parts of the organization to be successful. In fact, projects were probably the first of the many variations on matrix structures (Kerzner, 1984) which are now common in complex organizations. There is a need to link the project (that is, the project manager and team) to the rest of the organization through a designated individual, and quite often through a committee.

To achieve the base of support that is necessary to market a project and then support its initiation, planning, and eventual implementation, the proj-ect may be sponsored by an existing committee whose representation includes most, if not all, units of the organization who might be considered stakeholders in the project. If an appropriate committee does not already exist, or if the project is of sufficient importance to the organization, a committee structure may be established with the specific goal of providing support and direction to the project. Occasionally such a committee is the sponsor, and the project manager will report to it for purposes of the project, rather than to his or her usual supervisor.

Whatever the nature of the supporting committee structure, it is important that terms of reference be established that are clear to committee members, to the project manager, and to the project team. This is particularly important when special committees are established to advise or oversee projects. The formal terms of reference should include clear statements about the committee's decision-making mandates and procedures, its reporting channels, and the role of its chair. The terms "steering committee" and "advisory committee" are sometimes used interchangeably but, in fact, these two types of committees can and should have quite different roles. Quite often, a project steering committee is made up of individuals who have formal decision-making responsibility within the organization, where-as an advisory committee is established to provide stakeholder perspectives, usually without the authority to actually make decisions about the project. Setting up a project advisory committee is a means of including and informing project stakeholders. It can sometimes prevent stakeholders who are not supportive of the project mandate from obstructing the progress of a project. However, token stakeholder representation wastes time and other resources, and can produce cynicism and ill will if it appears that the recommendations of advisory groups are not taken seriously.

The sponsor of a project is the individual and/or group in the organizational structure who is responsible for the project and who has the authority or ability to validate, clarify, or if necessary, achieve alteration of its mandate. The reporting structure for a project should clearly spell out the authority and responsibility of the project sponsor, whether an individual or committee. In the case of committees, existing or specially developed terms of reference should be available to all those concerned with the project. The sponsor may be identified by the executive level, and may sometimes be a member of the executive team. Occasionally a person who has no interest in, or knowledge of, a particular project is appointed to sponsor a project. This is an undesirable situation that often leads to disillusionment of project team members and the project manager, and, not surprisingly, is a waste of the organization's resources. The skills of a project manager combined with cohesion and productivity of the project team can sometimes overcome the inherent difficulties of such a situation, but it is preferable that the sponsor and executive champion of a project believe in its value, concur with its objectives, understand the difficulties it is likely to face, and feel a commitment to supporting the project manager and team.

PROJECT MANAGER

In general, the role of a project manager is to

- lead and co-ordinate the activities of a project,
- recruit or develop the project team,
- keep the project moving forward by identifying and resolving issues and problems,
- manage the multiple communications processes and relationships required to keep the project moving forward,
- manage the project budget and other resources, and
- assure that project goals are achieved within the agreed upon time frame and resources.

If projects are relatively simple and grow from the grass roots of the organization, the role of project manager may be added to the regular responsibilities of a staff member with interests, knowledge, and leadership abilities relevant to the project. Occasionally, a project manager is seconded from regular responsibilities to lead a project on a part-time or full-time basis. This approach has the advantage of building support for the project from within the operating units of the organization, but can sometimes result in overload for the individual who is trying to maintain all regular responsibilities in addition to managing the project. In more complex projects a full- or part-time project manager may be seconded or even recruited to the role. However a project manager is chosen, it is of critical importance that the role and reporting channel for this individual be clearly defined. This is sometimes more easily said than done, because the project manager must obtain or communicate information important to the success of the project in a timely fashion; develop support for project activities; get agreement or commitment on scheduling issues that affect other departments; and maintain the necessary level of staffing support for the project. To do this, the project manager may need access to a variety of people and resources in different departments and at different levels of the organization. A project manager may be assigned to report to the same vice president as his or her departmental supervisor. Occasionally, a project manager will report directly to the chief executive officer or a board committee. Although such arrangements can be inherently stressful, they are recognized as a necessity by organizations that are successful in using a project management approach. A project can rarely remain on schedule and succeed if the project manager is confined by traditional bureaucratic hierarchy.

Good project managers need, and usually possess, many of the skills of successful line managers. However, skills in communication, consultation, persuasion, and negotiation assume greater prominence in project management where staff assigned or seconded to the project very often continue to report to, and have their performance assessed by, the manager of their home departments. The project manager gains authority from the project mandate and the degree of high-level organizational support that exists for the project. Developing commitment to the goals and demands of the project within the project team and the organization as a whole is often, however, a complex process that depends upon the integrity, the credibility, and the interpersonal and political skills of the project manager. Chapter 10 of this book deals with some of the issues and skills involved in developing shared commitment, behavioural norms, and high productivity among members of workgroups and teams. All of these apply to the work of project managers. In addition, project managers must be able to lead the team in structuring its goals and tasks and developing a work plan, in framing issues, and in resolving conflicts within the project team or between the team and other parts of the organization. Box 24.1 presents a list of steps that will serve as a useful guide to project managers. It was prepared by Nancy Rowan, a nurse who managed many projects within organizations and who now works as a consultant.

The project manager is responsible for managing and allocating project resources, and sometimes for obtaining them at the outset of the project, or throughout its life. She or he also manages, or facilitates management of, the many relationships that are affected by the project, including those involving other facets of the organization, and often including external stakeholders. Neglect of these many important relationships and failure to manage them along with other resources can result in major difficulties, delays, and costs for the project. Consulting firms that manage large projects now recognize this by assigning a very senior individual the responsibility for "relationship management" in a project.

PROJECT TEAM

The project team is made up of the project manager and all those individuals who have been recruited, seconded, or assigned to the project team or other roles critical to the project. The time, skills, and effort of project staff

Box 24.1
STEPS IN THE PROJECT MANAGEMENT PROCESS

Step 1. Project Initiation

- Analyzing the market
- Defining the scope
- Identifying the constraints
- Developing the conceptual framework
- Confirming the mandate
- Developing/negotiating the terms of reference
- Defining the organizational structure

Step 2. Planning the Project Work

- Establishing a shared vision
- Recruiting and training personnel for the project.
- Preparing a budget (financial integrity)
- Designing systems to assure a quality product (technical integrity)
- Establishing a communication and/ or marketing plan
- Establishing an evaluation plan
- Identifying the competition
- Identifying pockets of resistance
- Identify potential areas of conflict
- Identifying milestones
- Writing measurable objectives
- Identifying decision points and reporting intervals
- Identifying decision-making processes and criteria

- Establishing a detailed work plan

Step 3. Executing the Project Work

- Performing project activities
- Anticipating and managing operational problems
- Ongoing environmental scanning
- Adjusting priorities and schedules
- Tracking actual work
- Tracking and controlling costs
- Negotiating changes/commitments
- Managing conflict
- Reporting to stakeholders
- Monitoring performance
- Communicating with both internal and external audiences (formal and informal)
- Marketing the product

Step 4. Concluding the Project

- Evaluating outcomes
- Developing a final report
- Publishing results
- Terminating the project or re-establishing it in a new context
- Finalizing contracts or agreements
- Acknowledging participants
- Acknowledging stakeholders/ funders
- Planning for the continuance of the initiative (if indicated)

Source: Nancy Rowan BScN, MHSA. Used with permission.

are a major project resource. In some instances, a project manager is appointed and then has an opportunity to choose the individuals to be recruited or seconded to the project team. More often, people are assigned to the team because of their professional knowledge and skills, their previous experience in similar projects, or because they have uncommitted time. Occasionally, departmental managers decide to solve problems in a workgroup by loaning or transferring staff who are troublemakers to a project. These people can be an asset to a project if they have high levels of initiative and good interpersonal skills. Knowledge directly pertinent to a project is an asset and is, of course, required by a critical mass of members of the project team, but most projects can manage to absorb one or more individuals with generic skills, as long as they are willing to learn from others and have reasonably high interpersonal competence.

A mix of complementary technical and conceptual skills is required in most projects. Teams are brought together to implement projects precisely because the combined knowledge and skill of a group usually surpasses that possessed by individuals. A skilled project manager recognizes the need to share leadership within the project team so that the full potential of the team can be realized. Creation, modification, and implementation of the proj-ect work plan and schedule are among the many group problem-solving tasks faced by project teams. The team must communicate and agree about who is doing what, and it must become expert at identifying issues that affect the project in order to resolve them within the team, or to be able to communicate them and seek support for their resolution in various departments and at various levels of the organization. In addition to work done individually for the project by team members with particular knowledge and skills, the identification and resolution of issues is a central activity through out the life of a project. The initiative, creativity, and perseverance of proj-ect team members are decisive factors in the ability of project managers and teams to overcome obstacles and achieve their goals. The development of shared knowledge, behavioural norms, group history, and *esprit de corps* is also a critical success factor in the management and implementation of projects. Kanter (1989) has pointed out that the development process for projects is very knowledge-intensive, but also generates knowledge at a rapid rate. Projects frequently engender secondary innovations. Therefore, the cumulative expertise of a high-performance project team is an irreplaceable corporate resource and should be nurtured and protected as such.

OBJECTIVES AND WORK PLAN

A project is unlikely to succeed without clearly formulated objectives that are agreed upon by all stakeholders. It is sometimes necessary to revisit and revise project objectives. Recognizing when and why this may be necessary is a key skill of the project manager. Whether objectives remain the same, or are modified during the life of a project, it is necessary to be able to communicate about them clearly to stakeholders throughout the organization. The project objectives provide a high-level framework within which other project parameters such as budget and timelines are determined. They should specify what the project outcomes or deliverables are to be and provide guidance for the evaluation of project outcomes and effectiveness.

In its simplest form, a project work plan is a list of activities that specifies the dates each activity will begin and finish, and identifies the individual or group that has primary responsibility for assuring that the activity is completed properly and on time. This type of a work plan may be all that is necessary for an uncomplicated project. A Gantt Chart is commonly used to summarize activities, accountabilities, and time lines in simple projects. (Decker & Sullivan, 1992). An example is shown in Figure 24.1.

Figure 24.1

GANTT CHART FOR A GENERIC PROJECT

TASK/ACTIVITY	ACCOUNTABILITY	March	April	May	June	July	August	September
					TIME IN MONTHS			
Form Project Team	Executive Committee	▢						
Develop Work Plan	Project Team	▢						
Approve Work Plan	Executive Committee		▢					
Interview Consultants	Project Team		▢					
Select Consultants	Project Team/Executive Committee			▢				
Consultation with Stakeholders	Consultants			▢	▢	▢		▢
Focus Groups with Staff	Consultants			▢	▢			
Workload Study	Consultants				▢	▢		
Review Consultant's Report	Project Team						▢	
Develop Recommendations	Project Team						▢	
Approve Implementation Strategy	Executive Committee							▢
Initiate Phase II	Project Team							▢

Large projects that involve many stakeholders, large resource commitments, and that take place over extended periods of time, require the use of more elaborate project planning, scheduling, and monitoring technologies. A limitation of the Gantt Chart is that it does not show the interdependencies between activities, and does not distinguish between primary and supplementary activities. These limitations are overcome by the use of more complex network diagrams (Decker & Sullivan, 1992; Glasser, 1963) such as that shown in Figure 24.2.

In Figure 24.2, there are nine major activities (A1 through 9). Several of the major activities are comprised of sub-activities (S1, etc.). In this diagram, activities A1 through 3, including the sub-activities of each, will be taking place at more or less the same time. In order to complete Activity 4 on schedule, these three activities must be completed on time, and a delay in any one of them can result in a delay in beginning A4. In large and complex projects, person hours or days and their associated costs are budgeted to each activity and sub-activity. Even small delays can be costly and a major responsibility of the project manager is to monitor the completion of activities and to lead the development of contingency plans that may be necessary if unavoidable delays occur. The project sponsors would be notified of anticipated delays and any unexpected costs that can be expected to arise from them. Activities occurring in later phases of the project may have to be speeded up or done in different and less costly ways to compensate for delays in the early stages of the project. An array of computer software is now available to assist project teams in planning, scheduling, budgeting, and monitoring projects, and skills in using such tools will increasingly be seen as an important adjunct to more traditional managerial competencies.

An even more complicated skill is that of maintaining the commitment and morale of a project group, so that it can stay on schedule while responding positively and quickly to the inevitable obstacles that most projects encounter. If members of a project team continue to have other responsibilities within the organization, or if there is not clear and continuous direction and support from the project sponsors, this can be particularly difficult.

In the case example depicted in Box 24.2, the leadership and project management skills of a first-line nursing manager are recognized when she is asked to manage a project for the organization. This example highlights the way the project is structured and illustrates the type of matrix-reporting relationships that are common when projects are developed and supported using the human resources already available within the organization.

THE CULTURE OF PROJECTS

The noted management researcher and consultant Rosabeth Moss Kanter has discussed a number of differences between "mainstreams" (that is, the operational departments and functions of an organization) and "newstreams"(the channels and mechanisms set up to change the organization). She notes that "the operating logic of a newstream often conflicts with that

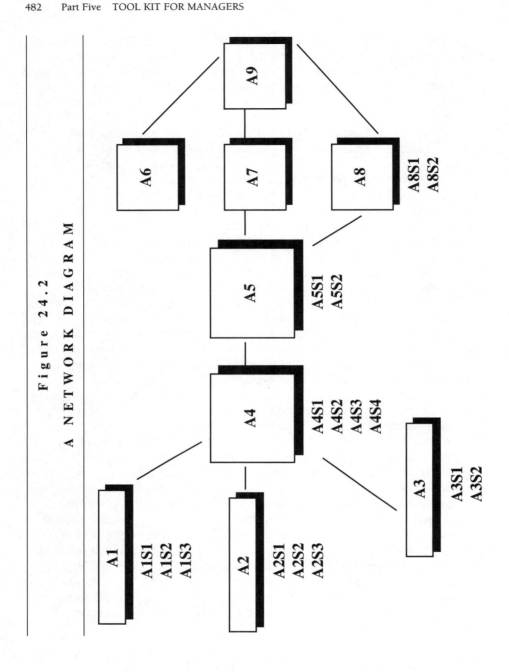

Figure 24.2

A NETWORK DIAGRAM

Box 24.2
A FIRST-LINE NURSING MANAGER IS ASKED TO MANAGE AN ORGANIZATIONAL PROJECT: A CASE EXAMPLE

Blue River Health Centre is a regional hospital of 300 acute-care beds, 100 continuing-care beds a number of continuing-care outreach services and various other ambulatory-care programs. The health centre received full accreditation when last surveyed by the Canadian Council on Health Services Accreditation two years ago, and will be surveyed again a year from now. The centre is going through a number of changes and its activity has been increasing as a result of changes at the provincial level and the recruitment of several new medical specialists to the community.

The senior management team at the health centre has decided to use a project management approach to plan and co-ordinate the activities required to prepare for and participate in the forthcoming survey. It has decided to ask Jane Murphy to be the project manager for an accreditation task force. Ms. Murphy has worked at the centre for eight years, formerly as a first-line manager, more recently as a program manager. She is highly regarded by her peers and the senior management group, and the high standard of care in her program is recognized throughout the health centre and in the community at large. The staff in her program area are highly motivated and have worked together for some time. They include several senior nurses who have previously acted in Jane Murphy's position while she was away on vacations or educational leave.

In her role as program manager, Ms. Murphy reports to the Vice President of Clinical Services. However, the accreditation task force has been structured to report to the Vice President of Organizational Development. Ms. Murphy will be seconded from her regular duties to act as a full-time project manager. An experienced administrative support person from the office of the Vice President of Organizational Development has been assigned to spend one quarter of her time supporting Ms. Murphy and the task force. The task force of eight people has been structured to provide leadership to the preparations for accreditation by linking with all major clinical and support departments and the medical staff. Members of the task force have been asked to participate in addition to their regular responsibilities, and it is expected that they will provide linkages to subcommittees in each department and program area. The role of the task force is to agree upon the activities that need to be accomplished, the timelines for these activities, and the individuals or departments that need to carry them out, and then to monitor and co-ordinate the activities for the health centre as a whole. Ms. Murphy will report on a day-to-day basis to the Vice President of Organizational Development, and will attend a meeting of the centre's senior management team every two months to report on the accreditation project. Following the survey visit of the accreditation team, the project will be finished and individuals in operational roles will assume any maintenance or follow-up activities that are necessary.

of the mainstream. Mainstreams and newstreams differ in performance criteria, predictability, and the need to shed the burden of the past" (Kanter, 1989, p. 202). She points out that creative projects, regardless of type, share the following characteristics:

- the need to move quickly when opportunity or inspiration strikes;
- missed deadlines and encounters with the unexpected;
- the constant need to justify the project, especially as new or more attractive options come up;
- extreme emotional swings, or frustrations and moments of despair alternating with clear highs;
- in joint efforts, the difficulty of keeping up with what everyone else on the project is doing and thinking; and
- an all-encompassing and absorbing project world.

These and other factors combine to produce a unique culture in each individual project and a project-oriented culture that characterizes some organizations. Recognizing the characteristics of newstream culture and the people who work within it is important, both to those who are a part of it, and to those who work in parallel or management roles. Projects and their culture will continue to be a part of organizational life for the foreseeable future. Nurses often possess the interpersonal and organizational skills that are critical to the success of projects, and many nurses have found exciting career opportunities in project management, or as members of project teams. These opportunities will continue to increase.

SUMMARY

- Projects are temporary management structures that are usually implemented when there is a need to rapidly diffuse an innovation or to make a major organizational change within a specified period of time.
- Projects can be initiated in a variety of ways and at various levels of an organization. To be successful, most projects will need approval or support from the senior level of the organization.
- The structural elements of a project include a sponsor and reporting mechanism, a project manager and project team, and usually some means of monitoring and evaluating the project. An executive champion and broadly-based organizational support can be critical to the success of projects.
- Projects require a clear mandate, in the form of goals, objectives, and deliverables.
- Project management requires many of the skills used by line managers, but is particularly dependent upon interpersonal, conceptual, and organizational skills.
- The work plan of a project is a tool for planning project activities, assigning responsibility for tasks, allocating resources, monitoring achievements, and identifying issues and problems. Planning and scheduling are of critical importance to most projects and can often be facilitated by the use of computer software designed to support project management.
- Projects usually develop a unique culture. A key feature of this culture is the acceptance of ambiguity and uncertainty as a fact of life within the project and the organization. To be successful, projects must often

be freed from the usual procedures and reporting channels of an organization. Organizations that hope to be successful in diffusing innovations and initiating change will need to develop a project culture that takes this requirement into account.

REFERENCES

Decker, P. J. & Sullivan, E. J. (Eds.). (1992). *Nursing administration: A micro/macro approach for effective nurse executives.*). East Norwalk, CT: Appleton & Lange.

Galbraith, J. (1982, Summer). Designing the innovating organization. *Organizational Dynamics, 10,* 5–25.

Glasser, J. J. (1963). Critical path method. In C. Heyel (Ed.). *The encyclopaedia of management.* 142–144. New York: Reinhold.

Kanter R. M. (1989). *When Giants Learn to Dance.* New York: Simon & Schuster.

Kerzner, H. (1984). Matrix information: Obstacles, problems, questions, and answers. In: D.I. Cleland (Ed.). *Matrix management systems handbook* (pp. 307–329). Toronto: Van Nostrand Reinhold.

Chapter 25

▼▼▼▼▼▼▼▼▼▼▼▼▼▼▼▼▼

Managing Conflict

PATRICIA E. B. VALENTINE

KEY OBJECTIVES

In this chapter, you will learn:

- Theory and concepts related to conflict.
- Conflict-management strategies, their uses, and outcomes.
- Typical responses to conflict by staff nurses and nurse managers.
- Reasons for applying conflict-management strategies, and potential outcomes.
- Gender as an issue in conflict management.

INTRODUCTION

The nature of work in health-care agencies is complex and constantly changing, and competition for funding resources is fierce. For these reasons, conflict in health agencies is inevitable. The importance of managing conflict was recognized by Mintzberg (1975) in the 1970s when he identified "disturbance handling" as one of ten key roles of effective managers. All nurse managers must be able to identify, understand, and use effective strategies for managing conflict.

The purpose of this chapter is to provide an overview of theory and concepts that underpin conflict management. Conflict assessment, management strategies, and their uses by staff nurses and nurse managers are discussed. The potential impact of gender on conflict management is introduced.

DEFINITION

Although there is no generally accepted definition of conflict, the one used in this chapter is by Thomas (1992). He defines conflict as "the process that begins when one party perceives that the other [party] has negatively affected, or is about to negatively affect, something that he or she cares about" (p. 653). Conflict stems from differences in thoughts, beliefs, attitudes, feelings, or behaviour of two or more parties.

FORMS OF CONFLICT

There are three forms of conflict: intrapersonal, interpersonal, and intergroup. In all three, tension is produced within an individual or party because of unmet needs, goals, or expectations.

Intrapersonal conflict occurs within an individual and is experienced, for example, when a nurse faces two competing demands, such as a need for patient teaching when staffing conditions do not allow adequate time for this important aspect of nursing care.

Interpersonal conflict occurs between two or more individuals or parties. An interdisciplinary group of health-care professionals may disagree over treatment plans for specific patients, for example, or over ethical dilemmas concerning "do not resuscitate orders" for seriously ill patients.

Intergroup conflict occurs between two or more groups; it often involves patient-care issues and personnel policies or procedures. Two groups, such as nurses and physicians, may vie for the same funds: the nurses want the money to increase staffing to improve the delivery of quality care, for example, while the physicians want to use the money to purchase the latest technological innovation.

MODELS FOR UNDERSTANDING CONFLICT

Two models for understanding conflict phenomena are the *structural model,* which attempts to understand conflict by viewing the underlying conditions that shape conflict, such as rules, roles, and relations; and the *process model,* which has as its focus the internal dynamics of specific conflict events. The two models are complementary: the structural model is useful for suggesting systemic changes, while the process model is more useful for managing an ongoing system and coping with crises (Thomas, 1976).

STRUCTURAL MODEL

Thomas (1976) developed a structural model that takes into account the context and its influences on the process of conflict and conflict management. This model is composed of four factors that influence how conflict is managed in organizations: behavioural predispositions of parties involved, social pressure, incentive structure of the organization, and rules and procedures.

Two parties in conflict come to any situation with behavioural predispositions emanating from their motives and abilities. Both parties are influenced by pressures in the immediate social environment. Both parties respond to conflict incentives in the situation, such as conflict of interest between them, and their investment in the relationship. And both parties interact in a context of rules and procedures that constrain their behaviour.

PROCESS MODEL

In the process model, the main subject of this chapter, conflict is described as a dynamic process with several stages that result in an episode of conflict. Researchers often use Thomas' (1992) model—which shows five stages: awareness, thoughts and emotions, intentions, behaviour, and outcomes—as a starting point for describing a conflict situation (see Figure 25.1).

An episode of conflict commences with one party's *awareness* of the conflict. Awareness leads to a variety of *thoughts and emotions* about the conflict episode and potential responses to it. The thoughts and emotions are based on normative reasoning and rational/instrumental reasoning that result in the development of *intentions*. These intentions, which are related to trying to cope with the conflict situation, result in some type of observable *behaviour*. There is a reaction from another person (other's reaction). The interaction may be prolonged because each party's behaviour stimulates the other party's response. As the interaction progresses, each party's thoughts and feelings about the conflict issue may change, which affects their behaviour accordingly. When interaction on the issue stops, *outcomes* are produced. The outcomes have consequences for both parties, such as mutual agreement, mutual avoidance, control by one party, or no resolution. The outcomes of a given situation determine whether a subsequent episode on the same issue will recur in the future.

ASPECTS OF CONFLICT

Initially, organizational conflict was viewed as destructive to organizational life. Managers were expected to control it at all costs by having rules or procedures for governing all situations (Etzioni, 1961; Fayol, 1949; Lewin, 1948; Weber, 1946). If conflict occurred, it was thought that a manager should confront it openly. During the 1960s and 1970s, the management literature began to suggest that conflict was not necessarily dysfunctional but could serve positive functions (Blake & Mouton, 1964: Coser, 1956), although there is sparse research to support this contention (Johnson, 1994). Currently, conflict is considered to be neither intrinsically good nor bad; it need not necessarily be eliminated but it must be effectively managed. An optimal level of conflict seems to be necessary for effective functioning of an organization.

Those who take a negative view argue that too much conflict can: 1. interfere with the climate of the organization; 2. decrease staff performance by dissipating energy; 3. impact negatively on morale; and 4. interfere with teamwork. Negative effects can produce ineffectiveness and inefficiency, and eventually result in organizational stagnation.

On the other hand, viewed positively, optimal conflict can: 1. unite a group by setting boundaries and strengthening a group's identity; 2. unify a group by distributing power; 3. help to balance a group by acting as a

F i g u r e   2 5 . 1

P R O C E S S   M O D E L   O F   C O N F L I C T   E P I S O D E S

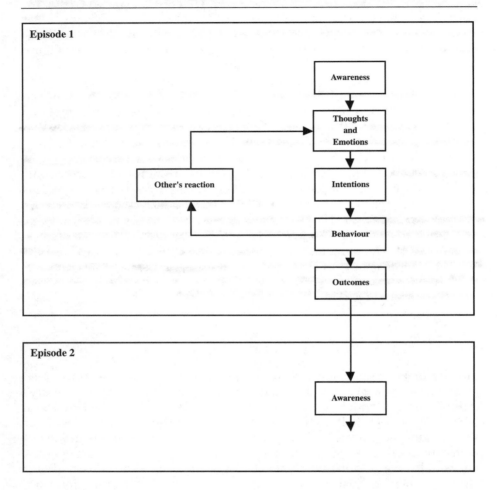

Source: Modified and reproduced by special permission of the Publisher, Consulting Psychologists Press, Inc., Palo Alto, CA 94303 from *Handbook of Industrial and Organizational Psychology*, Vol. 3 by M. D. Dunnette and L. M. Hough, Editors. Copyright 1992 by Davies-Black. All rights reserved. Further reproduction is prohibited without the Publisher's written consent.

testing ground for contrary interests; and 4. forge crucial relationships and teams (Huber, 1996). Growth, creativity, innovation, and change are stimulated by conflict (Coser, 1956).

CONFLICT-MANAGEMENT STRATEGIES

Since conflict first began to be studied, various conflict-management strategies have been delineated. Follet (1940) described three main ways of dealing with conflict: domination, compromise, and integration. Blake and Mouton (1964) developed a conceptual model that classified styles for handling interpersonal conflicts into five types, based on managers' attitudes toward production and people. Thomas (1976) honed this system by separating the conflict from the behaviours people used for handling it. Using different terms and slightly different meanings, Thomas developed five strategies—competing, compromising, avoiding, collaborating, and accommodating. The strategies were based on the intentions of a party; for example, these intentions could represent assertiveness (i.e., attempting to satisfy one's own concerns) or co-operativeness (i.e., attempting to satisfy another's concerns).

The Thomas-Kilmann conflict mode instrument (TKI) was developed to measure five ways of handling conflict (Thomas & Kilmann, 1974). Although several other conflict-handling instruments have been developed, the TKI has been the most widely used to measure nurses' strategies for handling conflict. Thomas and Kilmann's five strategies, therefore, will serve as the basis for describing these modes, their uses, and specific outcomes produced by the strategies. Additions from other management research literature will be included.

Competing (also known as "dominating," "coercing," "forcing," "telling") is a mode that is used when one party wins while another loses. It involves high concern for self and low concern for others (Rahim, 1986). Competing is power-oriented, with one party strongly defending its own stance and believing it to be the right one. Often an issue is forced onto the table through direct orders and voted on, with the minority losing. Competing is used when quick decisions are needed, for unpopular causes, for dealing with aggressive persons, when one has expertise that enables better decision-making, and as a defence against others who exploit non-competing behaviour (Hightower, 1986; Marriner, 1982; Rahim & Bonoma, 1979). Winning may be the goal. People who use competing successfully often avoid the truth, others' disagreement, or being challenged, even if wrong. They often respond aggressively when challenged. Decisions that are forced often produce unsatisfactory resolutions.

Compromising (also known as "sharing," "negotiating") is a mode used when each party relinquishes something to produce a decision acceptable to both parties (Rahim, 1986). Compromising, the "staple" (Huber, 1996, p. 422) of conflict management, involves democratic values. Compromising means taking a middle position and can often result in a "quick fix." It is frequently used for temporary resolution of complex issues, for inconsequential issues, when emotions have reached such a pitch that they require diffusion, or when goals are important but not worth major disruption.

Compromising is often used as a backup when collaborating and competing fail.

Avoiding (also known as "withdrawing") is a mode used when one party does not pursue his or her own concerns or those of the other party. It includes withdrawal and suppression (Robbins, 1982). It is allied with buck-passing, where issues may be postponed for a time or completely withdrawn. Avoiding is used as a "cool-down" mechanism. It is used for dealing with issues when the impact of confronting the other party is perceived to be more negative than attaining resolution of conflict (Rahim & Bonoma, 1979), more information is needed, issues are tactical, trivial, or pressing (Thomas, 1977), or there is no chance to satisfy the concern.

Collaborating (also known as "integrating," "problem solving") is a mode used when one party works with another party to find a mutually satisfying resolution. Collaborating includes co-operation between parties, candidness, information sharing (especially differences), to reach consensus. Confronting and problem-solving are part of this mode, and lead to creative solutions to issues (Rahim, 1986). Collaborating is used to develop an integrative solution to issues considered too crucial for compromise, to merge insights from different perspectives, to increase understanding by testing out various perspectives, to gain commitment to change, to work through disruptive emotional issues, and to spread responsibility while reducing risk taking. It is especially useful when time is not a consideration, and when long-term resolution of conflict is desired.

Accommodating (also named "obliging," "smoothing") is a mode used when one party deliberately neglects concerns to satisfy the concerns of the other. It involves focussing on similarities between parties while minimizing differences, and being self-sacrificing (Rahim, 1986). Accommodating may be used when one party realizes an error, the issue is more important to the other party, a point is relinquished to gain another point later on, one party is outmatched, preservation of harmony is crucial, and others need to learn from their mistakes. It is often considered appropriate for routine issues. However, its overuse may result in disappointment and resentment, especially if there is lack of reciprocation.

Research suggests that the modes of competing, compromising, avoiding, and accommodating usually result in temporary conflict management, but some frustration often remains in one or both parties (Thomas, 1976). In one study, subordinates perceived that supervisors handled conflict constructively when they used accommodative or collaborative techniques; competing and avoiding techniques were perceived to be the least constructive (Burke, 1970). Johnson (1994) suggested that collaborating is rarely used when a wide power differential exists between parties in conflict. Compromising and accommodating are frequently used when there are differences in power that permit one party to predominate.

Table 25.1 summaries the five strategies, the outcomes, and how nurses use them.

Table 25.1

SUMMARY OF CONFLICT-MANAGEMENT
STRATEGIES, OUTCOMES AND
RESEARCH FINDINGS

Conflict Management Strategies	Conflict Management Outcomes	Nursing Research Findings
Competing	win - lose assertive, uncooperative short-term resolution	• used infrequently by all nurses • *not* competing was strategy of choice used by nurse educators in one study
Compromising	no win - no lose moderately assertive, cooperative short-term resolution	• used predominantly by nurse managers
Avoiding	lose - lose unassertive, uncooperative short-term resolution	• used predominantly by staff nurses • used often by nurse managers
Collaborating	win - win fully assertive, cooperative long-term resolution	• no distinct pattern in usage by nurse managers • used infrequently by staff nurses
Accommodating	lose - win unassertive, cooperative short-term resolution	• used infrequently by nurse managers

NURSES' WAYS OF HANDLING CONFLICT

The TKI was used in six American studies to measure staff nurses' and nurse administrators' ways of managing conflict. In the study by Marriner (1982), the conflict-management profiles of 179 female and 3 male nurse managers were compared with the profiles of 339 practising middle- and upper-level managers, all male, in American business and government. All had previously been surveyed using the TKI. Marriner found that, compared with the middle- and upper-level managers who were predominantly male, the nurse managers as a group were slightly less competitive and collaborative, scored about the same on compromising and accommodating, and scored slightly higher on avoiding. In the nurse-manager group, collaborating and compromising were associated with effective conflict management, while avoiding and competing were allied with ineffective conflict management.

In Barker's (1984) study of 173 staff nurses in two Utah hospitals, avoiding was the most frequently used mode of dealing with conflict, and competing was the least frequently used (see Table 25.2). Barker concluded that infrequent use of competing and frequent use of avoiding may reflect the powerlessness associated with staff nurses' roles. Because associate degree nurses were the largest group in her sample, she suggested they may not be as educated in problem-solving and decision-making as other nurses. Since the small number of men in her study scored higher on competing, she speculated that male nurses may be more like their business counterparts, who tend to be more assertive and competitive than women.

In the western United States, Hightower (1986) carried out research on 160 predominantly (98%) female nurse managers occupying subordinate roles. Again, the most frequently used conflict-handling mode was avoiding (see Table 25.2). Hightower concluded that avoiding may be a response to the perceived risk attached to subordinate roles.

Washington (1990) studied 22 nurse managers and 38 staff nurses at a southwestern United States hospital. She found that avoiding was the most frequently used mode of staff nurses, while compromising was used most frequently by nurse managers (see Table 25.2). Competing was the mode least frequently used by both groups. She concluded that hospital nurses approach a conflict episode with concern for the other party uppermost in their minds; also, hospital nurses tend to avoid confrontation. She recommended that a future study should investigate the relationship between nurses' perceived power and their use of conflict-management strategies.

Cavanagh (1991) studied 145 staff nurses and 82 nurse managers in medical-surgical units in eight west coast American hospitals. Both groups used avoiding as their main way of handling conflict (see Table 25.2). Nurse managers, however, used compromising nearly as frequently. Cavanagh suggested that during high episodes of stress (cardiac arrest), where there is limited time for collaborating, or during differential power situations (physician-nurse), where confrontation could be threatening, avoiding may be functional.

Barton (1991) determined the impact of both the process and structural models on conflict management of nurses in a large teaching hospital in an American midwestern city (see Table 25.2). Of the 69 nurse managers at three levels—assistant head nurse (AHN), head nurse (HN), nurse administrator (NA)—she found that compromising was used most often. She gave no explanation for this outcome. The strategy of competing was the least used by AHNs. Barton correlated this finding with their liaison position and the need to avoid win/lose situations. AHNs also used avoiding more than the other managers, which she suggested may reflect their subordinate roles. Collaborating was the second most frequently used mode of AHNs and HNs. Barton suggested this may be due to middle managers' opportunity to work closely with subordinates. Since the most assertive mode (competing) and the most co-operative mode (accommodating) were used least often by all managers, she concluded they preferred a blend of co-operativeness and assertiveness.

Table 25.2

SUMMARY OF RESEARCH SHOWING STRATEGIES USED BY VARIOUS LEVELS OF NURSING STAFF TO RESOLVE CONFLICT (1—USED MOST OFTEN; 5—USED LEAST OFTEN)

	Competing	Compromising	Avoiding	Collaborating	Accommodating
Staff Nurses					
Barker (1984) n = 173	5	2	1	4	3
Washington (1990) n = 38	5	3	1	4	2
Cavanagh (1991) n = 145	5	3	1	4	2
Nurse Managers					
Hightower (1986) n = 160	4	2	1	3	5
Washington (1990) n = 22	5	1	2	3	4
Cavanagh (1991) n = 82	5	2	1	4	3
Barton (1991) n = 69*	5	1	3	2	4

* 32 assistant head nurses, 31 head nurses, and 6 nurse administrators

As Table 25.2 shows, generally nurses are unlikely to use competing as a strategy to resolve conflict. Compromising and avoiding were the most frequently used strategies of nurse managers. The most common way that staff nurses dealt with conflict was to avoid it. Collaborating was used as the fourth strategy in all studies of staff nurses. Most nurse managers used collaborating infrequently. Accommodating was also used infrequently by nurse managers, while accommodating and compromising were used almost equally by staff nurses.

How well do the most frequently used conflict-handling modes of staff nurses and nurse managers work in typical conflict situations in contemporary health-care organizations? Although competing is considered to be one of the more ineffective conflict-management strategies, its infrequent use by both staff nurses and nurse managers suggests they feel powerless, or have trouble taking a firm stand. The under-use of this strategy also suggests that competition may be viewed differently by nurses (women). Does concern for others stop them from using this mode?

The frequent use of compromising suggests nurse managers focus exclusively on practicalities rather than larger issues. The merits of crucial issues may be deflected by the gamesmanship of trading and bargaining. Nurse managers may feel they have to compromise because of their hierarchical position between the traditional decision-makers (administrators, boards, physicians), who are mostly men, and the subordinate workers (staff nurses, other health-care workers), who are mostly women.

Staff nurses' strong propensity to use avoiding suggests they may be reluctant to provide input into decisions because they feel they are always "walking on eggshells." Over-use of avoiding may result in decisions on crucial nursing issues being arrived at by default. The frequent use of this mode may also relate to a sense of powerlessness associated with staff nurses' roles. Nurses may feel that conflict is incompatible with the caring ideology of nursing.

The infrequent use of collaborating by most nurse managers and the under-use by staff nurses may mean they often fail to see differences as opportunities for joint gain. It may mean that in some health-care settings nurses are not encouraged to recognize collaborative possibilities. This may reflect the wide divergence in power between parties such as nurses and physicians who may find themselves in conflict.

The infrequent use of accommodating by nurse managers suggests they may have difficulty admitting they are wrong. Perhaps they have trouble building goodwill, fail to understand when to give up, or do not comprehend legitimate exceptions to rules. The under-use of this strategy may reflect the self-esteem of nurses or the overly bureaucratic nature of health-care settings.

ASSESSMENT OF CONFLICT SITUATIONS

When conflict occurs, the process for management or resolution needs to be identified and understood. Critical thinking, gathering information, and clearly defining the problem before intervening are important initial stages. Just as staff nurses assess patient situations, nurse managers need to assess organizational conflict situations. It is helpful for them to recognize their usual conflict-management strategies, and to know the five conflict-handling modes.

Because specific conflict-handling modes are useful in specific situations, nurse managers must be aware of the outcome of each strategy. Nurse managers need to choose conflict-management strategies that produce positive outcomes.

When conflict is identified, the following steps may be used to manage the situation:

- Diffuse strong feelings associated with an issue.
- Gather all facts before defining issue.
- Be aware of past personal approaches to conflict management.
- Determine whether the situation requires intervention.
- Determine whether intervention requires long- or short-term resolution.
- Be aware of research literature on effective conflict-management strategies.
- Intervene using the appropriate mode.
- Evaluate the outcome.

GENDER AS AN ISSUE IN CONFLICT MANAGEMENT

Health-care organizations are staffed predominantly by female workers; nurses make up the largest component of this work force. For the most part, however, nursing management literature lacks a gender perspective. Viewing health-care organizations through the lens of women's voices or from a "feminist standpoint" (Harding, 1987) is a contemporary perspective that warrants further attention. As Calas and Smircich (1996) indicated, feminist theories do not just concern issues about women; by using this perspective, "more inclusive organizational studies will be created" (p. 218).

Most nursing-management texts rely on organizational and administrative theories from traditional management research literature where research has usually been carried out on profit-motivated organizations. Also, such research has generally been carried out by males, on males, in male-dominated organizations. More recently, research has focused on women in male-dominated organizations (e.g., Hearn, Sheppard, Tancred-Sheriff, & Burrell, 1989; Mills & Simmons, 1994). However, there is sparse feminist research concerning women in human-service organizations, where women predominate.

A study of the culture of a Canadian hospital school of nursing revealed new aspects about nurses' (women's) distinctive orientation to the workplace (Valentine, 1995b). The school's work culture included blending home and work. Child bearing, child rearing, and household management were major aspects of the nurse educators' lives, and these posed dilemmas when nurses tried to fulfil career goals and to maintain family harmony. The bridging of work and home was a strong part of their reality, which also included a focus on staff, faculty, and student relationships. There was a striving for connection through food, social events, meetings, and supportive gestures. This study is consistent with other research and suggests that women tend to view the world through relationships rather than through rules (Gilligan, 1982). Women's identities are formed through affiliative personal relationships rather than impersonally.

There is minimal research literature on conflict in women's (Shakeshaft, 1987) or nurse's groups (Valentine, 1995a). The culture of women's organizations (Calas & Smircich, 1996; Gilligan, 1982; Nichols, 1996) suggests that women may have a different approach to conflict than men. As part of the larger study of the school, the process of conflict management also was investigated (Valentine, 1995b). Conflict was defined as "disharmony" by one key participant, suggesting there was a striving for harmony. Like the studies of staff nurses, the nurse educators' major mode of handling conflict was avoiding, with only one issue resolved through collaborating. Avoidance was viewed as a way of preventing open conflict. The nurse educators' explanation for the use of this mode was that they had to be exemplary role models for students by preventing the rupturing of relationships and sustaining the caring ideology that underpins nursing.

Conflict-management strategies were also examined as part of a study undertaken to investigate management processes among a group of female nurse educators/administrators who were working on a proposal to integrate nursing programs from several nursing-education institutions (Wood, Valentine, Richardson, & Godkin, 1994). These researchers found there were similarities in the group's conflict-management strategies and those described in traditional management literature. However, there also were significant differences.

This group rejected the strategy of competing, and deliberately favoured the mode of not-competing. They did this because competing meant destroying the collaborative relationships formed by the group. Compromising, on the other hand, was used because it included considerable discussion of issues until there was agreement; it meant compromising individual and institutional goals. Avoiding meant postponing potential conflict. It also meant issues were deferred to a later date, by which time they often had dissipated or become non-issues. Because consensus was one of the group's goals, avoidance proved to be an effective strategy. Collaborating was used infrequently. It was, however, used for dealing with the group's most critical issue, one that caused considerable anxiety and "heated" discussion.

CONCLUSION

Management of conflict is an essential management skill. Identifying, assessing, and appropriately intervening in conflict situations is crucial for optimal functioning of nursing organizations. Understanding the outcomes of various conflict-management strategies is essential for nurse managers. A review of nursing research literature on conflict management raises many questions that require thoughtful reflection by managers. Nurses continue to embrace the ideology of caring, which may influence the ways in which they perceive and handle conflict. A gender analysis of conflict situations could provide considerable insight into conflict management for a profession that is predominantly female.

SUMMARY

- Conflict is inevitable in all organizations.
- Conflict can be viewed negatively or positively.
- Knowledge of the five conflict-management strategies (competing, compromising, avoiding, collaborating, and accommodating) and their outcomes is essential to produce positive outcomes of conflict episodes.
- Two of the most frequently used conflict-handling modes are compromising for nurse managers and avoiding for staff nurses.
- A gender analysis of conflict management could provide useful insights into rationale behind conflict episodes and into use of specific conflict-management strategies.

FURTHER READINGS AND RESOURCES

Keenan, M., & Hurst, J. (1995). Conflict: The cutting edge of change. In P. Yoder-Wise (Ed.), *Leading and managing in nursing* (pp. 339-361). St. Louis, MO: Mosby. Keenan and Hurst outline Johnson's (1992) theory for managing unresolvable conflicts: issues that continue to recur after using appropriate conflict-management strategies. If a conflict is ongoing, seems to have two interdependent poles where choosing one requires incorporation of the other, and requires a "both/and decision," the section on polarity management in this chapter is worth reading.

Other references on the subject of conflict management include:

Hurst, J., & Keenan, M. (1986). Do you have any other ideas for improvement? *Nursing Success Today, 3*(1), 22–29.

Hurst, J., Keenan, M., & Minnick, J. (1992). Healthcare polarities: Quality and cost. *Nursing Management, 23*(9), 40–44.

Hurst, J., Keenan, M., & Sipp, R. (1993). Total quality management: A matter of quality polarity analysis and management. *The Health Care Supervisor, 11*(3), 1–11.

Johnson, B. (1992). *Polarity management: Identifying and managing unsolvable problems.* Amherst, MA: HRD Press.

Keenan, M., Hurst, J., & Olnhausen, K. (1993). Polarity management for quality care: Self-direction and manager direction. *Nursing Administration Quarterly, 18*(1), 23–29.

REFERENCES

Barker, G. (1984). *Conflict management behaviour of the staff nurse.* Unpublished master's thesis, University of Utah, Salt Lake City.

Barton, A. (1991). Conflict resolution by nurse managers. *Nursing Management, 22*(5), 83–84, 86.

Blake, R., & Mouton, J. (1964). *The managerial grid.* Houston: Gulf Publications.

Burke, R. (1970, April). Methods of managing superior-subordinate conflict: Their effectiveness and consequences. *Canadian Journal of Behavioral Science, 2,* 124–135.

Calas, M., & Smircich, L. (1996). Re-writing gender into organizational theorizing: Directions from feminist perspectives. In S. Clegg, C. Hardy & W. Nord (Eds.) *Handbook of organizational studies* (pp. 218–257). Thousand Oaks, CA: Sage.

Cavanagh, S. (1991). The conflict management style of staff nurses and nurse managers. *Journal of Advanced Nursing, 15,* 1254–1260.

Coser, L. (1956). *The functions of social conflict.* New York: Free Press.

Etzioni, A. (1961). *A comparative analysis of complex organizations.* New York: Free Press.

Fayol, H. (1949). *General and industrial management.* London: Sir Isaac Pitman.

Follett, M. (1940). Constructive conflict. In H. Metcalf & L. Urwick (Eds.), *Dynamic administration: The collected papers of Mary Follett Parker* (pp. 30–49). New York: Harper. (Originally published, 1926).

Gilligan, C. (1982). *In a different voice.* Cambridge, MA: Harvard University Press.

Harding, S. (1987). *Feminism and methodology.* Bloomington, IN: Indiana University Press.

Hearn, J., Sheppard, D., Tancred-Sheriff, P., & Burrell, G. (Eds.). (1989). *The sexuality of organization.* Newbury Park, CA: Sage.

Hightower, T. (1986). Subordinate choice of conflict handling modes. *Nursing Administration Quarterly, 11*(1), 29–34.

Huber, D. (1996). Conflict. In D. Huber, *Leadership and nursing care management* (pp. 407–430). Philadelphia, PA: W.B. Saunders.

Johnson, M. (1994). Conflict and nursing professionalization. In J. McCloskey & H. Grace (Eds.), *Current issues in nursing* (pp. 643–649). St. Louis, MO: Mosby.

Lewin, K. (1948). *Field theory in social science.* New York: Harper and Bros.

Marriner, A. (1982). Comparing strategies and their use managing conflict. *Nursing Management, 13*(6), 29–31.

Mills, A., & Simmons, T. (1994). *Reading organization theory: A critical approach.* Toronto: Garamond Press.

Mintzberg, H. (1975). The manager's job: Folklore and fact. *Harvard Business Review, 53*(4), 49–61.

Nichols, N. (1996). *Reach for the top: Women and the changing faces of work life.* Boston: Harvard Business.

Rahim, A. (1986). *Managing conflict in organizations.* New York: Praeger.

Rahim, A. & Bonoma, T. (1979). Managing organizational conflict: A model for diagnosis and intervention. *Psychological Reports, 44,* 1323–1344.

Robbins, S. (1982). "Conflict management" and "conflict resolution" are not synonymous terms. In D. White (Ed.), *Contemporary perspectives in organizational behavior* (pp. 299–310). London: Allyn and Bacon.

Shakeshaft, C. (1987). *Women in educational administration.* Beverly Hills, CA: Sage.

Thomas, K., & Kilmann, R. (1974). *Thomas-Kilmann conflict mode instrument.* Tuxedo, NY: XICOM.

Thomas, K. (1976). Conflict and conflict management. In M. Dunnette (Ed.), *Handbook of organizational psychology* (pp. 889–935). Chicago: Rand McNally College Publishing.

Thomas, K. (1977, July). Toward multi-dimensional values in teaching: The example of conflict. *Academy of Management Review, 22,* 142–149.

Thomas, K. (1992). Conflict and negotiation processes in organizations. In M. D. Dunnette & L. M. Hough (Eds.), *Handbook of industrial and organizational psychology* (pp. 651–717). Palo Alto, CA: Consulting Psychologists Press.

Valentine, P. (1995a). Management of conflict: Do nurses/women handle it differently? *Journal of Advanced Nursing, 22,* 142–149.

Valentine, P. (1995b). Women's working worlds: A case study of a female organization. In D. Dunlop & P. Schmuck (Eds.), *Women leading in education* (pp. 340–357). New York: State University of New York Press.

Washington, S. R. (1990). *Conflict management strategies utilized by nurses in the hospital setting.* Unpublished master's thesis, Texas Women's University College of Nursing, Denton, TX.

Weber, M. (1946). *From Max Weber: Essays in sociology.* Translated and edited by H. Gerth and C. Wright Mills. New York: Oxford University Press.

Wood, M., Valentine, P., Richardson, S., & Godkin, D. (1994). *Working in a collective way: The Edmonton experience.* Final report prepared for Alberta Foundation for Nursing Research. Unpublished document available Alberta Foundation for Nursing Research, Edmonton.

CASE STUDIES

Case Study #1

A patient is in early labour with her second child. Her doctor examines her and orders an oxytocin augmentation. He tells the nurse to call his office when he is needed for the delivery. After he leaves, the nurse explains the purpose of the augmentation to the patient. She reveals that this physician always augments his patients so they deliver during the day. She indicates that the patient can refuse, although it means the labour will last longer but will not be as intense. The patient opts for natural delivery. When the physician learns of this decision he explodes at the nurse manager, questioning the nurse's right to discuss this procedure with patients. The nurse manager placates him by apologizing and indicating she will make sure it does not happen again. However, she does not reprimand the nurse, but jokingly describes her interaction with the physician and suggests the nurse "go easy" with his patients.

In this situation, compromising was the conflict-management strategy used. The physician and the nurse both lose something: for the physician, the situation will likely recur; for the nurse, minimal support was received for being a patient advocate.

1. Is this strategy used to try to appease both parties, as a short-term resolution, or because the physician is perceived to be too powerful to suggest open discussion of the issue?
2. How could this situation be resolved differently?
3. Given the male bias in early research on conflict, what are the research implications for nursing as a female-dominated profession?

4. Can you identify several sources of conflict that may arise between physicians and nurses?

Case Study #2

During an extremely busy period in an emergency room, a female physician, who is examining a patient, steps from behind a curtain looking for a nurse. The physician motions to a nurse hurrying by, who says, "Can I help you?" When asked if she is looking after the physician's patient, the nurse replies that she is not, but indicates she will try to locate the patient's nurse. At this point, the physician turns around and exclaims sarcastically: "Oh, where is there another *waitress*!" Although the nurse is upset about the comment, she ignores it. However, it still bothers her several months later.

Avoiding is the strategy used in this situation. The nurse manager is not apprised of the exchange between physician and nurse, but the attitude expressed by the physician is not uncommon in health-care settings. Avoiding this and other slurs may lead to resentment that could eventually colour most interactions between nurses and physicians, to the detriment of patient care. The astute nurse manager will be aware of such attitudes, and get all parties to collaborate on working out a satisfactory resolution.

1. In such situations, what would you suggest?
2. What is it about the roles of staff nurses and their managers that has an impact on their conflict-management strategies?
3. Why do you think staff nurses tend to avoid conflict?
4. Do staff nurses have sufficient resources to effectively handle conflict episodes?

Case Study #3

When a staff nurse leaves for her assigned coffee break, she asks a colleague to assist one of her patients back to bed ten minutes later. The patient is expecting a telephone call momentarily, so she wants to remain in the bedside chair where she can more readily access the telephone. Upon returning from her coffee break, the nurse finds the patient slumped over in the chair, upset and crying; she claims no one came by to help her. The nurse apologizes. She angrily approaches the other nurse and asks why she failed to assist the patient back to bed. The nurse responds that she attempted to assist the patient but the intervention was refused. The nurse suspects her colleague is lying because, in the past, she has had reason to question her patient-care practices. Since this is not the first time this has happened, the nurse discusses the issue with the nurse manager.

Because this situation involves patient care, it requires collaborating to work out an effective long-term resolution. Both parties need to be brought together to confront the issue and work out a mutually acceptable solution. Candidness and co-operation are required to work out the differences; it may take more than one session but will be worth the effort. The situation also suggests that more attention to team building and more commitment to co-operation are needed on this unit. Although abundant research links collaborating to quality of working relationships, it may not be practical or useful in all situations, however. Nurse managers need to carefully assess whether the conflict-handling modes they frequently use are functional in the situations they face in health-care organizations.

1. What impact do you think the caring ideology has on nurses when dealing with conflict?
2. What is the role of managers when staff nurses are confronted by conflict situations?
3. Which conflict-handling modes do you use most frequently?
4. Try role playing how the nurse manager might go about using each of the different conflict-handling modes.

Chapter 26

▼▼▼▼▼▼▼▼▼▼▼▼▼▼▼

Working with Unions
JUDITH M. HIBBERD

KEY OBJECTIVES

In this chapter, you will learn:

- Major components of the system in which union-management relations operate, including collective bargaining.
- Rights and obligations of employers and employees.
- Typical terms and conditions of employment contained in a collective agreement.
- Grievance procedure.
- Steps managers may take to discipline an employee.
- Issues related to union-management relations, including bumping and professional responsibility committees.
- Ways of promoting effective employment relations.

INTRODUCTION

Most non-managerial health-care workers in Canada belong to unions and so administration of collective agreements is a key responsibility of managers. For nurse managers, there may be several union contracts to administer because health workers are often required under labour board rules to belong to predesignated categories for collective-bargaining purposes. Therefore, several unions may be operating independently in a particular patient-care area or community agency.

Effective administration of union contracts requires a basic understanding of the labour-relations system and how collective agreements are reached. Managers should also understand the goals and objectives of unions, the nature of the employment relationship, and the procedures for resolving union-management conflicts, especially grievance and disciplinary procedures. The purpose of this chapter, then, is to address these issues. With knowledge of these topics, managers should be able to develop appropriate skills and attitudes needed to establish constructive relations with union representatives.

Because local union representatives often attend workshops and labour schools sponsored by their unions, managers also need to be well-informed in the area of labour relations so that they may deal intelligently with union officials at work. Although there is a tendency to think of nurses' unions as somehow different from traditional blue-collar unions, the main difference is that nurses are apt to bring a broader range of issues to the bargaining table, including problems that focus on patient care.

FRAMEWORK FOR UNDERSTANDING COLLECTIVE BARGAINING BY NURSES

A collective agreement is a contract of employment. To understand the processes by which such a contract is reached, nurse managers need basic knowledge of the industrial relations system. Scholars frequently view the field of industrial relations from a systems perspective (e.g., Anderson, Gunderson, & Ponak, 1989; Craig, 1996). The Canadian industrial relations system is decentralized, somewhat like the health-care system, in that responsibility for employment relations rests with the provinces. Although the federal government has a labour code governing its own employees and certain national enterprises, each province establishes its own labour legislation. Consequently, there are eleven labour relations systems in the country, which means that procedures relative to collective bargaining tend to vary from province to province. This explains why nurses are entitled to strike in some provinces and not in others.

Environmental factors, such as the state of the economy and the legal system, can be expected to have an impact on the goals of the parties in collective bargaining. For example, during a recession, unions are more likely to give priority to job-security demands than to wage demands, and employers may try to secure wage concessions from unions, as Alberta's nurses discovered in 1988 (Hibberd, 1992).

Despite this, common elements of provincial industrial relations systems can be identified. In Figure 26.1, components of these systems that directly or indirectly influence collective bargaining by nurses are presented.

In the model shown in Figure 26.1, the principal participants in collective bargaining are the employers and their organizations, and nurses and their unions. But governments play a major part in labour relations in the health field; not only do they fund hospitals and community health-care agencies, they make the rules governing collective bargaining (i.e., the labour laws) and they are also responsible for protecting the public interest. Third parties include such people as conciliators, arbitrators, and lawyers called in to assist the main parties with processes. All parties at the collective-bargaining table have goals and special interests, and each draws on its own power resources to influence the process and outcomes.

The principal participants pursue their goals through a series of processes in which conflict, co-operation, and compromise are anticipated.

Figure 26.1

**FRAMEWORK FOR UNDERSTANDING
COLLECTIVE BARGAINING BY NURSES**

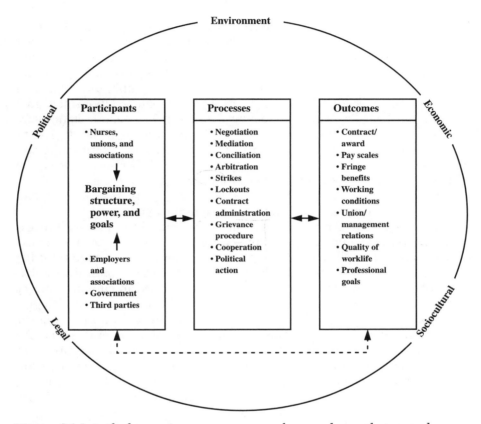

Figure 26.1 includes various processes and procedures that may be employed in reaching a collective agreement, such as negotiation, mediation, arbitration, strikes, lockouts, and the grievance procedure, to name a few. In the vast majority of cases, collective bargaining results in an agreement without conflict (Craig, 1996), and the principal outcome of these procedures is an employment contract, whether negotiated with or without third-party assistance or imposed by an arbitrator.

There are other possible outcomes in this system but the collective agreement, with its terms and conditions of employment, is the principal one. In addition to this contract between the parties, there are consequences for the continuing relationship of the union and employer. A long and bitter strike, for example, may have a lingering and negative impact on relationships in the workplace and can influence the goals that the parties pursue at the next round of bargaining. As collective bargaining recurs at periodic intervals, this framework may be viewed as a dynamic system in which component parts influence or are influenced by each other on a continuing basis.

THE UNION-MANAGEMENT RELATIONSHIP

The nature of relationships between employers and employees has been defined historically by past practices, common law, and labour statutes. Over the years, total employer domination over employees has been replaced with increasingly progressive laws protecting the rights of employees. All provinces have passed employment standards acts establishing minimum terms and conditions of work for all employees, as well as labour relations acts governing union-management relationships (Morris, 1991). Labour statutes are administered by labour relations boards (or in the case of Quebec, by labour courts), whose role is to oversee certification procedures, interpret the law, make decisions, and provide third-party assistance in disputes between the parties. Employees' rights are further protected by law in the areas of occupational health and safety, human rights, pay equity, workers' compensation, unemployment insurance, and tax and pension provisions.

The union-management relationship is formalized through the process of certification. The union applies to the labour relations board for the exclusive right to represent a defined group of employees. The union must file its constitution and bylaws, together with evidence that it represents a majority of a group of employees. Employers are entitled to submit contrary evidence to the labour boards, but they are prohibited from resisting legitimate unionizing activities. Once certified, the union notifies the employer of its intention to negotiate terms and conditions of employment, and the employer must then recognize the collective-bargaining relationship.

Successful union-management relations will depend a great deal on how the parties view each other. If they operate from a conflict viewpoint, then the collective agreement will be perceived as merely a temporary "peace treaty" (Giles & Jain, 1989). A more enlightened perspective is to recognize collective bargaining as "a joint decision-making process for determining terms and conditions of employment and spelling them out in collective agreements. It is grounded on a dependence or symbiotic relationship between employees and employers" (Fisher & Williams, 1989, p. 185). Such a definition implies a legitimate role for unions in framing the rules by which the parties relate to each other, and is more in keeping with the consultative approach to labour relations taken by professional employees such as nurses and teachers.

TERMS AND CONDITIONS OF EMPLOYMENT

Collective agreements in the health field are becoming more and more complex. Nevertheless, some standard provisions are common to most agreements, and these are listed in Box 26.1. The contract usually begins with a

---

Box 26.1

TYPICAL PROVISIONS OF NURSES' COLLECTIVE AGREEMENTS

---

1. Recognition of the parties and purpose of agreement
2. Definitions: nursing personnel covered by agreement
3. Union security: deduction of union dues or the Rand Formula*
4. Management rights
5. Grievance procedure
6. Seniority; promotion; layoff and recall
7. Hours of work; shift schedules; holidays; vacations
8. Fringe benefits: health-care benefits; sick leave
9. Compensation and premium payments

10. Committees: professional responsibility; occupational health and safety
11. Term of agreement: expiry date of contract
12. Appendices: letters of understanding; salary schedules

----

*A contractual arrangement in which the employer makes a payroll deduction of an amount equal to union dues from each member of the bargaining unit whether or not the employee is a member of the union.

---

preamble in which the parties recognize each other and state their intention to work together for the common purpose of providing health-care services. Each category of worker covered by the agreement is then defined. In many jurisdictions, first-line nurse managers are excluded from the bargaining unit (i.e., they are termed out-of-scope) by virtue of their managerial responsibilities. Where nurse managers are in-scope, they may face conflicts of interest as in the case of a grievance over the application of disciplinary measures. Unions have policies to deal with such situations that generally favour the grievor, although there may be informal discussions between union and nurse manager about the case.

It is important to keep in mind that provisions in the contract were jointly agreed to by the parties—albeit reluctantly in some cases and often in emotion-laden, marathon bargaining sessions. Nevertheless, if parties have ratified the agreement, they have a duty to honour it until such time that the contract is renegotiated.

MANAGEMENT RIGHTS— IMPLIED AND EXPRESSED

Historically, employers have gone to great lengths to protect their common-law prerogatives, and almost all collective agreements contain a management rights clause. The clause (or clauses) may take the form of a broad general statement or a detailed list of specific rights (Cohen, 1989); in either case, the nurse manager must be conversant with these express management rights. There is considerable debate in the labour relations literature on management rights. Unions argue that once parties enter a

Table 26.1

IMPLIED EMPLOYMENT RIGHTS AND DUTIES

Employer	Employee
• Provides work and pays compensation for labour • Responsible for safe workplace • Responsible for employees' conduct at work • Gives reasonable notice of termination in absence of just cause	• Co-operates with employer • Exercises reasonable skill and care • Obeys lawful directives • Is not excessively absent from work • Behaves in good faith, and does not disseminate confidential information

Adapted from H.J. Glasbeek, "The contract of employment at common law," in John Anderson and Morley Gunderson (Eds.), *Union Management Relations in Canada* (Don Mills, ON: Addison Wesley, 1982), pp. 47–77.

union-management relationship, unilateral discretion by the employer ceases and all decisions become negotiable. On the other hand, employers prefer a residual rights theory "based on management's assertion that all the rights and privileges that employers exercised before unionization must be considered to be reserved to them afterwards except for those specifically limited by the collective agreement" (Giles & Jain, 1989, p. 323).

Much of what goes on in the workplace, however, is not governed by union contracts because, as Giles and Jain (1989) point out, "collective agreements cannot possibly regulate even a small proportion of the issues, tensions, and relationships that spring from the social and physical setting" (p. 340). For this reason, managers need to be aware of the implied rights and duties derived from common law and past employment practices; these underlie all employment contracts, whether or not expressed in written contracts (McPhillips & England, 1989). Implied rights and duties, some of which are outlined in Table 26.1, serve as a guide to management practices when the collective agreement is silent on an issue, and they influence arbitrators' decisions when interpreting a collective agreement or judging the merits of a grievance.

The employment relationship is a fiduciary one; in other words, it is based on good faith and trust (McPhillips & England, 1989). While the employer retains the right to run the health agency, the employee has an obligation to co-operate with the employer. Any failure to fulfil these rights and responsibilities constitutes a breach of the employment contract.

Conflict between unions and management during the term of the collective agreement, whether or not over the question of management rights, may be resolved informally. More serious disputes may need to be formally resolved through the grievance procedure. Strikes and lockouts are dispute-resolution processes (see Figure 26.1), but in Canada they are not allowed during the term of the collective agreement (Sethi & MacNeil, 1989); for this reason, collective agreements must contain a grievance procedure.

GRIEVANCE PROCEDURE

A grievance is not only an allegation that one or more provisions of an agreement have been violated but is also a claim for redress (Gandz & Whitehead, 1989). There are three types of grievances: individual, group, and policy grievances. The type of grievance determines the level at which it can be initiated in the grievance procedure. A policy grievance affecting the union itself, for example, is usually filed directly with the chief executive officer of the agency, whereas an individual or group grievance must first be discussed with immediate supervisors. The subject of a grievance in Canada is confined to the contents of the collective agreement; in other words, there must be at least one clause in the union contract that relates to the complaint.

Although it is almost impossible to know the entire contract in detail, nurse managers must be thoroughly familiar with the grievance procedure. They must also know the scope of their authority in handling grievances; for example, they need to know at what stage humanresources personnel are to become involved in the process. A typical grievance procedure is presented in Table 26.2.

There is not much research on the incidence and pattern of nurses' union grievances. Research in other fields suggests that grievances may serve many functions: they are a means by which unions may communicate with employers; they permit one of the parties to challenge the rights or actions of the other party; they may be a form of continuous bargaining (i.e., a way of forcing a concession that could not be obtained through collective bargaining); or they may be politically motivated by self-serving individuals or groups either within the union or managerial ranks (Gandz, 1982).

Arbitrators have recognized the powerlessness and vulnerability of individuals who choose to challenge an employer's authority, and they uphold the principle of natural justice underlying the grievance procedure. A grievance allows a union member to appeal a manager's negative decision at increasingly higher levels of administrative authority, and ultimately to an independent arbitrator or arbitration board, without fear of punishment or dismissal. Even with the protection that a collective agreement affords, a nurse may feel too intimidated to complain. This is why unions have fought for the right to accompany their members throughout the grievance procedure, and to receive copies of all written communications about grievances.

The first-level manager plays a critical role at the first step of the grievance procedure. This step is an informal discussion during which the grievor and manager determine if a problem exists. This is where the facts of the situation are carefully and thoroughly investigated; where consultation is sought; and, ideally, where the problem is solved. If the decision is well founded at this point, the nurse manager can expect to be supported by senior administrators should the grievance advance through subsequent steps. To avoid the demoralizing experience of having a decision overturned at a more senior level of the organization, the nurse manager should consult the humanresources department and the next level of management

---

Table 26.2

A TYPICAL GRIEVANCE PROCEDURE

Complaint   A nurse discusses a complaint or concern informally with the
immediate supervisor and the complaint is satisfied or dismissed
within seven working days.

Step 1   The complaint becomes a grievance and is written on the union's
grievance form specifying: a. the nature of the grievance; b. the
articles in the collective agreement allegedly violated; and c. the
remedy sought; it is then submitted to the first-level nurse manager
within seven working days of the initial discussion.
A meeting may be held with the grievor, union representative, and
manager.
The nurse manager delivers a response in writing to the nurse
within seven working days.

Step 2   If the grievance has not been settled, it may be submitted in writing
to the department head within seven working days.
A meeting of all parties may be convened to discuss the grievance.
The director's decision is communicated in writing to the grievor
(copy to the union) within seven working days.

Step 3   If the grievance has not been settled, it may be submitted in writing
to the chief executive officer within seven working days.
A meeting of all parties may be convened. The chief executive
officer's decision is communicated in writing to the grievor (copy to
the union) within seven working days.

Step 4   If the grievance is not settled, either party may consider whether to
proceed to arbitration, or whether to abandon the grievance.
Decision to proceed to arbitration is communicated in writing to the
other party together with a name of a nominee to the arbitration
board within seven working days.

Arbitration   Final, binding decision is made.

Note: If the employer fails to respond within the specified time limits, the grievance automatically moves to the next step in the procedure. If the union or grievor fails to respond within specified time limits, the grievance is abandoned, unless there has been
prior mutual agreement to extend the time limits. At each step of the grievance, the employee may be accompanied by a union representative.

before dismissing or allowing a grievance. Senior administrators bring a
broader perspective to bear on the procedure and may have handled similar grievances in the past. Nevertheless, what seems like a clear-cut case to
unions and employers may be seen in a totally different light by an arbitration board. Indeed, it is often difficult to predict the outcome of arbitration.

GRIEVANCE ARBITRATION

At step four of the grievance procedure, either party may refer the dispute to an external arbitration board. Grievance arbitration should not be confused with interest arbitration, which is used to settle disputes arising out of collective bargaining. The two procedures are similar, but they deal with different types of disputes. Grievance arbitration deals with disputes arising out of the interpretation, application, or alleged violation of the terms of an existing collective agreement.

Fewer than two percent of written grievances proceed to arbitration, according to Gandz and Whitehead (1989), and so it is relatively rare for a nurse manager to have to take part in arbitration proceedings. However, if a grievance goes to arbitration, union and management each select a nominee to serve on the arbitration board. The nominees jointly select the chair, but if they cannot agree on this person, the provincial minister of labour will appoint the arbitrator. In some cases, the board consists of a sole arbitrator. A hearing is held, at which the parties may be represented by legal counsel. Witnesses may be called and cross-examined, and the parties will formally present their arguments (Gandz & Whitehead, 1989).

Arbitration is time-consuming and expensive; the parties are responsible for the expenses of their respective nominees and witnesses, and they share the fee of the arbitrator. By the time a grievance goes to arbitration, the parties are usually entrenched in their opposing positions and determined to win the case. The arbitration board's decision is final and binding on the parties, and can only be appealed under specific circumstances, such as if the arbitrator exceeds his or her jurisdiction or makes an error of law (Craig, 1996).

Appearing at an arbitration hearing is much like attending court, except that rules of evidence and procedure are not as rigorous, and the hearing may be held in a less formal setting than a law court. In preparation for serving as a witness for management, the manager and other witnesses must be well briefed on their roles at the arbitration hearing, preferably at a meeting with the lawyer or person presenting the case. Because of the potential for every grievance to become an arbitration case, managers must keep meticulous notes of each phase of the grievance process noting who attended each meeting, what main points were made, what the final decision was, and the underlying reasons for allowing or disallowing the grievance. Moreover, care must be taken with the content and language used in all written communications to the grievor because these will undoubtedly be filed as exhibits at the arbitration hearing. Even past performance appraisals may be submitted as an exhibit if the grievance involves the discipline of a nurse.

PROGRESSIVE DISCIPLINE

Occasionally, it will be necessary to discipline a staff member, and arbitrators in the past have expected employers to apply discipline in a progressive manner (Pearlman, 1991). One might well ask, as Eden (1992) does, whether application of negative sanctions is an appropriate corporate response to employee misconduct in light of contemporary trends in human-resource management. The objective of progressive discipline should be to correct behaviour, not to punish it (Cannon, 1980). Nevertheless, if the employee fails to respond to repeated warnings, the ultimate penalty could be dismissal. A typical disciplinary procedure appears in Table 26.3.

Discipline should be used to correct patterns of unsatisfactory behaviour, not to deal with occasional errors or misjudgements. On the other hand, gross misconduct such as sexual harassment of a patient would require immediate suspension so that an investigation could take place. Similarly, assaulting a patient would probably be considered just cause for dismissal. Where a staff member has demonstrated unsatisfactory behaviour in more than one area (e.g., absenteeism *and* failure to chart narcotic drugs), it would be necessary to apply discipline progressively to both problems. Moreover, a nurse manager has discretion to repeat a step, or to begin the procedure again if there has been a significant time lapse since an earlier disciplinary step. Whatever the situation, the problem must be communicated to the staff member immediately and in private, never in hallways or in earshot of patients and other staff. Discipline that is loudly applied in public is humiliating for the employee, and unprofessional on the part of the manager; it also undermines its objective, namely to effect a positive change in behaviour.

At every step of the disciplinary procedure, the nurse manager should be prepared for a grievance. The grievance procedure and the disciplinary procedure are similar processes in which increasing pressure is placed on the other party to bring about a change in thinking or behaviour. The disciplinary procedure, however, is the prerogative of management and is not usually spelled out in detail in the collective agreement. Even so, should the case go to arbitration, the employer will be required to show that there was sufficient cause to discipline the nurse, that the nurse understood the problem and was given opportunities and assistance to improve his or her performance, that there were no extenuating circumstances, and that the discipline was not arbitrary or unreasonable.

As in the grievance procedure, careful documentation is absolutely essential. All evidence that led to the discipline and relevant details of discussions and interviews must be recorded in the employee's file. Such data will likely be used at arbitration. Unions often negotiate time periods beyond which such documentation must be purged from the employee's file. Few managers look forward to using disciplinary measures, but if handled thoughtfully, objectively, and in a timely manner, both parties should emerge with their self-respect intact, and with respect for each other.

INSUBORDINATION

It will be remembered from Table 26.1 that an implied duty of employees, whether unionized or not, is to co-operate with lawful directives of the

Table 26.3
PROGRESSIVE DISCIPLINE

Step 1	**Informal discussion.** A private meeting is held between nurse manager and nurse to identify the problem, to discuss it, and to coach or counsel the nurse.
Step 2	**Verbal warning.** Assuming no improvement in behaviour, another meeting is held between nurse manager and nurse. Three points are made: a) the problem is identified and the desired change in behaviour stated; b) a time limit is set during which improvement is to occur; and c) the consequences of failure to improve are stated. The nurse must also understand that he or she has received a verbal warning.
Step 3	**Written warning.** At least 24-hours notice of a meeting is given to the nurse, who may be accompanied by a union representative. Discussion of the problem follows, with reference to previous verbal warnings. A letter is given to the nurse containing the same three points outlined in Step 2 above. Copies are filed in the employee's personnel record and with the union.
Step 4	**Suspension.** The procedures in Step 3 are repeated, but the letter states the length of the suspension, and whether it is to be with or without pay. The nurse must understand that the ultimate consequence of not responding to discipline in the specified amount of time will be dismissal. Copies are filed in the employee's personnel record and with the union.
Step 5	**Dismissal.** A final meeting is held, which includes representatives from the human resources department and the union. The letter terminating the nurse's employment contains a final pay cheque and relevant severance papers. Copies of the letter are filed in the employee's personnel record and with the union.

Note: The level at which discipline begins will depend upon the severity of the employee's misconduct or problem and the situation. Steps in the procedure may be repeated. A union representative may be present at each step of the procedure.

employer. Willful refusal to obey a lawful order is known as insubordination; employers consider insubordination a serious breach of the employment contract and just cause for discipline. It should be clear that effective management is impossible if the nursing staff no longer respect legitimate orders from the person in charge of a unit.

To be successful in disciplining a person for insubordination, a nurse manager will have to prove that:

- a valid order was given to the employee,
- the order was clearly communicated by a person having the authority to direct the employee, and

- the employee failed to comply with the order (Mrazek & Tumback, 1990).

It is important to note that these cases are not concerned with failure to comply with physicians' orders relative to patient care. Nurses are obligated under professional practice acts to question and, if necessary, to refuse to carry out a physician's order that they know to be erroneous and harmful to patients. Such disputes between professional colleagues fall outside the meaning and definition of insubordination because nurses do not normally report to physicians, but to someone in a line position in the formal structure of the health agency. The concern here is with orders given by nurse managers (as the employer's designate) to their staff members, and this includes patient-care assignments that an individual nurse might consider intolerable and unsafe.

Whether or not a nurse can refuse a legitimate order to care for patients is a complex question (Creighton, 1986; Huerta & Oddi, 1992; Northrop, 1987; Wahn, 1979), and nurse managers need to be clear where they stand in such situations. More importantly, a nurse manager must decide if the refusal to obey is serious enough to be defined as insubordination. For example, a nurse may try to avoid working with a particularly difficult client, or may simply forget to carry out a delegated task, neither of which really constitutes insubordination. The most reasonable response of a nurse manager would be to try to negotiate an acceptable compromise with the unwilling nurse, but the problem with this is that precedents can be set, and manipulative employees may be resented by other staff. The nurse manager must be sure of the facts before alleging insubordination.

An employee is entitled to refuse a supervisor's order when compliance:

- constitutes an illegal act,
- endangers the health or safety of the employee and co-workers, or
- causes irreparable damage to the interest of other employees (Mrazek & Tumbach, 1990), for instance, refusing to grant leave of absence to a union representative resulting in the loss of a union member's job at grievance arbitration.

This does not mean that the employee would necessarily escape discipline in such an event; rather, it means that arbitrators likely would rule in favour of the employee for refusing an order under any of these circumstances. There are, however, some requirements of employees who invoke any of these exceptional circumstances. The employee bears the onus of proving the case to the arbitrator, and for this reason the employee must, at the time the order is refused, explain the reason for refusal. As most employees would not be able to articulate their rights and obligations in a case of insubordination, it behooves the nurse manager to explain the seriousness of refusal to comply with a legitimate order, and to help staff articulate their reasons for refusing before administering discipline.

Nurses' refusal to undertake patient-care assignments has created some interesting jurisprudence. In the Mount Sinai case in which three nurses were disciplined for refusing to take an additional patient into an intensive

care unit (Sklar, 1979a, 1979b), arbitrators found the discipline to be justified on the basis that—notwithstanding the professional judgement and
legal liability of the nurses relative to patient safety—the health-and-safety
exemption listed above applies *only* to employees and co-workers, *not* to
third parties such as patients. In other words, the principle established is
that "heavy or excessive patient work-loads alone cannot be used as a basis
for refusal to carry out an assignment" (Mrazek & Tumbach, 1990). The reason for this is that the employer (including the nurse manager) is vicariously liable for any injuries to patients arising out of a nurse's inability or
failure to provide safe care to patients. Hence, employees should more appropriately observe the principle of "obey now, grieve later" (Mrazek &
Tumback, 1990).

The principle of "obey now, grieve later" reflects the duty of the employee to co-operate with the employer. Of course, it does not solve the
dilemma of the nurse who wishes to refuse a patient assignment on moral
and ethical grounds. Such situations can be avoided in part by frank discussions with nurses at the time they are hired, but there appears to be little to protect the conscientious objector (see Creighton, 1986; Peterborough
Civic Hospital and Ontario Nurses' Association, 1982). Similarly, nurses
who "whistleblow" are largely unprotected at the present time, although
there appears to be some movement toward policy changes in this area
(Fiesta, 1990; McKenna, 1989). Currently, if a nurse wishes to expose un-
lawful or hazardous working conditions to the media, he or she would attract discipline from the employer. Nevertheless, when all internal avenues
of protest have been exhausted, professional employees have a duty to their
clients to ensure that their safety and interests are properly served. Under
such circumstances, the first step would be to consult the professional
nurses' association.

DEVELOPING CONSTRUCTIVE UNION-MANAGEMENT RELATIONS

First-level managers, whether or not they are nurses, play key roles in promoting good relations between union and management. Although they may
regard the collective agreement as limiting their freedom to make decisions
and introduce change, the existence of a union contract requires managers
to be fair and impartial when supervising employees. Dealing with staff in
an equitable manner is essential if teamwork and co-operation are to flourish in the work setting. The contract provides a clear set of rules by which
such things as allocation of unpopular shifts and vacation times are decided. If properly administered, the collective agreement ensures standard
treatment of staff throughout the health agency, not solely on a particular
unit. If any clause in the collective agreement is unclear or unworkable, it
may become the subject of a grievance just to obtain clarification.
Alternatively, at the next round of collective bargaining, new wording for the
clause can be proposed by the employer. Collective agreements eventually

expire and, although terms and conditions continue until a new contract is signed, this open period allows both parties to negotiate improvements to the contract.

EFFECTIVE MANAGEMENT

Employment relations are more likely to be co-operative where there is effective management. On the whole, unions have little respect for ineffective managers and can readily find ways to create a hostile climate on a unit. For example, they might: challenge all management decisions whether related to the contract or not; file grievances; spend inordinate amounts of time on complaints; and file "professional responsibility forms." Under such circumstances, it becomes a great challenge to create positive relations with a union representative, especially if that person has leadership aspirations and is intent upon demonstrating militancy and developing a power base within the union. Most nurses promoted to a management position have at one time been members of unions, and so they are likely to understand the goals, values, beliefs, and internal organization of the nurses' union. An open-minded attitude toward unions will be a distinct advantage when working with union representatives, as will a willingness to listen to problems, investigate them, and negotiate solutions.

Collective agreements for nurses have become so complex that solving problems arising from their interpretation and administration should not be attempted without assistance. Health agencies have access to labour relations specialists, whether on site in the human resources department or externally from the health agency's legal firm, or from the provincial regional health authorities' association. Managers need to find out what the scope of their authority is with respect to contract administration and the grievance procedure in their own agency. Most health agencies have policies about reporting complaints and potential grievances, and so it is necessary to be aware of such internal guidelines.

ROLE OF UNION REPRESENTATIVES

Program areas or patient-care units typically have a local "shop steward" or union representative. These people may be elected, but usually they volunteer for these unpaid jobs within the union organization. They work closely with the union's employment relations officers and union leaders. Their role includes seeing that rights of union members are enforced; being available to union members during disputes and to attend their grievance or disciplinary meetings; helping write out grievances and prepare cases for arbitration; and collecting information for the union (American Nurses' Association, l985). Requests by the local union steward to leave the clinical area during a work day must not be unreasonably denied; nevertheless, such requests are negotiable, and the needs of patients and clients remain the prime factor in granting permission to leave the clinical area.

There is great variability in the degree to which union representatives pursue their roles and responsibilities. Some are aggressive in their approach to their duties, while others seem to be reluctant volunteers with little aptitude or enthusiasm for their roles. Nevertheless, unions have a duty of fair representation—that is, to represent all members of the bargaining unit fairly and without discrimination (Craig, l996). Human-rights legislation applies equally to employers and unions. In all but the most hostile cases, managers and union representatives are able to work out a mutually respectful and constructive relationship.

PROFESSIONAL RESPONSIBILITY COMMITTEES

In the late l970s, nurses began to demand ways and means of discussing their concerns about patient care with employers. After two major strikes in Alberta, nurses there obtained a clause in their collective agreement entitled "Professional Responsibility Committees" (PRCs). These committees are made up of equal numbers of managers and nurses, and they meet regularly. The committees have a great deal of potential for nurses to initiate needed changes affecting their work. They also provide a forum for the free flow of communication, ideas, and debate about nursing issues, as well as problems and events in the health agency in general.

In a recent study of the effectiveness of these committees, the majority of the managers and union members from the nineteen hospitals surveyed said that their PRCs were operating effectively. Nurses' concerns, rather than management concerns, dominated the agendas, and the type of problems referred to the PRCs included security issues, staffing levels, clinical protocols, and patient safety. Participants identified many concrete results from PRC meetings, such as new or revised policies (e.g., policies related to 'do not resuscitate' procedures, to smoking, or to staff abuse), systems improvement (e.g., security, parking, paging), and staffing improvements (e.g., float staff, job descriptions). Many of the participants commented that PRCs had improved the communication between management and union (Hibberd, 1996). Thus, PRCs have much potential as a forum for fostering union-management relations.

LAYOFFS AND BUMPING

One of the most stressful aspects of being a manager in the last few years has been dealing with the human consequences of regionalization and restructuring. Unions too have been affected by these trends, because regionalization has led to changes in bargaining units and the merger of previously competing unions (see Pedersen, 1997). In hospitals, restructuring and downsizing have led to widespread layoff of health workers, especially registered nurses. Unions have a vested interest in how health agencies go about laying off their members because of their highly cherished principle of seniority. Unions argue that because seniority is the most objective criterion for making decisions about employees' jobs, it should be the only criterion for determining who gets laid off. Seniority means that the longer an employee works for an employer, the greater the job security, and so if there are to be layoffs, the seniority principle ensures that members with the least seniority will be the first to be laid off and the last to be recalled to work. The application of seniority results in bumping, with many associated stresses and strains for employers and unions, as well as many grievances.

Bumping is defined as: "the procedure by which the employee with the greatest seniority who is about to be laid off is allowed to invoke her [or his] seniority rights so as to displace, or bump, a more junior employee from a job unaffected by the lay-off" (Brown & Beatty, 1994, 6:2330). This procedure can set off a chain of bumps. Generally, the senior employee must possess the skills and ability to do the desired job of the more junior employee. Ability to perform the work is a contentious issue between managers who try to protect the integrity of workgroups, particularly in highly specialized areas, and union leaders who want to defend the bumping rights of their members. Whether or not an employer can refuse a nurse's request to bump depends on the specific wording in the collective agreement, and on precedents set in previous arbitration rulings. Employers are generally expected to familiarize (i.e., provide orientation to) staff exercising bumping rights, but not necessarily to provide training where new knowledge and skills may be needed. For example, where hospital policy requires nurses to have qualifications beyond basic nursing preparation (e.g., in areas such as neonatal intensive care units or coronary care units), an employer may be entitled to restrict bumping just to nurses possessing those qualifications.

The practice of bumping is fraught with problems: what constitutes a layoff; whether a full-time nurse can bump a part-time nurse and vice versa; and whether seniority rights can be upheld in interorganizational mergers, are just a few. Moreover, there are various ways of effecting single bumps and chains of bumps. For example, it is possible for an employer and union to sit down together and work out a chain of bumps on paper, obtain agreement from all individuals, and then to announce a day on which the final bumps are implemented. This system avoids all intermediate bumping that goes on in the process of accommodating every nurse on the seniority list.

Displacement or relocation of nurses from one service to a similar or different service is highly disruptive for established workgroups, and creates tension, anxiety, distrust, disillusionment, and a deep sense of insecurity. Although sympathy is largely expressed for those whose jobs have been lost to individuals with greater seniority, nurses who initiate the bumping may suffer just as much pain (Smith, 1996).

Managers can do much to ease the tensions for everyone during such times, by ensuring that all bumping procedures are correctly followed; by paying attention to the needs of all staff whether they are coming, going, or staying; by ensuring that staff have the information they need to make optimal decisions; and, as Curtin (1996) suggests, by doing anything that increases people's sense of personal control.

CONCLUSION

The impact of restructure within Canada's health-care system is likely to place considerable strain on union-management relations, but it may also stimulate co-operation. Although relations between the parties can vary from outright hostility on the one hand to collusion or apathy on the other, nurse managers should try to promote constructive working relationships with unions rather than assume that the relationship is inherently adversarial. They can do this by recognizing the legitimacy of unions, and by fostering common goals such as promoting high standards of nursing service and job satisfaction among the staff.

SUMMARY

- Managers working in a unionized environment should have a basic understanding of the labour relations system.
- The collective agreement is a contract between employer and employees that outlines terms and conditions of employment, and the rules that govern relationships between the parties.
- Employers and employees have common law rights and responsibilities towards each other.
- Grievances provide the means by which employees may lodge complaints against employers who allegedly violate the collective agreement without fear of reprisal.
- Discipline is the means by which employers may deal with employees who fail to live up to their employment obligations.
- An employee who refuses to follow a manager's direction may be disciplined; three specific circumstances provide exceptions to this principle.
- Nurse managers can promote constructive union-management relations by becoming knowledgeable about the purpose of unions and the role of union representatives, serving on professional responsibility committees, and providing effective leadership and management.
- Laying off unionized staff results in bumping; managers need to develop strategies for minimizing the disruption and distress created by the relocation of nursing staff.

FURTHER READINGS AND RESOURCES

Julius, D. J. (1998). Managing in a unionized setting. Part I: The discipline process. *AORN Journal, 48*(5), 919–929. Part II: The grievance process. *AORN Journal, 48* (6), 1145–1151. These two articles provide a more detailed discussion of the discipline and grievance procedures than could be offered in this chapter. The reader should keep in mind, however, that the discussion is based on the U.S. labour relations system, although the two processes are treated similarly in Canada. Julius provides examples of disciplinary letters in Part I, and an example of a grievance form in Part II.

REFERENCES

American Nurses' Association (1985). *The grievance procedure.* Kansas City, MO: American Nurses' Association.

Anderson, J. C., Gunderson, M., & Ponak, A. (1989). *Union-management relations in Canada* (2nd ed.). Don Mills, ON: Addison-Wesley.

Brown, D.J.M., & Beatty, D.M. (1994). *Canadian labour arbitration* (3rd ed.). Aurora, ON: Canadian Law Book.

Cannon, P. (1980). Administering the contract. *Journal of Nursing Administration, 10* (10), 13–19.

Cohen, A. (1989). The management rights clause in collective bargaining. *Nursing Management, 20* (11), 24–34.

Craig, A. W. J. (1996). *The system of industrial relations in Canada* (5th ed.). Scarborough, ON: Prentice-Hall.

Creighton, H. (1986). When can a nurse refuse to give care? *Nursing Management, 17*(3), 16–20.

Curtin, L. L. (1996). Surviving "survivor syndrome." *Nursing Management, 27*(10), 7–8.

Eden, G. (1992). Progressive discipline: An oxymoron? *Relations Industrielles, 47* (3), 511–528.

Fiesta, J. (1990). Whistleblowers: Retaliation or protection? Part 2. *Nursing Management, 21* (7), 38.

Fisher, E. G., & Williams, C. B. (1989). Negotiating the union-management agreement. In J. C. Anderson, M. Gunderson, & A. Ponak (Eds.), *Union-management relations in Canada* (2nd ed.) (pp. 185–207). Don Mills, ON: Addison-Wesley.

Gandz, J. (1982). Grievances and their resolution. In J. Anderson & M. Gunderson (Eds.), *Union-management relations in Canada* (pp. 289–315). Don Mills, ON: Addison-Wesley.

Gandz, J., & Whitehead, J. D. (1989). Grievances and their resolution. In J. C. Anderson, M. Gunderson, & A. Ponak (Eds.), *Union-management relations in Canada* (2nd ed.) (pp. 235–260). Don Mills, ON: Addison-Wesley.

Giles, A., & Jain, H. C. (1989). The collective agreement. In J.C. Anderson, M. Gunderson, & A. Ponak (Eds.), *Union-management relations in Canada* (2nd ed.) (pp. 317–345). Don Mills, ON: Addison-Wesley.

Glasbeek, H. J. (1982). The contract of employment at common law. In J. Anderson & M. Gunderson (Eds.), *Union-management relations in Canada* (pp. 47–77). Don Mills, ON: Addison-Wesley.

Hibberd, J. M. (1992). Strikes by nurses. Part 2: Incidence, trends and issues. *Canadian Nurse, 88* (3), 26–31.

Hibberd, J. M. (1996) *Effectiveness of nurses' labour-management committees*. Final report to the Alberta Foundation for Nursing Research, Edmonton, Alberta.

Huerta, S. R., & Oddi, L. F. (1992). Refusal to care for patients with Human Immunodeficiency Virus/Acquired Immunodeficiency Syndrome: Issues and responses. *Journal of Professional Nursing, 8* (4), 221–230.

McKenna, I. (1989). Whistleblowing and criticism of employers by employees—The case for reform in Canada. In *Papers presented at the Conference Labour Relations into the 1990s*. School of Management, University of Lethbridge, September 10–12, 1987 (pp. 141–184). Don Mills, ON: CCH Canadian.

McPhillips, D., & England, G. (1989). Employment legislation in Canada. In J. C. Anderson, M. Gunderson, & A. Ponak (Eds.), *Union-management relations in Canada* (2nd ed) (pp. 43–69). Don Mills, ON: Addison-Wesley.

Morris, J. J. (1991). *Canadian nurses and the law*. Toronto: Butterworths.

Mrazek, M., & Tumback, D. (1990). Insubordination and incompetence—A nurse's dilemma. *AARN Newsletter, 46* (10), 18–19.

Northrop, C. E. (1987). Refusing unsafe work assignments. *Nursing Outlook, 36* (6), 302.

Pearlman, D. (1991). Progressive discipline: The grievance and arbitration process. In S. A. Ziebarth (Ed.), *Pinched: A management guide to the Canadian health care archipelago* (pp. 185–191). Ottawa: Canadian Hospital Association.

Peterborough Civic Hospital and Ontario Nurses' Association. (1982). 3 L. A. C., (3d), 21–54.

Pedersen, R. (1997). Nursing unions unite for 'stronger voice.' *Edmonton Journal,* Friday, September 26, B5.

Sethi, A. S., & MacNeil, M. (1989). Issues in contract administration and human rights. In A. S. Sethi (Ed.), *Collective bargaining in Canada* (pp. 317–340). Scarborough, ON: Nelson.

Sklar, C.L. (1979a). Saints or sinners? The legal perspective: Part I. *Canadian Nurse, 75* (10), 14–16.

Sklar, C. L. (1979b). Saints or sinners? The legal perspective: Part II. *Canadian Nurse, 75* (11), 16, 18, 20–21.

Smith, T. (1996). Two painful sides to bumping. *Canadian Nurse, 92* (7), 55.

Wahn, E. V. (1979). The dilemma of the disobedient nurse. *Health Care in Canada, 21* (2), 43–46.

CASE STUDY

Maureen Anderson is a patient care co-ordinator in a busy home-care program. The agency receives referrals from several hospitals and doctors' offices, as well as direct referrals from the community. Her staff consists of registered nurses who function as case managers, licensed practical nurses, home health aides, an occupational therapist (OT), physiotherapists (PT), and a respiratory therapist (RT). Ms. Anderson has been successful in hiring competent, self-directed professional staff, and loyal hardworking support staff. Although they all belong to various unions, she has never had a grievance, or an occasion to fire or discipline anyone.

In the last three months, however, she has received several complaints about one of her registered nurses, Nancy Reilly. One complaint was from the OT about an interaction he had observed between Ms. Reilly and a client. Another complaint from the RT indicated that Ms. Reilly had refused to assist with positioning a paralzsed patient for treatment. Two complaints from an active-treatment hospital cited lack of co-operation, and one complaint from a physician mentioned "unprofessional attitudes."

Maureen Anderson met with this nurse to discuss the complaints, but Ms. Reilly denied any problems, saying that everyone was really busy and tempers had been short lately. Five weeks later, Ms. Anderson decided to make one of her routine supervisory visits to a client's home. She timed this visit so that she could observe the care and talk to the client, in this case, Ms. Reilly's client. This particular client had multiple nursing-care needs and had been on the home-care service for many months. She was, therefore, familiar with all the staff. Ms. Anderson observed nothing unusual in Nancy Reilly's work. After Ms. Reilly left the client's home, Ms. Anderson remained to talk and, without prompting, the client proceeded to make a series of complaints about Ms. Reilly's rough manner, lack of punctuality, disorganization, and uncaring attitude.

On the basis of this visit, Maureen Anderson again called Nancy Reilly into the office to discuss her concerns. Ms. Reilly became upset and defensive, and the interview ended without agreement on any future plan of action. The next morning, Ms. Anderson received a telephone call from the nurses' union representative, alleging harassment and intimidation of Nancy Reilly, and violation of the clause in the collective agreement that allows Ms. Reilly to have a union representative accompany her at all steps of the disciplinary procedure.

1. What is the immediate problem facing Maureen Anderson?
2. What is the underlying problem for Ms. Anderson?
3. Identify the issues that should be addressed in this case.
4. What is the role of the union representative in this case, and why do you think Nancy Reilly turned to the union for help?
5. Comment on the way in which Ms. Anderson has handled the case thus far.
6. What would be an appropriate response by Maureen Anderson to the union representative?

Chapter 27

▼▼▼▼▼▼▼▼▼▼▼▼▼▼▼▼▼

Negotiating: A Basic Survival Skill

Lana Clark and Judith M. Hibberd

KEY OBJECTIVES

In this chapter, you will learn:

- Different types of negotiating and collective bargaining commonly used in health-care agencies.
- Three different styles of negotiation.
- Key principles that underlie the negotiating process.
- Four phases in the negotiating process.
- Common negotiating tactics and the rationale for using them.

INTRODUCTION

Many contributors to this book have noted that today's health-care system is characterized by rapid change, conflict, shrinking resources, and the need for precise, timely decisions. Managers often find themselves at the centre of action arising from this turbulent environment. The diverse expectations of multiple stakeholders often lead to incompatible interests or demands, and resolving these may require skilled intervention.

Although nurse managers may have opportunities to take part in formal negotiations such as collective bargaining, they are more likely to become involved in less formal, everyday types of negotiation, such as advocating for additional staff for a busy shift, or helping individual staff members settle disputes over the care of patients. Not only are managers increasingly required to engage in negotiations in various contexts, they are also expected to serve as mediators and to work with third parties using alternative dispute resolution processes (creating innovative and less formal ways of resolving conflict) (Grant, 1995).

It is imperative that contemporary nursing leaders learn the principles and process underlying the art and science of negotiation. Negotiation is replacing the traditional authority of the leader's coercive power (Biggerstaff & Syre, 1991) and is being recognized as a key strategy in successful conflict resolution (Smeltzer, 1991; Snyder-Halpern & Cannon, 1993). De-fined as "a process of communicating back and forth for the purpose of reaching a joint decision" (Fisher, Ury, & Patton, 1991, p. 32), negotiation has moved from a rarely-used technique to a basic survival skill for nurse managers.

This chapter provides an overview of the negotiation process and fo-cuses on the nature of what is encompassed in developing negotiation skills. First, however, there is a need to examine the differences between negotia-tion for collective agreements and day-to-day negotiation by managers.

TYPES OF NEGOTIATION

Day-to-day negotiation is a process that emphasizes the need to maintain long-term interpersonal relationships. It is an ongoing process built on trust, creativity, and co-operative decision-making. Going beyond the tra-ditional win-lose conflict resolution style and even the contemporary win-win style, day-to-day negotiation attempts to resolve conflict through communication, exchange of ideas, and commitment to a course of action.

In contrast, negotiation associated with collective bargaining has an identifiable time frame characterized by start and completion dates. More-over, rules, often specified in labour laws and associated regulations, gov-ern the process (see also Chapter 26). In collective bargaining, the parties are essentially required to negotiate together and, even if talks break off, they know that at some point they must return to the bargaining table. In this process, the objective is to attain a settlement, and there is little em-phasis on maintaining long-term relationships. Indeed, the atmosphere tends to be one that emphasizes the "we-they" component of the relation-ship, in contrast to the collaborative problem-solving environment associ-ated with the daily negotiation style.

WHY NEGOTIATE?

In the face of rapid change and shrinking resources, conflict in the Cana-dian health-care system is inevitable. As leaders, nurse managers increas-ingly encounter situations of conflict and the need to resolve these situations has become a significant challenge (Collyer, 1989). Approaches to resolving conflict are discussed extensively in published literature, and are also explored by Valentine in Chapter 25 of this book. Contemporary management theorists view conflict resolution as a critical process in searching for new methods or solutions to problems (Jones, 1993).

The collaborative approach to conflict resolution has been described in industrial research as the approach most likely to achieve successful out-comes (Citron, 1981). Marriner (1982) found that nurses who used collab-orating or compromising approaches were more likely to have successful conflict resolution. In comparison, avoiding or competing approaches were more frequently associated with unsuccessful resolution. A collaborative approach has been associated with the search for integrated solutions and empowerment of others (Kouzes & Posner, 1987), two outcomes that are highly valued within successful health-care organizations.

Negotiation in day-to-day practice is an effective interactive strategy that allows for the sharing of power and control (Barton, 1991) and emphasizes the need to maintain ongoing relationships (Fisher et al., l991). Because it promotes an environment that emphasizes collaboration, negotiation becomes a strategy for conflict resolution. Increasingly, managers use negotiation for securing the resources needed to support the effective delivery of health services. In addition, successful use of negotiation skills may enhance the team spirit of nursing and serve to benefit the organization, the patient, the nurse, and the nursing profession (Smeltzer, 1991).

WHEN TO NEGOTIATE?

Negotiation is a fact of life (Fisher & Ury, 1983). It can be used in any situation where there is a desire to affect the behaviour of others (Cohen, 1982). Whether it is used to determine the price of a new car, the time when a teenaged daughter should be home from a graduation party, or the details of a salary increment, negotiation can help to ensure an effective outcome for all parties. One of the major hurdles to the use of negotiation is the belief that negotiation is used only for collective bargaining. However, with their national best seller, *Getting to Yes,* Fisher and Ury (1983) helped to dismiss this belief and bring daily negotiation to the forefront in conflict resolution, and into the daily professional and home life of individuals and groups. Although every negotiation is different, the basic principles are consistent. Once the skill is learned, the daily negotiation process becomes easier with experience (Fisher et al., 1991).

HOW TO NEGOTIATE?

The actual "how to" of negotiation consists of two interrelated components: negotiating style and negotiating process.

STYLE

A negotiating style constitutes a method or manner of approach. The traditional negotiating style is well known and described by Fisher, Ury, and Patton (1991) as *"hard" positional negotiation.* This style is characterized in collective bargaining by the process in which each party takes a position on certain issues. There is generally a contest of wills where each side, through sheer power, attempts to change the position of the other party. Hard negotiation tends to strain relationships and may even destroy them during the bargaining process.

An alternative to "hard" positional bargaining is a style referred to as *"soft" bargaining* (Fisher et al., 1991). In this style, positions are still taken, but there is emphasis on being friendly, trusting the other side, making offers and concessions, and avoiding confrontation. Although this style emphasizes the building and maintaining of relationships, it often falls short of providing the best outcome for all parties.

A third negotiation style (Fisher et al., 1991) is that of *principled bargaining*. The five elements in this style are as follows:

- Separate the people from the problem.
- Focus on interests of the parties, not on positions.
- Establish precise goals at the start of negotiations.
- Work together to create options satisfactory to both parties.
- Negotiate successfully with opponents who are more powerful, refuse to play by the rules, or resort to "dirty tricks."

This style is based on a collaborative process that looks beyond the problem, focusing on interests and mutual gains. The situation of concern becomes depersonalized and energies are focused on issues rather than on defending positions. Because this style emphasizes the need to maintain on-going relationships and promotes trust and collaborative decision-making, principled bargaining is generally the style of choice for nurse managers.

PROCESS

Just as the foundation provides overall support for a house, principles are the base for all negotiation activities, whether they involve individuals or groups. In the literature on negotiation (Fisher et al., 1991; Jones, 1993; Roberts & Krouse, 1988; Smeltzer, 1991; Snyder-Halpern & Cannon, 1993), at least eleven key principles have been identified:

- Focus on the problem and not the individual or the individual's behaviour.
- Build rapport and maintain communication.
- Build trust.
- Explore interests and gather information.
- Maintain an "open mind" by searching for creative options (techniques such as brainstorming or the Delphi strategy may assist in this process).
- Focus on issues rather than taking positions. Once a position is taken, there is a tendency to defend the position rather than explore the underlying reason for a problem.
- Use facts and objective standards to shape solutions.
- Be aware of your own values and motives and attempt to understand the perspective of the other person/people.
- Emphasize mutual benefits versus forming options in terms of costs.
- Avoid "blaming" words, such as "you are late, as usual." Blaming tends to result in defensive behaviour.
- Promote co-operation instead of competition.

These principles are inherent in each of the four phases of the negotiation process: analyze, plan, negotiate, follow-up.

Phase 1: Analysis

Before initiating negotiation activities, it is imperative that the nurse manager analyze the context of the situation or problem. A thorough analysis will enhance the possibility of achieving a successful outcome in the shortest period of time. Six major components that should be considered in the analysis include:

1. *Delineation of the problem or issue.* This can be facilitated by separating personal characteristics and behaviour from the issues and identifying all factors contributing directly or indirectly to the problem.
2. *Identification of the individuals involved in the situation.* Who is directly involved and who are the other stakeholders? This information helps to ensure that the right people are involved in negotiation and that stakeholders are kept informed.
3. *Determination of personal factors that may affect the process.* As trust is a major component in the success of negotiation (Fisher et al., 1991), the nurse manager needs to determine the previous working relationships of the parties involved.
4. *Identification of the power distribution of both parties.* Power is of major consideration in any negotiation because an unequal balance of power may set up a win-lose outcome. One of the key principles in daily negotiation is to strive for collaborative decisions and to maintain relationships. Win-lose situations do not generally facilitate these outcomes.
5. *Collection of all necessary information.* The negotiation will be enhanced if all information is compiled in advance.
6. *Identification of the environment where negotiation will occur.* An individual's or group's power is thought to be enhanced when negotiation occurs in their territories. Selecting a neutral location will eliminate this possibility.

The determination of power distribution (Component 4) is essential to the analysis phase. One way to determine the power distribution of parties is known as BATNA (Best Alternative To Negotiated Agreement) and has been described by Fisher, Ury, and Patton (1991) and Keeney and Raiffa (1991). Simply stated, BATNA is a cut-off point; below that point there is no agreement and above it there is agreement (Keeney & Raiffa, 1991). Negotiating power related to BATNA depends primarily upon how attractive the option of *not* reaching agreement is to each party (Fisher et al., 1991).

Consider the situation where the nurse manager and a staff nurse are negotiating the nurse's request for a leave of absence when there is a shortage of qualified nurses. In this scenario, the nurse manager's BATNA is high and the staff member's is low. The alternative to a negotiated agreement is less critical to the nurse manager than it is to the staff member. However, the nurse manager who is aware of this unequal power distribution and who wishes to avoid a win-lose solution will need to approach this negotiation so that the outcome is not solely attributed to the manager's power.

Those who take the time to identify their own BATNA and to determine the BATNA of the other side are better prepared for negotiation. In situations of low BATNA, the nurse manager should make every effort to develop greater negotiating power. Developing BATNA may be accomplished through the exploration and refinement of other options than a negotiated agreement (Fisher & Ury, 1983).

Phase 2: Plan

During the planning phase, both parties determine a proposed course of action for negotiation. There may be joint discussions to determine meeting times and to arrive at a decision regarding the general approach to negotiation. In addition, individuals will plan their specific strategy and style based on the completed analysis of the problem. It would be foolhardy to attempt to negotiate an important objective without a well thought-out plan and some ideas about the negotiating techniques to employ.

Phase 3: Negotiation

In Phase 3, the actions of negotiation are implemented. In any negotiation, some techniques enhance the process and some inhibit it. The nurse manager needs to optimize enhancing techniques and minimize or eliminate restrictive techniques.

Techniques constructive to negotiation include:

- Open communication. This technique encourages participation by all involved in the process and allows for an interchange of ideas.
- Focus on the task or situation. This technique promotes communication and collaboration while minimizing power struggles. An environment of trust is likely to develop, which in turn facilitates more open discussion of options to resolve the problem at hand.
- Mutual responsibility. Communication that requires people to exchange ideas reinforces the belief that the participants can attain resolutions. Mutual responsibility is enhanced by focusing on the benefits of proposed solutions rather than emphasizing the costs.

Techniques that impede negotiation include:

- Divide and conquer. This tactic discourages group problem-solving and curtails open communication.
- Suppression. Pretending differences do not exist does little to promote collaborative decision-making or trust.
- Majority rule. Setting up competition for votes does not generally enhance successful resolution of differences.

- Blaming the other party or implying that the participants lack objectivity and rationality.
- Withdrawing before resolution is achieved.

In addition to these techniques, there is a range of tactics inherent in the negotiating process. Tactics are behaviours that can be used individually or in combination to influence negotiation. They may be used by either party. The advantages and disadvantages of each tactic need to be considered carefully before it is used so as not to compromise the negotiation process. Table 27.1 provides a list of some common negotiation tactics compiled from various sources in the literature (Cohen, 1982; Dolan, 1988; Fisher & Ury, 1983; Snyder-Halpern & Cannon, 1993).

Throughout Phase 3, there should be an exhaustive search for solutions or alternatives. The ultimate goal is to reach an agreement that satisfies those involved while also maintaining interpersonal relationships.

Phase 4: Follow-up

Once agreement has been reached, the final phase involves a process of evaluation to ensure successful resolution of the problem. The uniqueness of each negotiation process means that follow-up needs to be tailored to the specific situation. In this phase, there is a need to ensure that the plan of action successfully addresses the problem and that no further intervention is required.

WHAT TO NEGOTIATE?

Day-to-day negotiation can be used in any situation where two or more individuals need to reach an agreement on a particular issue. The negotiation process may be informal, such as in a discussion to change the uniform style worn on a particular unit, or the content of an orientation program to ICU, or the topics of a six-month inservice program. A more formal style in daily negotiation may be required in situations such as a grievance meeting or when the nurse manager needs to attain an increased operating budget for the unit or for capital equipment that was not included in the annual budget.

Regardless of the situation, the negotiating process described in this chapter provides a guide to help maximize the chance of a collaborative outcome and maintain the integrity of relationships. Although the steps are consistent, the formality and intensity of the negotiation meeting will vary with the situation.

SUMMARY

- Negotiating has become a basic survival skill for contemporary nursing and health-care managers.

Table 27.1

NEGOTIATING TACTICS AND THEIR USES

Tactic	Rationale for Use
Silence	Encourages the other party to continue to talk, thus revealing more information to you.
Answers that don't answer	Used to "buy" time or to subtly evade the need to answer a question directly.
Good guy/bad guy	Used to attain a specific result; there is a staged quarrel between two members on the same side, where one member takes a tough stand and the other appears to do a favour to other side by intervening.
Limited authority	A means of avoiding agreement by indicating that others with greater authority need to be involved in the solution.
Dumb may be smart	Used to buy time or to have the other side further articulate its perspective/concerns. Involves role playing and appearing not to understand the other party's point.
Nibbling	A means of getting more by breaking a large request into small parts so that it is easier to sell to the other side.
Package deal	Used to achieve concessions by grouping items together in a single offer.
Deadlines	A way to force the other party to make a decision by a designated time.
Trial balloon	Used to generate feedback by suggesting a position or idea without expressing commitment to the idea. Usually prefaced with a question such as "What if . . .?"
Change of pace	A means to postpone the need for a decision or to give the impression of a need to escalate the process.
Extreme demands	An attempt to eventually attain what is *really* wanted by beginning with options that are known to be extreme.

- Negotiating is an interactive skill for resolving conflict or making joint decisions. It can be used in any setting, with individuals or groups, and as an approach to personal or professional problem-solving.
- Negotiating, as used in collective bargaining, may result in the use of formal dispute resolution procedures; day-to-day negotiating is more likely to employ informal or alternative dispute resolution processes.
- The negotiation process has four phases, and involves principles, strategies, and tactics.

- Principled bargaining will be preferred by nurse managers because it emphasizes maintenance of relationships, promotion of trust, and collaborative decision-making.

REFERENCES

Barton, A. (1991). Conflict resolution by nurse managers. *Nursing Management, 22*(5), 83–86.

Biggerstaff, R. P., & Syre, T. R. (1991). The dynamics of hospital leadership. *Hospital Topics, 69*(1), 36–39.

Citron, D. (1981). Facing up to conflict. *Nursing Life, 1*(1), 47–49.

Cohen, H. (1982). *You can negotiate anything.* New York: Bantam Books.

Collyer, M. E. (1989). Resolving conflicts: Leadership style sets the strategy. *Nursing Management, 20*(9), 77–80.

Dolan, J. (1988). *Negotiating skills for attorneys: Workbook.* Boulder, CO: Career Track Inc.

Fisher, R., & Ury, W. (1983). *Getting to yes: Negotiating agreement without giving in.* New York: Penguin Books.

Fisher, R., Ury, W., & Patton, B. (1991). *Getting to yes: Negotiating agreement without giving in* (2nd ed). New York: Penguin Books.

Grant, A. (1995). Alternative dispute resolution, *Canadian Nurse, 91*(7), 53–54.

Jones, K. (1993). Confrontation: Methods and skills. *Nursing Management, 24*(5), 68–70.

Keeney, R. L., & Raiffa, H. (1991). Structuring and analysing values for multiple-issue negotiation. In H. P. Young (Ed.), *Negotiation analysis,* (pp. 131–152). Ann Arbor, MI: University of Michigan Press.

Kouzes, J. M., & Posner, B. Z. (1987). *The leadership challenge.* San Francisco: Jossey-Bass.

Marriner, A. (1982). Managing conflict: Comparing strategies and their use. *Nursing Management, 13*(6), 29–31.

Roberts, S. J., & Krouse, H. J. (1988). Enhancing self care through active negotiation. *Nurse Practitioner, 13*(8), 44–52.

Smeltzer, C. H. (1991). The art of negotiation an everyday experience. *Journal of Nursing Administration, 21*(7/8), 26–30.

Snyder-Halpern, R., & Cannon, M. E. (1993). A framework for the development of nurse manager negotiation skills. *Journal of Nursing Staff Development, 9*(1), 14–19.

CASE STUDY

At a small rural hospital, registered nurses and the two general practitioners with admitting privileges have been in a dispute over the on-call system at night. If the nurses need to consult a physician during the night, they often do not know whom to call. The workload of these doctors has become much heavier lately since one of their medical colleagues moved to the United States. Although the doctors cover for each other, they sometimes forget to inform the hospital of their whereabouts. The nurses may get an answering machine when they telephone the physicians' offices. Patients have started telephoning the hospital for medical advice at night when they are unable to contact their doctors.

The nurses' local union president has complained several times to the patient care co-ordinator about this situation. This management nurse has not been able to convince the doctors to set up a more systematic on-call roster. The doctors keep saying the nurses are worrying unnecessarily, and that if there is a problem, they can be sure of the doctors' support. However, the nurses have raised the issue with their professional responsibility committee in the expectation that the administrator, who usually attends these monthly meetings, will be able to prevail on the doctors.

One night, a man is brought into emergency with multiple injuries, and the nurse, unable to get hold of either physician, must make the decision to send the ambulance to the nearest city health centre, about 85 kilometres away. According to hospital policy, inter-hospital transfers by ambulance require physician authorization.

Two weeks later, the administrator schedules a meeting with both doctors, the patient-care co-ordinator, and a representative of the nursing staff (*not* the union president because the doctors have refused to meet with her). The two nurses decide to meet and plan their strategy in advance.

1. What should the nurses' BATNA be?
2. What do you expect the doctors' BATNA to be?
3. Assess the relative power of the stakeholders attending this meeting.
4. What role(s) do you expect the administrator to assume?
5. What strategies should the nurses use to foster a more collaborative relationship with the doctors?
6. If the doctors are not willing to negotiate seriously, are there any alternative approaches to the nurses' problem?

Chapter 28

▼▼▼▼▼▼▼▼▼▼▼▼▼▼▼▼▼▼

Issues in Managerial Communication

Donna Lynn Smith

KEY OBJECTIVES

In this chapter, you will learn:

- The nature and variety of communications activities that are expected of leaders and managers.
- How basic skills in interpersonal communication are the basis for developing specialized skills for managerial communication.
- Why good manners and common sense are important fundamentals of successful managerial communication.
- The importance of choosing the best medium of communication in a particular situation.
- The importance of interviewing skills as a basis for fact finding, problem solving, performance coaching, and career development, and some approaches managers can take to planning and conducting various kinds of interviews.
- Factors to consider when communicating with groups, colleagues, and people at senior levels of management.
- The importance of confidentiality, security, and awareness of legal issues regarding certain types of managerial communication.
- Some approaches that can be used when there is a need to communicate bad news or dissenting opinions.

INTRODUCTION

The ability to communicate effectively and to get along well with others are prerequisites for professional advancement in most work settings. As organizations of all kinds strive to improve their performance, and trends and gimmicks come and go, the importance of interpersonal skills and effective communications remains a constant theme. Leaders and managers, in particular, must be skilled communicators because the examples they set and the messages they convey have such an important impact on whether or not the organization is able to achieve its mission and goals.

When people in the community approach the health system as patients or clients, they and their families have a reasonable expectation that they will be listened to and respected. Legislation to protect human rights, to provide for the development and implementation of advanced directives, to protect persons in care, and to govern the relationships between employers and employees, all depend upon respectful and skillful communication to achieve their objectives. Through example and by helping their staff develop awareness and skills, leaders set the tone for courteous and dignified communication with members of the community.

Managers must use their communication skills to develop constructive and productive relationships with colleagues and workers. The ability to communicate well may be necessary to gain support for a course of action; to motivate, encourage, persuade, or to give recognition; to gather facts and opinions; to provide coaching or enact discipline; to negotiate; to assist in resolving conflict; or to convey information, sometimes of an unpleasant nature.

The purpose of this chapter is to focus upon some issues and skills of particular importance in communication by first-line or middle managers, and to offer suggestions to assist current and prospective nurse managers in accomplishing their professional and personal goals. The approach will be practical, rather than theoretical. Some basic rules prevail in most situations, but what may be an appropriate style and approach to communication in one organization, or at a particular time, may not be appropriate in another. Because of this, readers are encouraged to weigh the advice given in this chapter against the advice and example of leaders and mentors in their own organizational circumstances.

WHAT IS UNIQUE ABOUT MANAGERIAL COMMUNICATION?

Nurses have an opportunity to excel in the interpersonal aspects of management. Since the late 1960s, most basic nursing programs have placed significant emphasis on the development of interpersonal skills, and an understanding of factors that can improve or inhibit effective communication. Being able to convey respect for others, to listen effectively, to convey empathy, to offer support, to facilitate or participate constructively in problem solving, and to be sincere and genuine are of obvious importance in relationships with clients. They are also important in collegial relationships, and the ability to get along well with others is usually a prerequisite for professional advancement.

As a starting point for this chapter, it has been assumed that current or aspiring nurse managers already possess basic communications skills, and recognize the need to conscientiously use and improve upon them. However, skills that were originally developed for the purpose of establishing relationships with clients, their families, co-workers, and supervisors, will need to be refocused for the many different types and directions of communication that are at the heart of managerial roles. Managers continue to be required to communicate with clients and their families—when, for example, they monitor the quality of care, follow up on concerns or complaints, or assist in solving problems—and in these situations, they must be concerned about representing the organization to the public in a positive manner. In addition, managers are required to communicate with staff. Such communication may occur one on one or in small-group settings, for purposes of conflict resolution or performance coaching, for example, or it may take place in larger groups. With employees, managers also face such challenges as motivational communication regarding the mission, values, and current directions of the organization.

Nurse managers deal with and must help to resolve many types of problems. While the professional dimensions of their roles mean that they continue to be concerned about clinical problems and issues, the corporate aspects of their positions require an additional focus on the well-being of the unit or program as a whole and as a part of the total organization. Some problems are dealt with through direct personal intervention. In other instances, the best approach involves developing and empowering members of the work team so that they can prevent problems from arising, or can accept personal responsibility for finding solutions.

As the spokesperson for professional and organizational values, the manager must accept responsibility for defining problems and developing solutions. The manager must often weigh staff concerns and requests against the needs and wishes of clients. For example, if the nurses on an inpatient unit have been taking turns leaving fifteen minutes early on the evening shift, or going to coffee in friendship groups that leave the unit understaffed for periods of time, the manager will need to frame this as a problem and deal with it, in order to avoid a situation in which the unit does not have enough staff to respond appropriately to a clinical emergency. In a community health clinic, traditional working hours of 0800 to 1630 hours may be preferred by staff, but to better meet the needs of working families who need services at other times, the manager may be required to communicate the need and reasons for making a change to more "user-friendly" hours. Often it is possible to facilitate a solution that meets the needs of both clients and staff. However, in a situation where this cannot be achieved, the manager must make and communicate decisions that place the needs of clients first. In some cases, it will be necessary to obtain support from a supervisor or "champion" at a higher organizational level to achieve a solution.

PROFESSIONAL BOUNDARIES

It can be helpful to see the differences between therapeutic and managerial communications in terms of the boundaries of the various interpersonal relationships that managers must establish and maintain. Professional boundaries in clinical relationships have been defined as separating therapeutic behaviour from any other behaviour which, well-intentioned or not, could lessen the benefit of care to patients, clients, families, and communities (AARN, 1997). The relationships that exist between managers and the people they supervise share many elements with therapeutic relationships. In clinical roles, nurses are concerned primarily with managing the boundaries of their relationships with clients and colleagues appropriately. In addition to these concerns, managers must be concerned about maintaining appropriate boundaries in their relationships with staff, and with their own supervisors.

Sometimes managers fail to provide leadership or to make decisions that might be unpopular because they are eager to be accepted and liked by staff, or because they want to use a participative management style and feel that in doing so they should not take decisive action. However, these individuals must accept the fact that not only do they hold significant power to influence the well-being of clients, they also affect the degree of job satisfaction, the potential for career development, and even the livelihoods of those under their supervision.

In most organizations, policies stipulate that an individual cannot have a direct reporting relationship to his or her spouse; however, close friendships or other types of intimate relationships can also make it difficult for the manager to maintain an appearance of fairness towards all staff, or to provide objective performance ratings and recommendations that can affect career-development opportunities. To achieve credibility and be effective as a manager it is important to develop insight into one's own emotional needs and to recognize the boundaries that distinguish therapeutic, collegial, supervisory, and reporting relationships from close personal relationships. Boundary considerations also apply in mentoring relationships.

A mature and appropriate recognition of boundaries does not require that the manager be aloof, distant, or lacking in spontaneity. The ability of a manager to express warmth, sincerity, and humour, and to respect the individual qualities of others, is important in the creation of a climate where groups or units work productively and their members support one another. It has been suggested (Burns, 1953) that a joke is a shortcut to consensus in all societies. Leaders who have a sense of humour are appreciated by staff and can help themselves and others to manage stressful situations better. Respecting boundaries can help managers avoid the appearance of favouritism, or the pitfalls of judgement that close emotional bonds can sometimes create, but it need not prevent the development of reciprocal relationships of respect and fondness among managers and those who work with them.

GOOD MANNERS AND COMMON SENSE: FUNDAMENTALS OF EFFECTIVE MANAGERIAL COMMUNICATION

Sensitivity, courtesy, and discretion are the ingredients of good manners. These qualities are also fundamental to effective managerial communication and performance. As recently as the 1960s, the professional socialization of most nurses included instruction in manners, deportment, and dress. These factors are now considered matters of personal choice; nevertheless, social conformity has been shown to be an important factor in promotion to, and success in, managerial positions. Loyalty, the ability to accept authority, and the capacity to conform to a prescribed pattern of behaviour were identified by earlier writers as critical success factors for managers. In her classic study, *Men and Women of the Corporation*, Kanter (1977) points out that conformity pressures arise from the uncertainty surrounding managerial positions. When there is uncertainty and decisions must be made, personal discretion and being able to count on the loyalty of colleagues is very important:

> Discretion raises not technical, but human, social, and even communal questions: trust, and its origins in loyalty, commitment, and mutual understanding based on shared values. If conditions of uncertainty mean that people have to be relied on, then people fall back on the social bases for trust. (p. 49)

Trust is built in part on shared organizational experience, but in the past it was often also based on such factors as shared cultural and social backgrounds. In today's less homogeneous workplaces, where a variety of backgrounds and cultural perspectives may be represented, managers may need to encourage the use of empathy, respect, and cultural sensitivity in order to build trust.

Organizational cultures differ, and it is also important to be sensitive to the unique traditions and styles of particular organizations as they are communicated through formal corporate image-building, informal story-telling, and by successful role models. Newly appointed managers are wise to seek advice or coaching before they participate in important meetings, make presentations, initiate external or upward communications, or attend work-related social events. In a book addressed to aspiring executives, an industrial psychologist (Alihan, 1970) covered a range of topics including manners, relationships with clerical staff, receiving guests, conducting and participating in meetings, verbal and written communication, appearance, travel, and social functions. The following advice on courtesy is repeated here because it is of continuing relevance in many organizational settings:

> Courtesy under all circumstances, even when the tension seems unendurable, should be the young executive's number one guideline. This does not mean that he [sic] has to be servile or fawning. Far from it. It is simply that he must keep his resentments on a leash, his temper under control, and show a willingness to work hard and do his level-best at whatever his superior assigns to him without stepping out of line. (pp. 9–10)

Readers may be inclined to disagree with this advice on the grounds that the behaviour recommended might inhibit a free exchange of ideas or discourage the acceptance of individual moral responsibility among members of the management team. This is a legitimate concern that is is dealt with briefly in another section of the chapter. The point here is that within all organizations, managers are judged not only in terms of individual ability and performance, but by their ability to contribute to organizational goals and team performance. Viewed from the perspective of a senior manager, the type of courtesy described above contributes to economy of effort by enabling organizational activities and relationships to operate smoothly and predictably. Good manners and common sense are basic, and it is widely recognized that no amount of specialized knowledge or skill can compensate, in the long term, for deficiencies in these fundamental areas.

THE MEDIUM OF COMMUNICATION

Communication takes many forms and occurs on various levels. For example, values are best communicated through leadership behaviour, which includes written communication as well as many other types of interaction. Procedural instructions that need to be followed by many people are best communicated in writing. It is widely accepted that rewards and punishment are most effective when they occur in close proximity to behaviour, so recognition of work well-done or feedback about mistakes are most effective if communicated verbally and immediately. A well-known book entitled *The One-Minute Manager* (Blanchard & Johnson, 1982) is devoted to helping managers develop effective skills in providing such instant feedback. In each instance, the nature of a particular communication and the audience to be addressed should lead the manager to a carefully considered choice from among the many communications media available.

LEADERSHIP BEHAVIOUR

The most powerful form of managerial communication is the manager's own behaviour. As in therapeutic communication, the use of self is a valuable and important means of sending and receiving complex messages. For example, the manager's behaviour can either reinforce or discourage certain behaviours of colleagues and staff. If a manager spends more time on the concerns of "whiners" than attending to "star performers," a powerful message is being communicated. If all employees are treated similarly regardless of obvious performance differences, the "value" of mediocrity is communicated. By ignoring or tolerating instances of unkindness towards clients or colleagues, the manager communicates a lack of conviction about the values of respect for the dignity and rights of others. By failing to be accountable for reinforcing professional and corporate values, the manager abdicates leadership responsibility and demonstrates a lack of competence and confidence in the leadership role.

Body language can be more powerful than words in the communication process, particularly when this body language is not congruent with what is being said. For example, verbal expressions of concern or appreciation that are not accompanied by eye contact are likely to be experienced as empty or insincere. The strongest advocates of total quality management acknowledge that when leadership practices are not congruent with the values espoused in such programs, the programs themselves and their underlying values are likely to be perceived by employees as superficial "slogan-chanting." The phrase "walking the talk" is sometimes used to emphasize the need for leaders to match their words and actions to the values that they and the organization espouse.

INTERVIEWS

Interviews are a form of communication that managers use frequently. Many interviews are conducted for the purpose of information sharing. Unlike therapeutic interviews in which the purpose is to help clients identify and work through personal concerns and problems, information-sharing interviews conducted by managers are usually briefer and more content-focused (Northhouse & Northhouse, 1992).

Interviews conducted for the purpose of performance coaching or evaluation are a type of information-sharing interview that is a particular responsibility of managers. This type of interview has been discussed in Chapter 20 of this book.

Information-sharing interviews are also conducted for the purposes of fact finding. For example, the manager may have received a complaint from a client, a family member, or a staff member. Even if the problem has already been communicated in writing, it is usually wise to arrange for a private meeting in which to discuss it. Meetings with more than one person may have to be held in succession to obtain different perspectives and identify the differences in perceptions among various parties who might be involved, or have information to contribute. Inadequate fact finding can lead to premature or incorrect conclusions and actions. The consequences of poorly researched decisions are often costly in terms of time, relationships, and in more extreme instances, legal fees.

In other instances, an interview with one or more persons may need to be held to explore alternatives that could be considered in order to solve a problem. Often in an interview of this sort, the manager makes it clear at the outset that the purpose is to explore alternatives, but not necessarily to arrive at a decision. By making it clear that decision-making is a later, separate phase, it is sometimes possible to facilitate a freer and broader exchange of opinions and ideas. "Testing the water" in this way can help the manager understand what sort of decision or solution will be most appropriate and acceptable.

An interview may also be held to communicate a decision to one or more people. In this instance, the manager may do more talking than listening: firstly, describing the purpose for the meeting; secondly, communicating the decision; and finally, asking for and answering questions that explain it. The decision may not be a popular one and quite often in a meeting of this nature, efforts are made by the other party to debate, or change, the decision. This may not be possible, or even if it is, some further thought and consultation may be required. Therefore, in such an instance, the manager will usually choose to listen respectfully, indicate that he or she has understood the point, and then bring the interview to a conclusion with a promise to discuss the matter further, or to communicate a decision at another time. "Buying time" in this way provides the manager with an opportunity to obtain advice from a supervisor, a human resources consultant, or other experts, and to carefully consider the consequences of making one decision over another without the pressure and hazards of making and communicating a decision on the spot.

As these examples show, it is important for the manager to plan carefully for all interviews and meetings. The selection of time and place can be very important. For example, if it is likely that a staff member will be angered or upset with the information that is to be communicated, it may be wise to schedule such an interview at the end of the working day. If clients or their family members are asked about their satisfaction with care in a public area where their comments can be overheard, they may not feel free to give complete or honest information, particularly if there is any negative content in their message. If insufficient time has been scheduled, and important information is being shared by the other party, an interruption at an inopportune time may have negative consequences.

Interviews in which unpopular decisions or information will be communicated should be scheduled for a specific length of time, and the possible need for back-up support for the manager (e.g., from human resources, or even security) should be considered when the time is established. Occasionally, in such a situation the other party may become angry and abusive. No matter how acrimonious the other party in the situation becomes, the manager must remain in control of his or her own temper and maintain a courteous and respectful demeanour. This can and should be done, even if it is necessary to show the other person out of the office! Achieving this level of self-control can be difficult, but the nurse manager has the advantage of having learned the skills of non-defensive listening and therapeutic communication with angry or mentally-ill clients. Using these valuable skills in a confrontational situation may help to prevent additional accusations and problems.

All meetings or interviews do not have to end happily, and many do not. By taking the initiative, the manager can briefly summarize and bring a tense or acrimonious meeting to a matter-of-fact and business-like conclusion, leaving the door open for future discussions if appropriate. The manager who does not remain in control of the situation, and his or her own behaviour, risks a loss of credibility in the eyes of staff and colleagues, as well as a loss of self-esteem. Careful planning or even "rehearsing" with the assistance of a trusted colleague can help the manager reduce his or her own anxiety and approach interviews or meetings that are expected to be difficult with a greater sense of calm and confidence.

COMMUNICATING IN GROUPS

Managers must often communicate with groups of people. As a participant in groups convened by others, or as the chair or leader of a group or committee, the manager is called upon to make use of a number of communication skills.

A group meeting should only be convened during working time if there is a valid purpose and framework for its activities. In order to avoid wasting the valuable time of participants, careful planning and organization are necessary. This can be accomplished by using some of the following basic tools and strategies: 1. developing an agenda and a work plan; 2. ensuring that minutes are taken and circulated promptly; 3. ensuring that follow-up actions are recorded and that people know who is to carry them out; and 4. establishing a few concrete goals or outcomes for each meeting so that participants leave with a sense of accomplishment and the work of the group moves forward.

As leader of a program or unit, the manager has the responsibility to be effective in leading the working group. Helpful principles for establishing group or team values are suggested in a publication that the Einstein Consulting Group prepared for the American Hospital Association (Leebov, 1990). These principles are:

1. Respect people's differences.
2. Think positively.
3. Acknowledge co-workers.
4. Listen.
5. Pitch in and help out.
6. Live up to your end of the job.
7. Respect people's time and priorities.
8. Admit your mistakes.
9. Invest in other parts of your life.

If principles such as these are modelled by the leader and presented as norms for the behaviour of a working group, there is some likelihood that the common purpose and mutual accountability that are characteristics of effective teams will begin to develop. Where leadership skills and individual motivation are present, one or more teams can be developed from the baseline of skills in the work group so that, as Kastenbach and Smith (1993) suggest, they will enhance existing structures without replacing them. Communication skills provide the infrastructure for working effectively in groups and teams. Chapter 10 of this book presents more detailed information on this subject.

COLLEGIAL COMMUNICATION

There are many directions and styles of collegial communication. First-line nursing managers communicate downward to those they supervise, and upward to their own supervisors. Many lateral communications are also necessary. These take place between peers in a department or program, and with counterparts in other parts of the organization. Communication between nurse managers and their physician counterparts (that is, department heads or ward chiefs) is now recognized in progressive organizations as lateral and interdependent, with shared responsibility for successful outcomes.

LATERAL COMMUNICATION

The style of communication is determined by a number of factors, including the organizational culture, the objective of the communication, the personalities of the people involved, and the urgency to the matter to be discussed. In general, the purpose of lateral communication is to share information, to develop joint definitions of problems and ownership of responsibility for solutions, to give or obtain support, and to improve procedures for getting work done. Most lateral or collegial communication is informal in nature. Skilled managers keep personal notes of all of the meetings that they attend, including who was present, the main points of discussion, and what follow-up actions are to be taken and by whom.

UPWARD COMMUNICATION

Senior executives have demanding and often unpredictable schedules. The time they have for one-on-one communication with subordinates may be limited, not by choice, but by many competing demands. In many organizations, routine meetings are now looked upon with skepticism as being unaffordable and inefficient. With this in mind, the manager should plan and prepare for all but coincidental meetings with a director or vice president.

Preparation should focus on what needs to be accomplished. Is the purpose of the meeting to obtain endorsement for a proposed course of action, or to verbally report a serious incident and obtain direction about how to proceed? Is there a need to discuss a personal matter? It is helpful to distinguish in one's own mind between urgent and non-urgent matters. If time for discussion is limited, urgent matters should be prioritized, and arrangements may need to be made for another meeting when less pressing issues can be discussed.

Most senior executives routinely deal with incoming mail either early or late in the day. Incoming mail from, or relevant to, the responsibilities of a particular manager is often brought forward by the executive for discussion at the next available opportunity, or it may be answered with a brief comment or instruction. It is often helpful for managers to prepare succinct written background material to precede discussion of a developmental, innovative, or controversial issue. If this material is well-prepared, it can arouse interest, provide new or relevant information, present a rationale, and suggest a course of action. Short memos of this nature can set the scene for more effective use of valuable meeting time between executives and the managers who report to them. They also help to speed the decision process because without such material, the executive's initial response to a verbal request or proposal is often to ask for background information or to suggest that the manager consult with others or gather facts for a future discussion.

Other types of written communication can be less formal but equally considerate of the executive's time. For example, a short memo or an e-mail message could be used to advise the director that a staff member with many years of service is about to retire, and to invite the executive to make a presentation at the employee's farewell gathering.

In general, managers are advised to help their leaders "keep out of trouble" by providing them with important information in a timely fashion. Secretaries and administrative assistants are important allies in the communication process, and can offer assistance in locating and informing executives of urgent matters that arise unexpectedly, or of sensitive issues that may require immediate discussion.

In general, formal or scheduled communication with directors and vice presidents should be business-like, constructive in tone, have a clear purpose, and be as succinct as possible. It is not wise for the manager to assume that the role of the director or vice president is to listen to and sympathize with problems. Proposals, recommendations, or summaries of action taken or in progress are usually more welcome and appropriate.

Managers should expect to take responsibility for management of their own feelings. This may include taking the initiative in seeking professional assistance for personal difficulties, or to correct behaviour that is dysfunctional in the workplace. Clarkson (1992) offers excellent suggestions for overcoming negative communication behaviours that can be detrimental to professional effectiveness and career success.

Managers should also make use of informal opportunities to communicate with, and learn from, executives. These may include volunteering for committee work, task forces, or other special assignments; attending social events; or occasionally stopping by to report a small piece of good news.

CONFIDENTIALITY, SECURITY, AND LEGAL CONSIDERATIONS

Confidentiality and security have always been important issues in managerial communication, and the availability of new technologies has added to the complexities in this area. As recently as the mid-1980s, the major source of efficiency in written communication was use of a Dictaphone to produce tapes for transcription by a secretary into memos, letters, and reports. Now, electronic mail enables communication with individuals or groups by entering a message at one computer terminal to be read electronically at another. Facsimile (fax) transmission has turned telephone communication into a form of written communication. Verbal communication can now take place from a variety of locations via cellular phone, as well as by conventional telephone or face to face.

Although written communication may sometimes reiterate information that has already been conveyed in person, it is important that it be used in instances where a permanent or official record is indicated. In general, managers are well-advised to carefully consider the tone and substance of all their written communications, and to adopt a factual and businesslike approach. Freedom of information and privacy legislation is now being widely implemented and will have the effect of making the written communication generated within health organizations available to wider scrutiny than ever before.

Managers have a responsibility to assure the appropriate content and security of communications originating from their offices. To do this, it is necessary to have a clear understanding with support personnel regarding the general procedures for the office, and to provide more specific direction when needed. Friday (1992) offers advice regarding the type of material that should be protected, and its storage, transmission, and disposal.

Several kinds of material require special treatment. Notes or materials that the manager may want to remain privileged (that is, protected from possible disclosure in a court of law) need to be designated as having been prepared as personal reminders by the manager, or prepared exclusively for discussion with the agency's solicitor. If copies of such material are made, their privileged status will be lost. All materials pertaining to employee performance require special attention in preparation, transmission, and filing. Anecdotal notes and correspondence to employees must be handled according to the advice of the organization's human resource specialists. The existence of more than one personnel file for an employee can lead to serious labour-relations problems. A general principle to follow with regard to all written material is to circulate or distribute it only if directed to do so, and to treat all written material regarding client, legal or human resource matters as confidential.

The legislative framework within which communication takes place is generally designed to prevent harm to individuals. The law prohibits everyone from making written or verbal statements that have the potential to damage someone's reputation. Constitutional rights, human rights, and anti-hate legislation have been enacted to prevent or constrain other types of unacceptable communication. More specifically, provincial health-care legislation protects the confidentiality of client information.

Professionalism and skill in managerial communication require scrupulous distinction between facts and opinion. Managers should endeavour to learn as much as they can about the legal issues relevant to the types of communication for which they are responsible.

COMMUNICATING BAD NEWS

In some respects, the role of a first-line or middle manager is like that of a shock absorber in a vehicle—cushioning impacts from the road below, while functioning as one of many interconnected parts that keep the vehicle moving forward. These days, as health-care organizations experience transformation at unprecedented rates, communicating the purpose of changes and their effects on a unit, program, or individual staff members, is an important, and often difficult, task of first-line or middle managers. In more sophisticated organizations, resources may be developed and specialists made available to assist in this area. In smaller organizations, or after the specialists have made their contribution, the manager is left to reinforce the message and carry out the activities required to implement the organizational initiative.

During times of change, employees typically experience feelings of loss, insecurity, and anxiety. They may have honest intellectual objections to a course of action being taken by the organization. Their expressions of distress and anger may be directed at or through the manager, who is often the organization's most accessible representative. Leadership and communications skills become inseparable in such situations. Initially, the manager must listen non-defensively to staff reactions. However, it may be necessary to calmly communicate and reinforce the pertinent facts and the current reality. If change is occurring rapidly, there will be many unknowns. One of the manager's tasks will be to carry questions and concerns forward from the staff and to obtain and communicate additional information to them promptly as it becomes available.

At times, managers may be privy to more complete information than they are permitted to share. Managers may have participated in development or discussions of the corporate strategy, such as the budget or impending layoffs, but may have been instructed to keep what they know in confidence until an internal or external communications strategy can be implemented. An ethical perspective on lying, and on the dilemmas of concealment and revelation, is discussed in two books by Sissela Bok (1979, 1983). These and similar resources may help managers deal with issues of confidentiality in their work.

Despite uncertainty in changing times, the day-to-day work of the program or unit must continue. The manager must maintain a positive climate and be alert for signs of individual distress, intervening to set limits on extremes of behaviour that could disrupt the environment of care, or cause individual employees to feel harassed or embarrassed. Inexperienced managers should not hesitate to ask for the advice and support they may need in these difficult situations.

COMMUNICATING DISSENTING OPINIONS

While members of the management teams of most organizations are expected to be loyal representatives of corporate values, goals, and strategies, this does not necessarily require abandonment of critical thinking or humanistic values. In healthy and exemplary organizations, diversity is valued and cultivated. When concerted efforts are made to tap the intellectual and moral resources of employees, the result can be greater innovation, adaptability, and improved outcomes for the organization. In such a climate, managers in the "shock-absorber" role may experience greater uncertainty and ambiguity than their counterparts in organizations where supervisory relationships between corporate management and other levels are authoritarian and non-disclosing.

It is important and morally responsible for managers to reflect upon the consequences of the activities they are expected to perform, and to place them in the context of personal and universal values. If moral distress arises, it is important to clarify one's personal objectives and professional obligations before publicly expressing a view that is at odds with the corporate direction. Pronouncements about what is right or wrong, or other confrontational tactics, can lead to unexpected and sometimes harsh consequences, and should not be made on impulse. The skills of principled bargaining discussed by Fisher and Wry (1981) and Wry (1991) may be helpful to managers who want to express dissenting views or to influence decisions and events. In such situations, it is often useful to take some time for personal reflection, and to seek the advice and perspectives of trusted members of one's peer group or a mentor. Betraying confidences or refusing to carry out one's duties can have serious consequences, and the manager should be fully aware of them before considering such action. Sometimes expressing one's feelings or anxieties to a superior can provide an opportunity for receiving needed support or advice. Ultimately, a manager who experiences severe moral distress in the course of carrying out corporate directions will have to consider working in another environment or role.

CONCLUSION

Managers must engage in many communications activities with many different people. Some of these are straightforward, but many are complex. There is seldom a single best way of handling complicated communications challenges. It is important that managers possess a varied repertoire of communications skills, but also that they are able to convey a respectful and sincere interest in the people with whom they must communicate.

There is, however, one principle that should govern all professional communication, and particularly that of managers who are expected to set a positive example for their staff. This is the principle that good manners and courtesy should be present in *all* professional and managerial communication. Abiding by this principle does not require that the manager be insincere, or tentative about discussing problems when the need arises. It simply requires that a business-like, and where appropriate, therapeutic environment is maintained, despite differences of opinion, group tensions, or stressful circumstances. Colleagues appreciate a calm and respectful demeanor in their leaders; they also appreciate a sense of humour and the ability to empathize. Nurses who become managers often have an advantage in the interpersonal aspect of management because their basic professional education places great emphasis on the importance of interpersonal skills.

The world of health care is often fast-paced, and opportunities for lengthy communications with any individual or group are likely to be limited. This can be fortunate, since many complicated interpersonal situations are not likely to be solved during one or two interactions, but may require that a relationship be developed before "work" can be done to solve problems. A manager often feels, after a difficult communication session, that she or he was not effective or could have done better. Fortunately, in most instances there will be other opportunities to communicate with the same person, and it is often possible to develop confidence and improve the chances of success in a subsequent interaction by planning and preparing psychologically in advance.

Managers should expect to engage in reflection and learning throughout their careers. A willingness to seek and act on feedback about everyday communications challenges is one way of doing this. Role models and mentors can be of great assistance to nurse managers who want to become better communicators. There are many continuing-education opportunities and learning resources available to assist in the development of specific skills such as those used in formal negotiations, or in making presentations. For individuals and organizations, the domain of interpersonal communication remains one in which life-long learning is both professionally necessary and personally beneficial.

SUMMARY

- Effective managerial communication builds on the skills nurses learn as part of their basic education. Accepting a management position has the effect of multiplying the number and complexity of interpersonal roles and relationships.
- An awareness of the appropriate boundaries of professional relationships should be reflected in the manager's behaviour.
- Sensitivity, courtesy, and discretion are fundamental to effective managerial communication and performance.
- Organizations have different and sometimes unique cultures. It is important that in their communications, managers are aware and respectful of organizational norms.
- Of all the communications media available, the most powerful is leadership behaviour. Managers must be conscious of the messages they are sending through the choices they make and the way they conduct themselves.
- Managers often communicate with individuals or groups through interviews or meetings. Careful planning can help to ensure that the objectives of interviews or meetings are achieved and that a respectful and business-like atmosphere is maintained even when bad news must be communicated or an adversarial atmosphere exists.

- Organizations increasingly expect managers to communicate horizontally with their peers and colleagues to share information and solve problems. Managers must consciously build and maintain a collegial network within the organization.
- Individuals who hold senior positions in an organization are faced with many competing demands upon their time. To communicate effectively with people in senior positions, the manager must recognize the need to be considerate of the executives' time by accommodating to their schedules, and by being prepared, concise, and purposeful.
- Written communication usually becomes a permanent record, and is sometimes scrutinized by those outside of the organization in legal or labour-relations proceedings, or through the media. Therefore, written communication should always be factual, businesslike and courteous. Managers should consider having an experienced peer or a more senior manager review the material they write before it is circulated, particularly if it has the potential to be controversial.
- Communicating the purposes of organizational changes and their effects is an important and often difficult task of first-line or middle managers. In times of change or stress, the manager must maintain a positive climate through personal example, and by providing structure to the activities of the workgroup.
- Occasionally, a manager may feel uncomfortable about some of the messages she or he is expected to communicate, or about actions being taken by the organization. Betraying confidences or failing to carry out one's duties can have serious consequences and it is wise for a manager to consult with a more experienced colleague or mentor before considering such options.
- Interpersonal communication can be constantly improved upon through reflection and interaction with positive role models. However, managers should also seek continuing education and learning resources to develop some of the specific communications skills that may be required in their work.

FURTHER READINGS AND RESOURCES

Northhouse, P. & Northhouse, L. (1992). *Health communication: Strategies for health professionals.* (2nd ed.) East Norwalk, CT: Appleton and Lange. Health communication is defined in this book as the application of communications concepts and theories to transactions that occur among individuals on health-related issues. A comprehensive summary of communication models and variables is presented and a number of health-care relationships in which communication is significant are discussed. The sections on non-verbal communication, intervening, small-group communication, conflict resolution, and ethics in health communication make this book a valuable resource for managers.

Mintzberg, H. (1975). The manager's job: folklore and fact. *Harvard Business Review.* July-August, 49–61. This well-known article provides insight into the ways that senior managers often work and communicate. An awareness of this information can help newly appointed or junior managers to communicate appropriately and effectively with the executives to whom they report.

REFERENCES

Alberta Association of Registered Nurses (1997). *Professional boundaries: a discussion paper on expectations for nurse-client relationships.* Edmonton, AB: Alberta Association of Registered Nurses.

Alihan, M. (1970). *Corporate etiquette.* New York: Mentor.

Blanchard, K.H., & Johnson, S. (1982). *The one-minute manager.* New York: Berkeley.

Bok, S. (1979). *Lying: Moral choice in public and private life.* New York: Vintage.

Bok, S. (1983). *Secrets: On the ethics of concealment and revelation.* New York: Pantheon.

Burns, T. (1953). Friends, enemies, and the polite fiction. *American Sociological Review,* 18(6), 654–662.

Clarkson, I. (1992). Project the positive. *Canadian Nurse, 88*(9), 28–30.

Fisher, R., & Wry W. (1981). *Getting to yes: Negotiating agreement without giving in.* Boston: Houghton Mifflin.

Friday, R. (1992, October). How to safeguard your company's competitive edge. *Creative Secretary's Letter,* p. 15.

Kanter, R.M. (1977). *Men and women of the corporation.* New York: Basic Books.

Kastenbach, J.R., & Smith, D.K. (1993, March/April). The discipline of teams. *Harvard Business Review,* 111–120.

Leebov, W. (1990). *Positive co-worker relationships in health care.* Chicago: American Hospital Publishing Incorporated.

Northhouse, P. & Northhouse, L. (1992). *Health communication: Strategies for health professionals.* (2nd ed.) East Norwalk, CT: Appleton and Lange.

Wry, W. (1991). *Getting past no: Negotiating with difficult people.* New York: Bantam.

CASE STUDY

Lloy Jones is the care manager of a 40–bed unit in a progressive continuing-care centre. One of the residents on the unit, Mrs. Gerda Schmidt, is severely disabled as a result of a stroke. Gerda, who speaks only German, is unable to move independently, feed herself, or speak more than a few words. Gerda's children live in distant cities, and they have asked a close family friend, Margaret Anderson, to serve as Gerda's legal guardian for health matters. In consultation with Gerda's children and with the assistance of the social-services and pastoral-care departments of the centre, Margaret has arranged for a variety of supplementary services so that Gerda can have assistance with each of her meals, and a level of personal care and hygiene that goes beyond that provided by the centre (which includes, for example, one bath per week). Paid companions or volunteers are scheduled to spend time with Gerda each day, not only to assist her with this personal care, but also to help her to maintain her identity by reading to her, playing classical music for her, and accompanying her to activities.

Margaret has worked out a schedule that explains when these paid companion and volunteers will be present and what they will be doing, and she has posted it on the wall of Gerda's room. She has also posted a diagram showing how Gerda's hair should be arranged, and showing the meaning and pronunciation of several German words that the staff can use to communicate with Gerda.

Margaret has observed that the staff of the unit seem to consistently ignore the schedule and instructions; that they either duplicate the work of the supplementary caregivers, or pay no attention to Gerda at all while the paid companions or volunteers are present. Margaret has also noticed a number of recurring problems with Gerda's care. She is often incorrectly positioned in her chair; she may be put to bed by the staff before the paid companion arrives to feed her the evening meal; her mouth and teeth are frequently dirty, and incontinence pads are not put in a cupboard, but are stacked in plain view on the window sill. Gerda's hair is seldom arranged as shown on the diagram that Margaret has posted, and on some occasions Margaret has heard staff members shouting at Gerda as she approached from the hallway.

Margaret has mentioned her concerns about these problems to the staff members who are on duty, but the problems continue to occur. For several weeks she was hesitant to take her concerns beyond the front-line staff because she fears that retaliation may be directed toward Gerda if the staff become aware that she has complained. However, after many such instances, Margaret finally telephones Lloy Jones to arrange a meeting to discuss the co-ordination of Gerda's care.

1. What should Ms. Jones do to prepare for her meeting with Margaret? What goals and approaches are appropriate for this interview? How will Ms. Jones know if she has been successful in meeting her goals?
2. All of the following people or groups might be considered stakeholders in the situation that has developed. Following her meeting with Margaret, which of the following stakeholders should Ms. Jones interview or consult, and in what order?

   a. Gerda
   b. Registered nurses on the unit where Gerda resides
   c. Other staff of the unit where Gerda resides
   d. Representatives from the social-services and pastoral-care departments
   e. Senior administration of the centre

What goals should Ms. Jones have in mind as she approaches each of these consultations, and what communications skills could she use to achieve them?

3. In her interviews with staff, Lloy Jones detects an attitude of resentment toward Gerda and Margaret. Some staff express the opinion that it "isn't fair" that Gerda should have the attention of volunteers and paid companions when other residents don't have similar levels of support. One registered nurse, an opinion leader among the staff, suggests that Gerda is a "snob" and says that she doesn't blame the nursing aides for not wanting to care for her. What further communication activities will be required, and with whom, to address these attitude problems?

Chapter 29

▼▼▼▼▼▼▼▼▼▼▼▼▼

Writing as a Managerial Tool

JUDITH M. HIBBERD

KEY OBJECTIVES

In this chapter, you will learn:

- The importance of effective writing skills for influencing decisions in health agencies.
- Basic principles of successful business writing.
- Six common types of administrative documents and the general purpose of each.
- Resources and strategies for improving writing skills.

INTRODUCTION

Nurses spend much of their time documenting clinical information, completing forms, and recording data from interviews with patients and professional colleagues. This type of writing is highly structured and repetitive, and often does not require composition of a complete sentence, much less a whole paragraph. In managerial work, nurses may need to prepare many other forms of written communication, including formal letters, memoranda, reports, evaluations, briefs, and proposals. Many of these require considerable planning and different forms of presentation. Some documents written by a manager have legal implications and may end up as evidence in a courtroom or arbitration hearing.

Although they have post-secondary education, many health professionals do not write well and lack the confidence to write an original report. This is also true of managers, many of whom possess more than one university degree, so no one need be ashamed of experiencing difficulty putting ideas down on paper or into a word processor. Effective writing is a complex skill as well as an important managerial tool. A well-written memorandum or report submitted in a timely manner can be a powerful means of influencing policy decisions in health agencies.

Most of the principles of interpersonal communication discussed in the previous chapter by Smith also apply to written communications. However, when views, facts, arguments, and decisions are committed to paper, they become part of the permanent administrative record of a health-care agency. They serve as a paper trail for such events as development of a policy or introduction of change; moreover, a written message is not as susceptible as a verbal message to alteration when it passes from person to person. But if a written document is poorly constructed and the ideas not clearly developed, it may stand as lasting testimony to the writer's lack of skill or carelessness and could ultimately undermine his or her credibility and professional reputation.

The purpose of this chapter is to provide practical advice on writing the most common types of administrative documents. For those fortunate readers who do not suffer from self-doubt or the inability to express themselves in writing, the chapter will serve as a quick reference. For those who find writing difficult and time-consuming, and want to do something about it, the chapter may provide encouragement and tips on how to improve this essential managerial skill. Writing skills *can* be improved and, for many professionals, it becomes an ongoing developmental process of self-assessment, trial, error, and continuous learning. It is interesting to note that some of the best scholars often write multiple drafts of a single journal article, and then obtain several reviews as well as editorial assistance before submitting it for publication.

PRACTICAL GUIDELINES FOR WRITING ADMINISTRATIVE DOCUMENTS

Some general guidelines apply to all types of managerial writing, no matter what the specific type of document. These come under the headings of style, technical aspects, organization, and communications technology.

STYLE

The style of writing in administrative documents tends to be *more* formal than in personal letters and notes, and *less* formal than for term papers or articles published in peer-reviewed journals. The novice manager should review memoranda (or memos), reports, and other documents in the workplace to determine the level of formality generally adopted, because it varies from institution to institution. In fact, much can be learned about the culture of an organization from the standard of writing on display in memos and other communications posted on bulletin boards. For example, the tone of a memorandum and the way in which direction is given may suggest the particular values of the writer and his or her management style; it may even reflect the mood of the writer at the time of writing. When composing a memorandum, managers will think about the impression they wish to leave with the reader, and the extent to which their directives and communications are consistent with the organization's mission and culture.

A fundamental rule in writing is to make the tone sound genuine, and this is done simply by being oneself (Zinsser, 1985). It is possible to write in a formal manner without seeming pretentious or stuffy (Stewart & Kowler, 1991), and if you are someone who sets high personal standards, these will undoubtedly be reflected in your writings and will serve as a model for your staff. Business writing should be direct, simply expressed, and without clutter. Shorter sentences are better than longer ones. Language should be chosen carefully to promote uniform interpretation by your readers. Jargon and rhetoric should be avoided. Emotional undertones such as innuendoes and euphemisms should be rejected.

Zinsser (1985) is highly critical of contemporary business writing, saying that "we are a society strangling in unnecessary words, circular constructions, pompous frills and meaningless jargon" (p. 7). He suggests that every sentence should be stripped to its cleanest components, meaning that words that serve no function should be removed, long words replaced with shorter words, redundancies eliminated, and the active case substituted for the passive. Such plain writing may be difficult to adopt at first, but it is obvious that when giving direction to staff, for example, there is no room for ambiguity. If a communication is unclear and confusing, staff will waste time trying to interpret the message, and may even be misled by it.

The principle of unambiguous writing is especially true when issuing a policy (in which the reader is being told *what* to do) or a procedure (in which the reader is being told *how* to do it). In the case of policy and procedure manuals: "The writer must pay particular attention to the needs of the reader and use every technique available to communicate with accuracy, clarity, brevity so that the material can be readily understood. True sophistication in manual writing lies in expressing complex ideas in a simple manner" (Cryderman, 1996, p. 209). Thus, efficiency and effectiveness will be enhanced if there is clarity in the written rules and directives that guide staff in making routine and non-routine decisions at work.

TECHNICAL ASPECTS

Effective writing cannot be achieved without a good grasp of the basic rules and techniques of communicating in writing. This means that when drafting an administrative document, it is important to observe such things as proper grammar, syntax, spelling, and punctuation. One might expect such rules to be applied automatically in institutional writing, but common errors can often be found in all but the most highly scrutinized documents. Many excellent handbooks on style and grammar are available if you need to review basic elements of grammar, and some are listed at the end of this chapter.

Only a genius can write effectively without some basic tools, such as a dictionary, style manual, and thesaurus of synonyms and antonyms. These resources are standard office equipment for any manager, and have been incorporated into word processing packages. Consult these tools frequently, and keep hard-copy versions within reach of your desk both at work and at home; they will help you avoid embarrassing errors and may help to stimulate some creative writing. Increasingly, one can find resources for improving writing skills on the Internet; for example, direct access to the full version of the Merriam-Webster dictionary is available at the website: http://www.m-w.com/dictionary. Spellchecks on computers, however, are not infallible and they cannot pick up errors such as a wrong date, time, or place of a meeting.

It is sometimes tempting to dictate a letter and ask your secretary to sign it on your behalf. With the ubiquitous use of computers and word processors, managers may draft a dozen letters at home, then hand a disc with the files to a secretary to be formatted, printed, signed, and dispatched. With routine letters, this is a strategy for efficient management of time. However, failure to include your personal signature on non-routine letters that convey significant messages, or on announcements to key people in an organization, may offend the recipients and diminish the impact of the message. Moreover, you should read these important messages over; there may be mistakes, misinterpretations, or just plain bad writing that a secretary has not seen fit (or has not had the courage or ability) to change or improve.

All documents should be dated because institutional memories are short, and time can be wasted trying to establish the chronological order of events for historical records. If a report is lengthy and has undergone many drafts and changes, it may be money well spent to purchase the services of an editor to review consistency of style and format and give the document a finishing touch of quality.

ORGANIZATION

Another important consideration is the format, which may dictate the way your text is laid out on the page, and how ideas and points are organized throughout the document. Standardized formats exist for writing memoranda, letters, and incident reports and other short reports; most hospitals, nursing homes, and community health agencies use printed letterhead and printed forms for these communications. Non-routine reports and proposals are not generally as structured, so creativity and imagination will be needed to help you decide how to organize ideas and recommendations in these less standardized forms of writing.

Today, a variety of software programs allow the attractive and graphic presentation of ideas. Health-care agencies generally ensure that at least one clerical employee in the organization has the skills needed to handle graphics and produce professional-looking documents without incurring a great deal of expense and effort. Such people can help produce a well-designed title page for a report, discussion paper, or proposal. A professional-looking title page is likely to attract the reader's attention in much the same way that a succinct abstract or executive summary will determine whether the reader will read the full report or not. Such fine-tuning lends credibility to documents, and makes the job of the reader much easier. Even those who do not possess graphics software can produce a report that is neatly typed and well spaced on the page, or even attractively handwritten, if necessary. The overall appearance of any written document is important; it creates a supportive framework for the arguments, ideas, and information contained within the message.

Students often find it difficult to understand the importance of the appearance of their papers, and resist requirements that they produce written assignments in prescribed formats. Many are frustrated by a professor's insistence on the finer details, for example, of the *Publication Manual of the American Psychological Association* (APA) (APA, 1994), particularly when they lose marks for failing to observe rules of format and grammar. According to Harris and McDougall (1958), a grammatical error is a barrier to effective communication because it creates doubt in the reader's mind about the qualifications of the writer to speak as an authority on the subject under discussion. Similarly, they note that:

> A carelessly prepared manuscript creates the same kind of doubt. If the writer has chosen the wrong kind of paper, has failed to provide adequate margins, has not numbered his [sic] pages, or has neglected to place the title of the essay in the appropriate position on the first page, the reader is likely to feel either that the writer is ignorant of what constitutes a well prepared page or that he [or she] is not willing to take the necessary pains. To antagonize the reader at the outset is certainly not going to improve our chances of convincing him [or her] that what we have to say is sound (p. 100).

The final point in this excerpt is particularly true if the reader happens to be a teacher, or worse, an employer you wish to influence or, at least, impress. These days, you would also try to avoid the gender-biased writing demonstrated in the quotation above. Such writing was prevalent in the l950s and earlier, but it is not tolerated today in professional writing. Most reputable handbooks on style contain advice on how to keep your writing free of gender bias (see, for example, APA, l994, pp. 50–52).

COMMUNICATION TECHNOLOGY

There is little doubt that the growth of communications technology has quickened the pace of managerial work. Written information that would have taken days or even weeks to transmit a few years ago now can be obtained within minutes by fax or by e-mail. A letter can be sent instantaneously to hundreds of names on a list server all around the world. Responses to such communications are often immediate. You can also transmit lengthy documents by attaching files to letters, saving reams of paper in the process. Individuals can set up personal websites on the Internet and connect with people they may never meet but with whom they communicate on a daily basis. Groups of managers may be attached to a local area network for communication and exchange of information.

Communications technology has changed work lives—and not always for the better. People have come to expect instant gratification of their need for information. Failure of the technology to fulfil such expectations may create stress in the workplace and seriously affect routine operations. In one business where e-mail was introduced, the sudden and exponential use of it by employees created havoc and became a behavioural nightmare; it had to be banned for the best part of each day (Gwynne & Dickerson, 1997). One can easily become a slave to e-mail. After a few days away from work, managers may find a hundred or more e-mail messages and numerous copies of other people's e-mail awaiting their attention, in addition to the customary pile of items in their in-baskets. Responding to such a deluge of information can be time-consuming; managers may need to establish ways to control the torrent of information before it controls them.

Nevertheless, when used wisely, this technology improves efficiency and saves a great deal of time. For example, when the first edition of this book was written, all manuscripts were sent back and forth by courier or mail, as many contributors did not have access to e-mail. For this second edition, almost all communications and documents were transmitted electronically, with increased convenience and much lower cost.

E-mail messages should be written with the same kind of care as a hard-copy letter or memorandum in all but the most informal of messages. E-mail messages can be printed out and filed for future reference, and can be used by lawyers as evidence for or against a health agency in legal proceedings. Because access to e-mail is so easy and so quick, messages can be fired off rapidly before a person has collected his or her thoughts. This can be particularly devastating if a person writes in anger or frustration. After you hit the send button, the message cannot be retrieved, and the consequences may be regrettable and even harmful to individuals. Great care should be taken in responding to messages that have been sent to multiple e-mail users; an impulsive reply could end up on the monitors of the entire 'cc' (carbon copy) list.

It is a good policy to remain courteous at all times and to proofread e-mail messages before sending them because people expect high standards from professional workers. On the whole, the standard of e-mail writing tends to be informal (some would say lackadaisical); in many cases, the message is so poorly written and difficult to interpret that it would not be worthy of a passing grade for composition in junior high school.

RIGHT TYPE OF DOCUMENT

There are often no guidelines for helping a manager to select an appropriate type of written document, and there seems to be little in the nursing-management literature on forms of writing. How does a manager decide whether an issue or problem can be addressed with a memorandum, a letter, or a report, or whether it can be dealt with simply by a telephone call or an e-mail? Much will depend on the recipient of the written document, the nature of the problem or issue, whether or not the matter is routine, and the ultimate distribution of the document. If the recipient is an individual staff member, and the subject is related to performance, a future career, or a specific assignment, the document is most likely to be a letter. If the recipient is someone who has sent you a letter that requires a response—for example, a request for a reference—then you would certainly reply with a letter. If, on the other hand, the recipient is your entire staff, a memorandum would be the document of choice, especially if its purpose is to make an announcement or to communicate new information.

Routine reports to senior management generally follow a standard organization and may even be submitted on a form specifically designed for the purpose. The manager will have little difficulty deciding what type of document to send in the vast majority of circumstances, because most of the documents are used repeatedly. However, if a manager wishes to propose a major change in programming for clients, staffing, or some other kind of operational activity, a less standardized document will be required. Examples of proposals, discussion papers, and position statements can usually be quickly located by a telephone call to an executive secretary who, in the course of a career, handles dozens of different types of written documents and who can be a mine of information on how they should be written and presented, and what form they should take.

The remainder of this chapter is devoted to describing some of the most common administrative documents encountered by managers, the purposes of these documents, and suggestions on how they may be written to achieve the health agency's goals.

BUSINESS LETTERS

Writing letters is a common task of managers, particularly when the subject matter or the intended recipient is an individual. As an example, staff and former employees may request a letter of recommendation when applying for a job, or when applying for funding for education or research. References are generally written as letters unless, of course, you have been requested to complete a specific form. Disciplinary problems are generally dealt with by letter, with copies to the union (if any) and to the employee's file. A letter would be the document of choice when answering an advertisement for a job, when making complaints about patient services or treatment, or when writing to the editor of a newspaper. In other words, written communications that are sent outside the agency are most likely to be in the form of letters, and, if for no other reason than for good public relations, they should be presentable in appearance and well-written. A "covering" letter almost always accompanies such documents as discussion papers, reports, and briefs.

Business letters follow a standard format, are written on agency letterhead, and consist of the following elements:

- Address and telephone/fax number of sender (usually part of the letter-head).
- Date.
- Recipient's name, title, and address.
- Salutation.
- Text of the letter.
- Complimentary closure.
- Signature (with the sender's name and title, typed).

In addition to these elements, business letters may include a file number, placed under the date, and respondents are expected to quote this when replying. "Enc." placed under the sender's signature indicates that another document was enclosed with the letter, and "cc" followed by a name or names indicates the person or persons who received copies of the letter. Letters written on word processors generally include the name of the file where the letter is stored, in fine print in the bottom left hand corner.

MEMORANDA

Memoranda or memos are documents used exclusively for communicating information, announcements, instructions, policies, and decisions within organizations. They are internal documents and managers are likely to write more of them than any other type of administrative document. A memo is often shorter and less formal than a letter and, because it may be disseminated to a wide audience, it must be accurate, concise and coherent, and focus on only one topic. For example, it would not be helpful to send out a message about an upcoming fire drill in the same memorandum announcing the date of the next accreditation survey; the two events are apt to occur many weeks apart, and memos are often filed by subject matter.

As in the case of letters, there is a universal format for memos. Healthcare agencies often have a printed form, with the name of the hospital or nursing home at the top but without the address, in view of its internal usage. Individual departments may use specially printed memos that indicate the departmental telephone and fax numbers. The elements of any memorandum are as follows:

- Date:
- To:(person, group, or department)
- From:(name and title of sender)
- Subject:(Concise description of subject)
- Message.
- Signature (optional).

The first four elements are grouped together at the top of the page. The subject is given prominence, usually in bold type and underlined, and represents the title of the memo. The message, or body of the memo, consists of an introduction or a statement of the purpose of the memo, a discussion or explanation of the main points, and a conclusion and/or instructions. Figure 29.1 presents an example of a memo.

In no other type of document is it so important to attract and retain the reader's attention than in the first few sentences of a memorandum. The advice of Zinsser (1985) to those writing articles applies equally well to memos. He states that the first sentence is the most important: "If it doesn't induce the reader to proceed to the second sentence, your [memo] is dead. And if the second sentence doesn't induce [the reader] to continue to the third sentence, it's equally dead" (p. 65). Memos should be logically constructed so that each sentence leads directly into the next, "tugging" readers forward until they are safely "hooked" (Zinsser, 1985). In the sample memo in Figure 29.1, the first sentence will undoubtedly catch people's attention as parking problems are some of the most volatile in public organizations.

Unlike letters, memos do not need any form of greeting, salutation, or complimentary closure. Some people like to sign a memo; others will merely place their initials by their names at the top of the page. Memos are similar to letters in that the abbreviations related to enclosures (encs:), copies (cc:), and filing information may also appear at the bottom left hand corner of the page.

Most memos are no longer than a page, but this type of document is flexible and can also be used for short reports, investigations, or even proposals and recommendations. More complex reports from interdisciplinary bodies or task forces require a rather different approach, which will be discussed later.

PROPOSALS

The concept of a written proposal is closely associated with research, but it also applies to projects or even to purchase of a new piece of equipment. As almost any new program or change in process or procedure is likely to have financial implications not encompassed in the current budget, managers should develop the skills required to write a good proposal. Proposals are often the end product of much discussion among staff and managers about a problem or an idea, and may involve a preliminary investigation to collect information, literature review, and survey of similar health agencies.

There is no standard format for proposal writing because much will depend on the nature of the plan, the audience, and the resources required to carry out the project. If research is planned, the proposal must be prepared in the format required by review bodies, namely ethics committees and internal or external funding agencies. Guidelines for preparation of a research proposal may be found in introductory research textbooks, and examples of research proposals can usually be obtained from agency files or from people who have joint appointments with universities.

The details of proposal writing are discussed in relation to project management in Chapter 24, so they will not be repeated here. The main point,

Figure 29.1

EXAMPLE OF MEMORANDUM DIRECTED TO AN ENTIRE HOSPITAL

WESTBRIDGE COMMUNITY HOSPITAL
[Established June 1946]

MEMORANDUM

DATE: July 10, 1998

TO: Board Members, Executive Committee, Department Heads
All employees

FROM: George Middleton, P.Eng.
Director, Physical Plant

RE: **Temporary closure of the hospital parking lot**

The hospital parking lot will be closed for 60 hours from **Monday, July 20, 0700 hours to Wednesday, July 22, 1900 hours 1998.** This will allow us to resurface the lot and add 50 plug-in stalls at the north end. Additional lighting will be installed to address the personal security concerns of staff coming in and out of the hospital after dark.

I am pleased to announce alternative parking arrangements during this disruption. The Ozwiecki family, owners of the shopping centre opposite the hospital and long-term hospital supporters, have very kindly agreed to cordon off the north-west corner of their parking lot for exclusive use of hospital staff, patients, and visitors. Please park within the space designated for our use. I encourage you to use car pools during the day shift for these three days, as the designated shopping centre parking space is smaller than the hospital parking lot. There should be no difficulty finding a place to park on the evening and night shifts. Five temporary parking spaces will be created to the left of the Emergency Department doors for use by the handicapped, allowing them to enter the hospital through the Emergency entrance.

Expenditures for the improvement of the parking lot were approved by the Regional Health Authority as part of the hospital's 1998/1999 capital budget. These temporary parking arrangements have been planned to minimize any inconvenience to staff and the people we serve. I would like to thank you for your co-operation during this important capital-improvement project.

cc: Mr. Marko Ozwiecki

however, is that to obtain approval for innovative ideas, you must mount a good argument. An argument in this sense is not to disagree about something, but "to offer a set of reasons or evidence in support of a conclusion" (Weston, 1992, p. x).

A proposal usually starts with a problem statement, for example: "With the marked increase in clients attending outpatient clinics, the existing waiting room area and washroom facilities are now inadequate." The proposal would include supporting evidence such as figures on clinic attendance to illustrate the problem, and might include client comments about lack of privacy and waiting in line for the washrooms. Several possible solutions would then be suggested, with a specific recommendation. The cost of this specific recommendation (and possibly the comparative costs of other options) would be itemized.

In short, a proposal is a plan for addressing a problem or suggesting an innovative idea, and includes reasons why senior management should support the plan, methods to be used, human and financial resources required, time period required, and implications, strongly stated, for the health agency. Obviously, a proposal is a forward-looking document. If the proposed plan is implemented, there will undoubtedly be progress reports to write, as well as a final report. Unlike proposals, reports are retrospective documents whose intent is to account for events or projects that have already taken place.

WRITTEN REPORTS

There are many kinds of reports, but they all have two things in common: they are based on factual information that has been collected and presented in an organized form, and they supply needed information to the person or institution requesting the report (Stewart & Kowler, 1991). In all cases, the information sought is used as a basis for decision-making. A report is therefore an impartial, objective account of events, activities, or investigations, and may range from something as simple and routine as a narcotic count, to periodic summaries of operations or highly complex, confidential inquiries.

The majority of reports that a first-level manager must write are of a routine nature, and many are written on specially-designed forms, ensuring that there is consistency of reporting and adequacy of information. Facts from this kind of report may be entered into databases for accounting purposes. For example, the manager of an intensive care unit that is required to respond to all codes in the hospital may be required to submit a summary of such occurrences each month. Ultimately, a calculation of the cost per occurrence will assist with future planning of resources for this type of activity. Similarly, a manager may be required to explain variance between actual expenditures and budgeted expenditures from time to time, so total expenditures for a health agency can be closely monitored (refer to Chapter 22 for an example of a variance).

Other routine reports include personnel performance appraisals for which specially-designed forms may be used. Such forms usually do not require the manager to plan or organize the information sought, but merely to provide a mix of short answer and narrative responses to predesigned questions. On the other hand, if a special report is requested on the performance of a staff member who has been in some kind of difficulty, then the manager may have to plan and organize an original document.

Generally speaking, the less routine the report, the fewer the guidelines for writing it. However, most reports contain the following items in this order:

- Title page.
- Executive summary.
- Introduction and background, including review of relevant reports and literature.
- Methods used to collect data, and sources of information.
- Presentation of findings, analysis, and discussion.
- Conclusions and recommendations (these may be separate sections).
- Reference list.
- Appendices (terms of reference or authorization; letters; charts; data sheets; cost implications of various options recommended).

In summary, a report is an account of an investigation, an event, or a problem. Many reports are made verbally, leaving no permanent record, but written reports become part of the archives of an organization. Some are short-lived and soon discarded, while others are kept for years. The nature and scope of the subject and the person or group commissioning the report will determine the formality and detail to be included in the document. Whatever the nature of the subject, all written reports, whether a single page or more than 100 pages, consist of three main elements: an introduction, an investigation and discussion, and conclusions.

The points raised in the following case example show how managers plan and organize a report for which no standard format exists. Because interdisciplinary groups are increasingly involved in planning and decision-making in organizations, the example concerns a report prepared as the result of a task-force project.

CASE EXAMPLE

As a result of regionalization, the gynecology departments of two hospitals have been asked to merge their services on one site, using fewer beds and increasing the capacity for day surgery. Although an external consulting group is often asked to conduct a study in this type of situation, in this case an in-house group has been assembled to do the job. The task force consists of a gynecologist from each hospital, an anaesthetist, senior nurses from each service including the surgical suites, an administrator, and representatives from other disciplines, consumers, and the unions. Senior administration has drawn up the terms of reference for the task force, and named the person to chair the investigation.

The task at hand is somewhat like a feasibility study, and the group meets numerous times at the outset to plan strategy. Members collect a great deal of historical data on each service, such as types of surgical procedures performed, average occupancy rates, lengths of stay, number and categories of staff, outcome measures, budget performance, and a description of the physical plant. Interviews are held with key informants in each service. After analyzing the data, the task force proposes a series of options for, or ways and means of, accomplishing the goal of merging the services, and it must now prepare a report to present its recommendations to senior administration. As there is no paid assistant to write the report, one or two members of the task force agree to draft an outline. Various task-force members read and make comments on the draft, and some work on different sections of the report, but ultimately the finished product is the work of a few key members. Careful planning is essential because in this case, as in most projects, far more information has been collected than can be reported. The authors of the report will need to keep several points in mind.

Their *title* should be succinct and should accurately reflect the nature of the report. The name and monogram of the regional authority and the date of submission should appear on the title page. The names of everyone on the task force and of those who contributed to the writing of the report should be listed, if not on the title page, on the inside of the cover of the report.

The report should begin with an *executive summary,* which is a précis of the whole report, and is usually not longer than a couple of pages. It provides an overview of the salient points in a highly-readable format. Thus, an executive summary consists of the purpose or need for the study, a statement about what was done, the main conclusion, and the principal recommendations. Boards and administrators usually want to know the key points and main recommendations quickly, but they may not have time to examine the body of the report until a later time, or they may delegate detailed review of the report to an assistant. If the executive summary is well-written and clearly presented, there is a greater likelihood that the whole report will be read. Like an abstract in a research article, an executive summary serves as a "commercial" to attract the attention of readers.

The *introduction* should contain a brief contextual overview and history of the project, as well as a clear explanation of the reason the study was necessary. Reference may be made to trends and issues, to indicate that this project is consistent with what is going on elsewhere in the health-care system. A long, rambling introduction will ensure instant boredom, and the reader may then just flip through the report at random, perhaps missing much of the argument underlying the recommendations of the task force.

In this particular case study, the *literature review* may not be reported as a separate section of the report. Reference to current literature on mergers may be included in the introduction to the report as background information. Alternatively, a complete literature review might be included as one of the appendices. For this task force, there may not be many useful books or articles on the subject of merging gynecological services, but there may be unpublished reports from other agencies, and literature on related topics that may stimulate insights and creative thinking about the project. A report will have greater credibility if the authors provide evidence that the literature has been consulted.

The next section of the report should contains a description of *methods used to collect data* and be quite brief. Some questions to consider are: Did information come from records, or from interviews? If from interviews, how many people took part in the survey? How reliable and how valid were the methods used? What is the best way to present quantitative data: in figures, tables, or graphs? Any graphic representations must be appropriately labelled and readily interpreted by people unfamiliar with the material, and then only key points are elaborated upon in the body of the report.

Analysis, presentation, and discussion is an important part of the report because at least some readers will want know how the conclusions were reached. For example, if the task force concludes that merging the two services will not allow enough space for an increase in volume of day surgery, the data must support that conclusion. In other words, conclusions must flow directly from actual findings, not from preconceptions, self-interest, or any other unsubstantiated reason.

The *conclusions* and *recommendations* should be written boldly and without equivocation. These are often preceded by a summary of the project, but if the report started with an executive summary, this information does not need to be repeated at the end of the report.

It is important to be clear about the differences between a summary and conclusions; many a report has a section entitled "conclusion" that is, in fact, a brief reiteration of what has already been said. Conclusions are decisions about the investigation based on an analysis and interpretation of findings. For example, from analysis of the interview data, the task force may have concluded that the gynecologists are satisfied that their incomes will not be affected by a merger of the two departments. A consultant's assessment of the two surgical suites may have led to the conclusion that Hospital A will not be able to accommodate the surgical caseload of a combined gynecological service without major renovations to its operating rooms, and that Hospital B's surgical suite should be permanently closed.

In the same way that conclusions flow from findings, *recommendations* should flow directly from conclusions. As an example, a recommendation might be: "That the surgical suite in Hospital A be expanded by the addition of two new operating rooms." There are often many recommendations contained in a project, and these may include alternative solutions to a single fundamental problem. What are known as "serendipitous findings" may also be included here—some unrelated problem, for example, that simply turned up in the data collection but which the committee felt was important enough to warrant a separate recommendation (e.g., incompatible management practices in the two hospitals might interfere with the smooth merging of the two services).

References are all those published and unpublished documents that have been cited in the report. Alternatively, a *bibliography* may be preferred, as this is a list of all documents that have been used and consulted, whether or not cited in the report.

Finally, the *appendix* or *appendices* (plural) section is a convenient place to put copies of important correspondence, a glossary of terms, photographs, detailed tables that were too cumbersome to place in the body of the text, and the terms of reference or authorization of the task force. It is a good policy to keep appendices to a minimum in the interests of economy, as numerous copies of the report may need to be reproduced and circulated to interested policy makers and administrators.

LITERATURE REVIEW

In the previous section of the chapter, reference was made to reviewing the literature. A literature review is an extensive, thorough, and systematic examination of publications relevant to the project (Seaman, 1987). It should go almost without saying that managers need to subscribe to some key journals so that they can keep up to date with trends and issues in their field. They also need to have access to libraries and databases so they can, from time to time, review literature on various aspects of their work. The rate at which both administrative and clinical changes are occurring requires that managers demonstrate skill in assessing current literature. Moreover, there is a need to review the literature critically, weigh the strengths and weaknesses of research methods, and evaluate the findings of published research. For example, in developing care maps, professional staff need to be aware of the latest approaches to care and treatment of clients in a particular diagnostic category, and one of the first tasks would be to see what is being reported in the professional and research literature.

Literature review is a complex intellectual skill and takes much time to develop. Most undergraduate textbooks on research contain whole chapters on how to review the literature, and examples of literature reviews can be found as an integral part of most research articles, and as complete articles in administrative journals (see, for example, Hall & Donner, 1997). Whether writing a report, a brief, or a discussion paper, a manager's effectiveness in influencing decisions will be enhanced if these documents reflect a careful analysis of recent literature on the topic being addressed.

BRIEF

A brief is quite simply a short, concise report (Zilm, 1998), and may be delivered verbally or in writing. In the political world, one might read in the paper that the minister of some federal department has been "briefed" on latest developments in the portfolio. In this situation, an aide or advisor has

investigated the issue or problem, summarized the information, and identified options open to the minister for his or her public statements. Briefs in
the health-care system are more likely to be written, and due to their nature
are often biased in favour of (or against) a particular position. Indeed, they
may also include a formal position statement on the topic. Briefs are written with the intention of influencing decisions or public policy. To be effective they should be written clearly, persuasively, and succinctly, and they
should stick to the point, avoiding rhetorical digressions. Nurses' professional associations and unions often write briefs to governments to inform
the public-policy process, and to articulate their particular perspectives and
recommendations on a variety of issues affecting either nursing services to
the public or the work of nurses.

A manager may have cause to write a brief either as an individual or in
collaboration with other managers for the purpose of influencing policy decisions in health agencies. With the disappearance of functional departments, a brief can, for example, be a useful way to inform administrators of
the potential impact of organizational decisions on the practice of nursing.
Hence, the brief can be written from a nursing perspective or any other perspective. It must provide supporting evidence to strengthen whatever position is being taken. For instance, if an agency has no policy statement with
respect to physical or verbal abuse from staff and clients, a brief could be
written pointing out the need for such a policy. Evidence of recent abusive
incidents in the agency could be cited, together with information on the
policies that exist in other agencies. Again, reference to trends reported in
the literature on institutional policy advocating zero tolerance of abuse in
health agencies would strengthen the brief.

A brief can be written as a memorandum or as a mini report. Like all
reports, it should have an introduction that includes a clear statement of
purpose, a body of information and argument, conclusions, and recommendations. Unless the subject of a manager's brief is confidential, it can be
circulated among the staff as a means of informing them about the subject
of concern, and of securing their assistance and support.

NOTES TO FILE

The myriad of problems, issues, decisions, and events that managers deal
with on a daily basis places great demands on individual memories. Some
of these decisions and events should not be filed solely in managers' memories, but should also be stored in their paper or electronic files. The selec-
tivity of most memories can lead to disagreements about what was actually
said and what was perceived to have been said over the passage of time.
Should a problem wind up in court or arbitration, evidence drawn from
"notes to file" is likely to be more credible than evidence drawn from memory alone.

Managers can avoid the failure of their memories, besieged as they are
with a great deal of daily minutiae, by dictating or entering a note to the

relevant file. Notes to file are informal, personal records of events, decisions, discussions, or telephone conversations and they are frequently confidential and thus kept in a locked filing cabinet or drawer. A note to file must be made when a manager gives an individual staff member a verbal warning. The date, time, incident involved, what was said, and the staff member's response will all be recorded in such a note, along with plans for future follow-up. Depending on agency policy, such notes to file would also appear in the personnel file in the department of human resources. Similarly, if the manager receives a complaint from a patient or patient's relative, it would be wise to create a file and document the conversation. Thus, a diary of events is created on situations that have potential to become a more significant problem later on. Investing in a "DayTimer" or electronic diary is probably the most efficient means of keeping track of items that require a note to file. Notes to file can be of great assistance in recalling events and a great source of historical data when justifying decisions or writing more formal and public documents.

DISCUSSION PAPERS

In general, managers are more likely to be recipients of discussion papers than authors of them. Such documents can be important and informative, and they may require the manager to formulate a response to the points raised in the discussion. The subject of a discussion paper is most likely to be about an emerging issue or proposed public policy. For example, the Alberta government recently published a discussion paper on how regional health authority membership should be determined; the issue was whether members should be elected or appointed to regional health authorities. The purpose of a discussion paper in this case was to examine the issue from all points of view, without making any specific recommendations or favouring any particular position. Simply stated, the topic was presented in such a way as to stimulate discussion, and the public was invited to respond to the issues raised.

Unlike briefs, discussion papers are often lengthy and do not fall under a clear or universal format. Because the topics addressed are often new, one of the purposes of the paper may be to educate the reader. Hence, the body of the document may be didactic in tone, and careful attention may be given to defining the terms being used. In a recent discussion paper released by the Alberta Association of Registered Nurses (AARN) on professional boundaries (1997), the introduction is devoted entirely to an explanation of what is meant by professional boundaries. In the body of the paper, the nurse-client relationship is examined, using case studies to illustrate many aspects of the issue such as non-professional relationships, recognizing boundary signs, crossing professional boundaries, violations of professional boundaries, ethical implications, solutions, and options. After reading this paper, nurses and their managers should be able to discuss this subject with colleagues and describe professional-boundary problems or concerns. Subsequently, they could be expected to develop the standards that would guide their practice in the work setting.

Because of the novelty of the topic of discussion papers, there are often many attachments or appendices. In the AARN paper mentioned above, a glossary of terms is provided, and this is followed by references, a review of the literature, a summary of what is happening in other jurisdictions, and, finally, a list of various teaching resources.

SUMMARY

The purpose of this chapter is to provide practical advice on writing, and to discuss the most common types of documents managers have need to write, receive, or review. The following are key points to remember:

- Effective writing skills are essential for contemporary managers who spend considerable time documenting events and responding to requests for information.
- Managers who write well are likely to be more effective in influencing health-agency policies.
- Writing is a complex intellectual skill that can be developed with practice and critical self-appraisal.
- Four of the most common administrative documents a manager will write are letters, memoranda, proposals, and reports.

FURTHER READINGS AND RESOURCES

Gage Canadian Dictionary (rev.). (1997). Toronto: Gage Educational Publishing. This dictionary claims to be the only recognized Canadian dictionary, as distinct from British (e.g., Oxford), or American (e.g., Webster). An advantage to using this dictionary is that it gives both Canadian and American forms of spelling for many of its entries, with the version most commonly used in Canada placed first. Thus, if you are confused about which spelling to use, this dictionary will be helpful.

Gage Canadian Thesaurus (1998). Toronto: Gage Educational Publishing. If you know there is a word for what you are thinking about, but you just cannot extract it from your brain, then this sort of book can be helpful. Synonyms and antonyms for every entry are provided, and are invaluable if you have time to do crossword puzzles.

Messenger, W. E., & de Bruyn, J. (1986). *The Canadian writer's handbook* (2nd ed.). Scarborough, ON: Prentice-Hall. Although this reference book is twelve years old, it covers all important elements of correct writing. In it, you will find all that you need to know about the conventions of grammar, punctuation, spelling, usage of language in Canada, and more. This is one of the best examples of a basic guide to the technical aspects of writing.

Roberts, P. D. (1988). *Plain English: A user's guide.* London: Penguin. This book offers a great deal of information on the English language, and the author has a practical style of writing that is interesting yet plain, entertaining, and amply studded with personal observations and experiences. It covers such topics as dialects, and contains an excellent glossary of terms.

Sparks, S. M. (1997). Using the Internet for nursing administration. *Journal of Nursing Administration, 27*(3), 15–20. The author discusses the utility of the Internet for management purposes, and describes electronic mail, file transfer protocol, telnet, Gopher, and World Wide Web protocols. The Internet is a rapidly expanding information resource and managers are advised to develop skills in the use of search tools in order to find the information they need.

Weston, A. (1992). *A rulebook for arguments* (2nd ed.). Indianapolis, IN: Hackett. This little book is an introduction to the art of developing and assessing arguments. Anyone wishing to put forward a convincing position about why something should be done in a health agency, or why money should or should not be spent, will find this an indispensable resource. It offers a series of rules and principles, and deals with such ideas as arguments from authority, cause and effect, deductive arguments, and logical fallacies. It is invaluable for graduate students embarking on a research proposal.

Zilm, G. (1998). *The SMART way: An introduction to writing for nurses.* Toronto: Harcourt Brace. This book is an excellent investment for student nurses. Zilm outlines all you need to know about writing term papers, doing literature reviews, preparing résumés, and much more on how to improve writing skills. The author is a nurse, author, and editor, and has given dozens of workshops on her system. The acronym in the title stands for the five basic elements that affect all communications, whether oral, visual, or written. These are: Source (of communication); Message; Audience; Route; and Tone. Chapter 6 on the various Routes provides a much more comprehensive account of how to select and write the type of documents discussed in this chapter.

REFERENCES

Alberta Association of Registered Nurses. (1997). *Professional boundaries: A discussion paper on expectations for nurse-client relationships.* Edmonton: Author.
American Psychological Association. (1994). *Publication manual of the American Psychological Association* (4th ed.). Washington, DC: American Psychological Association.

Cryderman, P. (1996). Manuals that work: A focus on writing and regionalisation. In S. A. Ziebarth (Ed.), *Pinched: A management guide to the Canadian health care archipelago* (pp. 207–219). Nepean, ON: Pinched Press.

Gwynne, S. C., & Dickerson, J. F. (1997). Lost in the e-mail. *Time, 149* (16), 46–48.

Hall, L. M., & Donner, G. J. (1997). The changing role of hospital nurse managers: A literature review. *Canadian Journal of Nursing Administration, 10* (2), 14–39.

Harris, R. S., & McDougall, R. L. (1958). *The undergraduate essay.* Toronto: University of Toronto Press.

Seaman, C. H. C. (1987). *Research methods: Principles, practice and theory for nursing* (3rd ed.). Norwalk, CT: Appleton & Lange.

Stewart, K. L., & Kowler, M. E. (1991). *Forms of writing: A brief guide and handbook.* Scarborough, ON: Prentice-Hall.

Weston, A. (1992). *A rulebook for arguments* (2nd ed). Indianapolis, IN: Hackett.

Zilm, G. (1998). *The SMART way: An introduction to writing for nurses.* Toronto: Harcourt Brace.

Zinsser, W. (1985). *On writing well: An informed guide to writing nonfiction* (3rd ed.). New York: Harper & Row.

Chapter 30

▼▼▼▼▼▼▼▼▼▼▼▼▼

Career Planning for Leadership Roles

Gail J. Donner and Mary M. Wheeler

KEY OBJECTIVES

In this chapter, you will learn:

- What career planning and development is.
- Why career development is an important part of professional development.
- How nurse managers can use the career-development process to take control of their careers and their futures.

INTRODUCTION

In this a rapidly changing health-care environment there may be considerable anxiety and feelings of uncertainty among health-care providers about the future. Nurses and other health-care workers worry not only about providing quality care, but also about job security and their own marketability. Many nurses are asking themselves: "How can I plan my career?" "How can I remain employable?" "What are my opportunities today, and what will they be in the future?" and "Who can help me?" The majority recognize that they need to take control of their working lives and futures, but often they do not know where or how to begin.

Many factors influence an individual's ability to accept and cope with change, no matter whether the change is planned or unplanned, or whether it results from the employee's initiative or the employer's. These factors include clarity of goals, degree of control over the environment, trust in the initiators of change, good communication, and involvement in the change process.

Bridges (1990) notes that people and organizations go through three stages in the change process. The process begins with a recognition of the ending of the current state, or "what is," followed by a neutral zone that includes a letting go of the past. The third stage is the start of the new state, "what can be," and this is a new beginning. New beginnings involve testing the new situation, new energy and enthusiasm, renewed self-confidence and feelings of self-worth, a sense of inner realignment and new meaning, integration of the experience into everyday life and, finally, revitalization. Bridges found that human beings could not move into new roles with a clear sense of purpose and energy unless they let go of the way things were and of the self-image that fit the previous situation. (See Chapter 23 for more on Bridges' theories about change.)

Preparing employees to anticipate and respond to organizational change and enabling them to take greater responsibility for their career goals are critical elements in the maintenance of the viability of both the individual and the organization. Waterman, Waterman, and Collard (1994) see the development of self-reliant workers and a career-resilient work force as keys to the success of an organization. They define a career-resilient work force as a group of employees who are not only dedicated to the idea of continuous learning, but also stand ready to reinvent themselves to keep pace with change; who take responsibility for their own career management; and, last but not least, who are committed to the company's success. This definition of a career-resilient worker seems appropriate, relevant, and desirable for individual nurses and for the nursing work force as a whole.

The establishment of a career-resilient and self-reliant work force requires an organized program of career-development and planning assistance. Although best delivered as part of an organization's comprehensive professional development and education program, career-planning and development principles and strategies can also be implemented at the individual and/or work-unit level.

Career-development assistance is beneficial to employers and to employees in good times and in bad; it is only the objective that changes. In good times, when jobs are plentiful, nurses want to take advantage of the variety of opportunities, and employers want to retain staff. In bad times, when jobs are in short supply, nurses want to learn to control their futures and position themselves to cope with layoffs, job shortages, and competition, and employers want to help staff deal with uncertain futures. All of these circumstances demand career-planning and development skills.

Career planning must therefore be considered part of a nurse's professional development. It is congruent with the many definitions of professional practice that include autonomy, self-direction, and continuous learning. Career development embodies all of those qualities and must be integrated as part of the individual's quest for self-determination as a professional. This chapter outlines a model that provides nurses with a framework from which to grow and develop as professionals and build their careers in a comprehensive and satisfying way. It is a model that managers can use to assist their staff, as well as to plan their own careers.

CAREER PLANNING AND DEVELOPMENT MODEL

Career development is an iterative, rather than a linear, planning process that requires individuals to understand the environment in which they live and work, assess their own strengths and limitations, validate that assessment, identify career options, and develop a career plan. Stated more simply, it is a focused professional-development strategy. The following four-phase model was designed by the authors to help nurses take greater responsibility for themselves and their careers and prepare for changing organizations and new definitions of job security.

PHASE 1. SCANNING THE ENVIRONMENT

Scanning the environment includes taking stock of current realities and future trends at global, national, and local levels, not only within but beyond the health-care system and the nursing profession. Awareness of these realities and trends develops an appreciation for the skill expectations of employers, and for new and different potential future-employment opportunities. "Scanning" involves taking a critical look at the wider world in which we live and work, becoming informed, thinking in new ways, identifying opportunities, and assessing our potential to take on new challenges. It is necessary to recognize that in order to take advantage of new opportunities and new challenges, learning and the acquisition of new skills must become a never-ending process.

A scan of the environment indicates a number of trends and issues affecting workplaces today. Gutteridge, Leibowitz, and Shore (1993) summarize twelve challenges for the twenty-first century. These are: linking business strategy with the development of people, organizational downsizing, reorganizing, and restructuring; the reshaping of the work force; the evolution of new psychological contracts between organizations and employees; achieving a work/life balance; incorporating work-force diversity; focusing on quality; the empowerment of employees; new competency and skill requirements; the creation of organizations that support learning; the need to keep abreast of changing technology; and accommodating the trend towards globalization.

These issues are having, and will continue to have, a significant effect on the workplace and on the work force. As organizations move to restructure, everything changes—not only the work itself, but also the way in which work is organized. Part-time, contract, and project work are replacing long-term job security. Employees are being asked to identify their skills in order to meet the new objectives of organizations, rather than simply being asked to move to a new job. Positions are being declared redundant and long-time loyal employees are finding themselves in unfamiliar jobs, or even unemployed. The shape and size of the future health-care system, the services it will provide, the future role of hospitals within the system, the role of consumers, and the changing roles and types of health-care providers are issues that will profoundly affect the future of nursing and nurses.

Employer-employee relationships are changing. Noer (1993) found that in the past, relationships were assumed to be long-term, promotion was a reward for performance, and loyalty to an organization guaranteed a lifetime career. Experience, education, and long service propelled employees to the tops of organizations. In today's world, these relationships are situational, acknowledgement of contribution is reward for performance, and loyalty means responsibility and good work. Organizations are flat, growth is not hierarchical, systems are temporary, and careers are short-term. The new work relationships are temporary: employees do not contract for life and the organization does not assume lifelong care-taking responsibility.

These new expectations can be both overwhelming and frightening for people whose socialization was based on traditional work contracts and employment assumptions. To understand and integrate the new realities in their planning for the future, nurses must take responsibility for themselves and their careers, and must prepare for changing organizations and new definitions of job security. This challenge can be particularly onerous for nurses in management roles who are charged with the responsibility of helping their staff adapt to a changing environment, while at the same time coping with changes to their own roles and threats to their own job security (Donner, Wheeler, & Waddell, 1996).

At the end of Phase One, after a process of reading, listening, watching, and learning, both outside and inside their organizations, individuals are able to identify what employment skills will be required today and in the future. They can then go on to look at their own background and skills.

PHASE 2. SELF-ASSESSMENT AND REALITY CHECK

In health-care organizations and regulatory bodies, self-assessment may be the first step in performance management as part of quality-assurance programs. The nurse manager thus has a responsibility not only for her or his own self-assessment and reality check, but also for facilitating the independence and skill of staff in completing self-assessment as part of performance appraisal.

Conducting a thorough self-assessment is not an easy task, but it is a pivotal step in the career-development process. This step requires individuals to engage in considerable self-reflection and to ask themselves some hard questions. Scherer (1993) says that real value can only be given by people who know their own value. In order to assess the value of anything, it is necessary to complete an inventory. A self-assessment allows individuals to develop a personal profile, to build it, and to understand it; it is a task that requires adequate time and space to focus, concentrate, and look inwards. Those completing a self-assessment must be prepared to answer the question *"Who am I?"* honestly—including not just, "What do I do?" or "What is my job title?" but also "What do I value?" "What are my skills?" and "Where are my interests?" Values are the ideals that guide and give meaning to lives and work, skills are the abilities and behaviours used to produce results, and interests are the activities in which individuals like to spend most of their time and from which they gain pleasure.

Box 30.1

A SELF-ASSESSMENT QUESTIONNAIRE

Beliefs & Values

- How would you describe yourself?
- In what ways are you unique?
- What is important to you in your job and when you are away from work?
- What are your personal strengths/limitations?
- Who or what are the significant things in your life you need to consider at this time?

Employment

- What have you liked about your jobs? What have you not liked?
- What skills have you developed? What skills require further development?

- Are your values and interests congruent with those of your employer? How or how not?

Accomplishments

- In the past three to five years, what have been your most significant accomplishments at work and outside work? What skills did you acquire?

Reality Check

- What feedback have you received from your manager? Your peers? Others?
- What did these people have to say about your strengths/limitations?
- What three adjectives would these people use to describe you?

The responses to these questions should produce a tapestry, or a quilt, rich in colour and design. Answering the question *"Who Am I?"* includes reflecting on where the individual has been and where he or she is now. It is a journey of self-discovery, focusing on past and current strengths, successes, and potentials, and identifying individual uniqueness. It includes a list of accomplishments and challenges that have been faced both within and outside the workplace, the specific approaches that have been used, and an evaluation of the results.

Once the self-assessment has been completed, it requires validation. *"How am I seen by others?"* is therefore the next critical question to be considered. Careful career planning requires feedback, both formal and informal—not only from managers and peers, but also from friends and family, for work is only one part of a life story. On the job, this feedback may be provided through routine performance appraisals and through ongoing dialogue and discussion about current performance and future possibilities.

Many people find it difficult to ask for feedback, but career planning involves being open to new ideas and perspectives. It means listening to and accepting positive feedback and acknowledging those areas where change is needed. It includes seeking advice on new skills that may be required and learning how to develop them. Box 30.1 includes some questions that will guide those completing personal inventories in this phase of the process.

At the end of Phase Two, the nurse will have identified her or his strengths and limitations and targeted areas that require further development.

PHASE 3. EXPLORING CAREER OPTIONS

Restructuring has led to flatter organizations and fewer positions at the top. Completing a fast and furious upward trip is no longer the sole measurement of professional success. Those considering career success today must seek out opportunities that will build on their experience and ones that will increase their skills, thereby enhancing their options for future employment.

People can move, grow, and develop in organizations through a variety of career options, but before they do so, they need to formulate a career vision. A vision is another word for a dream, an image of potential, or a picture of where an individual wants to go. Those developing career visions must do some active daydreaming about an ideal day in the future, and develop an image of the nature of their ideal work and the ideal work environment. They must ask themselves not only "What do I want to do?" but also "Why do I want to do that?" "Where will it happen?" "With whom?" "How will the work environment be structured?" and "When will it occur?" Part of the process of choosing a career option is not only the articulation of the desired goal; it is also the visualization of what attaining that goal will look like. The vision needs to be clear, focused, defined, and realistic. Once a vision of a potential career option has been crafted, it is necessary for the individual to become committed to that vision and to do what is necessary to make it happen.

Kaye (1993) says that individuals should consider six career options: enrichment, lateral, realignment, vertical, relocation, and exploratory.

Enrichment focuses on making the current job better by increasing skill, variety, and challenge through seeking additional opportunities within the organization, continuing one's education, becoming involved in professional and community organizations, and other such possibilities. It may be defined as "growing in place."

A *lateral* option involves a change in job position, but not necessarily in status or compensation—it means moving *across* the organization. It is a way to keep challenged in an environment when there are limited "new" opportunities.

Realignment, or moving down, can be a response to dissatisfaction with current responsibilities, or may be necessitated by layoffs or dislocations. Self-determined realignment is a way to relieve job-related stress, or to create time to go back to school or to devote to family matters.

The *vertical* option is the traditional method of moving up within an organization. Even when employment prospects are limited, there are vertical opportunities, although they may require considerable strategic thinking and planning.

Relocation involves moving out of a particular department or organization, or even out of the profession. If a person's current position (or career) is not a "fit" with his or her interests or values, then moving out may be desirable. Since relocation is not always a matter of choice, however, Box 30.2 is included to assist employees to manage relocations resulting from circumstances beyond their control.

The *exploratory* option involves seeking other opportunities and workplace environments that require one's unique set of skills, interests, and values. It provides the individual with an opportunity to clarify choices. This option may confirm the benefits of a current position or career and put other options into perspective.

In choosing the most appropriate and realistic option, a person's skills must be considered, along with the various opportunities that exist for them within and outside the organization. By scanning the environment, individuals can determine where the opportunities are and where they may be in the future; through self-assessment, they determine where they may fit in the future.

Career options can also be used to develop both short- and long-term career goals and strategies. For example, obtaining a management position (vertical) may be a long-term career goal, but the short-term goal may be to develop leadership skills (enrichment), a prerequisite for any management role. A lateral move may be the desired option for a staff nurse wishing to remain at the bedside who has set a short-term goal to take a position that will expand and broaden skills and expertise. All career goals require a strategic career plan.

At the end of Phase Three, the nurse is able to describe an ideal career vision, has chosen a career option, and has begun to formulate some career goals.

PHASE 4. DEVELOPING A STRATEGIC CAREER PLAN

According to Barker (1992), vision without action is merely a dream, and action without vision simply passes the time; vision *with* action can change the world. Once the career option has been defined and career goals have been set, it is time for the individual to take action and to answer the question, *"How will I get there?"* As Hopkins (1986) says, "A goal is a dream taken seriously" (p. 23). The first step in taking a dream seriously is to articulate it. The second step is to set deadlines. The third step is to tell the dream to others. Those who feel comfortable in sharing career goals and asking for assistance enlarge their networks, thereby increasing their probability of success. The clearer the goals, the better and more successful their plan is likely to be.

This final phase in the career-planning and development process is where the career vision is grounded. Specific, time-framed, reachable, and relevant career goals are developed, and a plan for action is formulated.

A strategic career plan is a blueprint for action. Blueprints are concrete documents; that is, they are written down and visible for the author and

Box 30.2

WHAT WILL I DO IF I LOSE MY JOB TOMORROW?

In today's ever-changing work environment, the relocation career option may not be your choice but rather the choice your employer. Receiving a layoff notice can be one of the most unsettling times in a career. Those who are proactive and take control of their lives more often than not think creatively and are solution-focused. If you are concerned about the security of your position in the work force, you may wish to consider the following questions and work to develop a positively oriented job transition plan:

1. Support

- Can you identify a support group/person who could help you with the grieving process that occurs with job loss? Who would be able to challenge you to stretch and move forward?
- Have you ascertained what supports your organization would provide?
- Are you eligible for out-placement, financial, or career counselling services and employee-assistance programs?
- Does your province have a government program that provides practical support specifically to health-care workers who are laid off?
- Does your professional nursing association have a support network?

2. Financial Situation

- Have you recently done a thorough assessment of your financial situation? How much money do you need to live on monthly? How much money do you owe?
- Do you have an emergency fund put aside for a "rainy day"?
- Do you understand your employee benefits plan?
- If you had an option for early retirement, could you afford to take it?
- Do you know what the organization provides in the way of financial support through its severance packages? Do you have the name of an accountant or financial planner who could provide guidance on how to invest your compensation?
- Do you have a current copy of the *Employment Standards Act* from the Ministry of Labour that will define the minimum severance your employer must provide?
- Do you know how to access unemployment insurance?

3. Leaving the Organization

- If you had a choice, how would you like to leave the organization?
- If you received notice, who would you want to be with you?
- How has your organization traditionally given employees notice of layoff?
- How do management staff communicate their decisions to others in the organization?
- How much notice is given?
- Do you have any choice in how you would be informed?
- Do you know your collective agreement and understand how the layoff process could occur?
- If you are not part of a union, do you have access to the human resource policies and procedures that are used in your place of work? Do you know the name of an employment relations lawyer who could provide direction and guidance throughout the process?
- Does your nursing association have a legal-assistance program?

4. Taking Care of Self

- What components can you build into your plan that would focus on taking care of yourself?
- Have you considered joining a health club, participating in some relaxation sessions, or just taking some quality time for yourself? This might include going away to do some self-reflection and to plan your next move.
- If you should experience a period of unemployment, what rewards could you establish to help you celebrate successes and accomplishments along the way as you search for a new position? These might include making time to go for a walk, to go to the movies, or to meet friends for coffee.
- What other things could you do to maintain your health, your self-esteem and your relationships during a period of transition?

others to see. There are numerous ways to tackle the development of a strategic career plan. Box 30.3 provides a set of questions that may be useful in this endeavour.

At the end of Phase 4, the nurse has a plan on paper that includes goals, action steps, resources, time lines, and indicators of success. She or he has also begun to consult with others about the plan, and may ask, "What do others think? Do they have any more ideas or suggestions?"

SELF-MARKETING

Career planning never ends; it is not linear, but circular, and it changes along with the individual and the environment. The process is a way to help individuals find out more about who they are, what they like, and how they might find career satisfaction. Most importantly, career planning allows people to take control of their careers and their futures.

Once the strategic career plan has been developed, it needs to be put into action, and this requires self-marketing strategies and skills. When opportunities are scarce, competition is stiff. Those who wish to advance or change their careers must learn to represent themselves in the best way possible, using all available resources. They must move forward with confidence, having specified their goals, and identified those who can help. They do not need to represent themselves as someone other than who they are, or attempt to shape themselves into a mould they think that others want. They simply need to present their unique strengths in a positive and confident manner. They need to think of themselves as salespeople who are able to highlight the benefits and advantages unique to the product. In self-marketing, the individual is the product. If career planning is about taking control, then self-marketing is one way to get there.

A self-marketing plan includes personal resources, written materials, and interview skills. The following eight tips can assist in the development of a positive professional image.

Box 30.3

QUESTIONS TO ASK WHEN DEVELOPING A STRATEGIC CAREER PLAN

- What is my career option?
- What are my career goals?
- What action steps can I take to bring me closer to each goal?
- What resources can I use for each action step?

- When will I accomplish each action step?
- How will I know I have succeeded in reaching my career goal?

---

1. *Know yourself.*   You are your own best marketer. Every time you meet someone, you are presented with a new marketing opportunity. Keep a positive attitude, even on those days where it feels overwhelming. How you come across on paper and in person will only be as good as how you feel about yourself.

2. *Find and work with a mentor.*   Your mentor can provide you with information, advice, and support regarding your career plan and also give suggestions for individuals you should meet. Mentors have the potential to use both their informal and formal forms of influence to further your career.

3. *Network.*   In today's economic climate, you are more likely to get a position through your networks than by answering advertisements in the newspaper. To "network" is to build mutually beneficial relationships, where people work to help one another attain their goals. It is important to network effectively: who you know is often less important than who knows you.

4. *Form and use a support group.*   Surround yourself with individuals who support you, who expect the best from you. You need an environment that creates winners and supporters who will nurture, nourish, and care for you throughout the process. If you do not have a support group, find one or start one.

5. *Speak and write.*   Look for opportunities to profile yourself and your expertise through public speaking, presentations, and writing articles for professional journals or local community newspapers. Position yourself as an expert.

6. *Have and use a business card.*   When you meet key people, have a business card readily available so you are not fumbling for a pen and paper. Remember to include ways people can reach you by telephone, fax, and e-mail. Depending on where the card is to be used, this might be a personal business card rather than a business card provided by the employer.

7. *Develop a résumé and cover letter.*   The first impression a potential employer may have of you may be conveyed by your cover letter and résumé. They can be key factors in determining whether or not you get an interview. Both documents should be clear and concise (refer to Chapter 29 on writing skills). Remember they are a record of your accomplishments—the added value you bring to the job.

8. *Develop interview skills.* An employment interview, like any other communication event, is an opportunity to market yourself and your skills. The clearer you are about the fit between what you have and what the employer needs, the easier your interview will be. This means that you must be something of a detective. Learn as much as possible about the organization, the interviewer, the interview process, and the potential outcomes. Prepare for the interview, do your best, and always evaluate your performance afterwards. If you have not been to an interview in a while, read, learn, and practise these skills so you can present yourself with confidence.

Successful self-marketing is the presentation of one's knowledge, skills, and potential in the most positive and appropriate manner possible. All of the tools described above can be used to build a well-blended self-marketing strategy that looks professional and provides a competitive edge. Marketing is a challenge because, as with other steps in the career planning and development process, it must be tailored to the individual. As self-marketing is part of the process of personal and professional self-development, it is important to practise it consistently.

THE FUTURE: FOR HEALTH CARE, FOR ORGANIZATIONS AND FOR NURSES

While specific outcomes of the current phase of health-care reform are unclear, it is certain that the "new" system will be different. The traditional security that employees expected employers to provide is fast disappearing. The new paradigm focuses on the employee as a short-term contract worker who is flexible, adapts to change quickly, and is willing to take risks. There will be fewer long-term positions, and some workers may see self-employment as one way in which they can best make a contribution and ensure a long-term career. The majority of workers will undoubtedly choose to remain as employees, and will need to change their perspectives and skills in this new world of work. Entrepreneurial and intrapreneurial (within organizations) skills will be required to ensure that workers—both employees and self-employed—thrive in this new environment.

Health and social-service organizations are experiencing their greatest challenges in half a century—challenges from rising costs, new technologies, changing consumer expectations and government fiscal policies. The organization that survives into the twenty-first century will have a work force that understands and is prepared to meet the challenges ahead. That work force has the ability to anticipate and respond to rapid organizational change and take greater responsibility for the careers of its individual workers. Adaptability and self-management are key career competencies of the future. According to Noer:

> The only way you can provide security for yourself is by making sure that your work experience is as up to date as possible so that if tomorrow happens, you are able to go out and get another job because you have skills people want. That is the only way you have security. You are not going to get it from the company. It will never be that way again. (1993, p. 15)

SUMMARY

- Career development is part of ongoing professional development for both managers and staff.
- In a rapidly changing health-care environment, health workers worry not only about the quality of patient care, but also about their own job security and marketability.
- Career planning and development has four phases: scanning the environment; doing a self-assessment and reality check; exploring career options; and developing a strategic career plan.
- Taking control of career planning means learning how to market oneself.
- Self-marketing includes such activities as knowing oneself, acquiring a mentor; finding a support group; developing a résumé and cover letter; interviewing and being interviewed; and presenting one's knowledge, skills, and potential in the most positive manner.
- Due to uncertainties in current health work environments, it is wise for individuals to have contingency plans in case of layoff and unemployment.
- Job security is enhanced by acquiring and maintaining the type of knowledge and skills people in health agencies need and want.

FURTHER READINGS AND RESOURCES

Bridges, W. (1994). *Jobshift: How to prosper in a workplace without jobs.* Reading, MA: Addison-Wesley. Bridges provides the reader with an understanding of the new forces shaping tomorrow's work environment, and discusses in particular why today's organizations are moving away from the job as the best way to get work done. Insight into how tomorrow's "dejobbed" organization will work and how individuals will need to adapt their careers to the conditions that exist in "dejobbed" organizations is also highlighted. For individuals, this will mean shifting one's thinking from employee to independent worker. For organizations, it will mean helping people to refocus their energy on the work that needs doing and rethinking what they can do best. The book explores the new world of work, how organizations are responding, and how individuals will need to respond.

Donner, G., & Wheeler, M. (1998). *Taking control of your career and your future. For nurses by nurses*. Ottawa, ON: CNA Publications. Donner and Wheeler provide a framework to help nurses integrate career planning into their professional development and specific strategies to help them identify and achieve career success and satisfaction. The book addresses the diverse needs of nurses, and can be helpful for students about to embark on their nursing careers as well as those contemplating retirement, for staff nurses as well as those in management and education, for organizational workers as well as those considering a career in independent practice.

Moses, B. (1997). *Career intelligence, mastering new work and personal realities*. Toronto: Stoddart. Moses provides a perspective on what individuals need to do to manage their careers more intelligently. The author defines career intelligence as the ability to have a broad vision of oneself in the world, a vision that expresses who one is and what one wants to accomplish in life. It is a way of understanding one's self and the world in which one resides, and of "marrying" the two to take advantage of opportunities that come one's way. She notes that the workplace has become so complex that new rules for career success are needed: ensure marketability, think globally, communicate powerfully, keep learning, understand business trends, prepare for areas of competency (not jobs), and think lattice, not ladder.

REFERENCES

Barker, J. (1992). *Paradigms. The business of discovering the future*. New York: HarperCollins.

Bridges, W. (1990). *Transitions: Making sense of life's changes*. Reading, MA: Addison-Wesley.

Donner, G., Wheeler, M., & Waddell, J. (1996). *Career planning and development: An evaluation project*. Unpublished report, available from the authors.

Gutteridge, T. G., Leibowitz, Z. B. & Shore, J. E. (1993). *Organizational career development*. San Francisco: Jossey-Bass.

Hopkins, W. (1986). *A goal is a dream taken seriously*. King of Prussia, PA: The HRD Quarterly.

Kaye, B. (1993). *Up is not the only way: A guide to developing workforce talent*. Washington, DC: Career Systems Inc.

Noer, D. (1993). *Healing the wounds*. San Francisco: Jossey-Bass.

Scherer, J. (1993). *Work and the human spirit*. Spokane, WA: John Scherer & Associates.

Waterman, R. H., Waterman, J. A., & Collard, B. J. (1994, July/August). Toward a career-resilient work force. *Harvard Business Review*, pp. 87–95.

Notes on Contributors

▼▼▼▼▼▼▼▼▼▼▼▼▼▼▼▼▼▼▼▼▼▼▼▼▼▼

Sonia Acorn, RN, BN (McGill), MScN (Boston), PhD (Utah), is Professor, School of Nursing, University of British Columbia. She has extensive experience in nursing administration and currently teaches nursing leadership and management in the undergraduate and graduate programs at the University of British Columbia School of Nursing.

Donna Armann-Hutton, RN, BScN, MEd, is Director of Nursing at the Cross Cancer Institute, Edmonton, Alberta, where her leadership in implementing a professional nursing model is widely recognized. She has held several positions in health care, including clinical instructor in critical care, and Director of Nursing with the University of Alberta Hospitals. She is a surveyor with the Canadian Council of Health Services Accreditation, and is certified as an auditor/lead auditor in ISO9000 standards.

Elaine M. Baxter, RN, BSN (Alberta), MSN (UBC), is Program Manager (Medicine/Emergency/Psychiatry) at Surrey Memorial Hospital, Surrey, B.C., and Adjunct Professor, School of Nursing, University of British Columbia. She has an extensive background in a variety of work settings from teaching to community hospitals, in organizations from professional associations to a management consulting group, and in clinical settings including critical care, medicine, surgery, emergency, and psychiatry. She has also developed and taught management courses.

Elizabeth Broad, RN, BA, BScN, MN, is currently a Project Co-ordinator in Information Planning and Management for Alberta Health. She was a member of the AARN Ad Hoc Working Group on Health Information: Nursing Components, and has been a member of the Expert Working Group of the Canadian Institute for Health Information that is developing a minimum data set for long-term care. She has extensive experience in clinical nursing, nursing management, and in government, and is currently Co-ordinator of the Nursing Informatics course offered by Athabasca University.

John Church, BA (Hons), MA, PhD (Western Ontario), has spent the past twelve years conducting research on health policy and politics, with a specific emphasis on the development of regional and community-based models for the management and delivery of health services. He is currently Assistant Professor and Director of Graduate Training in the Department of Public Health Sciences, University of Alberta.

Lana Clark, RN, BScN (Alberta), MN (Calgary), is General Manager, Women's Reproductive Services and Children's Health, Saskatoon and District Health. She is a former Assistant Executive Director, Patient Care at the Royal University Hospital, Saskatoon. She has several years experience as a front-line manager and in senior nursing administration.

Germaine M. Dechant, BScN, MHSA, is the Executive Director of Child and Adolescent Services Association (CASA), an organization that provides community-based mental health services to children, adolescents and their families. She brings to this position a background rich in clinical work, teaching, research, management and senior administration, including a position as Chief Executive Officer of an urban community hospital.

Gail J. Donner, RN, PhD, is Professor and Associate Dean, Education, Faculty of Nursing, University of Toronto. Together with Mary M. Wheeler, she runs Donner & Wheeler and Associates. Well-known on the Canadian health-care scene, they speak, write, provide workshops and individual career counselling, and consult on career-development strategies in Canada and the United States.

Linda M. Doody, RN, MEd (St. John's), CHE, is a Nursing Consultant with the Department of Health in St. John's, Newfoundland. She is a certified member of the Canadian College of Health Services Executives, and is currently the board member for Newfoundland and Labrador. In her consulting role with the Department of Health, she carries out budget, staffing and operational reviews in health facilities throughout Newfoundland and Labrador. She has been extensively involved in policy direction as it relates to health-care reform in the province.

Phyllis Giovannetti, RN, BN, ScD, is Professor and Associate Dean of the Graduate Program in the Faculty of Nursing, University of Alberta. She was involved in some of the earliest North American efforts to develop nursing information, particularly in the area of nursing-workload measurement, nursing-resource utilization, and costs. A former president of the Alberta Association of Registered Nurses, she chaired the Canadian Nurses Association Planning Committee for the First Canadian Nursing Minimum Data Set Conference.

Moira Hennessey, BComm, is the Director of Hospitals, Health Centres and Nursing Homes with the Department of Health in St. John's, Newfoundland. In this capacity, she is responsible for the allocation and monitoring of expenditures to regional institutional boards. She also participates in budget, staffing, and operational reviews in health facilities, and has been extensively involved in policy direction as it relates to health-care reform in Newfoundland. Her previous work experience includes senior administrative responsibilities in community-based agencies and, private consulting work in health administration.

Judith M. Hibberd, RN, BScN (Toronto), MHSA, PhD (Alberta), is Professor Emeritus, Faculty of Nursing, University of Alberta, where she taught nursing management at both graduate and undergraduate levels. She has had wide experience as a first-line manager and senior administrator. Much of her research has focussed on labour relations and strikes in the health-care system.

Dennis Hutton is a registered engineering technologist and quality-systems consultant with many years of experience in developing, implementing and maintaining quality systems in business organizations, including, most recently, a large gas utility organization. He is a certified lead auditor for ISO9000 standards.

Noela J. Inions, RN, BScN, ORPG, LLB, LLM, has been an operating-room nurse, Corporate Counsel at the University of Alberta Hospitals, Associate Vice President, Medicine, at the Royal Alexandra Hospital, and Corporate Counsel for the Capital Health Authority in Edmonton. She is now a consultant in health law, undertaking projects in relation to health legislation, standards and outcome measures.

Philip Jacobs, DPhil [Economics], CMA, is a professor in the Department of Public Health Sciences, University of Alberta and is an affiliate professor with the Institute of PharmacoEconomics in Edmonton. His research is in the areas of health-care funding and economic evaluation of health-care interventions.

L. Jane Knox, RN, BScN (Saskatchewan), MN (Dalhousie), is a former community nurse (Ontario and Alberta), nurse educator, nursing association manager, and executive director of province-wide prevention services (Saskatchewan). She is Principal, Performance Audit, with the Saskatchewan Provincial Auditor. In this position, she audits the effectiveness of government management practices and recommends improvements in such areas as case planning, health-needs assessment, resource allocation based on health needs, performance indicators, and governance issues.

Stephanie Lawrence is the Co-ordinator of Communications and Marketing with the Canadian Council of Technicians and Technologists, as well as a freelance writer and editor. She is editor of two national technology newsletters and an associate editor with COMSYS, an Ottawa-based community development and health promotion firm. Stephanie has a BA in art history from Carleton University and a diploma in journalism from Algonquin College.

Bonnie L. Lendrum, RN, BScN, MScN (Toronto), is Planning Specialist at Hamilton Health Sciences Corporation, and an Assistant Clinical Professor in the School of Nursing, McMaster University. She brings both line and staff perspectives to the issues of design, measurement, and evaluation in her consulting role within the hospital. She is a member of a research team studying the effects of rapid organizational change on patient quality of care and staff quality of life.

Carl A. Meilicke, BComm (Saskatchewan), DHA (Toronto), PhD (Minnesota), is Professor Emeritus, University of Alberta. He was founder and first Director of the Program in Health Services Administration, University of Alberta (1968-1980). He was then seconded to the Alberta Department of Health as the first Associate Deputy Minister, Policy Development. He returned to the University of Alberta from 1982–1993 and taught in the Departments of Health Services Administration and Community Medicine. Throughout his career in health services administration, he maintained a special interest in the management of nursing services.

Leah Evans Parisi, RN, BScN (Ohio State), CRNA (Ohio State), MA (Lindenwood), EdD (Pepperdine), JD (Loyola Law School-Los Angeles), is a Professor, School of Nursing, McMaster University in Hamilton, Ontario. She teaches in the areas of management, law, and ethics, and is Co-ordinator of Studies and Co-ordinator of the Leadership/Management Distance Education Program. In the past, she has been a nurse anaesthetist, was founding Director of the UCLA graduate program in Nurse Anesthesia, has practiced medical malpractice and medical staff privileges defense law with the firm of Rushfeldt, Shelley, and Drake in Los Angeles, California, and has been Director of Critical Care and the Operating Rooms at St. Joseph's Hospital in Hamilton.

Carolyn J. Pepler, N, BNSc (Queen's), MScN (Wayne State), PhD (Michigan), is Consultant for Nursing Research at the Royal Victoria Hospital, Montreal, and Associate Professor, School of Nursing, McGill University. Her primary focus at the hospital is the development of a climate of inquiry and the promotion of clinical research. She also teaches successful research utilization courses for nursing staff at all local hospitals. In 1992, she was awarded the prestigious Canadian Nurses Foundation/Ross Laboratories Award for Nursing Leadership.

Ginette Lemire Rodger, RN, BScN (Ottawa), MAdmN (Montreal), PhD (Alberta), is President of Lemire Rodger & Associates. From 1981 to 1989, she was Executive Director of the Canadian Nurses Association, the Canadian Nurses Foundation, and the Canadian Nurses Protective Society. From 1974 to 1981, she was Director of Nursing at Notre-Dame Hospital in Montréal. She has worked in clinical nursing, management, education, and research, and has been recognized several times for her contribution to nursing administration.

Judith Skelton-Green, RN, BScN (McMaster), MScN (University of British Columbia), PhD (The Fielding Institute), has broad experience as a senior nurse executive in both educational and service settings. In these roles, she has made extensive use of change theory, tools, and strategies in start-up, rationalization, merger, and downsizing situations. She works as a consultant in health care, and as a faculty member at the University of Toronto.

Donna Lynn Smith, RN, BScN, MEd (Alberta), CHE, is currently Associate Professor in the Faculty of Nursing and Department of Public Health Sciences, University of Alberta where she teaches nursing management at both graduate and undergraduate levels. She has more than twenty years of leadership experience in a variety of health-care settings and in government, where she has established, led, participated in, and evaluated many innovative projects and programs. She is Director of the Service Integration Studies Unit in the Faculty of Nursing.

Jane E. Smith, BScN, MN (Alberta), is a graduate of the Vancouver General Hospital School of Nursing, and has held nursing positions in rural and urban acute-care settings. She has also worked as a police constable in the Vancouver City Police Department. Jane recently served as co-ordinator of a project to develop Interdisciplinary Case Management Education at the University of Alberta, and is currently undertaking doctoral studies.

Janet L. Storch, RN, BScN, MHSA, PhD (Alberta), is Director, School of Nursing, University of Victoria. She was previously Dean, Faculty of Nursing, University of Calgary, and is a former Program Director of the Health Services Administration Program at the University of Alberta. A noted teacher and author, she has written numerous articles on health-care policy and on ethical issues in health care and nursing.

Patricia E. B. Valentine, RN, BSN (UBC), MA (Calgary), PhD (Alberta), is Associate Professor, Faculty of Nursing, University of Alberta. She is interested in viewing nursing through a feminist lens. Her research shows that women bring different perspectives to organizational management and that this needs to be acknowledged both in management and nursing literature.

Susan VanDeVelde-Coke, BSc, MA, MBA, has held a number of administrative positions, including Vice-President (Nursing), Director of Nursing, and Assistant Director of Nursing at teaching centres in Canada and the United States. She has taught at Rush University, University of Washington, and University of Manitoba. She has served on the Canadian Nurses Association Board and on the editorial boards of *Heart and Lung, Canadian Journal of Nursing Administration,* and *Nursing Management.* She wishes to acknowledge the assistance of her husband, Dr. William Coke, in the preparation of her chapter.

Ardene Robinson Vollman, RN, BSN (Sask.), MA, PhD (Ottawa), is an Assistant Professor in the Faculty of Nursing, University of Calgary. She also holds an adjunct appointment to the Faculty of Medicine, Department of Community Health Sciences. Her interests are public health and health promotion of vulnerable populations.

P. Susan Wagner, RN, MSc (Nsg), is Professor, College of Nursing, University of Saskatchewan. She was elected by the public to the Saskatoon Regional Health Board in 1995, and served two terms as its chair. She has extensive background in community health boards, and her professional practice and research is in the evaluation of community programs.

Janet Walker, RN, BSN, MSN (UBC), is a Nurse Consultant and president of Walker Consultants. She is Adjunct Professor, School of Nursing, University of British Columbia, where she teaches nursing management and research, and has extensive management experience in acute-care organizations.

Mary M. Wheeler, RN, MEd, is President of Mary M. Wheeler & Associates, a consulting firm specializing in Organizational Transition Management. Together with Gail J. Donner, she also runs Donner & Wheeler and Associates. Well-known on the Canadian health-care scene, they speak, write, provide workshops and individual career counselling, and consult on career-development strategies in Canada and the United States.

Dorothy M. Wylie, RN, BScN, MA, MSc (HRD), held many senior management positions including that of Vice President of Nursing at the Toronto General Hospital. More recently, she was a consultant in organizational and management development and Associate Professor (part time), Faculty of Nursing, University of Toronto. Now retired, she continues in her capacity as Editor of the *Canadian Journal of Nursing Administration*.

Index

Nursing Management in Canada

READER REPLY CARD

We are interested in your reaction to *Nursing Management in Canada*, Second Edition, by Judith M. Hibberd and Donna Lynn Smith. You can help us to improve this book in future editions by completing this questionnaire.

1. What was your reason for using this book?
   __ university course   __ continuing education course
   __ college course   __ professional development
   __ personal interest   __ other _____

2. If you are a student, please identify your school, and the course in which you used this book:

   SCHOOL: _____

   PROGRAM: _____

   COURSE: _____

3. In what way did this book assist you in your course?

4. What did you like best about this book? What did you like least?

5. Please identify any topics you think should be added to future editions.

6. Please add any comments or suggestions.

7. May we contact you for further information?

NAME: _____

ADDRESS: _____

POSTAL CODE: _____   PHONE: _____

(fold here and tape shut)

MAIL ➤ POSTE
Canada Post Corporation / Société canadienne des postes

Postage paid
If mailed in Canada

Port payé
si posté au Canada

Business Reply

Réponse d'affaires

0116870399   01

0116870399-M8Z4X6-BR01

Larry Gillevet
Director of Product Development
HARCOURT CANADA
55 HORNER AVENUE
TORONTO, ONTARIO
M8Z 9Z9